Handbook of Normative Data for Neuropsychological Assessment

HANDBOOK OF NORMATIVE DATA FOR NEUROPSYCHOLOGICAL ASSESSMENT

Maura N. Mitrushina
Kyle B. Boone
Louis F. D'Elia

New York   Oxford
OXFORD UNIVERSITY PRESS
1999

Oxford University Press

Oxford   New York

Athens   Auckland   Bangkok   Bogotá   Buenos Aires   Calcutta
Cape Town   Chennai   Dar es Salaam   Delhi   Florence   Hong Kong   Istanbul
Karachi   Kuala Lumpur   Madrid   Melbourne   Mexico City   Mumbai
Nairobi   Paris   São Paulo   Singapore   Taipei   Tokyo   Toronto   Warsaw

and associated companies in
Berlin   Ibadan

Published by Oxford University Press, Inc.
198 Madison Avenue, New York, New York 10016

Oxford is a registered trademark of Oxford University Press

Library of Congress Cataloging-in-Publication Data

Mitrushina, Maura N.
Handbook of normative data for neuropsychological assessment /
Maura N. Mitrushina, Kyle B. Boone, Louis F. D'Elia
p. cm.
Includes bibliographical references and index.
ISBN 0-19-505675-2
1. Neuropsychological tests—Handbooks, manuals, etc. I. Boone,
K. B. (Kyle Brauer) II. D'Elia, Lou. III. Title.
[DNLM: 1. Neuropsychological Tests—standards. 2. Brain Damage,
Chronic—diagnosis. 3. Brain Injuries—diagnosis.   WL 103 M684h   1999]
RC386.6.N48M58   1999
616.8'0475—dc21
DNLM/DLC
for Library of Congress   98-13314

Since this page cannot legibly accommodate all the acknowledgments,
pages 511–512 constitute an extension of the copyright page.

9 8 7 6 5 4 3 2 1

Printed in the United States of America
on acid-free paper

With admiration and gratitude,
we dedicate this book to
those professionals whose
normative research efforts made
this volume possible.

Foreword

MURIEL D. LEZAK

Help has come at last! Here is the long-awaited neuropsychological test norms collection yearned for by many neuropsychology clinicians.

Any collection of test norms in a rapidly evolving discipline such as neuropsychology changes as the data are culled from the literature. Here we have the benefit of almost current norms (up to the date of delivery to the publisher) and the authors have the burden—which we hope they will accept—of providing us updates in the future.

This *Handbook* features 17 of the tests most commonly used by neuropsychologists (somewhat more than 20 if the tests that comprise the three Wechsler Memory Scale batteries are considered separately). Most of the norms were obtained by researchers other than the authors. What makes this collection so valuable is that for every test covered, the test user can find the most suitable norms (demographically, by ability level, and even—for some—by nationality or language, sexual preference, and/or medical or psychiatric status). Moreover, each norm set has been evaluated for its usefulness: its applicability to specific groups and considerations of sampling procedures and characteristics of the study. I suspect that test users who begin consulting this *Handbook* will become happily addicted.

Thank you, Maura, Kyle, and Lou.

Foreword

PAUL SATZ

It is indeed a felicitous occasion to write a foreword to this important and long-awaited book. The book represents the product of an idea that emerged gradually during the mid-1980s among a small group of fellows during their postdoctoral training in neuropsychology at the Neuropsychiatric Institute and Hospital at UCLA. I am also delighted to note that these fellows, now distinguished neuropsychologists and professors at UCLA, collaborated for so many years to bring this much-needed volume on norms to print. The original idea was Lou D'Elia's. Early in his fellowship he expressed concerns about the lack of published norms available for many of the tests used by neuropsychologists in clinical practice. Of equal concern was the dearth of information on demographics, methods, and procedures of studies reporting normative data on a particular test. These concerns were also shared by Allen Brandon and Kyle Boone who, along with Lou D'Elia, began to assemble laboratory norm books that provided some preliminary data from a few selected studies reporting normative data for a test.

Such efforts, often similarly crude and unsystematic, were occurring in other clinical settings in North America during the late 1980s and early 1990s. Spreen and Strauss (1998) referred to these products as "laboratory norm manuals." The problem with these norm manuals is that laboratories often used different study norms for a particular test without systematic review of the merits and usefulness of the test for different populations by gender, age, education, intelligence, and/or culture. With this state of affairs, test interpretation could vary depending, often unknowingly, on which norm was used and how appropriate it was for the client's demographics. I recall an early supervisory medical–legal case in which Lou D'Elia was surprised to learn that the plaintiff's expert had reported the presence of a severe memory impairment in a patient with relatively benign head injury based on performance on the Wechsler Memory Scale (WMS). This finding contrasted with our more comprehensive memory battery, including the WMS. Out of curiosity, Dr. D'Elia went to the UCLA library to try and figure out which study norm had been used by plaintiff's expert. This search yielded a surprising set of 18 normative studies, which included two of our WMS laboratory norms and the plaintiff expert's norms, the latter of which comprised a very small sample of Australian subjects who were administered a different form of the WMS! Had "the other side" done "norm shopping" figuring no one could possibly have access to all the norms and would not discover their possible deception?

This experience prompted Lou D'Elia's first systematic review and critique of studies reporting normative data on the WMS (D'Elia, Satz, Schretlin, 1989). This study also provided a methodologic and conceptual framework that was utilized by Kyle Boone and Lou D'Elia in conducting a comprehensive review of normative articles for various neuropsychological tests. With added efforts of Maura Mitrushina, who later joined the project, the authors completed the present review of all known published norms for 17 frequently administered neuropsychological tests in clinical practice.

The organization of this volume is clear and user-friendly and provides the clinician with easy access to which normative data best match the demographic characteristics of the patient. In addition to a review of conceptual and statistical issues fundamental to the art of assessment, the clinician is presented with all published and peer-reviewed normative studies for each test, with critical review of study strengths and weaknesses, related comments, and conclusion. Clinicians will find the data locator table an additional help in quickly accessing data for each study organized in ascending chronological order.

It is clear that this book will facilitate and strengthen the clinician's current efforts at test interpretation. It is also likely that the book will be favorably received by other medical, psychological, and legal disciplines who interact with patients complaining of cognitive problems associated with probable brain insult. However, the authors thoughtfully note that the interpretive effort in neuropsychological assessment requires clinical judgment that utilizes many sources of information including appropriate test norms, history, observations and knowledge of brain-behavior relationships. The authors' careful attention to various factors affecting test performance, and their review of philosophical and statistical issues relevant to testing, make this volume an excellent teaching resource for graduate classes in psychological and neuropsychological assessment.

The current volume should be viewed as a useful and necessary addition to two other Oxford publications (Lezak, 1995; Spreen and Strauss, 1998). The book by Lezak offers a comprehensive review of the history and psychometric properties of neuropsychological tests. Spreen and Strauss add some normative data to their extensive review of a large number of cognitive, behavioral, and personality tests. In contrast, a unique contribution of the current volume is in providing an *in-depth* review of comprehensive sets of normative data for *selected* tests most often used in neuropsychological assessment. It summarizes extensive data sets reported by Heaton, Ivnik, Yeudall, Bornstein, Van Gorp, and other neuropsychologists whose work has made this volume possible.

Preface

The *Handbook of Normative Data for Neuropsychological Assessment* that you now hold in your hands is our attempt to provide ready access to neuropsychological normative data and to evaluate their strengths and weaknesses. Because the interpretation of test scores profoundly affects the quality and utility of neuropsychological reports and research, we felt that a critical compendium containing all of the available normative data for commonly used tests was essential. Before this book's publication, only those lucky individuals with the time or staff to conduct exhaustive library searches, or with extensive professional subscription lists, could hope to be aware of more than a few normative reports for any specific test.

Although several books cover the intricacies of administration and scoring procedures for neuropsychological tests, and a few books contain some normative data, no previous volume has been exclusively devoted to the presentation and discussion of existing normative data for specific neuropsychological tests. Nor has any book provided a framework for judging studies that report normative data.

This *Handbook* was written to help guide the busy clinician, researcher, and graduate student to the most appropriate sets of normative data for comparison purposes. It provides normative data and critical reviews of the available normative reports for the most frequently administered neuropsychological tests, including the Trail Making, Color Trails, Stroop Color Word Interference, Auditory Consonant Trigrams, Boston Naming, Verbal Fluency, Rey-Osterrieth Complex Figure, Rey Auditory-Verbal Learning, Hooper Visual Organization, Seashore Rhythm, Speech Sounds Perception, Tactual Performance, Finger Tapping, Grip Strength (Dynamometer), Grooved Pegboard, and Category tests, as well as the Wechsler Memory Scale Battery (WMS, WMS-R, and WMS III).

ORGANIZATION OF THE BOOK

The book contains 20 chapters. The basic concepts of normative neuropsychology are addressed in the first three chapters. The first chapter provides an introduction to the practice and philosophy of neuropsychology as a clinical discipline. The second chapter is an overview of statistical methods and the use of statistical and methodologic concepts in neuropsychological practice. The third chapter explores the interface of neuropsychology with other professional/clinical disciplines.

The following 17 chapters review and present the normative data for specific neuropsychological tests. These chapters begin with a brief overview of the history and psychometric qualities of the test under discussion, which indicates whether there are different versions of the test and/or varying administration procedures. If more than one version of a test exists, then the differences in content, administration, and scoring are described. We purposely avoided an exhaustive review of the history and psychometric properties of the tests because this information is readily available in other Oxford publications, specifically the Lezak (1995) and Spreen and Strauss (1998) volumes.

The next part of the chapter is a summary of the findings from research that has examined the influence of demographic variables (such as age, gender, education, handedness, intellectual level) and administration procedures on test performance. The findings from this review highlight the critical variables needed to evaluate the normative reports for the test. These critical variables are broken down into two categories: (1) *subject variables* and (2) *procedural variables*.

Subject variables address such issues as:

"How broad are the utilized age-group ranges in data reporting?"

Optimally, studies report data across rather discrete age groupings (such as 20–24, 25–29, 30–34, 35–39, 40–44, 45–49, 50–54 years) rather than across one all-inclusive range (i.e., 20–54 years).

"What is the education and/or IQ of the study participants?"

Because education and IQ may have a dramatic impact on test performance, it is important to include this information so that data that closely match the education and/or IQ of the patient under study can be utilized.

"What was the sample size in each of the reported age or age/education categories?"

"Is the sample from which data were collected well described?"

For instance, the *age* of the subjects and the *country* where the study was conducted always must be reported. Depending on the test administered, other important variables may include gender and hand preference.

Procedural variables address such issues as:

"What version of the test was administered?"

"How was the test administered?"

"How was the test scored?"

"Did the data reported include mean and standard deviation scores?"

The next section of each of these chapters summarizes the status of the normative data for the test and answers the questions:

"How many studies are out there?"

"Which versions of the test have been the most frequently administered?"

"What demographic characteristics have been most frequently studied?"

The following section presents the data locator table, which summarizes the *subject* and *procedural variables* for each study organized in ascending chronological order. The table quickly highlights for the reader the most appropriate normative data, considering the demographic characteristics of the patient under study, as well as the test administration and scoring criteria that were utilized. The table also indicates the page number on which an extensive critical review of the study can be found. Therefore, readers have the option of reading the critical review of the normative data for a particular test, or simply using the data locator table to rapidly identify the appropriate data set for quick test interpretation.

The next section presents critiques of the studies with the strengths and considerations regarding use of each normative report discussed in some depth. Tables of normative data follow each study critique. The chapter concludes with a summary and offers suggestions for future research to improve the database for the test.

HOW TO BEST USE THE BOOK

The process of selecting the most appropriate normative report for interpretive purposes involves determining the "best fit" between your patient's demographic characteristics (e.g., age, years of education, IQ, handedness) and the demographic characteristics of the study sample. It is also critical to insure that the version of the test you administered is the same version used in collecting the normative data. Likewise, it is critical that the scoring procedures are identical.

As a general policy, before seeing a patient, we typically determine which normative data we are going to use to interpret his or her performance. This way we don't discover, after a patient has gone home, that the only reference data available utilized a different administration and/or scoring protocol than the version we used. Such "discoveries" undermine confidence in test score interpretation. Fortunately, however, the vast majority of normative reports do utilize standard administration and scoring procedures.

If your data have already been collected, an important variable to screen for initially is country of origin. If your patient was born and/or educated in the United States, then the most appropriate comparison data should have been collected from individuals born and/or educated in the United States. Another critical variable is age. Your patient's test scores must be compared to those of age-peers because performance on most neuropsychological tests changes as a function of age. Educational level and/or IQ are also important variables. Because they can have a tremendous impact on performance on most neuropsychological tests, your patient's IQ and/or educational characteristics should closely match the demographics of the normative comparison sample. Optimally, normative data are reported by age/education or age/IQ categories (i.e., performance of 20–25-year-olds with 12 years of education, performance of 20–25-year-olds with 13–15 years of education, performance of 20–25-year-olds with 16 years of education, etc.). Sample size is also critical because small sample size within any of the comparison categories (i.e., age, age/education) can undermine the stability of the normative data and reduce confidence in score interpretation. For some tests, gender and handedness must be considered. Ideally, the administration and scoring procedures utilized in assessing the patient should be identical to those used in collecting the normative comparison data.

If the data locator table suggests that more than one study could be appropriately utilized, then the reader is especially advised to read the critical reviews of the studies closely to help determine whether one dataset is more appropriate than the other. Close inspection of the details of the studies often leads to clear-cut conclusions.

HISTORY OF THIS PROJECT

This book originally grew out of the frustration I experienced in trying to locate appropriate normative data during the early years of my postdoctoral training. This frustration is familiar to anyone who has used normative data. Back in the "old days," it was fairly typical for practicing professionals to have access to, at most, one or two sets of normative data for any particular neuropsychological test. More often than not, graduate students and postdoctoral fellows and trainees were handed a manual of norms to be used in the clinic or laboratory. These "lab manuals" containing tables of normative data were passed from mentor to trainee (and vice versa) as if they were the Holy Grail. Early on, I began to ask, "Where did this data come from?" Sometimes a graduate student, postdoctoral fellow, or faculty member would "discover" a new set of norms for a particular test and a new table would magically appear in the lab manual. Applying the new reference data to the patient scores often yielded wildly different percentile performance interpretations from those based on the "standard" norms. This sent me to the biomedical library to search for the source of the data and to unearth the original research articles. Often, as I read the article, I discovered to my horror that the data had been collected from individuals not educated in the United States, that the sample size was extremely small (i.e., $n < 10$), or worse yet, that the data were generated from a different version of the test. If the same version of the test was being utilized, often the normative data had been collected by means of a nonstandard administration and/or scoring procedure! It was only after a thorough examination of how the studies were carried out—in terms of test administration, scoring, and demographic characteristics of the study participants—that one could begin to unravel the reasons why the use of one set of normative data yielded a different interpretation than use of another.

Those trips to the library resulted in the first article to summarize the available normative data for any neuropsychological test: "The Wechsler Memory Scale: A Critical Appraisal of the Normative Studies" (D'Elia, Satz & Schretlen, 1989). It was during the preparation of this article that our basic template for analyzing normative reports was developed.

The next question was: Why has no one gathered all this information together into a reference book? Fortunately I found two student colleagues in the same training program who shared my concern: Kyle Brauer-Boone and Allen D. Brandon. Kyle, Allen, and I eagerly returned to the library to collect the data necessary to produce a reference book. Soon we discovered why no such volume existed. It is hard to imagine now, but as recently as the late 1980s and early 1990s, the majority of neuropsychology-related professional journals still had not been referenced on computer. No subject category for "Norms" or "Normative Data" was listed in the key reference indices such as *Index Medicus* or *Psychological Abstracts*. As a result, most of the research papers were located by going through the various journals article by article. Gathering the necessary information proved to be a very large task, not one that I would recommend to a postdoctoral fellow at the beginning of his or her career. Yet that is exactly what we did. Hindsight is 20/20!

Allen Brandon withdrew from the project upon completing his postdoctoral fellowship. Private practice called. Only Kyle and I remained. The project slowly moved forward. Finding and cataloging the articles, then analyzing them by using the templates required much more work than we had imagined. About 4 years ago our friend and colleague, Maura Mitrushina, joined the project and with her considerable enthusiasm and efforts the project was completed.

FUTURE DIRECTIONS

The *Handbook* is as up-to-date as we could make it. In an imperfect world, we are certain that there will be omissions and errors. Accordingly, we have established a WEB site (www.normativedata.com) to post corrections/additions quickly and to make these updates and corrections to the book easily accessible. The WEB site was also created to alert users to all the available norms for any neuropsychological

test and to facilitate communication between researchers who develop normative data sets. We encourage our readers to e-mail us at this address to keep us abreast of their own normative projects.

We intend to update the *Handbook* every few years, and with subsequent editions, it will be expanded to include additional tests frequently used by neuropsychologists. For this initial outing, however, we decided to provide all the available normative data for 16 of the most frequently used neuropsychological tests as well as for the Wechsler Memory Scale battery. You will no doubt note some glaring test omissions. There was a method to our madness. For this edition, we decided not to include tests whose only normative data are reported in the test standardization manual (e.g., Wisconsin Card Sorting Test, California Verbal Learning Test, Wechsler Adult Intelligence Scale - III). Also, we wanted to get the book out before another 10 years passed! Almost all of the tests in this book continue to appear on lists of the most popularly utilized tests in neuropsychology. We also managed to sneak in some information regarding a couple of published tests that were developed in our laboratory that seem to be gaining popularity elsewhere (i.e., Color Trails Test, WHO-UCLA Auditory Verbal Learning Test).

We hope this book finds its place on the desks of professionals performing or reviewing neuropsychological assessments. We also hope it will be welcomed by teachers of assessment and psychological statistics, and will be helpful to graduate students learning to "interpret" test scores. Our goal is to help bolster confidence in the basis for clinical judgments and to strengthen the credibility of research and clinical findings.

Los Angeles, California   L.F.D.
March 1998

Acknowledgments

We wish to extend our deepest gratitude, appreciation, and thanks to all the authors whose normative and clinical comparison research is reviewed in this book. Without their work, this book would not have been possible. This volume is not intended to disparage the work of any author, as we strongly believe that each author has made an important contribution to knowledge through their research efforts.

Over the years several people have helped us with the preparation of this book. Their help took many forms, and included everything from help obtaining preprints of normative research articles or copies of previously unpublished normative data, to simple moral support. We offer each one our heartfelt thanks for every kindness and courtesy extended to us along the way: Jean Avezac, Izzy Baccarrdi, Julian Bach, Robert Bornstein, Virdette Brumm, Debora Burnison, Robert Butler, Janine Czarnetzki, Flo Comes, Lou Costa, Michele Croisier, Jeffrey Cummings, Doug Danaher, Dean Dellis, Jack Demick, Lois Desmond, Carl Dodrill, Linda Dukmajian, Robert Elliot, Gwenn Evans, Bee Fletcher, Travis Fogel, David Forney, Jennifer Forrest, Paula Fuld, Stephen Ganzell, Ismelda Gonzalez, Patricia Gross, Larry Herrera, Charles Hinkin, Stacey Horowitz, Robert Ivnik, Lissy Jarvik, Irene Kassorla, Ellen Kester, Glen Larrabee, Asenath LaRue, Stanislav Levin, James Loong, Enrique Lopez, Christine LoPresti, Lawrence Majovski, Gayle Marsh, James Marsh, Anahit Magzanyan, Mario Maj, Alfred Marohl, Joan McConnell, Susan McPherson, Fernando Melendez, Eric Miller, John Meyers, Robin Morris, Hector Myers, Linda Nelson, Tina Noriega, Lara Orchanian, Daniel Parks, Helen Paull, Eileen Pearlman, Marcel Ponton, Stephen Rebello, Mark Richardson, Linda Ringer, Eddie Rozenblat, Michael Salmone, Robert Sbordone, Jeffrey Schaeffer, Karen Schiltz, David Schretlen, Ola Selnes, Glenn Smith, Fabrizio Starace, Norton Stein, Tony Strickland, Donald Stuss, Donald Trahan, Craig Uchiyama, Doug Umetsu, Harry Van der Vlugt, Valdis Volkovskis, Wilfred Van Gorp, Lorne Yeudall, Travis White, Jane Williams, Bennett Williamson, and Betty Young.

Special thanks go to Muriel Lezak and Edith Kaplan who have been a constant source of encouragement and support from the very beginning of the project.

We extend our gratitude to Paul Satz who fostered in us appreciation for the complexity and excitement of the field of Neuropsychology.

The contribution of Dale Sherman in methodological accuracy of the book qualifies him a spot in heaven.

We also extend special thanks to Allen Brandon, who was an early collaborator on the book. Allen, your early efforts and great enthusiasm were deeply appreciated.

Dr. D'Elia offers his admiration and appreciation to his two coauthors, whose efforts brought this project to completion.

Endless thanks to our editor Jeffrey House, whose support throughout has been continuous and enthusiastic.

Finally, we would like to thank our families: M.M. thanks her children—big and little; K.B. thanks Rodney, Galen, and Fletcher; L.F.D. thanks his parents and family, especially Michael D. Salazar for their constant encouragement and support.

Contents

I. BACKGROUND

II. TESTS OF ATTENTION AND CONCENTRATION: VISUAL AND AUDITORY

III. LANGUAGE

IV. PERCEPTUAL ORGANIZATION: VISUOSPATIAL, AUDITORY, AND TACTILE

VI. MOTOR FUNCTIONS

VII. CONCEPT FORMATION AND REASONING

I

BACKGROUND

1

Introduction

Clinical neuropsychology is an applied science concerned with the behavioral expression of brain function and dysfunction (Lezak, 1995). Neuropsychologists are neurobehavior specialists who administer tests and test batteries that are typically tailored to answer specific referral questions. Ideally, a neuropsychological test battery consists of well-validated, reliable, standardized, and normed measures that serve to help elucidate and quantify behavioral changes that may have resulted from brain injury and other central nervous system disturbances. A neuropsychological examination provides a comprehensive evaluation of cognitive domains putatively associated with various brain substrates. The cognitive domains typically assessed include language, attention/concentration, visuospatial perception and constructional abilities, frontal systems/executive functions, and verbal and nonverbal learning and memory. Sensory and motor functions as well as general intellectual functioning are also routinely assessed. Findings from a neuropsychological examination can help highlight areas of functional strengths and weaknesses that may have focal or lateralizing significance. A neuropsychological evaluation is therefore considered an essential component in the diagnosis, treatment planning, and care of patients with suspected congenital or acquired brain dysfunction.

After administration of the test battery, the neuropsychologist is faced with making sense of a plethora of numerical and qualitative data. In order to make optimal use of the test data, the neuropsychologist must have an understanding of what constitutes "normal" performance on the tests before an opinion regarding the strengths and/or weaknesses of various neurobehavioral capacities can be offered.

To be meaningful, test scores must have an empirical frame of reference. Normative data provide this empirical context and represent the range of performance on a particular test of a group of medically/neurologically healthy individuals with relatively homogeneous demographic characteristics. These normative reference groups are considered the "gold standard" against which an individual's test performance is compared and contrasted.

However, while normative data are a critical starting point for the interpretative process, they do not provide the sole basis for the interpretation of test scores. Test data alone do not provide an adequate basis for making sound clinical judgments regarding cognitive functioning. As Lezak (1995) stresses, interpretation of the data obtained from a neuropsychological examination must take into account qualitative observations and the patient's history, background, present circumstances, motivation, attitudes, and expectations regarding self and the examination. A formal evaluation of the patient's emotional functioning and personality characteristics is also an intrinsic part of neuropsychological evaluation. All this information taken together provides a framework for an accurate understanding of a patient's cognitive strengths and limitations.

To illustrate the relationship between different sources of information, consider Figure 1.1.

As can be seen, no single section of the pyramid in Figure 1.1 should be used alone to form an opinion about neuropsychological functioning. All interpretative elements (raw data/norms, observations of test-taking behaviors, and medical history/presenting symptoms) must come into play in building evidence that forms the basis for a professional opinion. Further shaping the interpretative process, of course, is the neuropsychologist's clinical judgment, which is influenced by his or her education, professional experience, and research knowledge base.

The history (including medical, psychiatric, educational, vocational, and avocational) and presenting symptoms are important in understanding test data. A detailed medical/psychiatric history is an especially important source of information given that neuropsychological test performance can be greatly influenced by medical or psychiatric conditions. Documenting risk factors known to affect neuropsychological test performance is essential since an important task of neuropsychologists is to properly attribute

the contribution of peripheral nervous system, central nervous system, and medical and/or emotional dysfunction to the clinical picture.

It is also important to observe the qualitative process of performance leading to a specific score on a test. Reporting a score without revealing *how* it was obtained can sometimes be misleading. For illustrative purposes, assume that the criterion for passing a particular component of a driving test is that the car is in the garage. We look, and yes, the car is in the garage. Criterion met. The driver passed the test. Or did he? We interview an observer to the event and sadly learn that the person drove through the garage door to get there! Obviously not a stellar performance. Similarly, with neuropsychological testing, noting *how* an individual obtained a score can be quite illuminating. Consider two 75-year-old architects (patient A and patient B) who each obtain a score of 36/36 on the Rey-Osterrieth test. On a normative basis alone, performance scores for both patients would be considered within normal limits. But how did these two architects obtain the score? Patient A quickly recognized the overall gestalt of the drawing, drew a box, and filled in the details. Patient B failed to appreci-

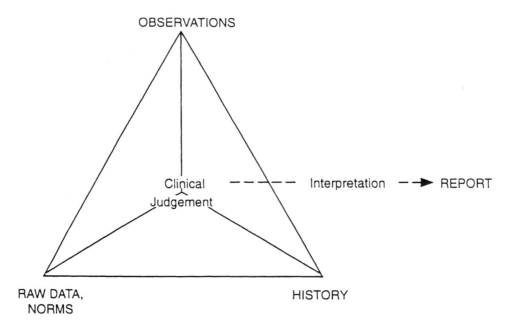

Figure 1.1. Graphic representation of the relationship between different sources of information contributing to decision-making process in neuropsychology.

ate the drawing's overall shape and built up the figure by accretion—taking eight minutes to do so with numerous erasures. Same score as patient A, but a dramatically different performance suggestive of a significant loss in spatial/constructional ability.

In observing a patient's test-taking style, it is important to assess attitude, effort, and motivation. In all evaluations one must ascertain whether patients are offering their best performance on the tests administered. Obviously, low test scores can be a product of lack of effort or deliberate failure. Unfortunately, only a few tests are available that permit neuropsychologists to assess malingering and level of test-taking motivation. However, the overall profile of scores across different measures and the consistency of successes and failures across measures addressing similar cognitive domains aid in determining the validity of test results. This issue is especially important in medical–legal evaluations due to identifiable secondary gain.

In neuropsychological practice, one examines the pattern of test performance within a functional domain to assure greater probability of accurate interpretation. No single test score is sufficient to render a judgment regarding brain dysfunction. For instance, a single score on a verbal memory test has little meaning unless interpreted in the context of the individual's pattern of performance on other tests which also assess verbal memory functioning.

The reason for this is quite simple. In most neuropsychological examinations one can expect to find an instance of unexplained performance deviation. This observed deviation may be due to an attentional lapse or to measurement error. Obviously, an occasional poor test finding, more or less in isolation, has less meaning than a pattern of poor test findings occurring within a specific cognitive domain. Also, it is important to keep in mind that no test is a perfect measure of what it purports to assess. Therefore it is often important to administer more than one test assessing a particular functional domain, especially if a lower than expected score is obtained on an initial examination of the functional capacity under study.

For instance, consider a neuropsychologist who administers the Grooved Pegboard Test as the only measure of motor functioning. The patient obtains a lower score for the dominant hand than the nondominant hand and the neuropsychologist regards this as evidence of left hemisphere dysfunction. The problem with this interpretation, of course, is that poor performance on the Grooved Pegboard Test might be due to factors other than a motor deficit, such as a "practice effect" which benefits the second hand to be tested. Poor dominant hand performance might also be explained by a patient's idiosyncratic approach and slow start on the task. Therefore, in this situation it would be important to administer other motor tests, such as finger tapping or grip strength, to document whether the original findings can be corroborated. Thus, more than one test should be administered when assessing performance within a specific functional domain so that the internal consistency of performance findings can be judged before offering an opinion about function.

In summary, failure to consider all aspects of the interpretative process will increase the probability of faulty inferences being drawn from the neuropsychological data obtained.

TEST NORMS

Despite the critical importance of having access to normative data to facilitate clinical interpretation of tests findings, there are relatively few large-scale normative reports in the literature. This is especially evident when one considers the large number of validation studies on the utility of neuropsychological tests in discriminating groups of patients with lateralized or focal lesions. To some extent, the relatively small body of literature regarding normative research is related to the formidable logistic problems and expense associated with the execution of such studies. However, the larger problem is that researchers generally have not been supported either financially or professionally in conducting normative research. Although test norms are essential to proper interpretation in clinical and research settings, major funding agencies have not favored such studies. The key problem is that these studies are inevitably descriptive, and descriptive studies are generally not considered "scientific" since no hypotheses are being tested. Until very recently, journal editors have generally been loath to publish normative reports, opting instead for more "scientific" works. As a result, a substantial number of normative datasets are imbedded in publications of clinical studies, making them difficult to locate. Since most researchers are employed in "publish-or-perish" environments, such research takes a low priority. These obstacles to normative research have remained in place despite the awareness that it is sorely needed, and indeed, essential. So, although neuropsychological assessment procedures are widely available, there is a relative scarcity of normative data for most tests.

For a few of the most popular tests (i.e., Trail-Making Test A & B, Rey Auditory-Verbal Learning Test), however, numerous reports are available which provide normative comparison data for performance across the greater part of the life span. The problem then arises for clinicians and researchers: which set of normative data to use? Large differences in reported scores among studies examining performance on the same test in groups of individuals that have nearly identical demographic characteristics, as well as vague descriptions of how the data were collected, compound the problem of identifying appropriate norms for comparison purposes. A frequent difficulty one encounters is that use of one set of norms may suggest that the patient is performing in the impaired range, while use of another normative sample may suggest that performance is within normal limits. Unfortunately, use of the wrong set of comparison data may pave the way for faulty inferences being drawn—perhaps also resulting in either unnecessary treatment or therapeutic neglect. To demonstrate this point, consider the hypothetical medical–legal case of a person born and educated in the United States (one year of college), physically healthy, 85 years old man who presents with complaints of memory difficulty. The patient would like to continue to handle his financial affairs, but his family is concerned about his competency to do so. In the course of evaluating the patient, you administer several memory tests including the Rey Auditory-Verbal Learning Test (AVLT). In the unlikely event that you were only interested in his performance score for trial 5, there would be seven published normative reports to choose from, which are presented in Table 1.1.

Let's assume that the patient's trial 5 score was 6/15 correct. Reliance on the Query and Megran (1983) "normative" data would suggest that test performance is in the average range (53rd percentile). However, close reading of that "normative" report would reveal that the data were collected on a sample of Veterans Administration (V.A.) patients hospitalized for a variety of physical complaints. Thus, overall performance scores of the comparison sample were probably artificially lowered because of hospitalization effects, chronic pain effects, and dysphoria. Therefore, applying the Query and Megran data would lead the examiner to conclude that the patient's performance was better than it probably was. Depending on which other remaining normative reports were utilized, the patient's score would fall in the low average (Geffen et al., 1990; 19th percentile), borderline (Rey, 1964, 5th percentile; Bleecker et al., 1988, sixth percentile; Mitrushina & Satz, 1991a, fourth percentile; Van Gorp et al., 1990, eighth percentile), or impaired range (Bolla-Wilson & Bleecker, 1986, first percentile).

Unfortunately, all the studies reporting trial 5 data for this age group suffer from small sample size ($n < 50$). In terms of selecting the "best study" for comparison purposes, those with the smallest sample size should probably be first rejected from consideration. This would eliminate from consideration the studies of Bleecker et al., Bolla-Wilson and Bleecker, and Geffen et al. Data from the Geffen et al. report should additionally be avoided due to cultural differences in comparing North American vs. Australian samples and also due to the fact that the educational level of the samples was low. As noted in Spreen and Strauss (1991), use of Rey's norms (reported in 1964, but collected in 1944) should be avoided because of test content and administration differences. Also, these data were collected over 50 years ago in Switzerland, raising serious concerns about cohort and cultural effects. Of the two normative reports remaining (Van Gorp et al., 1990; Mitrushina & Satz, 1991a), which incidentally both suggest that the patient's performance was borderline, the one by Van Gorp et al. would be selected

Table 1.1. Published Rey AVLT Normative Reports

Investigator	Age Group	N	Education	Trial 5	Trial 7	Length of Delay	Trial 8	Where Tested
Van Gorp et al., 1990	76–85	26	13.3 (3.6)	9.8 (2.7)				S.Calif
Mitrushina & Satz, 1991a	76–85	16	14.0 (3.6)	10.3 (2.4)	8.4 (3.5)			S.Calif
Geffen et al., 1990	70–86	10 males	11.1 (3.1)	8.2 (2.5)	6.4 (1.7)	20 min	5.6 (2.6)	S.Australia
Ivnik et al., 1992c	74–84	196	At least high school	Not reported		30 min	Tables indicate a score of 6 = 41–59th %tile	Minnesota
Query & Megran, 1983	70–81	23 males	11.4 yrs for ages 19–81	5.86 (2.04)				N.Dakota All VA Inpatients with physical complaints
Bolla-Wilson & Bleecker, 1986	70–84	10 males	Median for 51–84 age sample was 15(3) yrs	12.6 (2.2)				Maryland
Bleecker et al., 1988	80–89	11 males	18 (1.9)	9.2 (2.09)				Maryland
Rey, 1964	70–88	15	no info.	10.9 (2.9)				Switzerland

because of the larger sample size. The subject and procedural characteristics of these two studies are otherwise nearly identical. Finally, and most importantly, the demographic characteristics of the patient being evaluated matched well with the demographic characteristics of the participants in this normative study.

If one were interested in examining the delayed recall performance of this patient, only two studies would be available for normative comparison purposes (Geffen et al., 1990; Ivnik et al., 1992c). Geffen's report would be avoided in favor of Ivnik's for reasons of sample size and educational and cultural issues and the fact that the length of delay for the delayed recall condition was 30 minutes. However, if a better normative data match is not available, it should be considered that the greatest rate of forgetting occurs during the first 20 minutes. Consequently, the effect of variability in the length of delay between different norms from 20 to 30

minutes (even 45 minutes to 1 hour) on rates of forgetting is minimal. Because no normative study ordinarily allows a perfect fit to the demographic characteristics of the patient under study, the examiner should be aware of the specific limitations of any dataset used for inferential purposes.

Because patients are often evaluated more than once on the same test (often by different examiners), clinicians are urged to document the source of comparison data used to arrive at conclusions *within* the body of any report. This recommendation is especially relevant for tests with multiple and/or overlapping sets of normative data (D'Elia et al., 1989).

In addition to normative data, there is another set of data that can be used for comparison purposes when it is available. *Clinical comparison data* (aka: *abnorms*) represent the range of test performances of distinct groups of medically, psychiatrically, and/or neurologically compromised individuals with relatively homogeneous demographic characteristics.

Because of the general lack of clinical comparison data, however, neuropsychologists have largely relied on normative comparison data for interpretative purposes. As a result, interpretative comments have been limited to reporting how the patient under study differs from a healthy sample. Having the ability to discuss how a patient under study is similar to other *patient groups* would be a welcome addition to the field. The availability of clinical comparison data sets would permit such analysis.

TESTS

Standard and Experimental

Neuropsychologists use published, standardized measures that are well normed and generally accepted as standard tools of assessment in the field. There are several reasons why neuropsychologists must utilize standardized measures. Patients presenting for neuropsychological evaluation are frequently reevaluated over time, often by different examiners. As Figure 1.1 illustrates, the test data collected during the examination is an essential ingredient in forming a professional opinion regarding neuropsychological functioning. Since the written report of findings is a professional communication from one clinician to another, in order for the report to be meaningful and therefore useful to other professionals, the data presented in the report must have been obtained from tests that are familiar to, or can be easily referenced by, any clinician reading the report. The use of standard tests and standard administration/scoring procedures is especially critical in initial examinations of patients to establish a meaningful baseline. Baseline data are essential for subsequent comparison with retest data to document whether there has been improvement or decline in functioning. If tests are employed in the initial exam which are unique to the neuropsychologist administering them, then subsequent examiners will be unable to make comparisons between baseline and subsequent performance.

In a forensic context, the use of nonstandard tests and procedures impedes the fact-finding process. Unfortunately, it is not uncommon to review reports of medical–legal examinations that have relied heavily or exclusively upon findings from experimental measures as the basis for an opinion of neuropsychological impairment. Not surprisingly, the experimental measures employed almost always are purported to be tests of memory, attention/concentration, and/or frontal systems functioning—three cognitive domains that are especially sensitive to any brain insult, regardless of etiology. The use of experimental tests and the claims made to courts that the measures are at the "cutting edge" and provide objective evidence of impaired brain function often result in—at least for a while—increased business for the provider of this service. Rather than providing neuropsychological service, however, neuropsychologists conducting themselves in this way are practicing a form of modern day alchemy—they have found a way to turn their time into gold. Such practice not only harms the patient through mislabeling but also undermines the legitimacy of neuropsychological practice in the forensic arena.

Increasingly, neuropsychologists are being called upon to provide expert-witness courtroom testimony as to whether brain-behavior functioning is "intact", "impaired," or otherwise "compromised" after a brain insult (Satz, 1988; Matarazzo, 1990; Leckliter & Matarazzo, 1989). This development seems reasonable since neuropsychology is an applied science concerned with the behavioral expression of brain function and dysfunction. However, the days of being able to state in court, "*it is my professional experience that . . .*" without also providing the objective basis to support an opinion (i.e., normative data, clinical comparison data, history, medical records, symptoms, observations) are over. Neuropsychologists are now regularly asked by knowledgeable attorneys to produce the objective basis - particularly the normative data - for their opinions. This development stems in part from the scathing review of the field of neuropsychology for attorneys by Faust et al. (1991): *Brain Damage Claims: Coping With Neuropsychological Evidence*. Neuropsychologists must be prepared to state why they used a particular set of normative data for comparison purposes. Although this line of inquiry by attorneys is a relatively new development in the courtroom, the practice is sound and should be welcomed. Why? Let's look at what our professional rules of practice tell us. Principle 2.04(a) of our code of ethics (American Psychological Association, 1992) states that "Psychologists who . . . administer, score, interpret, or use assessment techniques are familiar with the reliability, validation, and related standardization or outcome studies of, and proper applications and uses of, the techniques they use." Principle 2.04(c) states, "Psychologists attempt to identify situations in which . . . assessment techniques or norms may not be applicable or may require adjustment in administration or interpretation because of factors such as individuals' gender, age, race, ethnicity, national origin, . . . disability, language, or socioeconomic status." Principle 2.05 states, "When interpreting assessment results, . . . psychologists . . . indicate any significant reservations they have about the accuracy or limitations of their interpretations." Finally, principle 2.07(a) states that "Psychologists do not base their assessment . . . decisions . . . on data . . . that are outdated for the current purpose."

Of course, experimental measures are occasionally used during the course of an evaluation. This is tolerated by our field because experimental test development is a natural evolution in a discipline that advocates and uses research to advance knowledge about clinical assessment and diagnosis. However, findings from experimental tests should be used only to supplement and support findings from standardized procedures that were also administered. Findings from experimental tests should never be used as the primary basis for forming opinions about impaired neuropsychological functioning. Serious professional and ethical concerns are raised when neuropsychologists substantially deviate from standard test administration and scoring procedures and/or rely heavily on experimental tests for clinical judgments.

When Is a Test Considered Experimental?

There are at least four levels of experimental tests (presented in the order from most experimental to least):

Level 1 tests have never been peer reviewed or published and are typically uniquely utilized by the neuropsychologist who developed them. Often normative data are sparse or nonexistent.

Level 2 tests, although never published, may have been reviewed by peers and used by a specific group of neuropsychologists conducting a multisite research study. Again, normative data may be sparse or lacking.

Level 3 tests often have been widely distributed to interested parties for experimental use; however, there have been no published studies utilizing these tests. Preliminary normative, reliability, and validity data are usually available.

Level 4 tests have been carefully described in peer-reviewed journals as having been included in a study where several other standardized tests were administered. Preliminary normative data are available, and there is also some information about the test's reliability and validity. These tests generally have not yet been formally published by a recognized test publisher/distributor but are made available by the author(s) to interested parties for research/experimental use.

Whereas findings based on level 1, 2, and 3 tests should be given little clinical weight and viewed with extreme caution, a level 4 test has at least undergone formal peer review before publication of the findings in a recognized professional journal. Therefore, although caution is warranted when discussing findings from a level 4 experimental test, the results may be used if they are buttressed by similar findings from more formal, standardized tests.

What Determines Whether a Test Is Considered "Standard?"

At a minimum, three of the following four criteria should be met before a test is regarded as being in standard use:

1. *The test must be readily available to the professional community and adequately normed.* Using this definition, however, it is possible for a test considered "standard" to slide into the "experimental" range when not adequately normed for the age group under study. For instance, the majority of our "standard" tests must be considered "quasi-experimental" when utilized in assessing adults over age 80, members of minority groups, or any individual who does not speak English or uses it as a second language: In each such case adequate normative data are often sparse or lacking. Fortunately, several research groups are currently addressing the need for norming within the upper age ranges (Ivnik et al.; Bornstein et al.; LaRue et al.; Ryan et al.), and for various cultural subsets (Ardilla et al.; Ponton et al.; LaRue et al.; Satz et al; Heaton et al.).

2. *The test stimulus and materials should be standardized. A manual describing test administration and scoring procedures and providing information on reliability and validity should be available.* The above requirements usually imply that the test has been formally published by a respected test publishing/distribution company. However, several tests that are considered "standard" have never been formally published. For instance, the Rey Auditory-Verbal Learning Test has never been formally published nor have the administration procedures been standardized. But most of the necessary information on norms, reliability, and

validity for this test can be found in the neuropsychological literature.

3. *Research using the test must have been peer reviewed and published in recognized professional journals.*

4. *The test has been reviewed in the* Mental Measurements Yearbook *and/or reviewed in more than one neuropsychological text by authors not connected with its development.*

In conclusion, neuropsychologists are responsible for choosing the particular tests utilized in attempting to answer referral or research questions, and for selecting the best possible clinical comparison data (both norms and "abnorms"). Being more accountable for what is done, and being able to elucidate *why* it was done, will not only serve to raise the credibility of neuropsychology as a distinct specialty but will also enhance the utilization of neuropsychological services within the medical and legal communities.

2

Statistical and Psychometric Issues

The administration, scoring, and interpretation of neuropsychological tests represent a major resource in the clinical practice of a neuropsychologist. However, accurate decision-making based on test results cannot be achieved without a clear understanding of the issues related to the measurement of psychological phenomena and the statistical properties of the tests. This chapter reviews basic statistical concepts of importance to neuropsychologists. No intent was made to provide a comprehensive review of statistics. The goal of this chapter is to help a novice understand and interpret psychometric data.

MEASUREMENT AND INTERPRETATION OF NUMERICAL VALUES

Measuring abilities and traits is an inherent part of clinical work. It facilitates decision-making by relating the performance of a given individual to an appropriate reference group or by uncovering a change in an individual's behavior over time. The nature of decision-making is specific to a given situation and includes a wide range of decisions, such as identifying cognitive strengths and weaknesses, choosing an appropriate course of cognitive rehabilitation, evaluating a patient's ability to function independently in an everyday environment, choosing an academic field and professional career, making diagnostic differentiation between disorders

that affect cognitive functioning, assessing the rate of improvement or deterioration in functional capacities, and making prognostic predictions.

The concept of measurement implies numerical representation of certain properties. Such physical properties as dimensions, intensity, speed, and gravity, which represent a core of scientific exploration, lend themselves to accurate and reliable measurements. In contrast to direct measurement of physical phenomena, psychological attributes such as cognitive abilities, personality traits, and emotional status cannot be measured directly. In order to assess these psychological constructs, we need to obtain a sample of behavior that can be quantified and represented in numerical scores. Well-validated psychological tests are designed to elicit behaviors that are representative of the underlying psychological constructs.

Numerical values derived from an individual's performance on a test are identified as raw scores and may represent the number of correct responses, time required for completion of the test, number of errors, rating of the quality of a drawing, or different combinations of the above criteria.

In contrast to physical measuring scales that have an absolute zero point, scaling of psychological measures does not start at the point of "no ability at all"—i.e., a raw score of zero on an arithmetic test does not indicate that the patient has no ability to solve arithmetic problems. If the test included basic operations of addition or subtraction of single digits, the patient would be likely to succeed on these items. As a result, we cannot infer that a patient who received a raw score of 50 on a test is twice as good in arithmetic as someone with a score of 25. Due to the lack of the absolute zero point in psychological measurements, ratios of scores are meaningless and most psychological tests are scored on an interval scale. Despite some disadvantages of the interval scale in comparison to the ratio scale, both of these scales provide measurements that lend themselves to advanced statistical analyses.

The raw score obtained on a test says little about an individual's level of ability or mastery of the subject. In order to interpret the raw score, it should be related to the content of the test or compared to the performance of a group of individuals on the same test:

1. Domain- or content-referenced interpretation indicates how proficient an individual is in the domain tapped by the task presented on the test. Content mastery is usually reported as a percentage of correct responses on the test.

2. Criterion-referenced interpretation relates an individual's performance on a test to an external criterion measure, such as a practical situation which requires skills assessed by the test. For example, expectancy tables tie different levels of test performance to expected practical outcomes.

3. Norm-referenced interpretation compares scores achieved by one individual to the performance of a respective group of individuals who have similar characteristics. This normative or standardization sample is assumed to be representative of a population from which it is drawn and is used as an external standard of performance for interpretation of individual scores.

There are several methods of relating individual performance to the norms:

a. Raw scores obtained on a test can be converted to age or grade equivalents which allow interpretation of a particular score in the context of expected performance for specific age or grade level. This method is highly useful in assessing the developmental standing of children in comparison to their peers, providing that a considerable and well-identified increment in ability with age and grade advancement is expected. However, this method loses its effectiveness when the rate of development becomes uneven and the relationship between levels of ability and developmental markers weakens.

b. Measures of relative standing of individual scores within a distribution provide an alternative method of evaluating individual performance. Percentile rank (*PR*) reflects the percentage of the standardization sample that scored lower than individual score (plus one-half of that portion of the standardization sample who achieved the same score as the individual being assessed). Percentile ranks are useful in providing the relative standing of a score; however, they indicate only the ordinal position of the individual score within the distribution. They do not show dispersion of the remainder of the distribution below that score and do not indicate the absolute amount of difference between scores. For example, percentile transformations magnify differences between individuals close to the center of the distribution and compress the differences at the extremes.

Let's consider a distribution of scores (*A*) representing the number of words recalled on the fifth trial of the Rey Auditory-Verbal Learning Test (RAVLT):

$$A = (5, 7, 8, 8, 9, 9, 9, 9, 10, 10, 10, 10, 10,$$
$$11, 11, 11, 11, 12, 12, 13, 15)$$

There are 21 observations in this distribution. An individual who obtained a score of 9 performed better than four individuals who received scores lower than 9, plus two out of four individuals (0.5) who achieved a score of 9. Relating this proportion of six individuals to the total number of 21 observations yields a percentile rank (*PR*) of 29, as follows from the formula:

$$PR_{(9)} = \frac{4 + (0.5)(4)}{21} \times 100 = 29$$

Similar calculations of percentile ranks for scores 8 and 7 in the above distribution yield $PR = 14$ and 5, respectively:

$$PR_{(8)} = \frac{2 + (0.5)(2)}{21} \times 100 = 14$$

and

$$PR_{(7)} = \frac{1}{21} \times 100 = 5$$

As follows from the above calculations, the difference in percentile ranks between scores 9 and 8 ($29 - 14 = 15$) is greater than the difference in percentile ranks between scores 8 and 7 ($14 - 5 = 9$). This example illustrates the main disadvantage of the percentile ranks: Whereas they reflect the relative position of an individual score respective to the standardization sample, they do not indicate the absolute differences between scores.

c. In order to accommodate the absolute differences between the scores, the interpretation of a raw score should be based on the relative standing of the score with respect to the mean for the distribution and the variability of the scores within the distribution. This can be accomplished through converting a raw score into a standard score. Most frequently used standard scores are z scores and T scores.

STANDARDIZATION OF RAW SCORES

Compare the distribution of RAVLT scores (A) used in the above example with another distribution of scores on this test (B), both of which range from 5 to 15 with a mean of 10:

A = (5, 7, 8, 8, 9, 9, 9, 9, 10, 10, 10, 10, 10, 11, 11, 11, 11, 12, 12, 13, 15)

B = (5, 5, 5, 5, 6, 6, 6, 7, 7, 8, 10, 12, 13, 13, 14, 14, 14, 15, 15, 15, 15)

Visual examination of these distributions suggests that the variability around the mean is much greater for distribution B. Therefore, a score of 7 would indicate very poor performance relative to distribution A and a much better performance relative to distribution B. In order to account for the degree of variability in the normative distribution, individual measurements are converted into z scores.

In another example, assessing recall of an individual on the fifth trial of RAVLT, we use a reference sample with mean of 10 (see graphs below). If the individual recalled seven words, comparison of the raw score with the mean for the reference sample ($X - M$) suggests that this individual's recall was three words below the expected score of 10 for his age. However, this does not tell us how low his or her performance was relative to the distribution of the normative sample.

If a high degree of variability is expected and the standard deviation for the reference sample is 6 (graph A), then a score of 7 falls halfway between a mean of 10 for the reference sample and a score of 4 representing 1 SD below the mean, which results in a z score of -0.5.

A)
$-1\,SD \quad X \quad\quad M$
|—|—|—|—|—|—|—|—|—|—|—|—|—|—|
1 2 3 4 5 6 7 8 9 10 11 12 13 14 15
Number of words

In reference to another sample with the same mean, but a much lower degree of variability reflected in a standard deviation of 1 (see graph B), a score of 7 lies 3 SD below the mean ($z = -3$). Therefore, the recall of seven words in relation to distribution B indicates much poorer performance than in reference to distribution A.

B)
$X - 1\,SDM$
|—|—|—|—|—|—|—|—|—|—|—|—|—|—|
1 2 3 4 5 6 7 8 9 10 11 12 13 14 15
Number of words

Thus, in order to account for the variability within the normative distribution, raw scores are standardized, i.e., converted into z scores which relate the difference between an individual score and the group mean ($X - M$) to the standard deviation for the reference group:

$$z = \frac{X - M}{SD}$$

A negative z score indicates that the raw score lies below the mean for the reference group, a positive z score represents higher performance than the mean for the group, and a z score of zero indicates that the raw score is equal to the mean of the reference group.

Z scores (standard deviation units) show not only how much an individual performance deviates from the mean of the sample, but also how likely it is that other individuals in the sample would achieve scores which are as high or as low as the person being tested.

The standardization of raw scores, e.g., their conversion into z scores, allows comparison of the relative standing of individuals across different tests in spite of the differences in the measurement scales or the means and standard deviations for these tests. A standardized distribution of z scores has a mean of 0 and a standard deviation of 1 because the mean is subtracted from each score and the result is divided by the standard deviation. It preserves the same shape as the distribution of the raw scores from which it was derived. Therefore, differences in standard scores are proportional to the differences in the corresponding raw scores.

In spite of the obvious advantages of using z scores over raw scores, some of the properties of z scores are viewed as undesirable: (1) z scores have fractional values which are carried to at least one decimal place; (2) half of the z scores in the standardized distribution are negative and half are positive, which leads to the zero-sum problem, i.e., corresponding values on both sides of the distribution cancel each other when totaled.

The parameter values of the standard distribution are arbitrarily designated. Therefore, they can be easily changed through simple arithmetic transformations of z scores. T score transformations overcome these disadvantages through multiplying z scores by 10 (thus eliminating fractional values) and adding a constant of 50 (which eliminates negative values and places all the scores on a scale from 0 to 100 with a mean of 50 and a standard deviation of 10):

$$T = 10z + 50$$

For example, a z score of -1.6 can be expressed in T scores as follows:

$$T = (-16) + 50 = 34$$

An example of a test which uses T score conversion is the Minnesota Multiphasic Personality Inventory (MMPI) and its recent revision. Clinically significant elevations on the scales are judged relative to a mean of 50 and standard deviation of 10, which equates the scale of measurement across all validity and clinical scales on this test.

STANDARD SCORES AND NORMAL DISTRIBUTION

Many biological measures and human characteristics are distributed so that the highest frequency of scores is observed around the distribution mean with a gradual decrease in the frequency further away from the mean which eventually tails off on both sides. Score distributions of many psychological tests approximate this model, which in its ideal hypothetical form represents a normal distribution. It is convenient to treat test score distributions as if they were normally distributed because the properties of this model are known:

1. The distribution of hypothetical score frequencies arranged from the lowest to the highest values is bell-shaped and symmetrical—i.e., the left and the right sides are mirror-images of each other.
2. The frequency is highest in the middle of the distribution; therefore the mean, median, and mode have the same values and divide the distribution into two equal parts.
3. The normal distribution stretches from minus to plus infinity; thus the "tails" of the distribution get closer and closer to the X-axis as they get farther away from the mean, but they never touch the X-axis.
4. The normal distribution is described by a specific mathematical formula.

Although the test score distributions do not perfectly match this model, if the number of cases were increased and smaller class intervals were used, the shape of the sample distribution would become relatively smooth and symmetrical, thus approximating the distribution of scores in the population from which the sample was drawn.

This assumption of normality of the test score distribution allows it to be converted into a distribution of z scores with a mean of 0 and a standard deviation of 1, which represents a standard normal distribution. The use of this conversion facilitates interpretation of the test scores because it allows comparison of a variety of otherwise not comparable distributions through equating their means and standard deviations. The proportion of cases comprising a certain area under the curve between two points along the z-axis is known, which permits conversion of z score units into percentiles. For example, it is known that 34.13% of all scores lie between $z = 0$ and $z = +1$. Since the mean of the distribution ($z = 0$) divides the distribution in half, we know that 50% of all scores lie below the mean. Thus, adding 34.13% of scores above the mean to 50% of scores below the mean suggests that the 84.13th percentile corresponds to a $z = +1$.

Figure 2.1 illustrates the corresponding conversion values for only selected z scores. The proportion of scores (i.e., the area under the standard normal curve) for each value along the z-axis can be easily determined using tables provided in any basic statistics textbook.

INTERPRETATION OF INFREQUENT (OUTLYING) SCORES

As follows from Figure 2.1, 68.26% of all scores fall within 1 standard deviation from the mean in both directions, 95.44% fall within 2 standard deviations, and almost all scores except for 0.0026% are included between −3 and +3 standard deviations from the mean.

This correspondence between the proportion of cases and z score values is important for interpretation of individual test performance, since such interpretation is based on the relative frequency of the score obtained by the individual being assessed with respect to the distribution of scores. For example, a test score falling above or below 2 standard deviations from the distribution mean is highly infrequent;

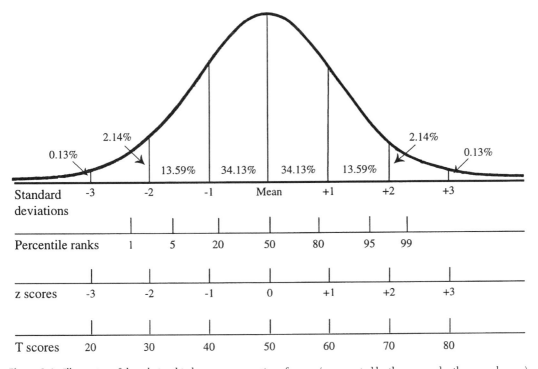

Figure 2.1. Illustration of the relationship between proportion of scores (represented by the area under the normal curve), percentile ranks, z scores, and T scores.

only 4.56% of the scores deviate that far from the mean in both directions. Therefore, individuals obtaining these infrequent scores may be viewed as outliers. The decision criteria for defining scores as outlying might vary from more conservative to more liberal in different clinical situations, depending on cost–benefit ratio of making false-positive vs. false-negative error.

Outlying scores can have different origins:

1. They might be due to the inherent variability in the population. Indeed, in any population, innate levels of a trait or ability range from a very low to very high, which is modeled by a normal distribution. Therefore, a certain proportion of extreme scores is a natural feature of the population.

2. There might be purely deterministic reasons accounting for too low or too high scores, such as:

Inadequate reliability of the measuring instrument

Variations in the test administration and scoring strategy

Errors in data recording or in calculating appropriate statistics

Demographic factors and physical handicaps affecting performance

Situational factors (e.g., external noise)

Sensitization and anxiety associated with the testing situation

Emotional factors and level of endurance (fatigue)

Response style and response bias

Motivational factors

Previous exposure to similar tests (practice effect)

3. Outlying scores may result from an execution error. In this case an individual score is foreign to the distribution used for comparison. For example, an elderly individual of low average ability might appear impaired when compared to a normative sample of highly functioning, independently living, relatively healthy elderly individuals. This bias in the normative sample, which is not representative of all func-tional and economic levels of the population for the respective age group, would result in an inflated mean and in upward "slippage" of the entire distribution. In order to avoid execution errors, a clinician should be highly sensitive to the appropriateness of the norms used for each individual being evaluated.

INTERPRETATION OF SCORES WHICH ARE NOT NORMALLY DISTRIBUTED

The interpretation of individual test scores respective to the normative distribution is based on an assumption of the normality of this distribution. In order to avoid interpretive errors, the basis for test score interpretation should be different if distribution is asymmetrical. Standardized distribution has the same shape as the original distribution of test scores, which is highly dependent on the characteristics of the individual items comprising the test.

If a test is designed in such a way that the majority of individuals can succeed on most of the items, test scores are compressed into a few discrete values at the upper extreme of the score range. There are only a few observations at the lower part of the score range. In this case, the distribution is negatively skewed and variability of scores falling within normal and above normal range is highly limited. The test has its highest discriminative power at the lower ability levels—i.e., it is most useful in identifying impaired individuals. For example, the distribution of scores on the Boston Naming Test and the Rey-Osterrieth Complex Figure (copy condition) in a sample of highly functioning individuals would acquire this shape.

In the case when test items present difficulty for the majority of subjects, the score distribution is positively skewed. Variability within the lower range of scores is highly limited, whereas the highest sensitivity is obtained in the upper part of the distribution. Such a test would be most appropriate for the selection of a few outstanding individuals from a large group of subjects. As an example, the distribution of scores for Raven's Advanced Progressive Matrices can be used.

In both of the above cases resulting in skewed score distributions, the use of z score conversions is inappropriate, since such conversions are based on the assumption of normality (particularly symmetry) of the distribution.

PSYCHOMETRIC PROPERTIES OF TESTS

In view of the proliferation of psychological tests with a high overlap in terms of abilities assessed by these tests, we are frequently faced with a dilemma: which test to select in a particular situation. All published tests have to meet the requirements outlined by the *Standards for Educational and Psychological Testing* (American Psychological Association, 1985). Yet, the choice of a test should be made in the context of a certain clinical situation. In choosing an appropriate test, one has to keep in mind several criteria for evaluating psychometric properties of the test.

Reliability

When measuring a certain aspect of individual's functioning, our main assumption is that the scores on a particular test would be consistent over repeated administrations. If an individual sometimes receives high scores and sometimes low scores on the same test, no inferences can be made regarding the level of ability which is measured by this test. In other words, we have to be assured that the test is a reliable measure of a stable construct such as a specific ability. However, a certain degree of variability is inherent in test performance. It is due to transient factors associated with the testing situation and the patient's state at the time of testing.

Thus, the score on a test reflects the contribution of the following two factors:

$$X = T + e$$

where:

X is the score on a test

T is a "true" score representing the actual level of ability measured by a test

e is an error of measurement reflecting random variability

With an increase in test reliability, a considerable proportion of the variability in the observed test scores is due to differences in the "true" scores. In other words, reliability can be expressed as the proportion of variance in test scores which is accounted for by the "true" differences between subjects on the ability being measured. Therefore, a reliability coefficient provides a measure of test reliability representing the ratio of "true" score variance to the total variance of the test scores:

$$r_{xx} = \frac{\sigma^2 T}{\sigma^2 T + \sigma^2 e}$$

Methods of Estimating Reliability of a Test

Several procedures have been developed to determine the reliability of a test by measuring the proportion of "true" variance vs. the proportion of "error" variance. Different methods define measurement error with respect to different sources of error. The four most common methods are described below:

1. The test–retest method assesses the consistency of test scores from one test administration to the next. It is measured as the correlation between the scores on the first test and the retest and reflects the stability of scores over time.

2. The alternate forms method assesses the correlation between scores obtained by the same subjects on the alternate forms of a test. This method is the closest approximation to the parallel tests model.

3. The split-half method involves splitting the test into two equivalent halves after a single administration of the test. There are different ways of splitting a test. The highest comparability of the two halves is achieved by an odd–even split in which one form contains all odd numbered items and the other all even numbered items.

4. The internal consistency methods estimate the reliability of a test based on the number of items and the averaged intercorrelations among test items. These methods are mathematically related to the split-half method. Coefficient α is the most general form of this method and represents the mean reliability coefficient which is obtained from all possible split-half comparisons. In essence, internal consistency estimates compare each item on a test to every other item.

There is no universally best method to evaluate test reliability. Each method has its advantages and disadvantages. The split-half reliability method overcomes theoretical and practical problems associated with the test–retest and alternate forms methods, such as difficulty in developing two equivalent forms of a test, carry-over effects, reactivity effects, and the effect of random variability on two test probes. However, the reliability estimate obtained by the split-half method varies depending on the arbitrarily chosen method of splitting. In addition, the split-half reliability coefficient underestimates the reliability of the full test and requires the use of a correction formula.

The level of reliability varies for different tests. Ideally, a highly reliable test would be preferred to a test with low reliability. However, many practical considerations might influence a clinician's test selection. The cost of error in a decision-making situation is another factor which needs to be considered in selecting an appropriate test for the given situation. Test reliability should be high when a patient's test performance is considered as one of the factors in making a final diagnostic determination. Tests with lower reliability might be acceptable in preliminary screening situations.

Typical levels of reliability attained by neuropsychological tests range from 0.95 to 0.80, which represent a high to moderate range of reliability. For a test with a reliability estimate of 0.80, 20% of the variability in the test scores is due to measurement error. Thus, tests with reliability below 0.80 introduce a considerable proportion of "noise" in the test scores which compromises their interpretability. For screening tests, low reliability between 0.80 and 0.60 would be acceptable, whereas reliability estimates below 0.60 are usually unacceptably low.

Standard Error of Measurement

The reliability estimate provides a relative measure of the accuracy of test scores. As any correlation, it is influenced by the variability of scores. In a sample with a heterogeneous score distribution, reliability will be higher than in a more homogeneous sample.

The reliability estimate does not indicate how much variability should be expected due to measurement error and how accurate the individual test scores are. Therefore, in addition to reporting reliability coefficients, test developers report the size of the standard error of measurement (SEM), which is useful in interpreting the observed scores for each individual patient. SEM is determined by the reliability of the test (r_{xx}) and the variability of test scores (σ_x):

$$SEM = \sigma_x \sqrt{1 - r_{xx}}$$

Since no test provides a perfect measure of ability, a certain degree of variability in the scores obtained by the same subject is expected. SEM indicates how much an individual's score might vary if he or she is retested repeatedly with the same test (assuming that there is no practice effect or fatigue effect). According to measurement theory, the scores obtained by one subject across an infinite number of retests with the same test would result in a normal distribution with the mean equal to this subject's "true" score and a standard deviation equal to the SEM.

Since in most clinical situations we have only one obtained score on a test, we may treat it as being an estimate of the theoretical "true" score. Using the SEM we can form a confidence interval around this score, which provides a range in which a subject's "true" score is likely to fall.

For example, a 70-year-old patient obtained a WAIS-III Full Scale IQ (FSIQ) of 110. According to the test manual, the size of the SEM for FSIQ for this age group is 2.19 (Wechsler, 1997). Since we know that 95% of all scores in a normal distribution fall within 1.96 standard deviations of the mean, the 95% confidence interval for this score will fall between 1.96 SEM below and 1.96 SEM above the obtained IQ score (110 ± 1.96 SEM). Calculation of a confidence interval by multiplying the SEM by 1.96 (2.19 × 1.96 = 4.29) suggests that we would expect 95% of the IQ scores obtained by this patient to fall in the range of 110 ± 4.29, or between IQs of 105.71 and 114.29.

If we want to increase the level of certainty in constructing a range in which a patient's true score is likely to fall, we can use the 99% confidence interval. In other cases, we might use lax confidence intervals which provide accuracy below the 95% level.

The drawback in using SEMs to determine the accuracy of the test scores is the fact that they do not always have the same size for all scores. They are smaller for the extreme scores and larger for moderate scores. Another limitation in using SEMs is that test scores are generally further away from the mean than "true" scores because of the tendency for regression toward the mean. In order to overcome this distortion, the confidence interval can be formed around the estimated "true" score, which is obtained from a regression equation.

Validity

When a test is used to assess a certain aspect of functioning, it is assumed that the test measures what it is supposed to measure and that the test is useful in making accurate decisions. Different validation strategies are used to understand the meaning and implications of the scores achieved on the test. Content and construct validity indicate whether a test is a valid measure of a specific ability. Criterion-related validity refers to the accuracy of decisions that are based on the test scores.

1. Content validity reflects the extent to which the behaviors sampled by the test are a representative sample of the ability being measured. It is not measured statistically, but is determined by agreement among expert judges with respect to a detailed description of the content domain that is measured by each test item.

2. Construct validity determines how well observable behaviors measured by the test represent underlying theoretical construct. This relationship can be established through high correlation of the test with other tests measuring the same construct (convergent validity) or through low correlation with the tests measuring different constructs (discriminant validity). If more than one method is used to measure several constructs, the correlations among these measures can be represented in a multitrait–multimethod matrix, which establishes whether the results of a certain test are determined by the construct being measured or by the method of measurement. Construct validity can be further assessed by correlating one test with many other tests using factor analysis. In this case, construct validity is established through the high loading of the test on the factors that represent those constructs presumed to be measured by the test.

Thus, content and construct validity represent two different strategies in determining that the test measures what it is supposed to measure: "Content validity is established if a test *looks* like a valid measure; construct validity is established if a test *acts* like a valid measure" (Murphy & Davidshofer, 1991).

3. The usefulness of a test in decision-making situations represents another aspect of test validity. Criterion-related validity reflects the relationship between test scores and measures of decision outcomes, i.e., criteria. Any measurable behavior can be used as a criterion. For example, the choice of a rehabilitation strategy can be evaluated using a measure of symptom reduction as a criterion, or the accuracy of a screening test can be assessed using a patient's psychiatric diagnosis as a criterion. The correlation between test scores and the criterion measure which is derived without using the test reflects the accuracy of predictions or decisions made on the basis of the test scores.

The criterion measures can be obtained *after* making decisions based on the test scores in a random sample of a population about which decisions are made (predictive validity), or *at the same time* when decisions are made in a preselected sample (concurrent validity). Whereas predictive validity is superior to concurrent validity in that it is a direct measure of the relationship between test scores and a criterion measure for the general population, it has a number of practical and ethical drawbacks. For this reason, the most practical and commonly used measure of criterion-related validity is concurrent validity, despite the fact that its coefficient underestimates the predictive validity.

Theoretically, an estimate of the correlation between test scores and a criterion measure obtained in a criterion-related validity study can range between -1 and $+1$. Validity coefficients for most of the tests are relatively low, ranging between 0.2 and 0.5. This is due to the imperfect reliability of the test and the criterion measure: Whereas a criterion is assumed to represent the "true state" of a patient, it is frequently based on subjective clinical judgment which is inherently unreliable.

If the correlation coefficient between a test and a criterion is 0.3, the proportion of the variance in the criterion that is accounted for by the test (r^2, or coefficient of determination) is 0.09. This means that only 9% of the variability in the criterion can be accounted for by the test scores. Although these numbers look discouraging, they should be interpreted in the context of other measures that contribute to the accuracy of decisions.

Decision Theory

In clinical practice, a clinician has to make decisions which range from applying a specific course of treatment to assigning a certain diagnosis. Since predictions based on the information available to the clinician are never perfect, each decision may have several possible outcomes. In the context of decision theory, the predictor and criterion values are reduced to only two categories, in spite of the continuous nature of these values. The comparison of predictions with the criterion values suggests that there are four possible outcomes of decisions: correct decisions include true-positive (*TP*) and true-negative (*TN*) outcomes, whereas incorrect decisions include false-positive (*FP*) and false-negative (*FN*) outcomes. Tests are used to maximize the number of correct decisions and to minimize the number of errors. The contribution of the criterion-related validity of a test to improvement in the accuracy of decisions depends on the base rate and selection ratio.

Base rates

The base rate reflects the proportion of an unselected population who meet the criterion standard. In a hypothetical example, assume that among 500 normal elderly, 9% would have scores below the cutoff for dementia of 24 on the Mini-Mental State Exam (MMSE). Assume that 80% of patients with the diagnosis of Dementia of Alzheimer's Type (DAT) score below a cutoff of 24. If 100 DAT patients were added to 500 intact elderly (total number of subjects 100 + 500 = 600), the base rate would be

100/600, or 17%. In this situation, the outcomes would be as follows:

$$100 \times 80\% = 80 \; TP$$

$$500 \times 9\% = 45 \; FP$$

$$500 - 45 = 455 \; TN$$

$$100 - 80 = 20 \; FN$$

Thus, follow-up of the subjects who score below the cutoff (80 *TP* + 45 *FP* = 125) will yield a hit rate of 80/125 = 64%. In other words, the diagnosis of DAT will be confirmed in 64% of those subjects who scored below the cutoff of 24 on this test.

In contrast to the above hypothetical example, in the general population the base rate for DAT is considerably lower than 17%. For example, if the base rate for DAT is 5%, then out of 600 subjects, 30 would be suffering from DAT and 570 would be intact with respect to this diagnosis. Assuming that 80% of DAT patients and 9% of the intact elderly score below the cutoff on the MMSE as was the case in the above example, the table of outcomes would look differently because of the lower base rate for DAT:

$$30 \times 80\% = 24 \; TP$$

$$570 \times 9\% = 51 \; FP$$

$$570 - 51 = 519 \; TN$$

$$30 - 24 = 6 \; FN$$

The ratio of true-positive scores to the total number of subjects scoring below the cutoff (24 *TP* + 51 *FP* = 75) will yield a hit rate of 24/75 = 32%, which is considerably lower than in the example with a higher base rate.

With a decrease in base rates, most of the population are "negatives"; "positives" become more rare, and, therefore, an attempt to identify this group will lead to an increase in the number of *FP* decisions. Low base rates also lead to a large number of *TN* decisions, since a majority of the population do not suffer from DAT. Following the same logic, in the case of high base rates, as the number of *TP* decisions increases, however, the frequency of *FN* errors also increases. An optimal base rate of about

50% minimizes decision errors and maximizes accurate decisions providing that the test which is used to assist in decision-making has sufficient validity.

In the general population, the base rates for certain disorders are usually low and most of the "red flags" represent false alarms. The base rates among the individuals referred for evaluation due to progressive symptomatology are higher and therefore, the expected number of false alarms would be lower.

Selection ratio

Another factor affecting the accuracy of decisions is the selection ratio, which is defined as the ratio of $TP + FP$ outcomes to the total number of subjects. Assume that a psychiatric ward has 30 beds for severely depressed patients. If only 32 patients are referred for hospitalization at any one time, the selection ratio would be high ($30/32 = 0.94$). The hospital cannot be very selective in this situation and most of the referred patients could be hospitalized. In another scenario, 100 patients could be referred for hospitalization at any one time due to severe depression. Since the selection ratio is low ($30/100 = 0.30$), a certain strategy needs to be used to identify those who are acutely suicidal for immediate hospitalization. When a selection ratio is low, a test with even modest validity can make a considerable contribution to the accuracy of decisions.

Incremental validity

The utility of a test has to be assessed in terms of an increase in the accuracy of decisions obtained using the test, which extends beyond the base rate or beyond information obtained from other sources. In other words, incremental validity reflects the unique contribution of a test to understanding the patient.

Incremental validity is affected by the base rate, selection ratio, and criterion-related validity of the test. When decisions are made at random, the frequency of different outcomes can be computed directly from the base rate and the selection ratio. The incremental validity of a test indicates the degree of improvement in the accuracy of decisions, i.e., frequency of TP and TN outcomes, beyond the random level, which are made using the test.

The incremental validity is highest when the base rate is moderate, selection ratio is low, and the criterion-related validity is high. Values of incremental validity for different combinations of base rates, selection ratios, and criterion-related validity coefficients are provided in Taylor-Russell (1939) tables.

Thus, the validity coefficient alone does not determine the usefulness of a test in each clinical situation. Test usefulness depends largely on the context in which the test is used.

Setting a cutoff

As pointed out above, in the framework of a decision theory approach, both the predictor (test) and criterion values are reduced to only two outcomes. Thus, the continuous nature of test scores is reduced to pass/fail, impaired/unimpaired categories, etc. The selection of a cutoff point dividing a sequence of test scores into these two categories is another factor affecting the accuracy of decisions. Through manipulating the cutoff, the frequency of a certain type of correct decision can be maximized at the expense of increasing the frequency of another type of error.

For example, test sensitivity or ability to correctly identify impaired individuals (which is expressed as a ratio of TP to all impaired individuals [$TP + FN$]), can be increased by fixing the cutoff at a small number of incorrect responses. This will reduce the frequency of FN errors but will increase the proportion of FP errors. In other words, this will assure correct identification of the majority of individuals with even mild impairment and very few misidentifications of impaired individuals as being intact. At the same time, this will yield a large number of intact individuals who will be misidentified as impaired. The costs of such misidentification include inappropriate treatment and psychological distress and adverse social/economic consequences for those individuals who are misidentified as impaired.

On the other hand, the test specificity or ability to correctly identify the absence of impairment (expressed as the ratio of TN to all intact individuals [$TN + FP$]) can be increased by setting the cutoff at a large number of incorrect responses. This will reduce the proportion of FP errors but will result in a large number of FN

errors. In other words, only those patients who have pronounced impairment will be identified as impaired, and very few intact individuals will be misidentified. However, many individuals with mild symptomatology will be missed. This will preclude timely therapeutic intervention which otherwise would allow stabilization or reversal of these patients' symptomatology.

Thus, manipulation of the cutoff affects the balance between sensitivity and specificity and results in different cost–benefit ratios. Based on the empirical evidence, the cutoff is usually set at the values which ensure a reasonable balance between sensitivity and specificity, so that only "borderline" patients will likely be misidentified.

3

Use of Methodological Concepts in Neuropsychological Practice

ASSESSMENT OF THE COGNITIVE COMPONENT OF MENTAL STATUS IN THE CONTEXT OF DIFFERENT CLINICAL DISCIPLINES

The notion of mental status has three components:

1. Mood and affect
2. Perception and content/process of thought
3. Cognitive status

Factors such as appearance, motor activity, insight, and motivation can be incorporated into these three components of mental status. Clinicians specializing in different disciplines approach the mental status evaluation from different perspectives.

For psychiatrists, the presence of the following symptomatology is of primary concern: affective symptoms (e.g., depression, mania, rapid cycling); perceptual disturbances (e.g., hallucinations); disturbance in content of thought (e.g., delusions); and disturbed process of thought (e.g., tangentiality, loosening of associations, flight of ideas). Assessment of cognitive status represents one of the aspects of psychiatric evaluation and includes brief appraisal of the level of consciousness, orientation, attention, memory, language, ability to follow verbal commands, calculations, abstract reasoning, fund of general information, and judgment.

Assessment of cognitive and affective components of mental status also constitutes part of a neurological evaluation which addresses higher cortical and limbic system functions. In addition, the neurological evaluation focuses on the integrity of the lower levels of the nervous system through assessing functions of the cranial nerves, motor systems, sensory systems, reflexes, coordination, station, and gait.

In the context of psychiatric and neurological evaluations, cognitive status is assessed by unstructured questioning or through administration of structured screening instruments, allowing quantification of a patient's cognitive status (e.g., Mini-Mental State Examination: Folstein et al., 1975). This assessment is brief (limited to 10–20 minutes) and, therefore, yields only a gross estimate of cognitive abilities.

In contrast, assessment of the cognitive component of mental status is the primary focus of neuropsychological evaluation, though affective state and content/process of thought are also attended to. The standardized neuropsychological instruments which are used in a comprehesive assessment of different cognitive domains are more sensitive to subtle functional deficits than the gross screening tools used in psychiatric and neurological evaluations.

STRATEGIES IN TEST SELECTION

A variety of instruments have been developed over the years to measure cognitive abilities.

Tests vary in their reliance on theoretical constructs, complexity of cognitive functions assessed, length and ease of administration, psychometric properties, relevant populations, and availability of norms.

Decisions regarding tests to use depend on the preferred approach. The fixed battery approach advocates the administration of a comprehensive battery of tests to all patients in invariant order. Any additional information is gathered after the battery is administered and results are analyzed, which prevents any bias in interpretation of the results. Clinical interpretation of the obtained data is compared to the information available from other sources for consistency. An example of such a data-driven approach is the Halstead-Reitan Battery.

In contrast, the flexible approach is based on a patient-centered model. The choice of tests is guided by the hypotheses formulated by the clinician after reviewing all available information about the patient. The battery is individually tailored for each patient to include measures used to test a priori hypotheses regarding possible patterns of cognitive dysfunction. Luria's (1980) view of neuropsychological evaluation is most descriptive of the hypothesis-driven flexible approach.

The advantage of the fixed battery approach is in systematic acquisition of data on a wide range of measures allowing comparisons across patients and across diagnostic groups, and building extensive databases for research purposes. The use of this approach overcomes the effect of base rates on test selection, thus minimizing the probability of error in the early stages of clinical decision-making. On the other hand, administration of an extensive battery to all patients, irrespective of their individual needs, leads to excessive testing and uneconomical expenditures of resources. In addition, the accuracy of the assessment is compromised if the fixed battery does not include tests sensitive to the deficits in specific functional domains suspected to be impaired in a given patient.

The flexible approach overcomes these shortcomings of the fixed approach. However, it is vulnerable to the effect of base rates and does not lend itself to across-patient or across-group comparisons given extensive missing data due to differences in tests administered.

In a compromise dictated by the realities of clinical practice and the economic environment, it is recommended that a screening battery specifically tailored for the respective diagnostic group or differential diagnosis in question (e.g., differential diagnosis of dementia in an elderly patient, or determination of learning disabilities in a child) be employed. Based on the pattern of weaknesses identified by this battery and on a priori–generated hypotheses, additional tests would be administered to specifically address extent and nature of the deficits. For further discussion of this issue, the reader is referred to Bornstein (1990).

SELECTION OF NORMATIVE REFERENCES AND APPLICATION OF STATISTICAL CONCEPTS TO THE INTERPRETATION OF CLINICAL DATA

Selection of the most appropriate tests alone does not assure accuracy in understanding the patient's cognitive profile. After the tests are administered and scored, the test scores need to be interpreted in reference to an appropriate set of norms. This section will expand on the issues of primary importance in test score interpretation, which were identified in the previous chapters of this book.

Because normative data are used for comparison purposes, the clinician or researcher must locate available norms that most closely match the characteristics of the patient or subject under study as well as match the administration/scoring procedures of the test utilized. It is well known that performance on most neuropsychological tests is highly related to the subject's age, intelligence level, education, and for a few tests, sex. The influence of these factors is even more apparent for neurologically normal individuals than for those who have cerebral dysfunction (Heaton et al., 1986).

Some investigators have argued that because the associations between age and education in relationship to neuropsychological scores are attenuated in a brain-damaged sample as compared to a normal sample, cognitive scores should not be adjusted for these factors in a clinical population (Reitan & Wolfson, 1995).

However, it is precisely because age and education relate to neuropsychological scores in a normal population, that test performance must be adjusted for these demographics in a patient population. For example, in a patient with acquired brain injury who previously completed 17 years of education, if his/her performance is adjusted for the high premorbid level of functioning, the resulting score will more accurately reflect how far this patient has dropped relative to premorbid functioning.

Regarding sex differences, males perform better on tests involving manipulation of spatial relationships, quantitative skills, and physical strength. Females perform better on certain verbal abilities. However, it is dangerous to generalize, because sex differences are not consistent even across tests within the same functional domain. For instance, males outperform females on finger tapping and grip strength (by about 40%), but females outperform males on the grooved pegboard task.

When you do happen to stumble across reference to a normative report in the discussion section of someone else's paper, you often encounter words to the effect that the data are based on biased samples (because the average FSIQ of the group is 120), with the conclusion that the data are "therefore of limited use." *There is no such thing as the best normative data* for *any* test, since only the clinician can determine what report is best applied given a specific patient and situation. *All* normative data are of limited use. The data are limited to use with patients whose demographic characteristics are similar and whose tests were administered and scored in the same way.

In order to choose the best set of norms for comparison purposes, it is therefore essential to know the subject characteristics and test administration procedures for the normative sample. *Subject characteristics* are specific identifiers regarding the subjects under study, such as their age, education, IQ and gender. *Procedural variables* represent details of test administration such as whether a 30-minute vs. a 1-hour delay was followed. In general, it is advised that selection of the normative data be based on careful review of the subject and procedural variables employed by the normative study, since the population to which the reported find-

Table 3.1. Subject and Procedural Variables to Consider When Trying to Locate an Appropriate Normative Comparison Data Set

---

Subject Variables:

Sample Composition Description

1. Age
2. Sample size
3. Education/IQ
4. Gender
5. Handedness (if appropriate)

Procedural Variables:

1. *Method of administration and scoring of the test* (for instance, if a memory test, it should be reported whether delayed recall and recognition conditions were administered)
2. *Mean, standard deviation, range* (base rate information is preferred as well)
3. *Testing history* (including order of testing)

---

ings apply may be either restricted or ambiguous. Important subject and procedural variables to consider can be found in Table 3.1.

In neuropsychological practice, once the appropriate normative data set has been identified, each raw test score is then compared to the distribution of performance scores on the same test obtained by a normative sample with similar demographic characteristics. With this comparison, one can determine whether the obtained test score was below average, above average, or just average relative to the normative group data (cf. Anastasi, 1988).

For instance, knowing that a medically healthy 76-year-old male obtained 18 out of 36 possible points on 3-minute delayed recall of the Rey-Osterrieth Complex Figure has little meaning by itself because the raw score conveys no information regarding the *expected* performance score. We have no idea whether this is a good, bad, or average score. Even knowing that 50% of the figure was recalled has little meaning, because there is no way to discern what percent recall would be expected. In this example, the subject (i.e., medically healthy 76-year-old male) and procedural variables are known (i.e., direct copy of drawing followed by 3-minute delay recall without warning, with scoring following Taylor's method) and are used to locate an appropriate normative sample. When the raw performance score is contrasted with the range of scores obtained by the normative sample, one can determine that a recall score of 18/36 is in the high average range (80th percentile) (in reference to the norms reported by Boone et al., 1992). In other words, we now know the subject's relative standing compared to the normative group (namely, that performance is better than 80% of all normals who took the test).

In order to more precisely judge the nature of performance on a test relative to the reference normative (e.g., standard) group, the raw score is converted to a standard score (typically a z score or T score, which is expressed in terms of *standard deviation units from the mean,* see Chapter 2). Such conversion not only permits one to determine the subject's relative standing compared with the normative group but also allows direct comparison of scores across different tests.

The development of "standard" measurement scales is especially important to neuropsychologists, since test scores collected while assessing the same functional domain are often expressed in different units of measurement. For instance, when assessing motor functioning, the Grooved Pegboard Test score is based on the number of *seconds* to complete placing metal pegs in all the grooved slots on the pegboard, the PIN Test score is based on the *number of holes punched,* the Dynamometer score is expressed in *kilograms,* and the Finger Tapping Test score in terms of the *number of taps* made in 10 seconds. The ability to convert each of these various scores to a common "standard score" equivalent, regardless of the previously expressed units of measurement (seconds, number of holes punched, kilograms, etc.) allows determination of a subject's relative standing in one distribution and also permits its comparison with relative standing in another.

The underlying assumption when using z scores or T scores is that the distribution of scores obtained by the normative sample follows what is known as the "standard normal distribution," which approximates the bell-shaped normal curve (see Chapter 2). Therefore, there is a fixed relationship between the standardized test scores, z scores, and percentile ranks. Table 3.2 illustrates the interrelationship between z

scores, percentile ranks, and corresponding WAIS-III IQ equivalents. A positive value z score will translate to a percentile rank of 50 or greater (refer to left side of the percentile rank column) and to a WAIS-III IQ of 100 or greater (left side of the WAIS-III IQ column). A negative value z score will translate to a percentile rank below 50 (use right side of column) and a WAIS-III IQ below 100 (right side of column).

Consider the following example: You have just assessed Mr. Smith's right (dominant) hand performance on the Grooved Pegboard Test, and you note that it took him 68 seconds to complete. Mr. Smith is 35 years old and has finished 11 years of formal schooling. He has lived almost his entire life in a large western Canadian city and only recently moved to the city where you evaluated his performance. After surveying the available normative data for possible comparison purposes (see Chapter 19), you decide that use of Bornstein's (1985) normative data for the Grooved Pegboard performance would be optimal. Examining the normative table you note that males in his age and education group performed the test with their dominant hand in 65.3 (8.5) seconds.

$$\frac{(68) - (65.3)}{(8.5)} = 0.32$$

Considering that higher scores on this test reflect poorer performance (since it took longer to complete placing all those pegs in the slots), you know that Mr. Smith has performed below the mean for the group ($z = -0.32$). Obviously, this z-score value will be converted to something less than the 50th percentile. And indeed, when you locate a z score of -0.32 in Table 3.2, the corresponding value (using the right side of the percentile rank column) is the 37th percentile.

Percentile ranks permit one to indicate whether the performance is very superior, superior, high average, average, low average, borderline, or impaired. By convention, neuropsychologists use the percentile cutoffs presented in Table 3.3 in describing performance levels.

Another method of psychological test interpretation involves comparing an individual's performance against some previously deter-

Table 3.2. Percentile Ranks and WAIS-III IQ Equivalent Scores for Corresponding Z-Scores

Standard Deviation or Z Score	Percentile Rank +SD	Percentile Rank −SD	WAIS-III IQ Equiv. +SD	WAIS-III IQ Equiv. −SD	Standard Deviation or Z Score	Percentile Rank +SD	Percentile Rank −SD	WAIS-III IQ Equiv. +SD	WAIS-III IQ Equiv. −SD
2.17–3.00	99	1	≥133	≤67	0.63–0.65	74	26		
2.96–2.16	98	2	130–132	68–70	0.60–0.62	73	27	109	91
1.82–1.95	97	3	127–129	71–72	0.57–0.59	72	28		
1.70–1.81	96	4	126	73–74	0.54–0.56	71	29		
1.60–1.69	95	5	124–125	75–76	0.51–0.53	70	30	108	92
1.52–1.59	94	6	123	77	0.49–0.50	69	31		
1.44–1.51	93	7	122	78	0.46–0.48	68	32	107	93
1.38–1.43	92	8	121	79	0.43–0.45	67	33		
1.32–1.37	91	9	120	80	0.40–0.42	66	34		
1.26–1.31	90	10	119	81	0.38–0.39	65	35	106	94
1.21–1.25	89	11			0.35–0.37	64	36		
1.16–1.20	88	12	118	82	0.32–0.34	63	37	105	95
1.11–1.15	87	13	117	83	0.30–0.31	62	38		
1.06–1.10	86	14	116	84	0.27–0.29	61	39	104	96
1.02–1.05	85	15			0.25–0.26	60	40		
0.98–1.01	84	16	115	85	0.22–0.24	59	41		
0.94–0.97	83	17			0.19–0.21	58	42	103	97
0.90–0.93	82	18	114	86	0.17–0.18	57	43		
0.86–0.89	81	19	113	87	0.14–0.16	56	44		
0.83–0.85	80	20			0.12–0.13	55	45	102	98
0.79–0.82	79	21	112	88	0.09–0.11	54	46		
0.76–0.78	78	22			0.07–0.08	53	47	101	99
0.73–0.75	77	23	111	89	0.04–0.06	52	48		
0.70–0.72	76	24			0.02–0.03	51	49		
0.66–0.69	75	25	110	90	0.00–0.01	50		100	100

mined cutoff score. The utility of cutoff scores is often compromised by the following factors:

1. The failure to account for base rates of the criterion condition ("abnormalcy"—the rates of occurrence of test scores that would be interpreted as falling in the impaired range) in the normative sample. For example, a score which occurs in less than 1% of a "normal" sample would carry greater clinical weight than a score which occurs in 15% of a "normal" sample (see Chapter 2). Generally, failure to account for base rates produces a high false-positive rate.

2. The failure to adjust for subject variables such as age, education, sex or cultural differences.

Some investigators suggest that many of the current cutoffs are too conservative (Fromm-Auch & Yeudall, 1983), thereby generating too many false negatives. However, their work has been done primarily with highly educated, high IQ samples, and of course, cutoffs based on average performers would generate a high false negative rate. Unfortunately, a large number of studies document unacceptably high false positive misclassification rates, placing normal subjects into impaired ranges across different tests which are interpreted using a cutoff criterion (see chapters on Halstead-Reitan Battery (HRB) tests in this book).

Table 3.3. Converting Percentiles to Performance Levels

Percentile	Level
≥98	Very superior
91–97	Superior
75–90	High average
25–74	Average
9–24	Low average
3–8	Borderline
≤2	Impaired

DIFFERENT LEVELS OF DATA INTEGRATION IN NEUROPSYCHOLOGICAL PRACTICE

As suggested in Chapter 1, a sole reliance on test scores and their normative references would frequently result in misinterpretation of a patient's cognitive profile. High vulnerability of such interpretation to erroneous outcome hinges on multiple sources of errors in different components of testing process. These sources can be identified as follows:

1. *Test Construction:* Error is inherent in test construction due to the fact that psychometric properties of the test are specific to the ability level of the subjects on which they were obtained; the values of item difficulty and item discrimination are sample-specific; the variance of errors of measurement is unequal across subjects with the consistency in performance of high-ability subjects being higher than corresponding values in average and low-ability subjects.

2. *Test Administration:* In spite of a meticulous description of procedures aimed at uniformity in test administration, an examiner's individual style and personal tempo, as well as idiosyncratic features of a subject's test-taking style, introduces variability in administration.

3. *Scoring:* Test authors define scoring criteria for each test item. At times, however, patients' responses are ambiguous and present a scoring dilemma. As a result, interrater reliability for the majority of the tests is less than perfect.

4. *Norms:* In using norms, error can be introduced by comparing individual performance to an inappropriate target population, outdated norms, or norms based on a low sample size.

5. *Interpretation:* Caution should be taken when performance on an individual test is interpreted as representative of a circumscribed cognitive ability. Cognitive abilities are highly interrelated, and performance on any test is dependent on the integrity of many different abilities and on the overall level of alertness.

Incorporating behavioral observations and qualitative performance indices in interpretation and decision-making process considerably improves the accuracy of attributions relating low performance scores to faulty cognitive mechanisms. Luria's approach to test interpretation heavily emphasizes the qualitative aspect of performance. This direction in neuropsychological practice was further promoted by efforts of Edith Kaplan. Her introduction of the WAIS-R as a Neuropsychological Instrument (WAIS-R-NI) (Kaplan et al., 1991a) attests to the importance of the qualitative performance indices even in the context of structured battery assessment. This movement toward attending to performance quality without compromising standardization of test administration procedures (or with minimal modification of the procedures) is also reflected in Lezak's (1995) distinction between *optimal* and *standard* testing conditions.

Based on a comprehensive review of recent developments in this area, Caplan and Shechter (1995) formulated the distinction between *testing* and *evaluation* as follows: "We view the former as a largely mechanical enterprise that, because of its rigidity, lends itself well to group or computer-based applications. Evaluation is, by contrast, an art applied on an individual basis that involves not only testing skills, but also professional creativity, observational expertise, flexibility, and ingenuity in the service of developing a multidimensional understanding of patients—their abilities and deficits, their emotional state, self-regulatory functions, the impact of environmental variables on test performance, and so forth" (pp. 359–360). The authors passionately advocate flexibility in testing procedures—specifically in the rehabilitation setting—to allow patients to maximally express their potential in test performance.

A similar appeal to "see beyond the test data" in offering an opinion on psychological functioning in the litigation setting was voiced by Matarazzo (1990). He proposed a distinction between psychological testing vs. psychological assessment; the latter incorporates historical information, medical history, and other relevant information in clinical decision-making process.

Based on the growing need to conceptualize the above issues, we want to outline the following levels of data integration in neuropsychological practice:

1. *Testing* refers to the psychometric aspects and addresses the quantitative appraisal of a patient's performance on different measures. It yields a score or a set of scores which allow comparison with normative data or with a patient's own scores across different tests and over time.

2. *Assessment* incorporates qualitative aspects of test interpretation in addition to psychometric determination of a patient's relative standing in reference to the normative data. It is reliant on behavioral observations to allow better understanding of the nature of difficulties in test performance and of dysfunctional cognitive mechanisms contributing to patient's low test scores.

3. *Evaluation* represents the most comprehensive level of integration, on which the psychometric and the clinical case-study approach are combined. The clinician integrates various sources of information in order to place interpretation of a patient's psychometric profile in the context of his/her history and current condition. Information is based on behavioral observations and an interview with the patient, in addition to the patient's test performance. Additional information can be obtained from medical and school records, interviews with significant others, schoolteachers, nursing staff, etc.

The following issues constitute the essence of a neuropsychological evaluation: the psychometric aspect of patient's performance across cognitive domains; qualitative interpretation of dysfunctional mechanisms; the patient's behavior and interaction with the clinician; effort/ motivation to perform on the tasks; other aspects of mental status including affective state; personality characteristics impacting information processing; demographic information including educational and occupational history; medical and psychiatric history; family history; current symptomatology, progression of symptoms and treatment; sources of social/financial support and living condition; patient's motivation to improve and future plans.

APPLICATIONS OF NEUROPSYCHOLOGICAL EVALUATION

The utility of psychological testing is in the midst of a heated controversy. Over the years, the psychometric approach has been criticized for being too mechanistic and biased against underrepresented groups. Neuropsychological evaluation is not limited to administration and interpretation of the tests; instead, it should provide a comprehensive picture of the patient, placing test performance in the context of expectations specific for this particular individual. This approach overcomes the flaws inherent in testing.

Clinical neuropsychology is a relatively young discipline which continues to shape itself in response to the pressing needs of clinical practice. With changing environmental demands, clinical neuropsychology redefines its objectives, its applications, and its relationship with other disciplines and revises its armamentarium.

At this time, clinical neuropsychology has a wide range of applications which include the following:

1. It is used in differential diagnosis of conditions involving cognitive dysfunction (for example, dementia of Alzheimer's type, vs. vascular dementia, vs. depression).

Traditionally, differential diagnostic questions addressed to a neuropsychologist were focused around organic vs. functional etiologies of disturbance. With growing evidence of neuropathological and chemical correlates of functional disorders, the organic vs. functional distinction becomes more vague.

One of the major tasks of neuropsychology in the past was localizing the lesion in the brain. With an advancement of neuroimaging techniques, this aspect of neuropsychology acquired only secondary importance.

2. Neuropsychological assessment is useful in defining baseline levels of cognitive functioning for longitudinal comparisons with follow-up data. For example, even subtle age-related decline in attention, decision-making, judgment, and visuospatial abilities in pilots might lead to their failure to respond adequately in a critical situation. In view of the tremendous responsibility for human lives imposed on pilots, early signs of age-related decline need to be identified through longitudinal comparisons of performance.

In another example, a baseline profile obtained on a child with suspected learning disability before entering primary school can be compared with the results obtained 1 year later. This defines the rate of acquisition of a particular skill and facilitates decision-making regarding the necessity of remedial intervention.

Longitudinal follow-up is also used to identify the rate of improvement or deterioration in cognitive status and response to treatment. For example, follow-up evaluations of a head injury patient help identify the rate of improvement with or without treatment in comparison to an initial evaluation taken a few weeks after the accident. This allows prediction of the extent of future recovery, nature and severity of residual deficits, and highest functional level to be achieved upon recovery. Availability of this information affords realistic expectations as to the limits of recovery, facilitates adjustment of patients and their families to possible changes in their lifestyle, and prompts reassignment of responsibilities within the family.

Similarly, rate and pattern of cognitive deterioration associated with dementia, as identified by follow-up probes, provide useful diagnostic and prognostic information.

3. Neuropsychological evaluation identifies cognitive strengths and weaknesses in patient's current functional status. This knowledge facilitates the selection of remedial techniques and rehabilitative strategies. It guides clinicians in their choice of rehabilitation strategy: either focusing on remediation of weaknesses or focusing on compensation for cognitive losses by utilizing intact abilities.

The pattern of strengths and weaknesses in neuropsychological performance can also shed light on the differential contribution of more recent, transient factors vs. long-standing factors in a patient's cognitive profile. This distinction is especially relevant for medical–legal evaluations.

4. Neuropsychological data are used in evaluating patients' employability and constitute a basis for determination whether they meet criteria for disability. Furthermore, these data are relied upon in determining patients' competence in handling their legal and financial affairs and their ability to function independently in an everyday environment. For example, a severe deficit in executive functions related to amnesia associated with Korsakoff's syndrome renders a patient totally dysfunctional and unable to maintain basic self-care and self-hygiene in spite of retaining a high level of psychometric intelligence. In such cases, the results of an evaluation identify the need for close supervision of the patient's everyday activities to protect the patient from inadvertent self-neglect and to help him/her structure and organize activities and, thus, improve the quality of his/her life.

II

TESTS OF ATTENTION AND CONCENTRATION: VISUAL AND AUDITORY

4

Trailmaking Test

BRIEF HISTORY OF THE TEST

The Trailmaking Test (TMT) is included in the Halstead-Reitan Battery (HRB) and was originally part of the Army Individual Test Battery (1944).

Part A is an 8″ × 11″ page on which the numbers 1 through 25 are scattered within circles. The patient is instructed to draw lines connecting the numbers in order as quickly as possible. Part B is a page with the numbers 1 through 13 and letters A through L within circles. The patient is instructed to draw lines connecting the numbers and letters in order, alternating between numbers and letters (e.g., 1-A-2-B, etc.). Specific administration procedures are provided in Reitan's (1979) *Manual for Administration of Neuropsychological Test Batteries for Adults and Children*. Two scores are obtained, reflecting the total time in seconds to complete each task. In the Reitan (1979) administration format, errors are not scored, but when they occur, the patient is alerted to the mistake and instructed to correct it, thus slowing overall performance time. The patient is presented with short sample items prior to the administration of each task. Detailed administration instructions and discussion of the test reliability and practice effects are provided in Lezak (1995) and Spreen & Strauss (1998). A children's version of the tasks (age 9–14) is available which incorporates fewer items. An oral version of the TMT has been developed for use with patients who have limited visual or motor skills (Abraham et al., 1996).

The Trailmaking Test (parts A and B) provides information regarding attention, visual scanning, and speed of eye–hand coordination and information processing. Part B also assesses the ability to alternate between sets of stimuli, an executive function. These abilities are known to be highly vulnerable to deterioration resulting from brain pathology of different etiologies. Thus, the TMT has enjoyed wide popularity as a sensitive measure of executive functioning, and as such is especially useful in documenting cerebral dysfunction in mild traumatic brain injury, in the differential diagnosis of dementia, and in detecting attentional/concentrational dysfunction in children and adults.

The manual for the Army Individual Test (1944) provides a 10-point scale for converting raw scores, with 10 the best score and 1 the worst. Reitan (1958) initially recommended use of this scaling method and suggested cutoffs for impaired performance based on the scaled scores. Given the significant association between TMT performance and age, IQ, education, and possibly sex, the use of single cutoff scores does not appear to be appropriate, as has been confirmed by several studies. Bornstein et al. (1987b) found that using a cutoff of ≥40 seconds on part A and ≥92 seconds on part B, 33% and 39% of a healthy elderly sample were misclassified as brain-damaged. Ernst (1987) found that use of cutoffs ≥39 and ≥92 seconds resulted in a misclassification rate of 48% for both Trails A and B. Bak and Greene (1980) reported that at least 40% of their elderly normal subjects were misclassified on part B. Dodrill (1987) documented an 11.7% and 13.3% misclassification rate when using cutoffs of ≥39 seconds on part A and ≥89 seconds on part B in a young control sample.

Bornstein and colleagues (1987b) note that 96% and 98% correct classification rate respectively, were obtained when cutoffs of ≥55 seconds and ≥137 seconds were used (but 46% and 40% of brain-damaged subjects were then misclassified with these cutoffs). The authors emphasize that cutoff scores may be useful, but only if considered in the context of other neuropsychological information obtained in a test battery and if age, education, and other appropriate adjustments are made.

Cahn et al. (1995) used cutoffs of ≥66 and ≥172 seconds for Trails A and B, respectively, in a study comparing a large sample of neurologically normal individuals with Dementia of Alzheimer's Type (DAT) patients. They report sensitivity and specificity indices of 69% and 90% for Trails A, and 87% and 88% for Trails B; the ratios of DAT patients to controls were 42/237 for Trails A and 30/235 for Trails B. The authors underscored the diagnostic effectiveness of Trails B, which was one of the few measures contributing to optimal differentiation between DAT and control subjects.

RELATIONSHIP BETWEEN TMT PERFORMANCE AND DEMOGRAPHIC FACTORS

The literature to date indicates that TMT performance is associated with age; increased age is related to poorer test scores. The association between age and TMT scores is present in both normals and patients but appears to be of a smaller magnitude in brain-damaged samples (Corrigan & Hinkeldey, 1987b). A number of studies have reported either significant correlations with age or significant differences across various age groups (Alekoumbides et al., 1987; Anthony et al., 1980; Bak & Greene, 1980; Bornstein, 1985; Davies, 1968; Gordon, 1972; Goul & Brown, 1970; Heaton et al., 1986, 1991;

Ivnik et al., 1996; Kennedy, 1981; Lyness et al., 1994; Parsons et al., 1964; Reed & Reitan, 1962; Salthouse & Fristoe, 1995; Stanton et al., 1984; Stuss et al., 1987), and two other studies, while not formally acknowledging the association between age and TMT performance, present their TMT data by age groupings and the mean scores of the groups obviously increase with age (Fromm-Auch & Yeudall, 1983; Harley et al., 1980).

The majority of the above studies document a greater association of age with performance on Trails B than on Trails A. This might be related to the finding reported by Salthouse et al. (1996) that some of the age-related variance in the Trails B measure is unique and independent of the age-related variance in the Trails A measure. This suggests that the requirement to alternate between letter and number targets imposes additional unique demands with increased age. On the other hand, Arnett and Labovitz (1995) found the difference in the physical layout of Trails A and B to have a significant effect on the time required for their completion.

In contrast, Yeudall et al. (1987) and Boll and Reitan (1973) detected no association between age and either part A or B. Yeudall et al.'s (1987) negative findings may be due to the restricted age range of their sample (range of 15 to 40); examination of other data sets suggests that declines with age appear to occur after age 40 (Goul & Brown, 1970; Stuss et al., 1987) or age 50 (Kennedy, 1981) for part A. The reason for Boll and Reitan's (1973) failure to document age effects is less obvious, but it could be due to small sample sizes in the very young and very old groups and problems in the linearity of the data (e.g., very young and very old subjects performing poorly). In spite of the reported nonsignificant correlations, the percent of subjects correctly classified as normal for the oldest age group (60–64) did fall precipitously compared to other age groups, suggesting that there was a decline with age in test performance at least in this age grouping.

Several studies have also documented a significant relationship between education and TMT scores in normal individuals, with higher education levels tied to better test performance (Alekoumbides et al., 1987; Anthony et al.,

1980; Bornstein, 1985; Bornstein & Suga, 1988; Finlayson et al., 1977; Gordon, 1972; Heaton et al., 1986, 1991; Ernst, 1987; Kennedy, 1981; Parsons et al., 1964; Portin et al., 1995; Stanton et al., 1984; Stuss et al., 1987); only two investigations failed to detect a significant correlation between education and TMT scores (Ivnik et al., 1996; Yeudall et al., 1987). Heaton and colleagues (1986), assessing the combined effect of age and education on TMT part B in normal subjects, documented a significant interaction, suggesting that for individuals less than 60 years old, lower levels of education are associated with greater amounts of age-associated impairment; for subjects more than 60 years old, the level of education has less of an effect than for younger individuals.

Another aspect of the age/education interaction in reference to Trails B performance was presented in a study by Richardson and Marottoli (1996). The mean performance for community-residing elderly subjects with less than 12 years of education was stable across younger-old (76–80) and older-old (81–91) age groups; it was considerably lower than for the better educated subjects in this study and well below expected in comparison to the Heaton et al. (1991) norms. However, for the subjects with 12 or more years of education, performance for the younger-old age group was superior to that of the older-old and was comparable to Heaton et al. (1991) norms.

The relationship between TMT scores and education in brain-damaged samples has been more equivocal, with some investigators documenting an association between education and TMT performance (Anthony et al., 1980) and others failing to detect a relationship (Finlayson et al., 1977) or reporting a statistically significant but clinically negligible association (Corrigan & Hinkeldey, 1987b).

Full Scale IQ has consistently been found to be related to TMT outcome in both patients and normal subjects, with higher intellectual levels associated with superior test scores (Anthony et al., 1980; Boll & Reitan, 1973; Corrigan & Hinkeldey, 1987b; Dodrill, 1987; Goul & Brown, 1970; Kennedy, 1981; Parsons et al., 1964; Warner et al., 1987; Wiens & Matarazzo, 1977). However, information regarding whether TMT data are more related to Performance IQ (PIQ) vs. Verbal IQ (VIQ) has been contradictory. For example, Yeudall et al. (1987) found a significant correlation between PIQ and both parts A and B but no relationship between TMT scores and VIQ. Conversely, Wiens and Matarazzo (1977) found a significant correlation between part B and VIQ but not PIQ. However, their data should be viewed with caution due to unexpected and unexplainable findings; specifically, a significant positive correlation was found between PIQ and Trails A (the higher the PIQ the *longer* it took subjects to complete the task), and the significant correlations were found for one control group but not a second one.

The literature on sex differences in TMT scores in normal subjects has generally indicated that there are no gender effects (Dodrill, 1979; Fromm-Auch & Yeudall, 1983; Heaton et al., 1986, 1991; Ivnik et al., 1996; Stuss et al., 1987; Yeudall et al., 1987). The three studies which found sex effects differed as to which sex performed better, and the differences in performance between the sexes were small: Davies (1968) found that men scored higher than woman on part B; Portin et al. (1995) reported superiority of men on part A; and Bornstein (1985) reported that women outperformed men on both test sections.

Multiple regression analyses of the effects of age, IQ, sex, and education on TMT scores in normal individuals by Greene and Farr (1985) suggested that age accounts for most of the variance, followed by FSIQ, for both part A and part B. Sex was a contributor to part B performance only, while education had a negligible association with both parts. In contrast, Heaton et al. (1991) found that while age accounted for the most test score variance on parts A and B, 16% to 27% of the unique test score variance was attributable to educational level; sex did not account for any appreciable test score variance. The relationship between FSIQ and TMT scores was not assessed in this study. Green and Farr (1985) and Heaton et al. (1991) data appear to be contradictory regarding the effect of education on TMT performance. However, the findings can be reconciled if the contribution of education to TMT scores is viewed as occurring through its association with IQ.

Hays (1995) reports a considerable effect of

intelligence level and age on TMT performance, demonstrated by multiple regression analysis of data collected on a sample of 661 psychiatric inpatients. The authors provide normal standard score conversions from raw scores and information derived from the regression analysis allowing correction of TMT scores for IQ and age.

METHOD FOR EVALUATING THE NORMATIVE REPORTS

In order to adequately evaluate the TMT normative reports, seven key criterion variables were deemed critical. The first six of these relate to *subject* variables, and the remaining dimension refers to *procedural* issues.

Minimal requirements for meeting the criterion variables were as follows:

Subject Variables

Sample Size

As discussed in previous chapters, a minimum of at least 50 subjects per grouping interval is optimal.

Sample Composition Description

As discussed previously, information regarding medical and psychiatric exclusion criteria is important. It is unclear if geographic recruitment region, socioeconomic status or occupation, ethnicity, handedness, and recruitment procedures are relevant, so until this is determined, it is best that this information be provided.

Age Group Intervals

Given the association between age and TMT performance, information regarding age of the normative sample is critical and preferably normative data should be presented by age intervals.

Reporting of IQ Levels

Given the relationship between TMT performance and IQ, information regarding intellectual level should be provided and preferably normative data should be presented by IQ levels.

Reporting of Education Levels

Given the association between educational level and TMT scores, information regarding highest educational level completed should be reported and preferably normative data should be presented by educational levels.

Reporting of Gender Distribution

Given a possible association between sex and TMT scores, it is preferable that information regarding sex distribution of the samples be cited.

Procedural Variables

Data Reporting

Means and standard deviations, and preferably ranges, for total time in seconds for each part of the TMT should be reported.

SUMMARY OF THE STATUS OF THE NORMS

Our review of the literature located 16 TMT normative reports for adults[1] published since 1965, as well as three interpretive guides for the Halstead-Reitan Battery (Gilandas et al., 1984; Golden et al., 1981b; Reitan & Wolfson, 1985). Hundreds of other studies have also reported control subject data and we have included discussion of eight of those investigations which involved some unique features, such as large sample size, retest data, elderly population, error analysis, etc.

Of note, few relevant manuscripts have emerged since the 1980s, perhaps due either to the publication of Heaton et al. (1991) comprehensive normative tables or to the escalating use in research and clinical practice of flexible neuropsychological test protocols which include newer tasks rather than traditional fixed neuropsychological batteries.

It should be noted that Russell and Starkey (1993) developed the Halstead-Russell Neuropsychological Evaluation System (HRNES), which includes TMT among 22 tests. In the context of this system, individual performance

[1] Norms for children are available in Spreen and Strauss (1998).

is compared to that of 576 brain-damaged subjects and 200 subjects who were initially suspected of having brain damage but had negative neurological findings. Data were partitioned into seven age groups and three educational/IQ levels. This study will not be reviewed in this chapter because the "normal" group consisted of the V.A. patients who presented with symptomatology requiring neuropsychological evaluation. For further discussion of the HRNES system see Lezak, 1995 (pp. 714–715).

There is a great deal of variability in the methodological aspects of studies summarized in this chapter. Sample sizes vary from 30 to over 700. Age represented in the studies varies from 15 to over 90 years, however, only six studies report data for older age groups. Sample compositions have been diverse and have ranged from neurologically normal individuals (according to stringent exclusion criteria), job applicants, medical/psychiatric patients, V.A. inpatients and outpatients, and homosexual/bisexual males.

The majority of studies report mean age, education, and gender distribution for the sample and/or for the age groups. Some studies report WAIS-R IQs or estimated intelligence level, handedness, occupational level, and ethnic composition.

Many studies present data divided into age groups. Few studies classify subjects into education or IQ groups or present data for males and females separately; two studies report data for males only, and one study presents data in age by education by sex cells. Geographical origin of the data also varies widely: British, Australian, and six Canadian datasets are presented in this chapter. The data are most commonly reported as time to completion for Trails A and B. Some studies present raw data converted to the T scores, error rate, percentile ranks, median time, or total time for $A + B$. One study provides regression equations to correct raw data for age and education. Few studies present classification rates for different cutoff criteria.

Test–retest data are reported in three studies with intertrial intervals ranging from 1 week to 24 weeks. Issues of reliability and/or practice effect are discussed in these studies.

Given that the use of the TMT has typically been within the context of the Halstead-Reitan

battery, the Reitan data and interpretation recommendations will be reported first, followed by a summary of the other interpretation formats, and then the normative publications presented in an ascending chronological order. The chapter will conclude with a review of TMT control data reported in various clinical studies.

Table 4.1 summarizes information provided in the studies described in this chapter.

SUMMARIES OF THE STUDIES

Interpretive Guides

Reitan and Wolfson (1985)

The authors provide general guidelines for TMT score interpretation in the form of "severity ranges" for part B only: "perfectly normal (or better than average)," "normal," "mildly impaired," and "seriously impaired." They list the test completion times (in seconds) which correspond to each severity range. No other information is provided such as score means or standard deviations, or any data regarding the normative sample on which these guidelines were developed. These cutoffs represent a substantial departure from cutoffs published earlier; the definition of normal performance here is approximately 20 seconds less than in the 1958 and 1979 guidelines.

Considerations regarding use of the study
The authors argue that these norms were meant as "general guidelines" and that "exact percentile ranks corresponding with each possible score are hardly necessary because the other methods of inference are used to supplement normative data in clinical interpretation of results of individual subjects" (p. 97). However, we maintain that more precise scores as well as separate normative data for different age, IQ, and educational levels are necessary to avoid false positive errors in diagnosis (Table 4.2).

Gilandas, Touyz, Beumont, and Greenberg (1984, p. 102)

The authors provide the percentile ranks associated with Davies (1968) TMT normative data and suggest that a percentile rank of 25 is "mild-

Table 4.1. TMT.L; Locator Table for the TMT

Study[°]	Age[°°]	N	Sample Composition	IQ,[°°] Educ.	Country/ Location
TMT.1 Davies, 1968 page 41	20–29 30–39 40–49 50–59 60–69 70–79	540 180 90 90 90 90	British subjects test scores were on 50 M and 40 F in each of 6 decade age groups. Mean times corresponding to several percentile ranges are presented	—	England
TMT.2 Eson et al., personal communication page 41	63.2 67.0 72.0 78.3	63 15 16 16 16	Older subjects. Data are provided for 4 age groups	—	—
TMT.3 Harley et al., 1980 page 42	55–79 55–79	193 160	V.A. hospitalized patients (w/chronic brain syndrome were included) Subjects in alcohol-equated sample. Both samples are divided into 5 age groups	Educ 8.8	Wisconsin
TMT.4 Fromm-Auch & Yeudall, 1983 page 43	15–64 25.4 (8.2) 15–17 18-23 24–32 33–40 41-64	193 32 75 57 18 10	111 M, 82 F volunteers described as nonpsychiatric & nonneurological. 83% are R-handed. Ss classified in 5 age groups	Educ. 8–26 years 14.8(3.0) FSIQ 119.1(8.8)	Canada
TMT.5 Bornstein, 1985 page 44	18-69 43.3 (17.1) 20–39 40–59 60–69	365	178 M, 187 F volunteers. 91.5% are R-handed. Data are presented in age by gender by education cells	Educ. 12.3(2.7) (5–20 years) < high school (HS) ≥ HS	Canada
TMT.6 Dodrill, 1987 page 45	27.77 (11.04)	120	60 M, 60 F volunteers. Data for various intelligence levels are presented	Educ. 12.28(2.18) FSIQ 100(14.3)	Washington
TMT.7 Ernst, 1987 page 45	65–75	110	51 M, 59 F volunteers. Time to completion and number of errors are provided	Educ. 10.3	Brisbane, Australia
TMT.8 Stuss et al., 1987 page 46	16–19 20–29 30–39 40–49 50–59 60–69	60 10 10 10 10 10 10	Canadian: English or French-speaking Ss; 55% male, 18% L-handed; 6 age groups represented. Data for test/ retest (1 wk) are provided	Educ. 14.3(2.62) >12 <12	Canada
TMT.9 Yeudall et al., 1987 page 47	15–20 21-25 26–30 31-40	225	Volunteers classified in 4 age groupings. 86% are R-handed 127M, 98F	Educ. 10–17 14.55(2.78) FSIQ 112.25(10.25)	Canada

continued

Table 4.1. *(Continued)*

Study°	Age°°	N	Sample Composition	IQ,°° Educ.	Country/ Location
TMT.10 Bornstein & Suga, 1988 page 49	55–70 62.7 (4.3)	134	Healthy elderly volunteers 49 M, 85 F. No history of neurological or psychiatric disorders. Data are divided by educational level	Educ. 5–10 years (n = 46) 11-12 years (n = 44) >12 (n = 44)	Canada
TMT.11 Stuss et al., 1988 page 49	16–29 30–49 50–69	90 30 30 30	Data are divided by three age groups for original test and 1 week retest. Expansion of the TMT.8 study	Educ./Range 14.1(1.34) 11-18 14.9(3.95) 5–20 13.2(2.38) 8–18	Canada
TMT.12 Van Gorp et al., 1990 page 50	57–85 57–65 66–70 71-75 76–85	156 28 45 57 26	Eldery Ss with no history of neurological or psych-iatric disorders. 61% F. 4 age groups presented	Educ. 14.4(2.86) FSIQ 117.21 (12.59)	California
TMT.13 Heaton et al., 1991 page 51	42.1 (16.8) 20–34 35–39 40–44 45–49 50–54 55–59 60–64 65–69 70–74 75–80	486	Volunteers; 65% of the sample were males. T-scores corrected for age, education, and sex are provided for 10 age groupings for M and F separately	Educ. 13.6(3.5) FSIQ 113.8 (12.3)	CA, WA, TX, OK, WS, IL, MI, NY, VA, MA, Canada
TMT.14 Selnes et al., a) 1991 b) personal communication pages 52, 53	25–34 35–44 45–54	453	Ss from MACS study. Sero-negative homosexual and bisexual males. Data are presented: a) for three age groups and three educational levels; b) age by education groupings	<College Col. >Col.	Los Angeles
TMT.15 Ivnik et al., 1996 page 53	56–59 60–64 65–69 70–74 75–79 80–84 85–89 90–94	359 54 81 65 57 53 27 17 5	167 M, 192 F; 332 R-handed; normal elderly volunteers. The article provides tables for age correction and a regression equation for education correction	MAYO FSIQ 106.2(14.0)	Minnesota
TMT.16 Richardson & Marottoli, 1996 page 54	81.5 (3.3) 76–80 81-91	101	All autonomously living elderly Ss, current drivers; 53 M, 48 F. Data are provided for Trail B for younger-old and older-old by two educational levels	Educ. 11.0(3.7) <12 ≥12	New Haven, CT

continued

Table 4.1. (*Continued*)

Study[*]	Age[**]	N	Sample Composition	IQ,[**] Educ.	Country/ Location
TMT.17 Goul & Brown, 1970 page 55	20–29 30–39 40–49 50–59 60–72	106 26 25 24 16 15	Ss were Canadian workers compensation non-brain-injured hospitalized patients. Data are stratified by five age groups	Educ. 6–13 yrs FSIQ 103.8(12.1) 110.1(8.9) 105.3(7.9) 112.7(8.6) 104.2(12.2)	Canada
TMT.18 Wiens & Matarazzo, 1977 page 58	23.6 24.8	48	All males, neurologically normal. Divided into two equal groups. Random sample of 29 were retested 14 to 24 weeks later	Educ. 13.7 14.0 FSIQ 117.5 118.3	Portland, Oregon
TMT.19 Anthony et al., 1980 page 59	38.88 (15.80)	100	Normal volunteers, Data are provided for Trails B only	Educ. 13.33(2.56) FSIQ 113.5(10.8)	Colorado
TMT.20 Bak & Greene, 1980 page 59	50–62 55.6 (4.4) 67–86 74.9 (6.0)	15 15	Participants were divided in two age groups; Ss were fluent in English & denied histories of neurological problems. 1st group had 9 F, 2nd group had 10 F	Educ. 13.7(1.91) 14.9(2.99)	Texas
TMT.21 Kennedy, 1981 page 60	20–29 30–39 40–49 50–59 60–69	150 30 30 30 30 30	Ss were employees of a mental health center. Five age groups are represented	Educ(est. IQ) 13.73(123.43) 13.53(127.10) 13.11(127.40) 11.59(123.30) 12.50(128.54)	Canada
TMT.22 Heaton et al., 1986 page 61	15–81 39.3 (17.5) <40 40–59 ≥60	553	356 M, 197 F. Data for the Trails B are reported; sample was divided into 3 age groups & 3 education categories; % of Ss classified as normal is provided	Educ. 13.3(3.4) <12(132) 12–15(249) ≥16(172)	CO, CA, WI
TMT.23 Alekoumbides et al., 1987 page 62	19–82 46.85 (17.17)	118	Ss were medical and psychiatric VA inpatients w/o cerebral lesions or histories of alcoholism or cerebral contusions. All Ss except for one were male	Educ. 1–20 years 11.43(3.20) FSIQ 105.9(13.5)	S. Calif
TMT.24 Bornstein et al., 1987a page 62	17–52 32.3 (10.3)	23	9 M, 14 F volunteers. Data on 3 week retest are provided	VIQ 105.8(10.8) PIQ 105.0(10.5)	

[*]The study number corresponds to the number provided in the text of the chapter.

[**]Age column and IQ/education column contain information regarding range, and/or mean and standard deviation for the whole sample and/or separate groups, whichever information is provided by the authors.

Table 4.2. TMT.R&W; Severity Ranges for Part B (Based on Time in Seconds).

	Perfectly Normal	0–60		Mildly	73–105
Normal			Impaired		
	Normal	61–72		Seriously	≥106

ly suggestive of brain damage," while scores at the 10th percentile and less are "moderately suggestive of brain damage."

Golden, Osmon, Moses, & Berg (1981b, pp. 22–23)

The authors provide recommendations regarding detection of laterality of brain damage:

part A is generally considered more a measure of right hemisphere integrity (i.e., visual scanning skills), where part B is more indicative of left hemisphere intactness (i.e., language symbol manipulation and direction of behavior according to a complex plan). Therefore when one part indicates impairment relative to the other part, a lateralized injury may be present. . . . Part A is considered to indicate greater impairment if the score on part B is less than twice the score on part A. Part B indicates greater impairment if its score is more than three times the score on part A. Tests in which the part B score lies between two times and three times the part A score suggest that performances on the two parts are essentially equal.

However, lateralizing properties of performance time ratios for two conditions have been repeatedly refuted in the literature (Hom & Reitan, 1990; Salthouse et al., 1996).

Normative Studies

[TMT.1] Davies, 1968

The author published TMT data on 540 British subjects as a part of her investigation of the influence of age on TMT performance. Test scores were obtained on 50 men and 40 women in each of six decade age groups. The reference Davies cited as containing a further description of her subject sample could not be located.

Mean times in seconds corresponding to 10th, 25th, 50th, 75th, and 90th percentile ranks for Trails A and B are provided for each age decade with the exception that the data on the subjects in their 20s and 30s were collapsed. Davies also reports optimal cutting points for young vs. middle-aged individuals. No significant sex differences were observed within any specific decade, although in the group as a whole, men performed slightly but significantly more quickly on part B.

Study strengths
1. The presentation of the data in 10- or 20-year age intervals.
2. Very large sample size and large Ns within each age subgroup, and fairly equal representation of males and females.

Considerations regarding use of the study
1. Lack of IQ and education data or description of exclusion criteria.
2. Lack of test score standard deviations.
3. Tested in England, which may limit generalizability for clinical interpretive purposes in the United States (Table 4.3).

[TMT.2] Eson, Yen, and Bourke, personal communication

The authors collected normative data for the TMT on a sample of 63 older subjects. Mean time in seconds and standard deviations are provided for four age groups with mean ages of 63.2, 67.0, 72.0, and 78.3, respectively. Sample sizes for each age group range between 15 and 16. No other information is provided such as exclusion criteria or demographic data.

Study strengths
1. Data provided on an elderly sample and stratified by age group.
2. Means and standard deviations are reported.

Table 4.3. TMT.1; Mean Time in Seconds Corresponding to 10th, 25th, 50th, 75th, and 90th Percentile Ranks for Trails A and B per Age Group

N	Age	A Percentile					B Percentile				
		10	25	50	75	90	10	25	50	75	90
180	20s+30s	50	42	32	26	21	129	94	69	55	45
90	40s	59	45	34	28	22	151	100	78	57	49
90	50s	67	49	38	29	25	177	135	98	75	55
90	60s	104	67	48	35	29	282	172	119	89	64
90	70s	168	105	80	54	38	450	292	196	132	79

Considerations regarding use of the study

1. No reported exclusion criteria or other demographic, IQ, or geographic data.

2. Age range or SD for each group is not reported.

3. Relatively low sample sizes (Table 4.4).

[TMT.3] Harley, Leuthold, Matthews, and Bergs, 1980

The authors collected TMT data on 193 V.A.-hospitalized patients in Wisconsin ranging in age from 55 to 79. Exclusion criteria included Full Scale IQ less than 80, active psychosis, unequivocal neurological disease or brain damage, and serious visual or auditory acuity problems. Patients with chronic brain syndrome *were* included. Patient diagnoses were as follows: chronic brain syndrome unrelated to alcoholism (28%), psychosis (55%), alcoholic (37%), neurotic (9%), and personality disorder (4%). Mean educational level was 8.8 years. The sample was divided into five age groupings: 55–59 ($n = 56$), 60–64 ($n = 45$), 65–69 ($n = 35$), 70–74 ($n = 37$), and 75–79 ($n = 20$). Mean educational level and percent of sample included in each of the diagnostic classifications are reported for each age grouping. The authors also

Table 4.4. TMT.2; Mean Time in Seconds and Standard Deviations (in Parentheses) for Trails A and B

N	Age	A		B	
15	63.2	38.9	(15.6)	115.3	(57.8)
16	67.0	42.1	(14.2)	134.9	(57.7)
16	72.0	46.2	(24.0)	145.2	(134.9)
16	78.3	80.1	(64.8)	234.8	(117.0)

provide test data on a subgroup of 160 subjects equated for percent diagnosed with alcoholism across the five age groupings. The "alcohol-equated sample" was developed "to minimize the influence that cognitive or motor/sensory differences uniquely attributable to alcohol abuse might have upon group test performance levels" (p. 2). This subsample remained heterogeneous regarding representation of the other diagnostic categories. Mean time in seconds, standard deviation, and ranges are reported for parts A and B for each age interval for the whole sample and for the alcohol-equated sample.

Study strengths

1. Large sample size and some individual cells approximate Ns of 50.

2. Reporting of IQ data, geographic area, age, and education.

3. Data presented in age groupings.

4. Means and standard deviations are reported.

Considerations regarding use of the study

1. The presence of substantial neurologic (chronic brain syndrome), substance abuse, and major psychiatric disorders in the sample.

2. Low educational level, though IQ levels are average.

3. No information regarding sex, but given the VA setting, it is likely that most or all of the sample were male.

Other comments

The scores for the two oldest age groups are identical in the whole sample and alcohol-equated group because these two groups did

Table 4.5. TMT.3; Mean Time in Seconds, Standard Deviations (in Parentheses), and Ranges for Trails A and B for Each Age Interval for the Whole Sample and for the Alcohol-Equated Sample

| Age | N | WAIS | | | Education | Trails | |
		FSIQ	VIQ	PIQ		A	B
Total sample							
55–59	56	98.57	99.39	97.00	10.1	67.04	175.5
		(11.43)	(12.92)	(10.65)		(29.75)	(99.98)
		80–129	77–131	72–129		25–160	60–676
60–64	45	98.58	101.27	95.00	9.8	63.67	158.67
		(9.93)	(11.42)	(9.82)		(24.30)	(55.11)
		80–121	78–123	78–116		26–114	70–275
65–69	35	97.51	100.37	93.66	8.7	87.89	219.43
		(11.18)	(12.51)	(10.20)		(75.60)	(120.60)
		80–130	80–135	68–120		27–470	80–678
70–74	37	100.41	102.95	97.24	8.8	95.24	237.16
		(9.92)	(11.81)	(10.08)		(64.17)	(126.90)
		82–125	80–133	75–114		35–353	83–606
75–79	20	101.75	101.40	102.15	6.5	85.80	225.15
		(10.18)	(11.40)	(9.95)		(43.64)	(81.16)
		81–119	77–117	83–119		28–180	100–410
Alcohol-equated sample							
55–59	47	99.00	100.00	98.00	10.1	65.89	178.43
		(11.73)	(13.02)	(11.13)		(28.21)	(107.29)
		80–129	77–131	72–129		25–140	60–176
60–64	33	96.00	99.00	93.00	9.3	71.82	174.97
		(9.43)	(11.33)	(9.30)		(23.08)	(52.68)
		80–117	78–123	78–112		26–114	80–275
65–69	23	99.00	102.00	95.00	8.8	88.78	210.26
		(12.06)	(13.06)	(11.52)		(88.34)	(135.24)
		80–130	80–135	68–120		27–470	80–678
70–74	37	100.00	103.00	97.00	8.8	95.24	237.16
		(9.92)	(11.91)	(10.08)		(64.17)	(126.90)
		82–125	80–133	75–114		35–353	83–606
75–79	20	102.00	101.00	102.00	6.5	85.80	255.15
		(10.18)	(11.40)	(9.95)		(43.64)	(81.16)
		81–119	77–117	83–119		28–180	100–410

not have overrepresentation of alcoholics, so they did not need to be adjusted (Table 4.5).

[TMT.4] Fromm-Auch and Yeudall, 1983

The authors obtained TMT data on 193 Canadian subjects (111 male, 82 female) recruited through posted advertisements and personal contacts. Participants are described as "nonpsychiatric" and "nonneurological." Eighty-three percent of the sample were right-handed and mean age was 25.4 (SD = 8.2, range = 15 to 64). Mean years of education was 14.8 (SD = 3.0, range = 8 to 26) and included technical and

university training. Mean WAIS FSIQ, VIQ, and PIQ were 119.1 (SD = 8.8, range = 98 to 142), 119.8 (SD = 9.9, range = 95 to 143), and 115.6 (SD = 9.8, range = 89 to 146), respectively. Of note, no subject obtained a FSIQ which was lower than the average range.

Mean time in seconds, standard deviations, and ranges for part A and B are reported for five age groupings: 15–17, 18–23, 24–32, 33–40, and 41–64, with sample sizes ranging from 10 to 75. The two oldest age groupings both had sample sizes less than 20. No sex differences were documented and male and female data were collapsed.

Study strengths

1. The large overall sample size and some individual cells approximate *N*s of 50.

2. Presentation of the data by age groupings.

3. Information regarding mean IQ, educational levels, age, gender, handedness, recruitment procedures, and geographic area.

4. Some psychiatric and neurological exclusion criteria.

5. Means and standard deviations are reported.

Considerations regarding use of the study

1. The high intellectual and educational level of the sample.

2. An age grouping of 41 to 64 with an *N* of 10 would not appear to be particularly useful.

3. Data were collected in Canada which may limit their usefulness for clinical interpretation purposes in the United States.

4. Essentially no differences in performance were noted between the 18–23-year-olds and the 24–32-year-olds, suggesting that use of a single age grouping for 18 to 32 would have been appropriate (Table 4.6).

[TMT.5] Bornstein, 1985

The author collected data on 365 Canadian individuals (178 males and 187 females) recruit-

ed through posted notices on college campuses and unemployment offices, newspaper ads, and senior-citizen groups. Subjects were paid for their participation. Participants ranged in age from 18 to 69 (mean = 43.3 ± 17.1) and had completed between 5 and 20 years of education (mean = 12.3 ± 2.7). Ninety-one and a half percent of the sample were right-handed. No other demographic data or exclusion criteria are reported.

Mean time in seconds and standard deviations for parts A and B are reported for three age groupings (20–39, 40–59, and 60–69), two educational levels (less than high school, greater than or equal to high school), and sex, resulting in a total of 12 separate groups. Individual group sample sizes ranged from 13 to 86. Significant correlations were obtained between TMT scores and age and education, suggesting that better performance was associated with younger age and more years of education. Females generally outperformed males on both parts A and B.

Study strengths

1. Very large overall sample size and several individual cells approximate *N*s of 50.

2. Stratification of the data by age, sex, and educational level.

3. This data set is unique in that it reports data for subjects with less than a high school education.

4. Information on handedness, recruitment procedures, and geographic area.

5. Means and standard deviations are reported.

Considerations regarding use of the study

1. Individual sample sizes of some cells were small (e.g., 13, 16, 17).

2. The lack of any reported exclusion criteria.

3. The data were collected on Canadian citizens, which may limit generalizability for their use in the United States.

4. The lack of IQ data. The concern over the lack of IQ data is somewhat mitigated by the fact that the mean education level was not unduly elevated (12.3 years), which might suggest that mean intellectual levels were within the average range (Table 4.7).

Table 4.6. TMT.4; Mean Time in Seconds, Standard Deviations (in Parentheses), and Ranges for Trails A and B

		Trails	
N	Age	A	B
32	15-17	23.4	47.7
		(5.9)	(10.4)
		15.2-39.0	25.4-81.0
76	18-23	26.7	51.3
		(9.4)	(14.6)
		12.0-60.1	23.3-101.0
57	24-32	24.3	53.2
		(7.6)	(15.6)
		11.8-46.0	29.1-98.0
18	33-40	27.5	62.1
		(8.3)	(17.5)
		16.0-52.7	39.0-111.0
10	41-64	29.7	73.6
		(8.4)	(19.4)
		16.5-42.0	41.9-102.0

Table 4.7. TMT.5; Mean Time in Seconds and Standard Deviations (in Parentheses) for Trails A and B for 3 Age Groupings and 2 Educational Levels for Males and Females Separately

	Education Groups							
	Males				Females			
	<HS		≥HS		<HS		≥HS	
Age	A	B	A	B	A	B	A	B
20–39	28.3	70.0	23.8	53.9	23.2	56.4	22.0	53.5
	(8.4)	(28.7)	(6.8)	(18.3)	(5.5)	(21.3)	(6.0)	(20.5)
		n = 21		n = 86		n = 13		n = 50
40–59	38.9	107.8	28.6	74.1	30.5	76.7	27.3	65.6
	(12.5)	(52.2)	(9.6)	(35.8)	(9.2)	(25.7)	(9.2)	(28.5)
		n = 13		n = 17		n = 22		n = 43
60–69	37.6	119.4	35.3	78.3	40.7	96.4	34.5	87.4
	(8.5)	(42.3)	(10.2)	(26.1)	(12.9)	(27.3)	(8.9)	(27.1)
		n = 16		n = 23		n = 22		n = 34

[TMT.6] Dodrill, 1987

The author collected TMT data on 120 subjects in Washington during the years 1975–1976 (n = 81) and 1986–1987 (n = 39). Half of the sample was female and 10% were minorities (six black, three native American, two Asian American, one unknown). Eighteen were left-handed and occupational status included 45 students, 37 employed, 26 unemployed, 11 homemakers, and one retiree. Subjects were recruited from various sources including schools, churches, employment agencies, and community service agencies and were either paid for their participation or offered an interpretation of their abilities. Exclusion criteria included history of "neurologically relevant disease (such as meningitis or encephalitis)"; alcoholism; birth complications "of likely neurological significance"; oxygen deprivation; peripheral nervous system injury; psychotic or psychotic-like disorders; or head injury associated with unconsciousness, skull fracture, persisting neurological signs, or diagnosis of concussion or contusion. Of note, one-third of potential participants failed to meet the above medical and psychiatric criteria, resulting in a final sample of 120. Mean age was 27.73 (±11.04) and mean years of education was 12.28 (±2.18). The subjects tested in the 1970s were adminstered the WAIS and the subjects asssessed in the 1980s were administered the WAIS-R; WAIS scores were converted to WAIS-R equivalents by subtracting seven points from the VIQ, PIQ and FSIQ. Mean FSIQ, VIQ, and PIQ scores were 100.00 (±14.35), 100.92 (±14.73), and 98.25 (±13.39), respectively. The IQ scores ranged from 60 to 138 and reflected a normal distribution.

Mean time in seconds and standard deviations for part A and B are reported as well as IQ-equivalent scores for various levels of intelligence. Between 10% and 15% of the sample were misclassified as brain damaged using a cutoff of 39 seconds for part A and 89 seconds for Part B.

Study strengths
1. Large sample size.
2. Comprehensive exclusion criteria.
3. Information regarding education, IQ, occupation, sex ratio, age, handedness, ethnicity, recruitment procedures, and geographic area.
4. IQ equivalent scores provided.
5. Data for different IQ levels provided.
6. Means and standard deviations are reported.

Considerations regarding use of the study
1. Undifferentiated age range (Table 4.8).

[TMT.7] Ernst, 1987

The author obtained TMT data on 110 primarily Caucasian (99%) residents of Brisbane, Australia, aged 65 to 75. Fifty-nine were female and

Table 4.8. TMT.6; Mean Time in Seconds and Standard Deviations (in Parentheses) for Trails A and B for the Whole Sample and for Different Intelligence Levels

N	Age	Education	FSIQ	VIQ	PIQ	Trails A	Trails B
120	27.73 (11.04)	12.28 (2.18)	100.00 (14.35)	100.92 (14.73)	98.25 (13.39)	25.37 (9.17)	66.02 (34.17)

N	FSIQ	Trails A	Trails B	FSIQ	Trails A	Trails B
7	130	20	50	>89	<30	<76
18	125	21	47	80-89	30-39	76-103
34	120	20	48	70-79	40-49	104-180
64	115	22	49	<70	>49	>180
93	110	23	53			
101	105	24	56			
75	100	25	60			
60	95	26	62			
48	90	26	68			
33	85	28	82			
19	80	30	99			
10	75	33	135			
	70	39	159			

51 were male, and mean educational level was 10.3 years; men and women did not differ in years of education. Subjects were recruited primarily through random selection from the Queensland State electoral roll ($n = 97$), with the remainder ($n = 13$) solicited through senior-citizen centers. Exclusion criteria included history of significant head trauma or neurologic disease. Nearly one-half of the sample were diagnosed with at least one chronic disease (hypertension = 33, heart disease = 9, thyroid dysfunction = 7, asthma = 5, emphysema = 2, diabetes = 1) for which they were receiving treatment and which was described as well controlled. Sixty-six of the subjects were receiving medications, primarily for the diseases listed above.

Test administration was according to the Reitan instructions. All subjects were administered the Trailmaking Test first, followed by either the Tactual Performance Test or Booklet Category Test. Using the standard cutoffs of 39 seconds and 92 seconds, 48% and 48% of all subjects were misclassified as impaired for Trails A and B, respectively. Gender differences were not significant for TMT performance; however, education was significantly related to performance on Trails B. There were no significant effects of chronic disease or medication intake.

Study strengths
1. Large sample size in a restricted age range.
2. Presentation of the data by sex.
3. Information regarding education, geographic recruitment area, recruitment procedures, and ethnicity.
4. Information regarding test administration order effects.
5. Means and standard deviations are reported.

Considerations regarding use of the study
1. Approximately half of the subjects had at least one chronic illness, and over half were taking prescribed medications.
2. No information regarding IQ.
3. Low mean educational level.
4. Data were collected in Australia and may be unsuitable for clinical use in the United States (Table 4.9).

[TMT.8] Stuss, Stethem, and Poirier, 1987

The authors collected normative data on 60 Canadian English- or French-speaking subjects

Table 4.9. TMT.7; Mean Time in Seconds and Standard Deviations (in Parentheses) for the Trails A and B and the Number of Errors for Each Condition

N	Sex	Trails	
		A	B
51	Male	40.5	98.2
		(21.1)	(52.9)
	Errors	0.3	0.8
		(0.6)	(1.1)
59	Female	42.3	108.7
		(14.4)	(79.2)
	Errors	0.3	0.7
		(0.5)	(0.9)

who were recruited through personal contacts or employment agencies and were paid for their participation. Test administration was conducted in each subject's native language. Subjects were tested twice at 1-week intervals. Exclusion criteria included abnormal vision (even after correction); history of substance abuse; presence of medical, neurological, and/or psychiatric disorders; and current use of any psychotropic medication (Stuss, personal communication). Ten subjects were assigned to each of six age ranges: 16–19, 20–29, 30–39, 40–49, 50–59, and 60–69. Fifty-five percent of the sample were male, and 18% were left-handed. Mean years of education were 14.3 (SD = 2.62). Data are provided regarding handedness, sex distribution, and education (means, standard deviations, ranges, frequency of subjects with less than/equal to and greater than high school education) for each age interval.

Mean times in seconds and standard deviations for the two parts of the TMT for the first, second, and combined testing sessions are reported for each age interval. Mean times and standard deviations are also provided for males, females, those with less than or equal to 12 years of education, and those with greater than 12 years of education collapsed across age groupings.

Older subjects and those with a high school education or less performed significantly poorer than younger subjects or those with some college or university education. Educational level was somewhat irregularly distributed across age groups, and the authors suggest that the normative data be used with caution. A practice effect was present but the authors question the clinical relevance of the improvement. No significant sex differences in performance were present.

Study strengths
1. Presentation of the data by age groupings, education groupings, and sex.
2. Extensive information on educational level.
3. Description of sex, handedness characteristics, geographic location and recruitment procedures.
4. Adequate exclusion criteria.
5. Information regarding practice effect.
6. Means and standard deviations are reported.

Considerations regarding use of the study
1. Small sample sizes within each age group.
2. Variability in mean educational levels across the age groups; of importance, the 50–59-year-old group had the lowest mean educatonal level and the lowest mean test scores and largest standard deviations relative to the other age groups.
3. Lack of IQ data.
4. Unknown influence of language differences.
5. Data were obtained in Canada and may be of limited usefulness for clinical interpretive purposes in the United States (Tables 4.10 and 4.11).

[TMT.9] Yeudall, Reddon, Gill, and Stefanyk, 1987

The authors obtained TMT data on 225 Canadian subjects recruited from posted advertisements in workplaces and personal solicitations. The participants included meat packers, postal workers, transit employees, hospital lab technicians, secretaries, ward aides, student interns, student nurses, and summer students. In addition, high school teachers identified for participation average students in grades 10 through 12. Exclusion criteria included evidence of "forensic involvement," head injury, neurological insult, prenatal or birth complications, psychiatric problems, or substance abuse.

Table 4.10. TMT.8a; Mean Time in Seconds and Standard Deviations (in Parentheses) for Trails A and B for the First Administration, Retest 1 Week Later, and 2 Testing Probes Combined: The Data Are Presented for 6 Age Groups Separately

| | | | | | | | | | Trails | | | | |
| | | Sex | | Hand | | | | A | | | B | | |
N	Age	M	F	R	L	Educ	Comb	Test1	Test2	Comb	Test1	Test2
10	17.3 (0.95) 16–19	5	5	8	2	12.3 (0.95) 11–13	21.8 (7.0)	21.8 (5.3)	22.2 (8.7)	45.4 (17.2)	49.0 (21.2)	41.8 (13.1)
10	23.0 (2.67) 20–29	6	4	6	4	16.2 (1.39) 14–18	17.3 (5.1)	18.5 (5.1)	16.2 (5.0)	37.8 (12.1)	41.6 (11.4)	34.0 (12.7)
10	33.9 (2.88) 30–39	5	5	7	3	16.7 (3.86) 10–20	20.1 (4.6)	21.9 (6.3)	18.4 (2.9)	46.5 (12.6)	46.3 (13.7)	46.8 (11.4)
10	44.2 (3.12) 40–49	6	4	9	1	15.5 (2.88) 10–20	27.9 (8.2)	29.2 (9.0)	26.5 (7.5)	64.3 (19.7)	64.1 (16.3)	64.4 (23.0)
10	55.3 (2.98) 50–59	6	4	9	1	11.7 (2.41) 8–16	35.6 (20.9)	38.5 (18.2)	32.7 (23.8)	77.3 (42.8)	83.1 (44.3)	71.4 (41.3)
10	63.7 (3.13) 60–69	5	5	10	0	14.3 (2.00) 12–17	33.6 (11.8)	37.3 (14.7)	29.9 (8.9)	70.3 (21.7)	73.3 (20.3)	67.3 (23.2)

TMT data were gathered by experienced testing technicians who "motivated the subjects to achieve maximum performance" partially through the promise of detailed explanations of their test performance.

Means and standard deviations for time in seconds to complete parts A and B are presented for four age groupings (15 to 20, 21 to 25, 26 to 30, and 31 to 40) for males and females combined and separately. Information regarding

Table 4.11. TMT.8b; Data for Trails A and B for the Whole Sample Stratified by Gender and Education

	N	Trails A	Trails B
Males	33	25.80 (14.85)	58.40 (30.97)
Females	27	26.32 (10.08)	55.10 (21.27)
≤ High School	27	28.56 (15.06)	63.58 (32.33)
> High School	33	23.98 (10.37)	51.63 (20.44)

percent right handers, mean years of education, and mean WAIS/WAIS-R FSIQ, VIQ, and PIQ is reported for each age grouping, and age by sex grouping. For the sample as a whole, 88% were right handed and had completed an average of 14.55 (SD = 2.78) years of schooling. The mean FSIQ, VIQ, and PIQ were 112.25 (SD = 9.83), 114.77 (SD = 10.34), and 108.50 (SD = 10.34), respectively.

No significant correlations were found between age or education for Trails A; a significant correlation emerged for age and Trails B ($r = 0.27$), but no significant relationship was documented between education and Trails B. Significant correlations emerged between Trails A and B and PIQ, but not VIQ. No significant sex differences were observed for Trails A or B. The authors recommend use of the combined age group norms for Trails A and the separate age-grouped norms for Trails B.

Study strengths

1. Large sample size and individual cells approximate Ns of 50.

2. Grouping of data by age.

3. Data availability for a 15- to 20-year-old age group.

4. Adequate medical and psychiatric exclusion criteria.

5. Information regarding handedness, education, IQ, sex, occupation, recruitment procedures, and geographic area.

6. Means and standard deviations are reported.

Considerations regarding use of the study

1. The sample was atypical in terms of its high average intellectual level and high level of education.

2. The data were obtained on Canadian subjects, which may limit their usefulness for clinical interpretation in the United States due to possible subtle cultural differences (Table 4.12).

[TMT.10] Bornstein and Suga, 1988

As a part of their evaluation of the effect of educational level on neuropsychological test performance in the elderly, the authors report TMT data on 134 healthy elderly Canadian volunteers aged 55 to 70 according to three educational levels: 5–10 years ($n = 46$), 11 to 12 years ($n = 44$), and greater than 12 years ($n = 44$). Nearly two-thirds of the sample were female ($n = 85$). The average age for the sample was 62.7 (±4.3), and the mean ages of the three educational groups were comparable (62.3, 62.9, and 63.0, respectively). Exclusion criteria included history of neurological or psychiatric disorder.

Significant group differences in both TMT A and B performance were obtained across the three education groups, which was due to the group with 5 to 10 years of education performing significantly more poorly than both of the other education groups (which did not differ from each other). Mean time in seconds and standard deviations for parts A and B are reported for the three education groups.

Study strengths

1. Large sample size and individual cells approximate Ns of 50.

2. Reporting of data by three education groups; the study is unique in terms of representation of subjects with less than 12 years of education.

3. Information regarding sex, age, and geographic area.

4. Means and standard deviations are reported.

5. Minimally adequate exclusion criteria.

Considerations regarding use of the study

1. No information regarding IQ.

2. Greater than 12 years education too large a category.

3. Data collected in Canada, which may limit generalizability for use in the United States (Table 4.13).

[TMT.11] Stuss, Stethem, and Pelchat, 1988

In a subsequent publication, Stuss and colleagues increased the size of the sample and

Table 4.12. TMT.9; Mean and Standard Deviations (in Parentheses) for Time in Seconds to Complete Trails A and B for 4 Age Groupings and for the Total Sample

N	Age	Educ.	%Right Hand	FSIQ	VIQ	PIQ	Trails	
							A	B
62	15–20	12.16 (1.75)	79.03	111.75 (10.16)	111.18 (10.92)	108.30 (10.47)	24.75 (8.19)	49.17 (15.21)
73	21–25	14.82 (1.88)	86.30	109.79 (9.97)	110.48 (10.43)	105.88 (11.20)	24.53 (7.93)	50.36 (12.96)
48	26–30	15.50 (2.65)	89.58	113.95 (10.61)	114.40 (11.45)	110.28 (8.72)	24.49 (7.22)	51.94 (15.75)
42	31–40	16.50 (3.11)	90.48	116.09 (9.51)	117.76 (9.32)	109.72 (11.45)	25.74 (7.53)	59.35 (17.12)
225	15–40	14.55 (2.78)	85.78	112.25 (10.25)	112.60 (10.86)	108.13 (10.63)	24.81 (7.75)	52.05 (15.36)

Table 4.13. TMT.10; Mean Time in Seconds and Standard Deviations (in Parentheses) for Trails A and B for Three Education Groups

N	Education	Age	Sex M	Sex F	Trails A	Trails B
46	5–10 8.5	62.3	17	29	38.9 (11.5)	102.0 (39.5)
44	11–12 11.7	62.9	16	28	33.6 (10.3)	82.5 (34.5)
44	>12 15.0	63.0	16	28	34.0 (10.7)	80.9 (30.9)

°Note: education range and mean education are provided for each group.

collapsed the subjects into three age groupings of 30 subjects each: 16–29, 30–49, and 50–69. Sex distribution was essentially equal across groups. Mean years of education for the youngest to oldest groups were 14.1 (SD = 1.34, range = 11–18), 14.9 (SD = 3.95, range = 5–20), and 13.2 (SD = 2.38, range = 8–18), respectively (compare to TMT.8).

Mean times in seconds and standard deviations for the two parts of the TMT for the first and second testing sessions are reported for each age interval. In addition, the combined data from the two testing sessions (Stuss, personal communication) are presented in a boxplot form which displays data variability. The boxplot depicts the mean, median, 25th and 75th centiles, and interquartile range. The authors call attention to the skewness and lack of normal distribution of the test data, which they suggest have implications for test score interpretation.

Study strengths
1. Increased sample size per age interval.
2. Adequate exclusion criteria.
3. Information regarding education, sex, and handedness.
4. Data regarding retesting at 1-week intervals.
5. Presentation of the data in boxplot format to show skewness.
6. Means and standard deviations are reported.

Considerations regarding use of the study
1. Considerations remain the same as for the initial report except for the improvement in sample size (see TMT.8) (Table 4.14).

[TMT.12] Van Gorp, Satz, and Mitrushina, 1990
The authors present TMT data for 156 healthy elderly subjects ranging in age from 57 to 85 recruited from an independent living retire-

Table 4.14. TMT.11; Mean Time in Seconds and Standard Deviations (in Parentheses) for Trails A and B Divided into 3 Age Groups, for 2 Testing Sessions 1 Week Apart

N	Age	Sex M	Sex F	Hand R	Hand L	Educ.	Trails A Test1	Trails A Test2	Trails B Test1	Trails B Test2
30	22.43 (2.67) 16–29	16	14	22	8	14.1 (1.34) 11–18	21.48 (6.44)	19.68 (7.32)	48.77 (18.66)	42.18 (15.54)
30	40.63 (2.97) 30–49	14	16	26	4	14.9 (3.95) 5–20	27.58 (9.43)	22.95 (6.23)	61.30 (17.88)	61.52 (22.79)
30	61.77 (3.0) 50–69	14	16	28	2	13.2 (2.38) 8–18	36.73 (13.68)	29.30 (14.73)	76.97 (30.52)	67.10 (28.37)

ment community in California. The data were collected as a part of their investigation of neuropsychological processes in normal aging. Information regarding general medical status was collected. Subjects with a history of neurological or psychiatric disorder or substance abuse were excluded. Sixty-one percent of the sample were females. Mean years of education was 14.14 (SD = 2.86) and mean FSIQ (WAIS-R Satz-Mogel format) was 117.21 (SD = 12.59).

Mean times in seconds and standard deviations to complete Trails A and B were listed for the sample as a whole and for four age groups: 57–65, 66–70, 71–75, and 76–85. Sample sizes for each age group ranged from 26 to 57. Mean Verbal and Performance IQs and standard deviations for each age range are listed. Mean VIQs were consistently within the high average range except for a mean VIQ for the 71–75-year-olds within the superior range. Mean PIQs were within the high average range for the 57–65-year-olds and 76–85-year-olds. Older subjects (greater than or equal to 70) did not differ significantly from younger subjects (less than 70) in VIQ, PIQ, or years of education.

Study strengths
1. Large sample size with some individual cells approximating *N*s of 50.
2. Small age range within each age grouping.
3. Use of exclusion criteria.

4. Information on IQ, educat geographic recruitment area.
5. Means and standard devia ported.

Considerations regarding use of the study
1. High mean IQs of the sample.
2. Relatively high educational level.
3. Unexplicably, part B performance was lower in the 66–70-year-olds relative to the 71–75-year-olds, and there appeared to be considerably more variation in performance in the 66–70 age grouping. Given that increasing age is associated with a worsening of performance, the data for the 66–70-year-old group is problematic (Table 4.15).

[TMT.13] Heaton, Grant, and Matthews, 1991

The authors provide normative data on the TMT from 486 (378 in the base sample and 108 in the validation sample) urban and rural subjects recruited in several states (California, Washington, Colorado, Texas, Oklahoma, Wisconsin, Illinois, Michigan, New York, Virginia, and Massachusetts) and Canada. Data were collected over a 15-year period through multicenter collaborative efforts; the authors trained the test administrators and supervised data collection. Exclusion criteria included history of learning disability, neurologic disease, illnesses affecting brain function, significant head trauma, significant psychiatric disturbance (e.g.,

Table 4.15. TMT.12; Mean Time in Seconds and Standard Deviations (in Parentheses) for Trails A and B for Four Age Groups and for the Sample as a Whole

				Trails	
N	Age	VIQ	PIQ	A	B
28	57–65	117.20 (11.33)	109.20 (11.56)	41.50 (7.38)	84.40 (24.60)
45	66–70	114.80 (17.03)	111.47 (16.83)	43.20 (14.98)	105.20 (43.43)
57	71–75	122.88 (11.38)	115.08 (11.94)	50.08 (12.88)	97.79 (30.40)
26	76–85	110.55 (11.25)	101.00 (8.78)	59.73 (15.95)	153.09 (62.60)
156	57–85	117.65 (13.53)	110.62 (13.49)	48.70 (14.47)	107.55 (45.63)

schizophrenia), and alcohol or other substance abuse. Mean age for the total sample was 42.06 ± 16.8, and mean educational level was 13.6 ± 3.5. Sixty-five percent of the sample were males. The majority of the subjects were administered the WAIS; mean FSIQ, VIQ, and PIQ were 113.8 ± 12.3, 113.9 ± 13.8, and 111.9 ± 11.6, respectively.

The TMT was administered according to procedures outlined by Reitan and Wolfson (1985) with the exception that attempts to complete Trails B were limited to 10 minutes. In those situations in which Trails B was stopped at 10 minutes, the time score was prorated by dividing 300 seconds by the number of items completed and then multiplying the resulting figure by 25. Subjects were generally paid for their participation and were judged to have provided their best efforts on the tasks. For Trails A, 30% of score variance was accounted for by age, while 16% was attributable to educational level; sex accounted for a negligible amount of unique variance in performance (1%). A total of 35% of test score variance was accounted for by demographic variables. For Trails B, 34% of score variance was accounted for by age, while 27% was attributable to educational level; again sex accounted for a negligible amount of unique variance (1%). A total of 45% of test score variance was accounted for by demographic variables. The normative data, which are not reproduced here, are presented in comprehensive tables in T-score equivalents for test-scaled scores for males and females separately in 10 age groupings (20–34, 35–39, 40–44, 45–49, 50–54, 55–59, 60–64, 65–69, 70–74, 75–80) by six educational groupings (6–8 years, 9–11 years, 12 years, 13–15 years, 16–17 years, 18+ years). For the sample as a whole, mean time in seconds for part A was 29.0 ± 12.5 and for part B was 75.2 ± 42.8.

Study strengths
1. Large sample size.
2. *T* scores corrected for age, education, and sex.
3. Comprehensive exclusion criteria.
4. Information regarding IQ and geographic recruitment area.

Considerations regarding use of the study
1. Above-average mean intellectual level (which is probably less of an issue given that these are WAIS rather than WAIS-R IQ data)

Other comments
1. The interested reader is referred to 1996 critique of Heaton et al. (1991) norms, and Heaton et al.'s 1996 response to this critique.

[TMT.14a] Selnes, Jacobson, Machado, Becker, Wesch, Miller, Visscher and McArthur, 1991

The investigation used subjects from the Multi-Center AIDS Cohort Study (MACS). The article presents results of seronegative homosexual and bisexual males in Los Angeles for the purpose of establishing normative data for neuropsychological test performance based on a large sample. Subjects with history of head injury with loss of consciousness greater than 1 hour, and who reported drinking ≥21 drinks per week in the previous 6 months were excluded.

The majority of sample consisted of Caucasian subjects. Percent of African-American subjects ranged from 3.4 to 4.1 for different age groups. Percent of left-handers ranged from 11.3 to 14.9.

Study strengths
1. The overall sample size is large and all individual cells have more than 50 subjects.
2. Normative data are stratified by age and education.
3. Information on ethnicity and handedness is reported.
4. Means, SDs, as well as scores for the percentiles 5 and 10 are presented.
5. The paper reports demographic composition for each age and education cell separately.
6. Some exclusion criteria.

Considerations regarding use of the study
1. All male sample.
2. No information on IQ is reported.
3. High educational level of the sample.
4. The *N*s for the age and education groupings are unknown (Table 4.16).

Table 4.16. TMT.14a; Data for the Sample Stratified by Age and Education

			TMT Trials					
			A				Percentiles	
				Percentiles				
Age	Mean Age	Education	Mean (SD)	5th	10th	Mean (SD)	5th	10th
By Age:								
25-34	31.0	16.1	19.0	27	24	49.5	80	74
	(2.6)	(2.2)	(5.9)			(17.1)		
35-44	39.3	16.4	20.8	32	29	52.5	83	78
	(2.9)	(2.3)	(5.5)			(18.6)		
45-54	48.5	16.7	23.1	37	35	53.9	87	79
	(2.6)	(2.6)	(7.3)			(20.3)		
By Education (<College, College, >College):								
<Col.	36.1	13.7	22.8	31	30	51.8	87	79
	(7.4)	(1.2)	(7.1)			(20.7)		
Col.	35.6	16.0	19.2	32	25	51.4	83	75
	(7.2)	(0.0)	(5.8)			(17.1)		
>Col.	38.4	18.6	20.1	30	28	50.2	79	73
	(7.8)	(1.3)	(5.5)			(15.8)		

[TMT.14b] Selnes and Miller, personal communication

Ola Selnes and Eric Miller provide an update to the data reported in their 1991 paper (TMT.14a), reflecting ongoing data collection from their longitudinal epidemiological study of HIV infection. They now present the data in a combined age and education grouping. All data are from healthy HIV-negative gay and bisexual males (Table 4.17).

[TMT.15] Ivnik, Malec, Smith, Tangalos, and Petersen, 1996

The study provides age-specific norms for the TMT obtained in Mayo's Older Americans Normative Studies (MOANS) projects. The total sample consisted of 746 cognitively normal volunteers over age of 55; however, only 359 volunteers participated in TMT testing. Mean MAYO FSIQ (which differs somewhat from standard WAIS-R FSIQ) for the whole sample was 106.2 (±14.0) and mean Mayo General Memory Index on the WMS-R was 106.2 (±14.2). For a description of their samples the authors refer to their earlier publications. Subjects were independently functioning, community dwelling persons who were recently examined by a physician and had no active neurologic or psychiatric disorder with the potential to impact cognition.

Age categorization utilized the midpoint interval technique. The raw score distribution for each test at each midpoint age was "normalized" by assigning standard scores with mean of 10 and SD of 3, based on actual percentile ranks. The authors provided tables of age-corrected norms for each age group (see below). The procedure for clinical application of these data are described in the original article (Ivnik et al., 1996) as follows: "first select the table that corresponds to that person's age. Enter the table with the test's *raw score*; do not use corrected or final scores for tests that might present their own age- or education-adjustments. Select the appropriate column in the table for that test. The corresponding row in the leftmost column in each table provides the MOANS Age-Corrected Scaled Score . . . for your subject's raw score; the corresponding row in the right-most column indicates the percentile range for that same score."

Further, linear regressions should be applied to the normalized, age-corrected MOANS

Table 4.17. TMT.14b; Distribution of TMT Scores by Age and Education for MACS HIV-1 Seronegative Participants

	Age Group		
	25–34 (N = 107)	35–44 (N = 93)	45–60 (N = 42)
<College Education			
Trailmaking, Part A	21.7 (8.8)	23.1 (5.0)	25.1 (5.7)
Trailmaking, Part B	53.3(18.4)	49.6(23.6)	52.6(22.2)
College Education			
Trailmaking, Part A	18.3 (4.4)	18.4 (5.3)	22.2 (8.5)
Trailmaking, Part B	49.5(16.2)	51.8(20.7)	50.9(16.1)
>College Education			
Trailmaking, Part A	17.5 (3.7)	20.9 (5.5)	21.9 (6.9)
Trailmaking, Part B	46.3 (16.3)	53.3(14.7)	54.6(15.5)

Scaled Scores (A-MSS) derived from the tables, to adjust patient's score for education. Age-and-education-corrected scores for the TMT (A&E-MSS) can be calculated as follows:

$$A\&E-MSS_{TMT} = K+(W_1 \circ A - MSS_{TMT}) - (W_2 \circ Education)$$

Where the following indices are specified for the two parts of the TMT:

	Trails A	Trails B
K	1.99	3.38
W_1	1.10	1.06
W_2	0.21	0.29

Education should enter the formula in years of formal schooling.

Study strengths
1. Demographic characteristics of the sample are well described including sex, education, ethnicity, IQ levels, and handedness.
2. The data were stratified by age group based on midpoint interval technique.
3. The innovative scoring system was well described. The authors developed new indices of performance.
4. The sample sizes for most groups are large.
5. Restricted age range in each cell.
6. Adequate exclusion criteria.

Considerations regarding use of the study
1. The measures proposed by the authors are quite complicated and might be difficult to use in clinical practice.
2. Smaller sample sizes for groups over 80 years.

Other comments
1. The theoretical assumptions underlying this normative project have been presented in Ivnik et al. (1992a,b).
2. The authors cautioned that validity of the MAYO Indices depends heavily on the match of demographic features of the individual to the normative sample presented in this article.
3. Correlations of Trails A and B with age were 0.30 and 0.53, whereas correlations with education and sex were negligible (Table 4.18 and 4.19).

[TMT.16] Richardson and Marottoli, 1996

The authors report data for 101 autonomously living elderly subjects who comprise a subsample of a cohort of participants in "Project Safety," a study on driving performance conducted in New Haven, Connecticut. Individuals with a history of neurologic desease, excessive use of alcohol, or those who were at risk for dementia based on the MMSE scores, were excluded.

The sample consisted of 53 males and 48 females with a mean age of 81.47 (±3.30) and mean education of 11.02 (±3.68) years. The

Table 4.18. TMT.15a; Demographic Description of the Sample Used in TMT Testing

Characteristics	N
Age Groups	
56–59	54
60–64	81
65–69	65
70–74	57
75–79	53
80–84	27
85–89	17
90–94	5
95+	0
Education	
≤7	2
8–11	33
12	135
13–15	87
16–17	67
≥18	35
Sex	
Males	167
Females	192
Race	
Caucasians	358
Blacks	1
Handedness	
Right	332
Left	17
Mixed	10
Total	359

Trails B part was administered and scored according to the standard instructions provided in the test manual.

The data were divided into two age groups of younger-old (76–80) and older-old (81–91) and two education groups. The results indicated that the mean performance for subjects with less than 12 years of education was stable across younger-old (76–80) and older-old (81–91) age groups; however, it was considerably lower than for the subjects with >12 years of education and well below expected in comparison to the Heaton et al. (1991) norms. For the subjects with 12 or more years of education, performance for the younger-old age group was superior to that of the older-old and

was comparable to the norms published by Heaton et al. (1991).

Study strengths
1. Data for a relatively large sample of very elderly subjects are presented.
2. Information on age, education, gender, and geographic location is reported.
3. Exclusion criteria are described.
4. The data are classified into two-age-by-two-education groups.
5. Means and standard deviations are reported.

Considerations regarding use of the study
1. Only the Trails B part of the test was administered.
2. No information on intelligence level is provided.
3. Sample sizes for each age-by-education cell are relatively small (Tables 4.20 and 4.21).

Control Groups in Clinical Studies

[TMT.17] Goul and Brown, 1970

The authors tested 103 (or 106) Canadian workers compensation board non-brain-injured patients who had been hospitalized at least 3 months. These data were collected as a part of the authors' analysis of the effects of age and intelligence on TMT performance. Subjects had negative neurological histories and included amputees, burn victims, and patients with lumbosacral fusions. Educational levels ranged from 6 to 13 years of formal schooling; no means are reported. Subjects were classified into five age groups: 20–29, 30–39, 40–49, 50–59, and 60–72. Individual group sizes ranged from 15 to 26. Mean WAIS FSIQs for the five groups were 103.8 (SD = 12.1), 110.1 (SD = 8.9), 105.3 (SD = 7.9), 112.7 (SD = 8.6), and 104.2 (SD = 12.2), respectively.

TMT part A and B data are presented in terms of mean time in seconds, standard deviations, ranges, medians, and recommended cutoff scores for the five age groups. Performance declined significantly with age. Contrary to the expectations, IQ was found to be significantly *positively* correlated with TMT scores.

Table 4.19. TMT.15b; Age-Corrected Norms for Each Age Group (A-MSS): The Procedure for Applications of These Data are Described in the Text

Scaled Score	Age Group 56–62 A	Age Group 56–62 B	Age Group 63–65 A	Age Group 63–65 B	Age Group 66–68 A	Age Group 66–68 B
2	>74	>225	>74	>228	>106	>240
3	62–74	188–225	65–74	200–228	74–106	210–240
4	59–61	156–187	61–64	189–199	64–73	190–209
5	55–58	141–155	56–60	155–188	58–63	155–189
6	49–54	117–140	50–55	132–154	50–57	132–154
7	41–48	97–116	45–49	104–131	46–49	107–131
8	37–40	88–96	39–44	92–103	40–45	97–106
9	34–36	78–87	36–38	83–91	37–39	85–96
10	30–33	64–77	31–35	73–82	32–36	75–84
11	27–29	60–63	29–30	63–72	29–31	69–74
12	25–26	55–59	26–28	58–62	27–28	61–68
13	22–24	49–54	23–25	51–57	25–26	54–60
14	20–21	42–48	22	45–50	22–24	47–53
15	18–19	39–41	19–21	42–44	21	43–46
16	17	36–38	17–18	38–41	20	41–42
17	16	34–35	16	34–37	18–19	34–40
18	<16	<34	<16	<34	<18	<34
N	160	160	206	206	152	152

Scaled Score	Age Group 69–71 A	Age Group 69–71 B	Age Group 72–74 A	Age Group 72–74 B	Age Group 75–77 A	Age Group 75–77 B
2	>110	>240	>110	>250	>110	>263
3	93–110	230–240	108–110	240–250	108–110	250–263
4	76–92	220–229	90–107	235–239	94–107	240–249
5	63–75	212–219	81–89	225–234	81–93	237–237
6	56–62	160–211	64–80	212–224	71–80	234–236
7	47–55	137–159	55–63	157–211	57–70	168–233
8	42–46	104–136	46–54	138–156	46–56	145–167
9	38–41	91–103	41–45	105–137	42–45	124–144
10	34–37	80–90	36–40	84–104	36–41	92–123
11	31–33	72–79	32–35	78–83	33–35	81–91
12	29–30	63–71	29–31	69–77	30–32	73–80
13	26–28	55–62	27–28	64–68	27–29	67–72
14	23–25	50–54	25–26	53–63	25–26	53–66
15	21–22	43–49	22–24	45–52	23–24	45–52
16	20	41–42	20–21	41–44	20–22	41–44
17	18–19	34–40	18–19	34–40	19	34–40
18	<18	<34	<18	<34	<19	<34
N	134	134	125	125	111	111

Scaled Score	Age Group 78–80 A	Age Group 78–80 B	Age Group 81–83 A	Age Group 81–83 B	Age Group 84–86 A	Age Group 84–86 B
2	>110	>263	>115	>315	>115	>315
3	108–110	250–263	112–115	263–315	112–115	263–315
4	94–107	240–249	94–111	250–262	94–111	250–262
5	83–93	237–239	84–93	240–249	84–93	240–249
6	73–82	234–236	75–83	234–239	75–83	234–239
7	59–72	180–233	64–74	183–233	64–74	183–233
8	53–58	145–179	58–63	158–182	58–63	158–182
9	43–52	135–144	53–57	142–157	53–57	142–157
10	40–42	101–134	43–52	115–141	43–52	115–141
11	36–39	92–100	40–42	104–114	40–42	104–114

continued

Table 4.19. (*Continued*)

Scaled Score	Age Group 78–80		Age Group 81–83		Age Group 84–86	
	A	B	A	B	A	B
12	32–35	82–91	36–39	94–103	36–39	94–103
13	29–31	70–81	31–35	82–93	31–35	82–93
14	26–28	66–69	28–30	70–81	28–30	70–81
15	23–25	45–65	23–27	66–69	23–27	66–69
16	21–22	41–44	22	45–65	22	45–65
17	19–20	34–40	21	41–44	21	41–44
18	<19	<34	<21	<41	<21	<41
N	89	89	81	81	81	81

Scaled Score	Age Group 87–89		Age Group 90–97		Percentile Ranges
	A	B	A	B	
2	>115	>315	>115	>315	<1
3	112–115	263–315	112–115	263–315	1
4	94–111	250–262	94–111	250–262	2
5	84–93	240–249	84–93	240–249	3–5
6	75–83	234–239	75–83	234–239	6–10
7	64–74	183–233	64–74	183–233	11–18
8	58–63	158–182	58–63	158–182	19–28
9	53–57	142–157	53–57	142–157	29–40
10	43–52	115–141	43–52	115–141	41–59
11	40–42	104–114	40–42	104–114	60–71
12	36–39	94–103	36–39	94–103	72–81
13	31–35	82–93	31–35	82–93	82–89
14	28–30	70–81	28–30	70–81	90–94
15	23–27	66–69	23–27	66–69	95–97
16	22	45–65	22	45–65	98
17	21	41–44	21	41–44	99
18	<21	<41	<21	<41	>99
N	81	81	81	81	

Study strengths

1. Presentation of the data by age groupings.
2. Information on mean IQ and standard deviation for each age grouping.
3. Information on educational level and geographic area provided.
4. Means and standard deviations are reported.

Considerations regarding use of the study

1. Subjects were medical patients with extensive hospitalizations.
2. Lack of data regarding education means.
3. Some variability in IQs across age groups.
4. Small sample sizes in the upper age ranges.
5. Data were collected in Canada, raising

Table 4.20. TMT.16a; Demographic Characteristics of the Sample

	Total Sample	Younger Old	Older Old
N	101	50	51
Age	81.47 (3.30)	78.80 (1.07)	84.08 (2.56)
Education	11.02 (3.68)	10.44 (3.86)	11.59 (3.45)
MMSE	26.97 (2.55)	26.56 (3.03)	27.37 (1.92)
% Female	47.5%	46.0%	49.0%
% White	90.1%	82.0%	98.0%
% Black	9.9%	18.0%	2.0%

Table 4.21. TMT.16b; Means and Standard Deviations for Time in Seconds to Complete Trails B by the Sample Divided Into 2 Age Groups by 2 Education Groups (in Years of Schooling)

	Age			
	76–80		81–91	
	Education			
	<12	≥12	<12	≥12
N	26	24	18	33
Trails B	197.17	119.17	195.47	137.30
	(71.03)	(33.47)	(69.70)	(55.93)

questions regarding their usefulness for clinical interpretive purposes in the United States (Table 4.22).

[TMT.18] Wiens and Matarazzo, 1977

The authors collected TMT data on 48 male applicants to a patrolman program in Portland, Oregon, as a part of an investigation of the WAIS and MMPI correlates of the Halstead-Reitan battery. All subjects passed a medical exam and were judged to be neurologically normal. Subjects were divided into two equal groups which were comparable in age (23.6 vs. 24.8), education (13.7 vs. 14.0) and WAIS FSIQ (117.5 vs. 118.3). TMT mean time in seconds and standard deviation are provided for each group. A random subsample of 29 of the applicants was readministered the TMT 14 to 24 weeks following the original administration. Means and standard deviations for TMT times in seconds for both the original testing and retest are reported. None of the 29 original subjects obtained scores lower than Reitan's suggested cutoff for part B; however, one subject fell below the recommended cutoff for part A on *second administration*. Correlations between test performance and IQ scores were somewhat nonsensical. In the first group, significant negative correlations were obtained between part B performance and FSIQ and VIQ, but no significant correlations were obtained between the second control group and IQ measures. In group 1 a significant negative correlation was noted between part A and

Table 4.22. TMT.17; Mean Time in Seconds, Standard Deviations, Ranges and Medians for Trails A, B and Total Time for A + B Combined

N	Age	FSIQ	VIQ	PIQ	Trails		
					A	B	A + B
26	20-29	103.8	102.6	104.7	36.1	85.7	121.8
		(12.1)	(12.6)	(13.0)	(10.0)	(38.7)	(42.2)
		Range			19–62	47–245	72–290
		Median			35.0	76.0	111.5
25	30-39	110.1	106.4	113.7	35.5	79.6	114.0
		(8.9)	(11.3)	(8.9)	(9.4)	(20.4)	(25.3)
		Range			19–58	32–115	51–173
		Median			34.0	80.0	115.0
24	40-49	105.3	105.8	104.5	40.0	105.2	145.0
		(7.9)	(9.1)	(9.2)	(13.3)	(42.2)	(48.5)
		Range			16–70	51–225	72–277
		Median			38.0	99.5	142.0
16	50-59	112.7	111.2	111.6	45.3	103.2	148.4
		(8.6)	(11.5)	(9.0)	(13.6)	(43.3)	(53.0)
		Range			22–68	58–190	80–253
		Median			46.0	98.5	140.0
15	60-72	104.2	103.2	105.4	68.9	158.8	227.7
		(12.2)	(13.2)	(11.6)	(21.2)	(49.5)	(63.2)
		Range			35–120	88–272	123–347
		Median			68.0	147.0	219.0
106	total	107.0	105.6	107.9	42.9	101.7	144.3
		(10.6)	(11.8)	(11.2)	(17.3)	(46.2)	(58.6)

FSIQ, and a significant *positive* correlation was documented between part A score and PIQ; again, no significant correlations were obtained between part A scores and IQ measures in the second control group.

Study strengths
1. Information on test/retest performance.
2. Adequate medical exclusion criteria.
3. Information regarding educational level, IQ, sex, and geographic recruitment area.
4. Means and standard deviations are reported.

Considerations regarding use of the study
1. High IQ level.
2. High educational level.
3. All-male sample (Table 4.23).

[TMT.19] Anthony, Heaton, and Lehman, 1980

The authors amassed TMT data on 100 normal volunteers from Colorado as a part of a cross-validation of two computerized interpretive programs for the Halstead-Reitan battery. Subjects had no history of medical or psychiatric problems, head traumas, brain disease, or substance abuse. In addition, for 85% of the controls, normal EEGs and neurological exams were obtained; in the remaining 15% of the subjects it appears that this information was not available. Mean age was 38.88 (SD = 15.80) and mean years of education were 13.33 (SD = 2.56). Mean WAIS FSIQ, VIQ, and PIQ were 113.54 (10.83), 113.24 (11.59), and 112.26 (10.88), respectively. TMT data are presented

in terms of mean times in seconds and standard deviations for part B only.

Study strengths
1. Large sample size.
2. Adequate exclusion criteria.
3. Information regarding education, IQ, age, and geographic recruitment area is provided.
4. Means and standard deviations are reported.

Considerations regarding use of the study
1. The large undifferentiated age grouping.
2. The IQ range is high average.
3. No information is available regarding sex ratio.
4. Data on Trails B only (Table 4.24).

[TMT.20] Bak and Greene, 1980

The authors gathered TMT data on 30 right-handed Texan subjects as a part of an investigation of the effect of age on performance on the Halstead-Reitan Battery and the Wechsler Memory Scale. The participants were equally divided into two age groupings: 50 to 62 and 67 to 86. Subjects were fluent in English and denied history of central nervous system (CNS) disorders, uncorrected sensory deficits, or illnesses or "incapacities" which might affect test results; subjects in poor health were excluded. The mean ages of the two groups were 55.6 (SD = 4.44) and 74.9 (SD = 6.04), respectively. Subjects in the first group were born between the years 1916 and 1929, and subjects in the second group were born between 1892 and 1912. Nine individuals in the first group were

Table 4.23. TMT.18; Means and Standard Deviations for Times in Seconds for Two Equal Groups of Subjects, and Data for the Original Testing and Retest 14–24 Weeks Later for a Random Subsample of 29 Subjects

						Initial Test		Retest	
N	Age	Education	FSIQ	VIQ	PIQ	A	B	A	B
24	23.6 (21–27)	13.7 (12–16)	117.5 (8.3) (105–139)	117.4 (8.4)	115.4 (10.5)	23.83 (6.61)	56.42 (12.79)		
24	24.8 (21–28)	14.0 (12–16)	118.3 (6.8) (108–131)	116.4 (6.9)	118.2 (8.6)	20.54 (4.43)	51.04 (11.46)		
29	24 (21–28)	14 (12–16)	118	116	118	21.76 (5.65)	54.17 (12.54)	21.72 (5.86)	51.28 (12.29)

Table 4.24. TMT.19; Sample Description and Data for Part B

N	Age	Education	FSIQ	VIQ	PIQ	Trails B
100	38.88	13.33	113.54	113.24	112.26	68.58
	(15.80)	(2.56)	(10.83)	(11.59)	(10.88)	(32.72)

female, and 10 subjects in the second group were female. Four WAIS subtests were administered (Information, Arithmetic, Block Design, Digit Symbol); the mean scores on these measures suggested that IQ levels were within the high average range or higher.

Mean times in seconds and standard deviations for part A and B are presented for the two groups. Significant differences in performance were documented between the two groups on both parts of the test.

Study strengths

1. Data on a very elderly age group rarely found in other published normative data.
2. Adequate exclusion criteria.
3. Information regarding education, IQ, sex, handedness, fluency in English, and geographic recruitment area is provided.
4. Means and standard deviations are reported.

Considerations regarding use of the study

1. The high IQ level.
2. High educational level.
3. The older age grouping spans nearly two decades and may be too broad for optimal clinical interpretative use.
4. Small sample sizes (Table 4.25).

[TMT.21] Kennedy, 1981

The author collected TMT data on 150 Canadian subjects as a part of his analysis of effects of age on TMT performance. Participants were employees of a mental health center "who represented diverse work roles" randomly selected from five age groups: 20–29, 30–39, 40–49, 50–59, 60–69.

Subjects were excluded who reported histories of "central nervous system disorders, illnesses, or incapacities which would bias test results"; exclusion criteria were not further specified. Mean years of education were 13.73, 13.53, 13.11, 11.59, and 12.50, respectively; the 50–59-year-olds were significantly less educated than the 20–29-year-olds and the 30–39-year-olds. The Ammons Quick Test was used as an estimate of intelligence level; average estimates for the five goups were 123.43, 127.10, 127.40, 123.30, and 128.54. Males and females were equally represented in each grouping.

The mean time in seconds and standard deviations for Trails A, B, and A + B for each group are provided. Performance decreased significantly with age, and significant negative correlations between TMT test scores and education and IQ suggested that lowered education and IQ are adversely related to test performance.

Table 4.25. TMT.20; Mean Time in Seconds and Standard Deviations (in Parentheses) for Trails A and B for 2 Age Groups. WAIS Data Are Presented in Raw Scores

N	Age	Education	Trails A	Trails B	WAIS Info	WAIS Arith	WAIS Blk Design	WAIS Digit Sym
15	50–62							
	55.6	13.7	32.53	81.67	20.13	11.87	34.33	54.67
	(4.44)	(1.91)	(12.58)	(30.76)	(3.38)	(1.92)	(6.79)	(12.19)
15	67-86							
	74.9	14.9	41.60	109.00	21.07	13.60	28.07	39.47
	(6.04)	(2.99)	(10.33)	(38.84)	(3.84)	(2.97)	(5.36)	(12.11)

Study strengths

1. Large sample size, although the individual cells had only 30 subjects per cell.

2. Presentation of the data in terms of age groupings.

3. Reporting of education, IQ estimates, sex and geographic area.

4. Means and standard deviations are reported.

Considerations regarding use of the study

1. Very high mean intelligence scores.

2. Some variability in educational level across groups which may have led to some unusual findings; inexplicably, the 60–69-year-olds performed either as well as or slightly better than the 50–59-year-olds.

3. Vague exclusion criteria.

4. Lack of reference to ethnicity/language issues and the fact that data were obtained on Canadians, possibly reducing its generalizability for clinical interpretive use in the United States (Table 4.26).

[TMT.22] Heaton, Grant, and Matthews, 1986

The authors obtained TMT data on 553 normal controls in Colorado, California, and Wisconsin as a part of an investigation into the effects of age, education, and sex on Halstead-Reitan Battery performance. Nearly two-thirds of the sample were male (males = 356, females =

197). Exclusion criteria included history of neurologic illness, significant head trauma, and substance abuse. Subjects ranged in age from 15 to 81 (mean = 39.3 ± 17.5), and mean years of education was 13.3 (±3.4) with a range of 0 to 20 years. The sample was divided into three age categories (less than 40, 40–59, and greater than or equal to 60 years) with Ns of 319, 134, and 100, respectively, and into three education categories (less than 12 years, 12 to 15 years, and greater than or equal to 16 years) with Ns of 132, 249, and 172, respectively.

Testing was conducted by trained technicians, and all participants were judged to have expended their best effort on the task. The TMT mean time in seconds for part B is reported for the six subgroups, as well as percent classified as normal using Russell et al.'s (1970) criteria. Approximately 30% of test score variance was accounted for by age and approximately 20% of test score variance was associated with education level. Significant group differences in TMT scores were found across the three age groups, and across the three education groups, and a significant age-by-education interaction was documented. No significant differences in performance were found between males and females.

Study strengths

1. Large size of overall sample and individual cells.

Table 4.26. TMT.21; Mean Time in Seconds and Standard Deviations (in Parentheses) for Trails A, B, and Total Time A + B for 5 Age Groups°

N	Age	Education	IQ Estimate	Trails		
				A	B	A + B
30	20–29 25.77	13.73	123.43	25.03 (8.94)	59.58 (28.78)	84.62 (33.11)
30	30–39 34.34	13.53	127.10	28.88 (9.70)	70.28 (27.79)	99.13 (34.57)
30	40–49 45.79	13.11	127.40	29.68 (7.67)	78.80 (26.81)	108.48 (30.32)
30	50–59 53.74	11.59	123.30	37.73 (19.01)	96.01 (39.25)	133.74 (55.98)
30	60–69 64.24	12.50	128.54	35.22 (12.36)	95.02 (34.62)	130.23 (40.67)

°Note: age range and mean age are provided for each group.

2. Information regarding sex, geographic area, age, and education.

3. Minimally adequate exclusion criteria.

4. Data grouped by age and also by educational level.

Considerations regarding use of the study

1. No reporting of data for part A.

2. No reporting of TMT score standard deviations.

3. Mean scores for individual WAIS subtest scaled scores reported but not overall IQ scores (Table 4.27).

[TMT.23] Alekoumbides, Charter, Adkins, and Seacat, 1987

The authors report data on 118 medical and psychiatric inpatients and outpatients without cerebral lesions or histories of alcoholism or cerebral contusion, from V.A. hospitals in Southern California, as a part of their development of standardized scores corrected for age and education for the Halstead-Reitan battery. Among the 41 psychiatric patients, nine were diagnosed as psychotic and 32 were neurotic. In addition to psychiatry services, patients were also drawn from medicine ($n = 57$), neurology ($n = 22$), spinal cord injury ($n = 9$), and surgery ($n = 6$) units. Mean age was 46.85 ± 17.17 (ranging from 19 to 82), and mean years of education was 11.43 ± 3.20 (ranging from 1 to 20). Frequency distributions for age and years of education are provided. Mean WAIS FSIQ, VIQ, and PIQ were within the average range (105.89 ± 13.47, 107.03 ± 14.38, and 103.31 ± 13.02, respectively); means and standard deviations for individual age-corrected subtest

scores are also reported. All subjects except one were male; the majority were Caucasian (93%), with 7% African-American. The mean score on a measure of occupational attainment was 11.29.

No differences were found in test performance between the two psychiatric groups and the nonpsychiatric group, and the data were collapsed. Mean time in seconds and standard deviation to complete parts A and B are reported. In addition, regression equation information to allow correction of raw scores for age and education is included.

Study strengths

1. Large sample size.

2. Information regarding IQ, age, education, ethnicity, sex, occupational attainment, and geogprahic area.

3. Regression equation data for computation of age and education corrected scores.

4. Means and standard deviations are reported.

Considerations regarding use of the study

1. Data were predominantly collected on medical and psychiatric inpatients.

2. Undifferentiated age range (mitigated by the regression equation information).

3. Nearly all-male sample (Table 4.28).

[TMT.24] Bornstein, Baker, and Douglass, 1987a

The authors collected TMT test-retest data on 23 volunteers (14 women, nine men) who ranged in age from 17 to 52 (mean = 32.3 ± 10.3) as a part of an examination of the short-

Table 4.27. TMT.22; Mean Time in Seconds for Trails B, and Percent Classified as Normal Using Russell et al.'s (1970) Criteria for Each Age and Education Subgroup

N	Age	Education	Trails B	% Normal	WAIS SS Mean[*]
319	<40		58.5	91.5	11.9
134	40–59		78.3	74.6	11.2
100	≥60		116.8	33.0	9.7
132		<12	102.2	54.6	9.5
249		12–15	69.7	79.9	11.2
172		≥16	57.9	89.5	12.9

[*]Mean scaled scores for WAIS subtests.

Table 4.28. TMT.23; Sample Description and Data for Trails A and B

						Trails	
						A	B
N	Age	Education	FSIQ	VIQ	PIQ		
118	46.85	11.43	105.89	107.03	103.31	48.60	120.49
	(17.17)	(3.20)	(13.47)	(14.38)	(13.02)	(23.79)	(78.90)

term retest reliability of the Halstead-Reitan Battery. Exclusion criteria consisted of a positive history of neurological or psychiatric illness. Mean Verbal IQ was 105.8 ± 10.8 (range = 88 to 128) and mean Performance IQ was 105.0 ± 10.5 (range = 85 to 121).

Subjects were administered the Halstead-Reitan Battery in standard order both on initial testing and again 3 weeks later. Means, standard deviations, and ranges for time in seconds to complete parts A and B for both testing session are provided, as well as raw score change and standard deviation, median raw score change, and mean percent of change. For part A, no significant correlations between mean change and age or education or between mean percent of change and age or education were documented. For part B, no significant correlations between mean change and age or education or between mean percent change and education were found; however, a significant correlation did emerge between mean percent of change and age.

Study strengths
1. Information on short-term (3-week) retest data.
2. Information on IQ level, age, and gender.
3. Minimally adequate exclusion criteria.

4. Means, standard deviations and ranges are reported.

Considerations regarding use of the study
1. Undifferentiated age range.
2. Small sample size.
3. No data on educational level (Table 4.29).

CONCLUSIONS

The trailmaking tasks have been quite popular as an essential component of neuropsychological test batteries and as a measure of information processing efficiency administered in the context of a general psychological evaluation. In spite of the high sensitivity of these tasks to attentional/concentrational and executive problems, as well as psychomotor slowing, it would be misleading to view these tests as *the test for organic brain pathology*. For example, patients with memory deficits associated with temporal lobe pathology may perform normally on the Trailmaking Test, and if the Trailmaking Test is administered in isolation, the serious processing difficulties of this population will be overlooked.

Most commonly, the clinical use of the Trailmaking Test is based on a norm-referenced in-

Table 4.29. TMT.24; Means, Standard Deviations (in Parentheses), and Ranges for Time in Seconds to Complete Trails A and B for Two Testing Sessions 3 Weeks Apart°

				Test		Retest		Raw Score Change		Median Raw Score Change		Mean % of Change	
N	Age	VIQ	PIQ	A	B	A	B	A	B	A	B	A	B
23	32.3	105.8	105.0	25.6	52.1	21.5	47.4	3.1	6.9	3	6.5	13	9
	(10.3)	(10.8)	(10.5)	(6.8)	(15.1)	(5.6)	(16.5)	(4.9)	(11.4)				
				17–41	34–97	15–35	25–73						

°Raw score change and standard deviations, median raw score change, and mean percent of change are also reported.

terpretation of completion time for each condition. Use of the TMT cutoff criteria for brain impairment is now quite infrequent (Spreen & Strauss, 1998). Since performance on the TMT (especially part B) is highly affected by age and possibly by education and intelligence level, it is of the utmost importance to interpret individual scores with reference to the *relevant* normative data. Similarly, in future investiga-

tions, the optimal format for data reporting is in age by education and/or by intelligence level cells.

A large body of studies addresses the clinical utility and psychometric properties of the TMT. However, issues related to the different information-processing aspects of the two parts of these tests have not been sufficiently addressed.

5

Color Trails Test

BRIEF HISTORY OF THE TEST

Because of their ease of administration and sensitivity to brain damage, trail-making tasks have long been among the most widely used measures in neuropsychological practice (Lezak, 1995). There are currently two commercially available trail-making tasks: the original Trail-Making Test which was developed in 1944 (see Chapter 4) and the newer Color Trails Test, published in 1994.

The Color Trails Test is available in adult and child formats from PAR, Inc. (see Appendix for ordering information). Preliminary normative data for the children's version of Color Trails can be found in Williams et al. (1995).

The Color Trails Test was created in response to a request made in 1989 by the World Health Organization (WHO) for development of a test that would be similar to the Trail-Making Test (1944) in terms of its sensitivity and specificity yet allow broader application in cross-cultural contexts. The WHO also wanted a test with standardized, equivalent, multiple forms for test–retest purposes. Because the original Trail-Making Test (TMT) uses English alphabet letters as part of the test stimuli, its use in non-English-speaking countries was limited. Additionally, although the TMT had been translated into other languages, its basic linguistic and phonological properties continued to limit its application in special-needs contexts

(e.g., language disorders, specific reading disorders, or illiteracy).

The WHO also wanted *standardized* test stimuli to insure the new test's reliability (Maj et al., 1993). Because of the TMT's popularity and its availability in the public domain, it became perhaps the most frequently photocopied neuropsychological test of the 20th century. Poor photocopy quality often blurred the target stimuli, and it was not uncommon to discover TMT protocols in which the stimuli closest to the edge of the page had been cut off due to improper placement of the original on the photocopy machine. Successive generations of photocopies yielded slightly smaller or slightly larger versions of the test, thereby changing the distance between stimuli. Because the *time to complete* score obtained for the test reflects not only visual scanning and psychomotor speed, but also the distance traveled *between* stimuli, the problem of not having a standardly utilized version of the TMT would necessarily hamper the comparability of research and clinical findings. Therefore, it was important to develop a format of the test that would also discourage photocopying (D'Elia et al., 1994).

The Color Trails Test (CTT) retains the same psychometric properties as the TMT but substitutes the use of color for the use of English (or any other) alphabet letters. Specifically, the CTT uses numbered, colored circles and universal sign language symbols. Instructions may be administered verbally or nonverbally by using only visual cues.

Like the TMT, the Color Trails Test is a paper and pencil test that is administered in two parts, 1 and 2. Color Trails 1 is presented on an 8½" × 11" page on which are scattered the numbers 1 through 25, printed within colored circles. All even-numbered circles are printed with a bright yellow background and all odd-numbered circles with a vivid pink background. These background color differences are perceptible even to colorblind individuals. The individual is instructed to quickly draw a continuous line connecting the numbers in consecutive/sequential order. The incidental fact that color alternates with each succeeding number is not highlighted or discussed with the subject since attention to color sequence is not necessary for completion of Color Trails 1.

Color Trails 2 introduces a divided attentional component, requiring attention to the alternating and sequencing of the stimuli. For Color Trails 2, the number 1 circle is printed against a vivid pink background; however, the numbers 2 through 25 are presented twice: once with a vivid pink background and once with a bright yellow background. For Color Trails 2, the subject has to again quickly connect up the numbers in sequence; however, he or she must do so in an alternating color sequence (e.g., pink 1, yellow 2, pink 3, yellow 4, etc.). Therefore, there is always a distractor number that must be avoided that is printed against a color background that is not appropriate to the sequence. Before Color Trails 1 and Color Trails 2 are administered, practice trials are administered to insure that the subject understands the task.

The decision to use numbers and colors was based on the fact that both are universal symbols that place limited demands on language production or knowledge. In cross-cultural pilot tests of the Color Trails, it was found that individuals in poor Third World countries in Africa, Asia, and South America, with little or no formal education, know and recognize the Arabic numbers 1 through 25—perhaps because they have to barter for goods and services (Maj et al., 1991). In developing the test, it was hypothesized that the alternating shift between number and color sequences would require more effortful executive processing than the shift between numbers and letters of the alphabet. Specifically, in the United States, the English alphabet is learned at a very early age. Not only are students taught to recite the alphabet, but to sing it as well. As such, the alphabet sequence is strongly encoded. Indeed, it is not unusual to observe a premorbidly high-functioning individual presenting with a history of moderate brain injury who is able to call upon sufficient brain reserve capacity (Satz, 1993) to complete TMT Part B within a nominally "normal" time limit. Interestingly, these individuals have been occasionally observed to hum or sing the alphabet (although almost inaudibly) while solving part B. Removal of reliance on the English alphabet to solve Color Trails 2 effectively eliminates this potential performance confound.

Use of colors also permitted the development of identical, equivalent forms of the test for repeat administration in longitudinal research. Currently there are four versions of the Color Trails Test (i.e., forms A, B, C, and D). Form A is the standard test form on which normative data were collected. Therefore, form A is the only form that should be utilized for clinical evaluation. The subsequent forms were created by printing a mirror-image version, a 90° rotated version, and a 90° mirror-image version of form A. This method of creating alternate forms insured that the distance traveled between stimuli was standard for all forms. The alternate forms (i.e., forms B, C, and D) are considered experimental, and should only be used in research settings.

The scoring of the CTT differs from the TMT to allow quantification of the cognitive slippage that often occurs following mild brain injury. For instance, following mild cerebral insults, patients commonly present with reports of subtle changes in sequencing, planning, and their ability to inhibit specific responses. They frequently complain that it takes extra effort to perform most tasks they formerly completed without much thought or effort. Unfortunately, current approaches to characterizing performance on most neuropsychological tests only allow empirical quantification of gross errors, but not the more subtle forms of cognitive slippage frequently described by these patients.

The Near-Miss score was developed to allow empirical quantification of this type of cognitive slippage. This response occurs when a subject initiates an incorrect response but self-corrects before actual connection to a distractor circle. Reporting Near-Miss scores allows the examiner to comment upon the degree to which a patient is susceptible to distractors. Other scoring criteria include quantification of prompts, number-sequence errors, and color-sequence errors.

In the course of preparatory work for the World Health Organization cross-cultural study on the neuropsychiatric aspects of HIV-1 infection, Maj et al. (1993) evaluated the Color Trails Test in comparison to translated versions of the Trail-Making Test at four world sites: Munich, Germany; Bangkok, Thailand; Naples, Italy; and Kinshasa, Zaire. The results of the evaluation suggested that the Color Trails Test is not only sensitive to HIV-1-associated cognitive impairment but is more culturally fair than the Trail-Making Test. The sensitivity of the test was found to "hold" across different cultures.

RELATIONSHIP BETWEEN COLOR TRAILS PERFORMANCE AND DEMOGRAPHIC FACTORS

There are currently three normative reports regarding the Color Trails Test. Analyses conducted on the CTT data obtained from the U.S. standardization manual revealed that increasing age adversely affects performance on both Color Trails 1 and Color Trails 2. Increasing education was found to enhance performance on Color Trails 2, but not on Color Trails 1. Gender, and the interactions between gender and age, were not significantly related to CTT performance scores after the effects of age were removed (D'Elia et al., 1994). Ponton et al. (1996), in examining the normative data from their Hispanic sample, also found a negative performance association between increasing age and CTT 1 and 2 test scores. They also found a positive performance association between increasing education and CTT 2 scores, and for CTT 1 scores as well. No gender effects were found. Similarly, Hsieh and Riley (1997), in examining the normative data from their

Chinese sample, found a negative performance association between increasing age and CTT 1 and 2 test scores and a positive performance association between increasing education and CTT 1 and CTT 2 scores. No gender effects were found in the Chinese sample.

In summary, research suggests that performance on the Color Trails tests is enhanced by education and negatively affected by increasing age. No gender effects have been reported.

METHOD FOR EVALUATING THE NORMATIVE REPORTS

Our review of the literature located a normative report for Spanish-speaking adults (Ponton et al., 1996), a normative report for Mandarin speaking mainland Chinese (Hsieh & Riley, 1997) and the U.S. standardization manual (D'Elia et al., 1994).

In order to adequately evaluate the CTT normative reports, five key criterion variables were deemed critical. The first four of these relate to *subject* variables and the last to *procedural* variables.

Minimal requirements for meeting the criterion variables were as follows:

Subject Variables

Sample Size

As discussed in previous chapters, a minimum of at least 50 subjects per grouping interval is optimal.

Sample Composition Description

Information regarding medical and psychiatric exclusion criteria is critical. It is unclear if geographic recruitment region or recruitment procedures are important, so until this is determined, it is best that this information be provided.

Age Group Intervals

Given the association between age and CTT performance, information regarding age of the normative sample is critical. At a minimum, normative data should be presented by age in categories that are narrowly defined.

Reporting of IQ and/or Education Level

Given the association between educational level and CTT scores, information regarding highest educational level completed should be reported. The education categories should be narrowly defined. Optimally, normative data should be categorically reported by age *and* education level. It is unclear if IQ is relevant, so until this is determined, it is best that information on IQ be provided.

Procedural Variables

Data Reporting

Means and standard deviations, and preferably ranges, for total time in seconds for each part of the CTT should be reported.

SUMMARY OF THE STATUS OF THE NORMS

In terms of subject variables, the standardization manual and the Ponton et al. (1996) study provide performance data grouped by age and education categories. The Hsieh and Riley study presents data separately for age and for education.

Although the total sample for the U.S. standardization study is 1,528, unfortunately the manual does not indicate the sample size within each of the 30 age/education categories. The sample size for each of the age and education categories reported by Ponton et al. (1996) is small. Similarly, the sample size for each of the age categories reported by Hsieh and Riley is small.

For both the standardization and Ponton et al. (1996) studies, the younger age group categories are generally narrowly defined and therefore adequate. However the older age group categories tend to be very broad. Hsieh and Riley report age data in 10 year increments, however also provide data according to the age groupings found in the U.S. standardization manual. Regarding procedural variables, all studies report means and standard deviation scores. Only the U.S. standardization manual reports data regarding error and near-miss responses, and data for prompts. The standard-

ization manual and the Hsieh and Riley study provide data on the interference index. The Ponton et al. (1996) and D'Elia et al. (1994) normative data were collected from subjects residing in the United States. The Hsieh and Riley data were collected from subjects residing in the mainland People's Republic of China.

Table 5.1 summarizes information provided in the studies described in this chapter.

SUMMARIES OF THE STUDIES

This section presents critiques of the normative studies for the Color Trail Test (1994). The studies are reviewed in chronological order.

Normative Studies

[CTT.1] D'Elia, Satz, Uchiyama and White, 1994

This is the original standardization of the Color Trails Test. The manual reports normative data from a sample of 1,528 healthy, normal individuals residing in a variety of settings in diverse regions of the United States. Participants were excluded if there was a history of head trauma, neurological disorder, or substance abuse. The data were collected during the course of several norming studies with distinct samples, including medically and psychiatrically normal participants from a longitudinal cardiovascular epidemiological study that has been ongoing since 1960; medically and psychiatrically normal pilots from four major U.S. commercial airline manufacturing corporations undergoing a yearly medical examination as part of a nationally mandated Federal Aviation Administration/ Equal Employment Opportunity Commission (FAA/EEOC) study to obtain normative data on neuropsychological functioning of pilots across the age span; medically and psychiatrically normal residents living in an independent retirement community in Southern California; medically and psychiatrically healthy HIV-negative bisexual and homosexual men participating in a multicenter epidemiological study; and medically and psychiatrically healthy African-American men living in Los Angeles with no history of drug/alcohol abuse participating in a

Table 5.1. CTT.L; Locator Table for CTT

Study	Age	N for Age/ Education Category	Sample Composition	Education	Country/ Location
CTT.1 D'Elia et al., 1994 page 68	18–29 30–44 45–59 60–74 75–89 °n =1,528 Total sample	° ° ° ° °	Medically & psychiatrically healthy adults residing in a variety of settings Sample is 88% male	Data are stratified at each age category by 6 education Categories: <8 years, 9–11 years, 12 years, 13–15 years, 16 years, ≥17 years	USA
CTT.2 Ponton, et al., 1996 page 70	16–29 30–39 40–49 50–75	42 66 27 45	180 female, 120 male medically & psychiatrically healthy Hispanics	Data are stratified at each age category by <10 and >10 years of education	Southern California USA
CTT.3 Hsieh & Riley, 1997 page 70	30–39 40–49 50–59 60–69 70–83	43 39 33 32 30	Urban-dwelling Mandarin-speaking adults, 93 males and 84 females	Data collected on individuals with 1–17 years of education; however, data reported by age categories only	Mainland China

larger study of the neuropsychological, medical, and psychosocial consequences of poly-drug abuse and HIV.

The data are stratified by age and education. There are five age categories: 18–29, 30–44, 45–59, 60–74, 75–89. For each age category, data are reported for performance of those with 8 years of education or less, 9 through 11 years, 12 years, 13 through 15 years, 16 years, and 17 years or more.

The sample is primarily male; women comprise only 12% of the sample. The manual reports that "Gender and the interactions between gender and age were not significantly related to CTT raw scores after the effects of age were removed, explaining between 0.4% to 2.4% of the variance. Therefore, the relatively small proportion of women in the normative sample does not constitute a threat to either the validity or the utility of the CTT" (D'Elia et al., 1994).

Spanish-language administration instructions and preliminary normative data for Hispanics are provided in the manual. The preliminary normative data are from a sample of healthy, normal Hispanics living in Southern California, participating in a large, ongoing normative study. The Hispanic data are reported separately, since all participants in this subsample were educated outside the United States and are primarily Spanish speaking, or Spanish was their first language. Data for Hispanics are presented by four age categories: 17–29 years, 30–39 years, 40–49 years, and 50–75 years.

The normative data contained in the standardization manual are not reproduced here, and the interested reader is referred directly to the publication for further information.

Study strengths

1. Sample composition is well described in terms of exclusion criteria.

2. Performance is reported by age *and* education intervals.

3. Data reporting includes means and standard deviation scores for each age/education interval.

4. Age-group intervals are generally adequate.

Considerations regarding use of the study

1. Sample size within each of the 30 age/education categories not indicated.

2. No information on the IQ of the participants is reported, although the data are presented by age/education intervals.

[CTT.2] Ponton, Satz, Herrera, Ortiz, Urrutia, Young, D'Elia, Furst and Namerow, 1996

This study presents normative data stratified by age and education for Spanish-speaking adults' performance on the Neuropsychological Screening Battery for Hispanics (NeSBHIS), which contains the Color Trails Test. This is the initial report from an ongoing project. The sample consists of 300 volunteers (180 female, 120 male) recruited from fliers and advertisements posted at community centers and churches in Los Angeles County (Santa Ana, Pasadena, Pacoima, Montebello, and Van Nuys). The sample was primarily right-handed (95%). Regarding language, 210 were monolingual Spanish, and 90 were rated by the examiner to be bilingual. The average duration of residence in the United States was 16.4(14.4) years; however, 55% of the total sample had lived in the United States less than 15 years, and "half of those subjects had less than 6 years of residence in this country" (p. 97). Sixty-two percent of the sample were born in Mexico, 15% in Central America, and 23% in other Latin countries. Exclusion criteria included a history of neurological disease, psychiatric disorder, alcohol or drug abuse, or head trauma. Participants ranged in age from 16 to 75 years old (mean = 38.4[13.5] years). Whereas the 30–39 and 40–49 age groupings are adequate, the 16–29 and 50–75 interval groupings are quite broad.

The data are reported by age and education groupings. The tables separately present data for males and females.

Study strengths
1. Sample composition is well described in terms of exclusion criteria.
2. Educational levels are reported.
3. Mean and standard deviation scores are reported.
4. Age-group intervals are generally adequate for younger sample (<50 years).

Considerations regarding use of the study
1. Sample size is generally small per age/education interval.
2. Age-group interval too broad for older sample (50–75 years).

Other comments
1. IQ scores are not reported; however, scores are reported for Raven's Standard Progressive Matrices Test at each age/education level. Raven's test is used to provide an estimate of nonverbal intelligence.
2. Although the data are reported by gender, there does not appear to be a significant gender effect (Table 5.2 and 5.3).

[CTT.3] Hsieh and Riley, 1997

This report provides normative data on tests of attention and concentration collected in the People's Republic of China. The normative sample consisted of 177 (93 male, 84 female) urban-dwelling, Mandarin-speaking subjects recruited across a broad range of educational and occupational categories. The data are stratified by age categories and by education categories. The age categories are 30–39, 40–49, 50–59, 60–69, and 70–83 years old. The education categories follow the Chinese system of primary (1–6 years), middle school (7–9 years), and high school (10–12 years). The vast majority of adults over the age of 60 had fewer than 6 years of education.

Study strengths
1. Data reporting includes means and standard deviation scores.
2. Age group intervals are adequate.

Considerations regarding use of the study
1. Sample composition description does not sufficiently address study inclusion/exclusion criteria.
2. Sample sizes are generally small.

Other comments
1. Years of education per age group are presented in a table.
2. Performance is reported separately for age and for education categories. CTT data would generally be more useful if they were partitioned by an age/education category (Tables 5.4–5.6).

CONCLUSIONS

Research to date suggests that the Color Trails Test holds promise for cross-cultural and longi-

Table 5.2. CTT.2a; Means and Standard Deviations for Performance of Females Stratified by Age and Education

	Age Group			
	16–29		30–39	
	Years of Education			
	<10	>10	<10	>10
	Sample Size			
	N = 12	N = 30	N = 22	N = 44
Color Trails 1	49.33	34.43	49.62	34.96
	(30.75)	(12.69)	(13.76)	(11.91)
Color Trails 2	128.58	80.03	114.05	84.48
	(45.19)	(23.43)	(49.80)	(27.40)
Raven's Total	38.33	42.73	34.77	42.48
	(13.24)	(10.28)	(13.82)	(9.70)

	Age Group			
	40–49		50–75	
	Years of Education			
	<10	>10	<10	>10
	Sample Size			
	N = 16	N = 11	N = 25	N = 20
Color Trails 1	56.38	34.09	70.28	44.20
	(14.16)	(6.44)	(44.10)	(15.73)
Color Trails 2	134.06	79.46	146.72	99.20
	(54.15)	(28.42)	(62.21)	(25.75)
Raven's Total	29.19	41.36	23.36	42.30
	(12.49)	(9.52)	(7.63)	(10.38)

tudinal research as well as the clinical assessment of non-English-speaking adults and adults with limited education, English as a second language, and language and reading disorders. Because the Color Trails Test only recently made its appearance on the scene, research regarding it effectiveness in clinical and research settings is only just starting to emerge.

There are four equivalent forms that have been developed for the Color Trails Test (forms A, B, C & D). Currently only form A of the Color Trails Test has been normed for clinical use. Even though all four forms are physically equivalent to each other, future research is needed to establish the psychometric and normative equivalence of the alternate forms. Future research should also focus on establishing the reliability and equivalence of the alternate forms in samples of both normal subjects and patients

with specific neurobehavioral dysfunction (e.g., clinical comparison data; aka "abnorms"). Future normative studies with any form of the test should report data regarding error and near-miss responses, data for prompts and information regarding the interference index, in addition to reporting the time to complete the test. For instance, no age-and-education-corrected normative data are available for Hispanics regarding the occurrence of near-miss and error responses, nor information regarding prompts and the interference index. The Chinese study reports information regarding the time to complete CTT 1, CTT 2, and the interference index, but no information regarding prompts, near-miss, or errors.

Normative data are needed for English-speaking and non-English-speaking individuals with low or no education. Hsieh and Riley

Table 5.3. CTT.2b; Means and Standard Deviations for Performance of Males Stratified by Age and Education

	Age Group			
	16–29		30–39	
	Years of Education			
	<10	>10	<10	>10
	Sample Size			
	N = 11	N = 25	N = 13	N = 18
Color Trails 1	49.27	37.28	49.23	39.28
	(15.70)	(13.20)	(10.92)	(10.44)
Color Trails 2	100.64	88.36	116.31	84.33
	(20.38)	(26.39)	(39.35)	(17.11)
Raven's Total	35.09	42.68	38.08	46.28
	(10.00)	(11.86)	(10.44)	(7.76)

	Age Group			
	40–49		50–75	
	Years of Education			
	<10	>10	<10	>10
	Sample Size			
	N = 12	N = 17	N = 18	N = 6
Color Trails 1	59.08	36.88	53.06	55.17
	(15.22)	(8.12)	(20.00)	(21.86)
Color Trails 2	129.17	91.24	136.22	113.83
	(39.64)	(16.12)	(34.71)	(39.78)
Raven's Total	28.58	45.94	31.78	42.50
	(13.84)	(6.62)	(8.63)	(10.17)

Table 5.4. CTT.3a; Sample Size for Each Age/Education Category

	Education		
Age	1–6 yrs	7–10 yrs	11–17 yrs
30–39	6	14	22
40–49	6	19	14
50–59	6	15	12
60–69	22	6	4
70–83	28	2	0
Total	68	57	52

Table 5.5. CTT.3b; Effect of Age on Test Performance

	30–39 (n = 43)	40–49 (n = 39)	50–59 (n = 33)	60–69 (n = 32)	70–83 (n = 30)
Color Trails 1	42.05	50.97	56.76	129.66	162.97
	(15.69)	(20.66)	(27.63)	(80.99)	(98.55)
Color Trails 2	89.95	104.74	138.58	225.31	306.47
	(37.47)	(35.65)	(67.75)	(103.06)	(188.38)
Interference Index	1.24 (0.80)	1.28 (0.97)	1.59 (1.17)	0.98 (0.73)	1.01(0.75)

Table 5.6. CTT.3c; Effect of Education on Test Performance

	Years of Education		
	0–6 (n = 96)	7–9 (n = 59)	10–17 (n = 22)
Color Trails 1	132.9 (92.45)	55.6 (30.42)	48.2 (25.5)
Color Trails 2	243.1 (154.3)	128.0 (77.17)	97.9 (39.9)
Interference	1.12 (0.73)	1.28(1.08)	1.56 (1.11)

(1997) provide preliminary data for low-educated Chinese adults above age 59. Fortunately they are continuing to collect normative data in China and are also sampling older, highly educated urban Chinese. As a result, the sample sizes will grow to allow reporting by age/education categories. Reporting the data by age/education categories would allow performance comparison across cultures.

In general, the age categories need to be narrowed for reporting data for older adults. We would recommend that future studies follow the WAIS-III age-group category groupings as an example.

Normative work still needs to be done regarding Hispanic individuals' performance on the Color Trails Test above age 75 years. Fortunately, Ponton and colleagues continue to collect normative information on their Neuropsychological Screening Battery for Hispanics (NeSBHIS), and therefore a larger normative database will accumulate, allowing a sample size more appropriate for inferential purposes with Hispanics. In their initial report of Spanish speaking individuals, the sample size for the age-and-education-corrected groups was quite small. Yet comparison of this preliminary performance data with that found in the U.S. standardization manual for the CTT at the same age and education levels does not suggest a significant difference in performance. This finding, coupled with the findings of Maj et al. (1991, 1993), further supports the notion that the CTT may be a more culturally fair test.

6

Stroop Test

BRIEF HISTORY OF THE TEST

The Stroop Test measures the relative speeds of reading names of colors, naming colors, and naming colors used to print an incongruous color name (e.g., the color *red* is used to print the word "blue"). The last task requires one to override a reading response. This conflict interference situation has come to be called *the Stroop Effect*.

The Stroop Test has traditionally been viewed as a measure of executive functioning involving cognitive inhibition (Boone et al., 1990), and specifically, the ability to inhibit an overlearned response in favor of an unusual one (Spreen & Strauss, 1998) and "to maintain a course of action in the face of intrusion by other stimuli" (Comalli et al., 1962, p. 47). Factor analyses of sets of executive measures suggests that the Stroop Test has more in common with timed executive measures, such as verbal fluency (FAS), and measures of information processing speed, such as Digit Symbol, than executive tests involving set shifting (Wisconsin Card Sorting Test) or divided attention/working memory (Auditory Consonant Trigrams) (Boone et al., in press).

Initial lesion studies indicated that poor performance on the interference section of the Stroop Test was associated with left frontal lobe pathology (Perret, 1974), while subsequent functional imaging studies have found Stroop performance to be associated with perfusion of

the right anterior cingulate (Bench et al., 1993; Liddle et al., 1992; Pardo et al., 1990), and right prefrontal polar cortex and right orbitofrontal cortex (Bench et al., 1993). Poor performance on the Stroop Test has been found to be associated with frontal systems dysfunction secondary to closed head injury (Trenerry et al., 1989), discrete frontal lobe lesions (especially left frontal lobe; Perret, 1974; Regard, 1981 in Spreen & Strauss, 1991), frontotemporal dementia (Pachana et al., 1996), frontal lobe seizures (Boone et al., 1988), white-matter hyperintensities (Fukui et al., 1994; Ylikoski et al., 1993), depression (Boone et al., 1995; Trichard et al., 1995), schizophrenia (Brebion et al., 1996; Buchanan et al., 1994; Schreiber et al., 1995), and late-life psychosis (Miller et al., 1991).

In addition, Stroop scores are also lowered in damage not confined to anterior brain areas, such as left and right cerebrovascular accident (Trenerry et al., 1989) and Alzheimer's disease (Binetti et al., 1996; Koss et al., 1984; Pachana et al., 1996). Stroop performance is impaired in both left and right cerebral damage but may be particularly pronounced with left-sided damage (Perret, 1974; Trenerry et al., 1989), although this may be an artifact of coexistent aphasia. Specifically, Nehemkis and Lewinsohn (1972) found that patients with left cerebral damage with aphasia performed particularly poorly on the Stroop, while patients with left cerebral damage without aphasia actually performed better than patients with right hemisphere dysfunction.

The Stroop Test paradigm is among the oldest in experimental psychology. Interest in the relative speeds of color naming and reading color-words has been active for over a century. In 1883, as a result of a suggestion by Wilheim Wundt (who founded the first psychological laboratory in Leipzig, Germany), America's first psychologist, James Cattell (then a student of Wundt) began conducting what would later become the earliest published study (1886) examining the relative speeds of color naming and color-word reading. Over 40 years later, the first published report of the conflict/interference situation (e.g., where one must name the color of the ink used to print the word when the color and color name are incongruous) originated in the Marburg, Germany, laboratory of Erick Rudolf Jaenasch (Jensen & Rohwer, 1966).

Some years later, John Ridley Stroop, then a graduate student working in the Jesup Psychological Laboratory at George Peabody College for Teachers, began his doctoral research examining interference in serial verbal reaction in which he developed and used the color-word interference test that now bears his name (Stroop, 1935).

Stroop's original studies employed three cards, all with white backgrounds:

1. *An achromatic color word reading card*—consisting of a series of 100 words for colors printed in black ink.
2. *A chromatic color-word naming card*—consisting of a series of 100 color names printed in a color of ink incongruent with the word.
3. *A pure color card*- consisting of a series of 100 squares of solid color printed in different colors.

For all cards, *five* colors and/or color words were used (red, blue, green, purple, and brown). The words and the colors were generally arranged in a 10″ × 10″ grid of evenly spaced rows and columns. As Stroop notes: "The colors were arranged so as to avoid any regularity of occurrence and so that each color would appear twice in each column and in each row, and that no color would immediately succeed itself in either column or row. The words were also arranged so that the name of each color would appear twice in each line." For the chromatic color-word naming cards, "no word was printed in the color it names but an equal number of times in each of the other four colors: i.e., the word 'red' was presented in blue, green, brown, and purple inks; the word 'blue' was printed in red, green, brown, and purple inks, etc. No word immediately succeeded itself in either column or row" (p. 648). An alternate form was also created by printing all the cards in the reverse order.

In three experiments, Stroop examined *four* different tasks using the above three mentioned cards. Using cards 1 and 2, experiment 1 examined the differences in rates of *reading* color word names (task 1) when the word was printed in black ink vs. when printed in an incongruous ink color (task 2). Using only cards 2 and 3, experiment II examined the differences in rates of verbally identifying squares of color (task 3) vs. *naming* ink colors against the distraction of incongruous color words (task 4). For experiment III, Stroop modified his test, shortening the cards to 10 columns and *five* rows (so that there were only 50 responses required per card instead of 100) and using colored swastikas on the pure color card instead of solid square color patches. For experiment III, Stroop administered each of the four tasks separately on different days. Stroop never administered all three cards in the same testing period; this procedure did not become standard until the time of Thurstone's (1944) investigations of perception using the Stroop paradigm.

As testimony to its popularity, the Stroop has been translated into several languages, including Chinese (e.g., Chen & Ho, 1986), Czechoslovakian (e.g., Sovcikova & Bronis, 1985), German (e.g. Perret, 1974), Hebrew (e.g., Ingraham et al., 1988), Swedish (e.g., Hugdahl & Franzon, 1985) and Japanese (e.g., Fukui et al., 1994; Toshima et al., 1992; Toshima et al., 1996; Yamazaki, 1985), among others.

The major problem with the Stroop literature is the presence of numerous versions of the task. The following is a summary of the variations:

Stimulus Cards

1. Color and shape of items: Cards have contained three, four, or five colors presented as either squares, or rectangles, or circles, or dots, or swastikas, etc.

2. Number of items: Various stimulus cards have contained 17, 20, 22, 24, 27, 50, 100, 112, and 176 items.

3. Size and presentation of stimuli cards: The size of the stimulus cards has varied from small flash cards to wall charts, and some studies have used a tachistoscopic, slide, or computer presentation.

4. Stimuli background: Although most investigators have used stimulus cards with a white background, others have used cards with a black background, or a color different from both the color ink of the word and the color name (super-stroop; Dyer, 1973).

5. Number of stimuli cards: Various versions of the test require the use of two, three, or four cards.

Administration Procedures

1. Scanning orientation: Some versions require the examinee to scan across rows from left to right, whereas others require the examinee to read down columns.

2. Stimuli sequence: Some versions present word reading followed by color naming and vice versa.

Method of Scoring

Total score: Determination of the total score has ranged from the number of correct responses made in 45 or 120 seconds to each card, the total time to complete each card, a difference score (color-interference minus color naming or reading), to the total number of errors made in 45 seconds.

Current Administration Procedures

At present, there is no one recognized standard version of the Stroop Test. There are, however, three versions of the test that are commercially published: Charles Golden's Stroop (1978), Max Trenerry's Stroop (1989), and Peter Comalli (1962) and Edith Kaplan's Stroop (personal communication). Charles Golden's and Max Trenerry's versions of the Stroop are available from Psychological Assessment Resources, Inc., and Peter Comalli and Edith Kaplan's Stroop is available from The Boston Neuropsychological Foundation. The Stroop available from the Boston group can be used as a Comalli et al. (1962) version (reading words, naming colors, naming colors with incongruous color names), or as the Comalli and Kaplan version (naming colors, reading words, naming colors with incongruous color names). Carl Dodrill (1978a) and Otfried Spreen and Esther Strauss (1991) have also developed versions of the Stroop, which can be obtained by writing to their respective laboratories. (see Appendix 1 for ordering information)

The Stroop versions reviewed in this chapter will be limited to the five formats which are commercially published or readily available from the authors. These versions differ in format and will be briefly described below.

Comalli/Kaplan Stroop, 1962 and Personal Communication

The Comalli and Kaplan Stroops use the same three cards originally developed by Comalli et al. (1962), although Comalli and Kaplan differ in the order of presentation of cards 1 and 2. All three cards are 9¼" × 9¼" with 100 stimuli per card arranged in a 10 × 10 grid against a white background. At the top of each card is an additional row of 10 practice items. The color-name reading card consists of color words (*red, blue, green*) printed in black ink and presented in random order. The color naming card consists of rectangles (5⁄16" by 3⁄16") of colors (red, blue, green) arranged in random order. The third card presents color words printed in an ink whose color is different from the color designated by the word. For each card, subjects are instructed to proceed line by line down the page either reading words or naming colors as quickly as they can. Each line is scanned from left to right, mirroring English reading format. The time to complete the 100 items on each card is recorded, along with the number of errors made. Near-miss responses (i.e., self-corrected errors) are also recorded. The Comalli-Kaplan Stroop scoring protocol also allows for independently tracking the response times for the first half of each card separately from the last half.

In the Comalli et al. (1962) administration format, the word-reading card is presented first, followed by the color-naming card, and then the interference card.

The Kaplan alteration in the test administration format occurred by happenstance when a research assistant mistakenly reversed the order of cards 1 and 2. In thinking about the mistake, Edith Kaplan decided the error might have been fortuitous. As a result, she decided to permanently make the modification in card order presentation in her laboratory for the following reasons: (1) administering the color-naming card first allows an immediate check on whether the subject is color-blind, a condition which would invalidate the use of the test, and (2) more importantly, administration of the Word-Reading task *immediately before* the Interference task (in which the subject must now inhibit a reading response) may exert a priming effect on the degree of interference, whereas presenting the Color-Naming card before the Interference task (in which the subject is again expected to identify color) may serve to minimize the "stroop effect" (personal communication).

Demick, Kaplan, and Wapner (personal communication) have more recently proposed a process-oriented scoring system for the Stroop that utilizes the identification of specific verbal errors (reflecting both deviant responses to items, e.g., inappropriate color responses, and deviant responses to sequence, e.g., inserted linguistic words or phrases); nonverbal behaviors serving as cognitive devices (e.g., nodding, body rocking); and expanded temporal measures (e.g., time per line, time between utterances). Based on exploratory studies (Demick & Wapner, 1985; Demick, Salas-Passeri, & Wapner, 1986), they have documented that while various developmental groups may not differ with respect to achievement measures (e.g., total time), they are distinguishable on the basis of more process-oriented measures (e.g., relative to young and middle-aged adults, older adults used significantly more inefficient strategies, such as gazing across the cards to identify specific patterns and/or using fingers as if counting in succession to modulate responses,

to meet task demands; on a downward extension of the Stroop for preschoolers, 4 and 5-year-olds employed a range of nonverbal strategies to maintain serial organization, while 3-year-olds failed to do so).

Dodrill Stroop, 1978a

The Dodrill version of the Stroop consists of two alternate administrations of one stimulus card containing 176 color-words (*red, green, blue,* and *orange*) randomly printed in 11 columns of 16 color-words. Each color-word is printed in an incongruous color (e.g., the color-word *blue* is printed in green ink, etc.). In the first administration, subjects read the color-words as they scan down the columns. In the second administration, subjects name the color of ink the words are printed in. Time to complete each card is noted. Two scores are generated: the total time to complete part I (which is essentially an estimate of the examinee's reading speed) and difference between the total times for part II minus part I, "which reflects an estimate of the degree of interference induced by the test" (Dodrill, 1987, p. 6).

Golden Stroop, 1978

This version of the Stroop uses three 8½" × 11" pages. Each page has 100 items presented in five columns of 20 items. Page 1 consists of the words *red, green,* and *blue* presented randomly, printed in black ink. Page 2 contains blocks of *XXXX*s printed in either red, green, or blue ink. Page 3 is the "Stroop effect" card and contains color-words printed in a noncongruent color (i.e., the word *blue* is printed in red ink, etc.). For each page, the examinee is required to scan the columns vertically, starting on the left side of the page and moving to the right. The score is the number of correctly identified items per page within 45 seconds. Errors are not counted.

Trenerry et al. Stroop, 1989

This version of the Stroop consists of two cards: form C and form C-W. Form C contains 112 color-words (*red, blue, green,* and *tan*) randomly arranged in four columns of 28 color-words. Each color-word is printed in an incongruous ink color (e.g., the word *tan* is printed in red, etc.). Form C-W follows the same format as for form C; however, there is a different random order of color-words.

For form C, the examinee is requested to read the words as quickly as possible as he/she scans down the columns. For form C-W, the examinee is instructed to name the color ink the color-word is printed in as quickly as possible, again as he/she scans down the columns. A maximum of 120 seconds is allowed to complete each task. The score for each task is the number of correct responses (or number of items completed) minus any incorrect responses.

Although the Dodrill version relies upon a difference score between the reading and interference cards, a discriminant analysis conducted by Trenerry and colleagues demonstrated that the data from form CW alone provided the sharpest classification accuracy, and thus the score from form C-W is the only one used for interpretation purposes.

Victoria Stroop, 1991 (as Reported by Spreen & Strauss, 1991)

The Spreen and Strauss version of the Stroop (also known as the Victoria version) uses three 21.5×14 cm cards presented in the following order: part D, part W, and part C. Each card has six rows of four items. Part D contains colored dots (red, green, blue, and yellow), and on this card the task is to name the colors as quickly as possible. Part W has the words "when," "and," "over," and "hand" printed in red, green, blue, or yellow ink, and the examinee must name the color ink each word is printed in as quickly as possible. On part C the color-words *red, green, blue,* and *yellow* are printed in incongruous-colored ink (e.g., the word *red* is printed in green ink, etc.), and the examinee must name the color ink the color-word is printed in as quickly as possible. Rows are scanned from left to right as the subject works down the page. Time to completion and the number of errors are recorded for each card. For further information regarding this version of the Stroop, please see Spreen and Strauss (1991, pp. 52–56).

Jensen and Rohwer (1966) provide a detailed and fascinating review of the Stroop Test and its many reincarnations, and Dyer (1973), Golden (1978) and MacLeod (1991) review applica-

tions and research findings subsequent to Jensen and Rohwer's report. Lezak (1995, pp. 373–376) also provides an overview of the test for the interested reader.

RELATIONSHIP BETWEEN STROOP TEST PERFORMANCE AND DEMOGRAPHIC FACTORS

While some studies have found no significant age effect on the Stroop Test (Graf et al., 1995) or an age effect that was equaled by the effect of health status (Houx *et al.,* 1993), others have found significant or nearly significant age-related decrements in Stroop performance (Boone et al., 1990; Cohn et al., 1984; Comalli et al., 1962; Daigneault et al., 1992; Feinstein et al., 1994; Ivnik et al., 1996; Jensen & Rohwer, 1966; Klein et al., 1997; Libon et al., 1994; Panek et al., 1984; Spreen & Strauss, 1998; Swerdlow et al., 1995; Trenerry et al., 1989; Whelihan & Lesher, 1985). Older individuals show declines in performance on the color interference section of the Stroop, but also in color naming (Cohn et al., 1984). Of interest, younger and older groups may show a different pattern of performance on color interference, with younger subjects performing the first half of the task faster than the second half, and older subjects demonstrating the opposite pattern (Klein et al., 1997).

One study reported that more highly educated subjects perform better on the Stroop Test (Houx et al., 1993); however, other studies have not been able to document a significant relationship between education and Stroop performance (Trenerry et al., 1989).

The literature on gender differences in Stroop performance is equivocal, with some studies observing differences (Martin & Franzen, 1989) and others finding none (Connor et al., 1988; Houx et al., 1993; Jensen & Rohwer, 1966; Swerdlow et al., 1995; Stroop, 1935; Trenerry et al., 1989), and others reporting a female advantage confined to color naming (Golden, 1978; Stroop, 1935; Jensen & Rohwer, 1966; Strickland et al., 1997) or word reading (Strickland et al., 1997)

Spreen and Strauss (1998) suggest that there is a relationship between Stroop performance and intellectual level, although Trenerry and colleagues (1989) indicate that Stroop scores are not strongly related to IQ in brain-damaged subjects.

A recent examination of the relative contribution of IQ and demographic factors to Comalli Stroop color-interference performance in a large sample of healthy, older subjects found that age and FSIQ accounted for 15% and 13%, respectively, of unique test score variance; education and gender did not contribute to test performance (Boone, in press). Similarly, Ivnik et al. (1996), using Golden's (1978) version of the Stroop, found that age strongly influenced Stroop performance, accounting for 13% of the test's raw score variance on the Word-Reading card, 29% on the Color-Naming card, and 27% on the Interference card. Education accounted for 8% of the performance variance on the Word-Reading card, 3% on the Color-Naming card, and only 2% on the Interference card. Gender accounted for less than 4% of the performance variance on any card, "suggesting that sex-corrections were not needed" (p. 263).

The literature taken as whole suggests that age and IQ are substantial contributors to Stroop performance. Gender appears to have a minimal relationship to Stroop scores. It is doubtful that educational level has an impact on test performance over and above that accounted for by IQ.

METHOD FOR EVALUATING THE NORMATIVE REPORTS

Our review of the literature located two Stroop manuals (Golden, 1978; Trenerry et al., 1989), as well as six normative reports, and 13 clinical studies reporting control data on the Stroop Test. The manuals are for the Golden and Trenerry Stroop versions, while the normative studies are for the Kaplan (Demick & Harkins, 1997; Schiltz, personal communication; Strickland et al., 1997), Golden (Ivnik et al., 1996), and Victoria versions (Regard, 1981, in Spreen & Strauss, 1991; Spreen & Strauss, 1991). Among the control data studies, six provide data for the Comalli version (Boone et al., 1990, 1991; Boone, in press; Comalli et al., 1962;

Eson, personal communication; Stuss et al., 1985), two present data for the Kaplan version (D'Elia, Satz, & Uchiyama, unpublished data; Selnes & Miller, personal communication), three report data for the Golden version (Connor et al., 1988; Daigneault et al., 1992; Fisher et al., 1990), and two present data for the Dodrill version (Dodrill, 1978a; Sacks et al., 1991).

In order to adequately evaluate the Stroop Test normative reports, eight key criterion variables were deemed critical. The first six of these relate to *subject* variables, and the remaining two dimensions relate to *procedural* variables.

Minimal requirements for meeting the criterion variables were as follows:

Subject Variables

Age-Group Interval

Given the consistent evidence of a significant decline in performance with advancing age, Stroop data should be presented in age groupings.

Sample Size

As discussed in previous chapters, a minimum of at least 50 subjects per group interval is optimal.

Reporting of IQ

Some data suggest that IQ may be nearly as predictive of performance as age, although this finding needs to be replicated in additional studies. For the time being, Stroop normative data probably does not need to be presented by IQ group intervals but information on the IQs of normative samples should be provided.

Reporting of Educational Levels

Data on the relationship between education and Stroop performance is equivocal, and thus until this issue is firmly resolved, information regarding the educational level of the normative samples should be included.

Reporting Gender Composition

Data on the relationship between gender and Stroop performance is also equivocal, and thus until this issue is definitively resolved, information regarding the gender composition of normative samples should be provided.

Sample Composition Description

As discussed in other chapters, information regarding medical and psychiatric exclusion criteria is important; it is unclear if geographic region, ethnicity, occupation, handedness, fluency in English, or recruitment procedures are relevant, so until this is determined, it is best that this information is provided.

Procedural Variables

Description of Test Stimuli and Administration Format Used

There are several different versions of the Stroop Test, and each version differs regarding administration and scoring procedures. Therefore, normative data sets must indicate the precise test stimuli and administration format. (For the purposes of this chapter, only those studies which met this criterion were reviewed.)

Data Reporting

Means and standard deviations, and preferably, ranges, for time in seconds for each card are important. In addition, it is advantageous for data to be provided for number of errors (corrected and uncorrected).

SUMMARY OF THE STATUS OF THE NORMS

In terms of subject variables, all studies provide information on age and all but three present data by age groupings (Boone et al., 1991; Dodrill, 1978a; Stuss et al., 1985). Data on IQ is reported much less frequently, appearing in only six publications (Boone et al., 1990, 1991; Boone, in press; Regard, 1981, in Spreen & Strauss, 1991; Sacks et al., 1991; Stuss, 1985); data are stratified by IQ and age in one report (Boone, in press). Educational level is indicated in all but three reports (Eson, personal communication; Golden, 1978; Regard, 1981, in Spreen & Strauss, 1991); one publication presents data by educational levels (Selnes & Miller, personal communication) and another provides a correction for education (Ivnik et al., 1996). Gender is indicated in all reports but five (Comalli et al., 1962; Eson, personal communication; Golden, 1978; Regard, 1981 in Spreen & Strauss, 1991; Spreen & Strauss, 1991), and two reports present data for an all-male sample (D'Elia, Satz, & Uchiyama, unpublished data; Selnes & Miller, personal communication).

Cell sample sizes are generally adequate in six studies (Daigneault et al., 1992; D'Elia, Satz, & Uchiyama, unpublished data; Dodrill, 1978a; Ivnik et al., 1996; Schiltz, personal communication; Selnes & Miller, personal communication; Trenerry et al., 1989). Medical and psychiatric exclusion criteria are judged to be adequate in a majority of studies (Boone et al., 1990, 1991; Boone, in press; Daigneault et al., 1992; D'Elia, Satz, & Uchiyama, unpublished data; Dodrill, 1978a; Schiltz, personal communication; Selnes & Miller, personal communication; Strickland et al., 1997; Trenerry et al., 1989). Geographic recruitment area is indicated in 15 reports (Boone et al., 1990, 1991; Boone, in press; Comalli et al., 1962; Connor et al., 1988; Daigneault et al., 1992; D'Elia, Satz, & Uchiyama, unpublished data; Dodrill, 1978; Fisher et al., 1990; Ivnik et al., 1996; Sacks et al., 1991; Schiltz, personal communication; Selnes & Miller, personal communication; Strickland et al., 1997; Stuss et al., 1985); most of the data were collected in the United States although some data were collected in Canada (Daigneault et al., 1992; Stuss et al., 1985; and it is assumed that the Regard, 1981, Spreen & Strauss samples were also obtained in Canada) and Australia (Sacks et al., 1991). Ethnicity is reported in seven studies (Boone et al., 1990, 1991; D'Elia, Satz, & Uchiyama, unpublished data; Dodrill, 1978; Ivnik et al., 1996; Selnes & Miller, personal communication; Strickland et al., 1997), occupational status is indicated in only four publications (Daigneault et al., 1992; D'Elia, Satz, & Uchiyama, unpublished data; Dodrill, 1978a; Ivnik et al., 1996), and handedness is described in only three reports (Boone et al., 1991; Ivnik et al., 1996; Regard, 1981, in Spreen & Strauss, 1991). Language and/or fluency in English is reported in six studies (Boone et al., 1990, 1991; Boone, in press; Daigneault et al., 1992; Selnes & Miller, personal communication; Stuss et al., 1985), and recruitment procedures

Table 6.1. Stroop.L; Locator Table for Stroop Test

Study/Version	Age	N	Sample Composition	IQ, Education	Country/Location
STROOP.1 *Golden* Golden, 1978 page 83	15–45 46–64 65–80	— — —	— — —	— — —	U.S.
STROOP.2 *Trenery* Trenerry et al., 1989 page 84	18–49 x = 30.34 (8.57) 50–79 x = 62.68 (7.93)	106 50	43 males 63 females 26 males 24 females Non-neurological Non-psychiatric	14.68 (2.44) 14.70 (3.24)	U.S.
STROOP.3 *Victoria* Regard, 1981, in Spreen & Strauss, 1991 page 84	20–35 x = 26.7	40	Right-handed	average IQ	Canada
STROOP.4 *Kaplan* Schiltz, personal communication page 85	18-20	50	28 males 22 females College students No head injury with loss of consciousness Native English-speaking	13.36(0.63) range = 13–15	S. CA
STROOP.5 *Victoria* Spreen & Strauss, 1991 page 85	50–59 60–69 70–79 80+	19 28 24 15	Healthy volunteers	13.2 (3.1)	Canada
STROOP.6 *Golden* Ivnik et al., 1996 page 86	56–59 60–64 65–69 70–74 75–79 80–84 85–89 90–94	54 81 65 57 52 27 16 4	165 males 191 females 355 white 1 black 329 R hand 17 L hand 10 mixed hand Non-neurol. Non-psych.	≤7 = 2 8-11 = 34 12 = 133 13-15= 86 16-17= 66 ≥18 = 35	MN
STROOP.7 *Kaplan* Demick & Harkins, 1997 page 87	20–39 40–59 60–74 75+	231 24 M, 32 F 21 M, 34 F 23 M, 31 F 38 M, 28 F	community-dwelling individuals in good health	Education: high school plus some college	Boston, MA
STROOP.8 *Kaplan* Strickland et al., 1997 page 89	19–41 30.17 (6.34)	42	15 males 27 females Black Non-neurolog. Non-psych. No substance abuse	14.76 (2.2)	S. CA
STROOP.9 *Comalli* Comalli et al., 1962 page 91	17–19 25–34 35–44 65–80	18 14 16 15	17–44 yr-old, college students 65–80 from community old age club		MA
STROOP.10 *Dodrill* Dodrill, 1978a page 92	27.34 (8.41)	50	30 males 20 females 49 white 1 nonwhite	11.96 (2.01)	WA

continued

Table 6.1. *(Continued)*

Study/Version	Age	N	Sample Composition	IQ, Education	Country/ Location
			9 students 26 unemployed 15 employed Non-neurolog.		
STROOP.11 *Comalli* Eson, personal communication page 92	63.2 67.0 72.0 78.3	15 16 16 16	—	—	NY
STROOP.12 *Comalli* Stuss et al., 1985 page 93	29.2 (12.0)	20	13 males 7 females English/French	12.5 (2.0) 106.6(13.4)	Canada
STROOP.13 *Golden* Connor et al., 1988 page 93	18–32	40	17 males 23 females	college students	WV
STROOP.14 *Comalli* Boone et al., 1990 page 94	50–59 60–69 70–79	25 21 15	25 males 36 females 51 white 4 black 3 Asian 3 Hispanic Fluent English Non-neurol. Non-psych. Non-substance abuse	14.34(2.63) 113.79(13.51)	S. CA
STROOP.15 *Golden* Fisher et al., 1990 page 94	72.9 (8.3)	36	13 males 23 females no ocular dis.	14.6 (2.7)	S. CA
STROOP.16 *Comalli* Boone et al., 1991 page 95	35.8(13.7)	16	7 males 9 females 19% lt. hand. 14 white 2 Asian Fluent English No substance abuse Non-neurolog. Non-psych.	15.2(2.8) 2 learn dis 109.1 (10.9)	S. CA
STROOP.17 *Dodrill* Sacks et al., 1991 page 96	22.4(5) Range = 18–32	12	male normal vision	13.7(2.3) 109.1(9.5)	Australia
STROOP.18 *Golden* Daigneault et al., 1992 page 96	20-35 27.71(4.05) 45-65 56.62(5.29)	70 58	38 males 32 females 30 males 28 females French lang. No substance abuse Non-neurol. Non-psych. Unskilled blue collar to professional	12.36(2.09) 12.11(3.63)	Canada
STROOP.19 *Kaplan* D'Elia et al., unpublished data page 97	40–49 50–59	118 79	White male pilots Passed med exam	16.1(1.9) 15.6(2.0)	U.S.

continued

Table 6.1. *(Continued)*

Study/Version	Age	N	Sample Composition	IQ, Education	Country/Location
STROOP.20 *Kaplan*	30–39		Gay/bisexual male		S. CA,
Selnes & Miller, personal	13–15 years ed	64	Native English		PA
communication	16 years ed	93	No Alcohol abuse		
page 97	>16yrs ed	95	no head inj/LOC		
	40-49		90% non-Hispanic white		
	13–15 years ed	49			
	16 years ed	65			
	>16yrs ed	116			
STROOP.21 *Comalli*	<65		53 males	14.57(2.55)	S. CA
Boone, in press	average IQ	33	102 females		
page 98	high average IQ	23	Non-neurol.		
	superior IQ	35	Non-psych.		
	≥65		no substance abuse		
	Average IQ	20	Fluent English		
	High average IQ	16			
	superior IQ	24			

are specified in 10 datasets (Boone et al., 1990, 1991; Boone, in press; Connor et al., 1988; Daigneault et al., 1992; D'Elia, Satz, & Uchiyama, unpublished data; Dodrill, 1978; Fisher et al., 1990; Ivnik et al., 1996; Schiltz, personal communication).

Regarding procedural variables, test stimuli and procedures are described in all reports. (They would not have been included in the chapter if they did not.) Means are presented in all datasets, although standard deviations are not reported in two studies (Comalli et al., 1962; Golden, 1978). One study only provides data for the color-naming trial (Stuss et al., 1985), and five studies only report data for the color interference trial (Boone et al., 1991; Boone, in press; Daigneault et al., 1992; Sacks et al., 1991; Schiltz, personal communication). Two studies provide cutoff scores (Dodrill, 1978a; Trenerry et al., 1989), and one study presents data for the first half and the second half of the color interference trial separately (Schiltz, personal communication). Several studies report error scores as well as time scores (Boone et al., 1990; D'Elia, Satz, & Uchiyama, unpublished data; Regard, 1981, in Spreen & Strauss, 1991; Spreen & Strauss, 1991;), two reports provide data on practice effects (Connor et al., 1988; Sacks et al., 1991) and one presents information on alternate forms (Sacks et al., 1991).

Table 6.1 summarizes information provided in the studies described in this chapter.

SUMMARIES OF THE STUDIES

Published manuals for the Stroop Test will be reviewed first, followed by normative studies, concluding with Stroop control data reported in various clinical studies.

Manuals

[STROOP.1] Golden, 1978 (Golden Version)

The test stimuli and administration procedures developed by Golden are well specified. Primarily utilizing previously published normative reports, the "norms" presented in this manual have largely been empirically derived by calculating how many items the subjects in other studies would have obtained if the test were discontinued after 45 seconds. In addition to including data from his own studies (sample sizes unknown), Golden utilized normative data provided by Stroop (1935), Jensen (1965), and Comalli et al. (1962) to generate the "norms." No information is provided regarding demographic, IQ, or other characteristics of Golden's own normative samples.

Using the tables in the manual, all raw scores can be converted to *T* scores. For subjects younger than 17 and older than 45, age corrections need to be applied before the *T*-score conversion can be made. The manual cautions that the age corrections for adults over age 65 and children under age 17 are considered to be "experimental."

The normative data contained in Golden's manual are not reproduced here, and the interested reader is referred directly to this publication for further information.

Study strengths

1. The Stroop cards developed by Golden and test administration procedures are well described in the manual.

2. Mean scores are reported for number of items completed.

3. Some of the data are presented by age-group intervals, although the age ranges within each grouping are broad (15–45, 46–64, 65–80) and of questionable clinical utility.

Considerations regarding use of the study

1. A major problem with Golden's use of other published normative data to generate his norms is that the Stroop formats and procedures used by the other investigators all differed from Golden's version (e.g., in other formats, subjects scanned from left to right while in his version subjects scanned the stimuli vertically from top to bottom; other versions required subjects to complete the entire stimulus cards rather than stopping at 45 seconds, used colored rectangles rather than employing colored *X*s, used a wall chart presentation rather than standard page presented up close to the subject, etc.).

2. No information is provided regarding the number of subjects in Golden's sample.

3. No information on exclusion criteria is available for Golden's sample.

4. The gender, educational, and IQ levels of Golden's sample are not reported.

5. No standard deviations are provided.

[STROOP.2] Trenerry, Crosson, DeBoe, and Leber, 1989 (Trenery Version)

This manual presents the standardization data for this version of the Stroop Test. The sample consisted of 156 adults ranging in age from 18 to 79, divided into two age groups: 18 to 49 (*n* = 106) and 50 to 79 (*n* = 50). Exclusion crite-

ria included history of neurological disorder, major psychiatric illness, or physical handicaps which might affect performance. The younger group averaged 30.34 ± 8.57 years of age, 14.68 ± 2.44 years of education, and contained 43 males and 63 females. The older group averaged 62.68 ± 7.93 years of age, 14.70 + 3.24 years of education, and contained 26 males and 24 females.

Test administration procedures are carefully specified. Means and standard deviations for number of items completed, number of incorrect responses, and color scores are provided for the Color task. Similarly, means and standard deviations for number of items completed, number of incorrect responses, and color-word scores are reported for the Color-Word task. In addition, optimal cutoff scores are provided for each score for each age grouping, and percentile ranks for raw scores are also reported for each age grouping. This is a proprietary test, and the normative data are available in the test manual. A significant age effect on performance was detected, but no relationship between education or gender and test performance was observed.

Study strengths

1. Cell sample sizes are adequate.

2. Minimally adequate exclusion criteria.

3. Information provided for each age grouping on mean age, education, and gender distribution.

4. Test stimuli and administration procedures are specified.

5. Means and standard deviations reported for each age grouping on a wide range of scores, as well as optimal cutoff scores and percentile ranks.

Considerations regarding use of the study

1. The age-group intervals are quite broad.

2. No information regarding IQ.

3. High educational level of the sample.

Normative Studies

[STROOP.3] Regard, 1981 (as Reported in Spreen & Strauss, 1991) (Victoria Version)

Stroop data were obtained on 40 right-handed young adults of average intelligence. Average

age was 26.7 (range = 20–35). The Victoria Stroop Test stimuli and procedures were employed. Means and standard deviations are reported for time and errors.

Study strengths
1. Homogeneous age grouping.
2. Information regarding IQ, handedness, and average age.
3. Test stimuli and procedures are described.
4. Means and standard deviations for time and errors are reported.

Considerations regarding use of the study
1. Fairly small sample size.
2. No information regarding educational level, gender, fluency in English, geographic recruitment area (assumed to be Canada), or exclusion criteria (Table 6.2).

[STROOP.4] Schiltz, Personal Communication (Kaplan Version)

The sample consists of 50 (28 male, 22 female) native English-speaking subjects recruited from the UCLA undergraduate introductory psychology courses during 1988–1989. These were healthy normal adults aged 18 to 20 without histories of head trauma or loss of consciousness. The average number of years of education for the group was 13.36 ± 0.63 years (range = 13–15 years).

All students were required to participate in ongoing research as a part of their coursework, and students self-selected to the various studies based on the written descriptions of the studies. The Comalli stimulus cards and Kaplan administration procedures (i.e., color naming, word reading, color interference) were used as part

of a larger neuropsychological battery assembled for the purpose of collecting norms. All subjects were tested individually. Total battery length was 55 minutes, and the Stroop was administered about 30 minutes into the protocol.

Means, standard deviations, and ranges in seconds are reported for the first half of each stimulus card as well as for each card in total. Performance time on the second 50 items can be calculated by subtracting the time to complete the first half of the card from the total time to complete the whole card.

Study strengths
1. The sample size is adequate for the restricted age interval.
2. Exclusion criteria were minimally adequate.
3. Data on gender composition, educational level, geographic area, and recruitment procedures are reported.
4. Test stimuli and administration procedures are specified.
5. Means for time in seconds and standard deviations are reported.
6. Data provided for the first half of each card as well as total.

Considerations regarding use of the study
1. No data on IQ (Table 6.3).

[STROOP.5] Spreen and Strauss, 1991 (Victoria Version)

These authors collected Stroop normative data on 86 healthy older subjects aged 50 to 94; average age was 68.5 ± 10.78. Mean years of education was 13.2 ± 3.1 years. The Victoria Stroop Test stimuli and administration procedures were used. Means and standard deviations are reported for time and errors for four age groupings: 50–59 (n = 19), 60–69 (n = 28), 70–79 (n = 24), and 80+ (n = 15).

Study strengths
1. Data presented by narrow age groupings.
2. Information provided regarding mean age and mean educational level.
3. Test stimuli and procedures are well described.
4. Means and standard deviations reported for time and errors.

Table 6.2. Stroop.3

	Ages 20–35
Naming Color of Dots (D)	
Time	10.10 ± 2.01
Errors	0.03 ± 0.16
Naming Color Print of Noncolor Words (W)	
Time	12.00 ± 2.49
Errors	0.03 ± 0.16
Naming Color Print of Color Words (C)	
Time	19.25 ± 5.18
Errors	0.23 ± 0.53

Table 6.3. Stroop.4

	First Half	Total
Color naming	23.02 ± 3.28	51.14 ± 6.79
	(range = 16–30)	(range = 37–67)
Word reading	17.62 ± 2.78	38.46 ± 5.10
	(range = 13–25)	(range = 30–54)
Interference	43.22 ± 9.23	89.40 ± 17.76
	(range = 27–74)	(range = 58–132)

Considerations regarding use of the study

1. Unclear exclusion criteria (subjects are described as "healthy").

2. No information regarding IQ, gender, fluency in English, and geographic recruitment area (assumed to be Canada).

3. Small cell sample sizes (Table 6.4).

[STROOP.6] Ivnik, Malec, Smith, Tangalos, and Petersen, 1996 (Golden Version)

This study presents normative data for performance on the Golden (1978) version of the Stroop Test obtained on 356 individuals between the ages of 56 and 94, who participated in the ongoing MOANS study, a project to develop normative data for elderly individuals on various neuropsychological tests. The data are derived from a population of "almost exclusively Caucasian older adults who live in an economically stable region of the United States" (the area surrounding Rochester, MN). All subjects were community dwelling and had no active neurologic or psychiatric disorder and had undergone recent physical exams.

Data are reported in discrete age ranges (re-produced below along with demographic data). Age categorization utilized the midpoint interval technique. The raw score distribution at each midpoint age was "normalized" by assigning standard scores with a mean of 10 and a standard deviation of 3, based on actual percentile ranks. The authors provided tables of age-corrected norms for each age group. The procedure for clinical application of these data is described in the original article (Ivnik et al., 1996) as follows: "first select the table that corresponds to that person's age. Enter the table with the test's raw score; do not use 'corrected' or 'final' scores for tests that might present their own age- or education-adjustments. Select the appropriate column in the table for that test. The corresponding row in the left-most column in each table provides the MOANS Age-Corrected Scaled Score . . . for your subject's raw score; the corresponding row in the right-most column indicates the percentile range for that same score."

Mean and standard deviation scores for performance by age are not reported; however, the raw performance score can be easily translated

Table 6.4. Stroop.5

	Age Groupings			
	50–59	60–69	70–79	80+
Naming Color of Dots (D)				
Time	13.74 ± 2.58	12.71 ± 1.90	15.00 ± 5.07	18.87 ± 4.67
Errors	—	—	0.08 ± 0.28	0.20 ± 0.56
Naming Color Print of Noncolor Words				
Time	16.58 ± 3.34	16.32 ± 3.33	19.04 ± 5.10	24.13 ± 5.13
Errors	—	0.04 ± 0.19	—	0.13 ± 0.35
Naming Color Print of Color Words				
Time	28.90 ± 7.62	31.82 ± 9.86	38.83 ± 13.29	61.13 ± 30.94
Errors	0.42 ± 0.77	0.36 ± 0.68	0.71 ± 1.16	2.73 ± 2.46

to percentile performance scores (and standard scores) by using the data tables. Performance by age and education level have to be empirically derived by using the following equation:

$$A\&E-MSS_{Stroop} = K + (W1 \circ A - MSS_{Stroop}) - (W2 \circ education)$$

where K = a constant for each test

$W1$ = a weight to be applied to the age-corrected MOANS scaled score

$W2$ = a weight to be applied to the person's education

For the Stroop Test, the values are as follows:

	K	W_1	W_2
Word	3.47	1.10	0.34
Color	1.88	1.10	0.23
Interference	1.38	1.09	0.19

Analyses did not suggest a performance correction was necessary for gender.

Study strengths
1. Minimally adequate exclusion criteria.
2. Information regarding age, education, gender, handedness, ethnicity, recruitment procedures, and geographic area is reported.
3. The data are stratified by age group based on the midpoint interval technique.
4. The sample sizes for the five age groupings spanning 56 to 79 exceed ns of 50.
5. The test version and scoring procedures are specified.

Considerations regarding use of the study
1. The requirement to use an equation to derive age and education scores may be cumbersome.
2. No information on IQ (Tables 6.5 and 6.6).

[STROOP.7] Demick and Harkins, 1997 (Kaplan Version)

The sample consists of 231 individuals recruited in Massachusetts who participated in a study assessing relationships between field dependence-independence (FDI) cognitive style and driving behavior. Participants were community-dwelling individuals who in telephone screening denied any history of major impairment in

Table 6.5. Stroop.6a; Demographic Description of the Sample

	N
Age Groups	
56–59	54
60–64	81
65–69	65
70–74	57
75–79	52
80–84	27
85–89	16
90–94	4
Education (years)	
<7	2
8–11	34
12	133
13–15	86
16–17	66
>18	35
Sex	
Males	165
Females	191
Race	
Caucasian	355
Black	1
Handedness	
Right	329
Left	17
Mixed	10

perception, cognition, or motor execution, and described themselves as having good overall health; corrected visual problems were allowed. The average educational level of the sample was high school plus some college courses completed.

The Comalli cards and Kaplan administration procedures (i.e., color naming, word reading, color interference) were employed. Means, standard deviations, and ranges for time in seconds, errors, color difficulty factor (total time on B/total time on A), and interference factor (total time on C minus total time on B) are provided for four age groupings (20–39 years, 40–59 years, 60–74 years, 75+ years).

Study strengths
1. Overall sample size is large and individual cell sizes exceed n of 50.

Table 6.6. Stroop.6b; Age-Corrected Norms for Each Age Group (A-MSS): The Procedure for Applications of These Data Is Described in the Text

	Age Group									
	56-62			**63-65**			**66-68**			
Scaled scores	Word	Color	C/W	Word	Color	C/W	Word	Color	C/W	Percentile
2	<60	<41	<17	<58	<39	<16	<58	<32	<16	<1
3	60–63	41–42	17–18	58	39–40	16	58	32–40	16	1
4	64–65	43–44	19–20	59	41–43	17	59	41–42	17	2
5	66–72	42–50	21–23	60–68	44–48	18–21	60–68	43–47	18–21	3–5
6	73–77	51–54	24–25	69–76	49–53	22–23	69–74	48–51	22	6–10
7	78–82	55–59	26–28	77–81	54–58	24–26	75–80	52–57	23–26	11–18
8	83–88	60–64	29–30	82–86	59–61	27–29	81–85	58–59	27–29	19–28
9	89–93	65–66	31–34	87–91	62–64	30–32	86–91	60–63	30–31	29–40
10	94–101	67–71	35–38	92–98	65–70	33–36	92–97	64–69	32–35	41–59
11	102–107	72–75	39–40	99–103	71–73	37–39	98–103	70–72	36–38	60–71
12	108–111	76–81	41–43	104–109	74–80	40–42	104–109	73–78	39–42	72–81
13	112–116	82–85	44–47	110–115	81–82	43–45	110–115	79–81	43–44	82–89
14	117–122	86–88	48–49	116–122	83–86	46–48	116–122	82–85	45–47	90–94
15	123–125	89–91	50–55	123–125	87–89	49–51	123–125	86–87	48–50	95–97
16	126–129	92–93	56–57	126–127	90–92	52–54	126–127	88–90	51–52	98
17	130–139	94–104	58–62	128–132	93–104	55–62	128–131	91–104	53–60	99
18	>139	>104	>62	>132	>104	>62	>131	>104	>60	>99
N	160	160	160	206	206	206	152	152	152	

	Age Group									
	69–71			**72–74**			**75–77**			
Scaled scores	Word	Color	C/W	Word	Color	C/W	Word	Color	C/W	Percentile
2	<44	<24	<16	<42	<24	<4	<42	<23	<4	<1
3	44–46	24–30	16	42–45	24–30	4–6	42–45	23	4–6	1
4	47–50	31–41	17	46–48	31–39	7–15	46–48	24–26	7–13	2
5	51–59	42–45	18–19	49–56	40–41	16–17	49–54	27–39	14–15	3–5
6	60–71	46–48	20–21	57–63	42–44	18–20	55–63	40–43	16–17	6–10
7	72–79	49–52	22–24	64–76	45–49	21–22	64–72	44–48	18–21	11–18
8	80–83	53–57	25–27	77–81	50–53	23–26	73–80	49–51	22–25	19–28
9	84–87	58–60	28–29	82–85	54–58	27–28	81–84	52–55	26–27	29–40
10	88–94	61–65	30–32	86–93	59–63	29–31	85–91	56–60	28–30	41–59
11	95–98	66–71	33–35	94–96	64–67	32–33	92–96	61–65	31–32	60–71
12	99–103	72–76	36–39	97–100	68–71	34–36	97–98	66–70	33–34	72–81
13	104–111	77–81	40–44	101–105	72–74	37–40	99–105	71–73	35–38	82–89
14	112–120	82–85	45	106–111	75–80	41–44	106–110	74–80	39–42	90–94
15	121–125	86–87	46–50	112–115	81	45	111–115	81	43–45	95–97
16	126–127	88–90	51–52	116–122	82–84	46–49	116–122	82–84	—	98
17	128–131	91–104	53–60	123–130	85–90	50–52	123–130	85–90	46	99
18	>131	>104	>60	>130	>90	>52	>130	>90	>46	>99
N	134	134	134	124	124	124	111	111	111	

	Age Group									
	78–80			**81–83**			**84–86**			
Scaled scores	Word	Color	C/W	Word	Color	C/W	Word	Color	C/W	Percentile
2	<41	<23	<4	<41	<23	<4	<41	<23	<4	<1
3	41–44	23	4–6	41–44	23	4	41–44	23	4	1
4	45–48	24–26	7–13	45–47	24–25	5–6	45–47	24–25	5–6	2
5	49–52	27–39	14	48–52	26–30	7–10	48–52	26–30	7–10	3–5
6	53–63	40–41	15	53–63	31–39	11–15	53–63	31–39	11–15	6–10

continued

Table 6.6. *(Continued)*

	Age Group									
	78–80			81–83			84–86			
Scaled scores	Word	Color	C/W	Word	Color	C/W	Word	Color	C/W	Percentile
7	64–70	42–45	16–20	64–69	40–42	16	64–69	40–42	16	11–18
8	71–76	46–48	21–22	70–74	43–45	17–19	70–74	43–45	17–19	19–28
9	77–82	49–51	23–25	75–80	46–49	20–22	75–80	46–49	20–22	29–40
10	83–88	52–57	26–28	81–86	50–53	23–25	81–86	50–53	23–25	41–59
11	89–93	58–60	29	87–91	54–56	26–28	87–91	54–56	26–28	60–71
12	94–96	61–65	30–32	92–96	57–59	29–30	92–96	57–59	29–30	72–81
13	97–98	66–71	33–36	97–98	60–64	31–32	97–98	60–64	31–32	82–89
14	99–104	72–75	37–39	99–104	65–71	33–38	99–104	65–71	33–38	90–94
15	105	76–80	40–43	105	72–78	39–40	105	72–78	39–40	95–97
16	106–109	81	44	106–109	79–80	41–43	106–109	79–80	41–43	98
17	110–114	82	45	110–114	81	44	110–114	81	44	99
18	>114	>82	>45	>114	>81	>44	>114	>81	>44	>99
N	88	88	88	79	79	79	79	79	79	

	Age Group						
	87–89			90–97			
Scaled scores	Word	Color	C/W	Word	Color	C/W	Percentile
2	<41	<23	<4	<41	<23	<4	<1
3	41–44	23	4	41–44	23	4	1
4	45–47	24–25	5–6	45–47	24–25	5–6	2
5	48–52	26–30	7–10	48–52	26–30	7–10	3–5
6	53–63	31–39	11–15	53–63	31–39	11–15	6–10
7	64–69	40–42	16	64–69	40–42	16	11–18
8	70–74	43–45	7–19	70–74	43–45	17–19	19–28
9	75–80	46–49	20–22	75–80	46–49	20–22	29–40
10	81–86	50–53	23–25	81–86	50–53	23–25	41–59
11	87–91	54–56	26–28	87–91	54–56	26–28	60–71
12	92–96	57–59	29–30	92–96	57–59	29–30	72–81
13	97–98	60–64	31–32	97–98	60–64	31–32	82–89
14	99–104	65–71	33–38	99–104	65–71	33–38	90–94
15	105	72–78	39–40	105	72–78	39–40	95–97
16	106–109	79–80	41–43	106–109	79–80	41–43	98
17	110–114	81	44	110–114	81	44	99
18	>114	>81	>44	>114	>81	>44	>99
N	79	79	79	79	79	79	

2. Data are presented by age groupings.

3. Probably adequate exclusion criteria.

4. Information regarding gender, overall educational level, and geographic region is provided.

5. Test stimuli and procedures are indicated.

6. Means, standard deviations, and ranges are provided.

Considerations regarding use of the study

1. No information regarding intellectual level.

Other comments

1. Theoretical issues concerning the Stroop (e.g., process versus achievement measures, identification of a cognitive style) are discussed (Tables 6.7 to 6.10).

[STROOP.8] Strickland, D'Elia, James, and Stein, 1997 (Kaplan Version)

Stroop data were collected in Southern California on 42 African-American subjects (15 males and 27 females) aged 19 to 41 with no remarkable histories of neurologic, psychiatric, sub-

Table 6.7. Stroop.7a

| Measure | 20–39 Age Grouping | | |
	M	SD	Range
Number of Errors: Card A	0.5	0.8	0.0–3.0
Number of Errors: Card B	1.4	1.5	0.0–6.0
Number of Errors: Card C	3.5	2.9	0.0–14.0
Total Time(s): Card A	45.0	6.7	28.0–65.0
Total Time(s): Card B	62.1	12.0	41.0–91.0
Total Time(s): Card C	109.4	29.5	70.0–233.0
Color Difficulty Factor (Total Time on B/Total Time on A)	1.4	0.3	0.8–2.3
Interference Factor (Total Time on C – Total Time on B)	47.3	24.6	14.0–151.0

M Age = 24.2 Years; SD = 6.2 Years; N = 56; 24 M, 32 F.

Table 6.8. Stroop.7b

| Measure | 40–59 Age Grouping | | |
	M	SD	Range
Number of Errors: Card A	0.3	0.9	0.0–5.0
Number of Errors: Card B	0.9	1.3	0.0–7.0
Number of Errors: Card C	1.3	1.8	0.0–8.0
Total Time(s): Card A	43.7	8.8	32.4–85.0
Total Time(s): Card B	59.2	11.5	36.0–93.0
Total Time(s): Card C	104.5	20.6	63.0–155.0
Color Difficulty Factor (Total Time on B/Total Time on A)	1.4	0.2	1.0–2.0
Interference Factor (Total Time on C – Total Time on B)	45.3	15.4	17.0–82.0

M Age = 48.9 Years; SD = 5.5 Years; N = 55; 21 M, 34 F.

Table 6.9. Stroop.7c

| Measure | 60–74 Age Grouping | | |
	M	SD	Range
Number of Errors: Card A	0.5	0.9	0.0–4.0
Number of Errors: Card B	1.7	2.0	0.0–11.0
Number of Errors: Card C	2.8	3.5	0.0–13.0
Total Time(s): Card A	48.5	11.2	25.0–86.0
Total Time(s): Card B	69.4	14.1	46.0–123.0
Total Time(s): Card C	142.4	26.2	88.0–204.0
Color Difficulty Factor (Total Time on B/Total Time on A)	1.4	0.3	0.8–2.2
Interference Factor (Total Time on C – Total Time on B)	73.0	23.1	32.0–142.0

M Age = 68.9 Years; SD = 3.8 Years; N = 54; 23 M, 31 F.

Table 6.10. Stroop.7d

Measure	75+ Age Grouping		
	M	SD	Range
Number of Errors: Card A	0.6	2.1	0.0–16.0
Number of Errors: Card B	2.1	2.2	0.0–8.0
Number of Errors: Card C	3.2	4.7	0.0–29.0
Total Time(s): Card A	50.2	9.1	33.0–76.0
Total Time(s): Card B	77.6	19.0	44.0–133.0
Total Time(s): Card C	156.6	49.8	66.0–344.0
Color Difficulty Factor (Total Time on B/Total Time on A)	1.5	0.3	1.0–2.7
Interference Factor (Total Time on C – Total Time on B)	79.0	40.4	2.0–216.0

M Age = 80.7 Years; SD = 3.6 Years; N = 66; 38 M, 28 F.

stance abuse, or cardiovascular disease. Mean age for the whole sample was 30.17 ± 6.34 years; mean age of the males was 31.93 ± 5.26 years and for the females 29.19 ± 6.75 years. Mean educational level for the sample was 14.76 ± 2.24 years.

The Comalli stimulus cards and Kaplan administration procedures (i.e., color-naming, word reading, color interference) were employed to obtain Stroop data. Mean times in seconds and standard deviations are provided for each of the three cards. Errors and near-miss (i.e., self-corrected errors) responses were tabulated. Women demonstrated significantly better performance than men on cards 1 and 2. There was a similar trend noted on card 3.

Study strengths
1. Adequate exclusion criteria.
2. Information regarding gender, ethnicity, age, educational level, and geographic area.
3. Information regarding test stimuli and test administration procedures is provided.
4. Means and standard deviations for time in seconds, errors, and self-corrected errors is provided for each card.

Considerations regarding use of the study
1. Small sample size.
2. Undifferentiated age range.
3. High educational level of the sample.
4. No information regarding IQ (Table 6.11).

Control Groups in Clinical Studies

[STROOP.9] Comalli, Wapner and Werner, 1962 (Comalli Version)

These authors provide data (on the Comalli Stroop version) for 235 subjects aged 7 to 80 apparently in Massachusetts as a part of their study of the effects of aging on the Stroop task. For the purposes of this review the data on the 63 adult subjects will be reported. The adult subjects were divided into four age groupings: 17–19 (n = 18), 25–34 (n = 14), 35–44 (n = 16), 65–80 (n = 15). The 17- to 19-year-olds were undergraduate students, the 25-to-34- and 35-to-44-year-old groups were drawn from an evening college, and the 65–80-year-old group was drawn from a community old-age club.

Mean time in seconds for each card are charted in a graph for each age group; no standard deviations are provided.

Table 6.11. Stroop.8

	Time	Errors	Near-Misses
Color-naming	59.26 ± 17.57	0.43 ± 0.74	1.28 ± 1.29
Word reading	43.62 ± 7.17	0.24 ± 0.53	0.50 ± 0.67
Color interference	109.98 ± 23.42	1.05 ± 1.82	2.74 ± 2.07

Study strengths

1. Data presented in narrow age groupings.
2. Good description of test stimuli and administration procedures.
3. Information on geographic recruitment area.
4. Mean time in seconds reported.

Considerations regarding use of the study

1. No exclusion criteria.
2. No information regarding gender or IQ, and cursory data on educational level is only provided for the 17–19-year-olds.
3. Small individual cell sizes.
4. No standard deviations reported (Table 6.12).

[STROOP.10] Dodrill, 1978a
(Dodrill Version)

Dodrill collected control data on 50 subjects in the state of Washington as a part of his investigation of the cognitive correlates of epilepsy. Thirty were male and 20 were female, and mean age and educational level were 27.34 ± 8.41 and 11.96 ± 2.01, respectively. Forty-nine were Caucasian with one listed as non-Caucasian. Nine were students, six were housewives, 20 were unemployed, and 15 were employed. Subjects were recruited through employment facilities, churches, a community college, a public high school, a volunteer service agency, and semisheltered workshop. Subjects underwent a detailed neurological history and subjects with diseases or other conditions affecting the nervous system were excluded.

The Dodrill version of the Stroop was administered. Means and standard deviations are reported for time in seconds to complete part I and part II. In addition, means and standard deviations are provided for part I + part II, and part II minus part I. Using a cutoff of 93/94 seconds on part I, 70% of controls were correctly

Table 6.13. Stroop.10

Part I	88.62 ± 17.23
Part II	225.80 ± 59.44
Part I + part II	314.32 ± 71.04
Part II − part I	137.18 ± 50.74

classified. A cutoff of 150/151 seconds for part II minus part I resulted in a 74% correct classification rate.

Study strengths

1. Adequate sample size ($n = 50$).
2. Information on age, education, gender, occupation, geographic area, ethnicity, and recruitment procedures is provided.
3. Test stimuli and procedures are specified.
4. Mean time in seconds and standard deviations are reported.

Considerations regarding use of the study

1. No information on IQ.
2. Apparently adequate exclusion criteria although some controls were recruited from sheltered workshops.
3. Undifferentiated age range (Table 6.13).

[STROOP.11] Eson, Personal
Communication (Comalli Version)

Eson provides Stroop data on 63 older subjects in four age groupings reflecting the following mean ages: 63.2 ($n = 15$), 67.0 ($n = 16$), 72.0 ($n = 16$), and 78.3 ($n = 16$).

The Comalli test stimuli and administration procedures were utilized. Means and standard deviations are reported.

Study strengths

1. Large overall sample size, and while individual cell sizes are small, these *n*s are for very restricted age ranges.
2. Test stimuli and administration procedures specified.
3. Mean time in seconds and standard deviations are reported.

Considerations regarding use of the study

1. No information on exclusion criteria, education, gender, IQ, or other characteristics (Table 6.14).

Table 6.12. Stroop.9

	Age Groupings			
	17–19	25–34	35–44	65–80
Word reading	40.5	39.4	42.6	45.1
Color-naming	56.1	60.9	57.9	68.9
Color interference	103.0	106.2	109.9	165.1

Table 6.14. Stroop.11

	Ages			
	63.2	67.0	72.0	78.3
Stroop A	46.9 ± 11.4	51.8 ± 18.6	53.4 ± 20.3	67.9 ± 23.3
Stroop B	64.9 ± 16.2	71.2 ± 18.4	71.6 ± 20.4	83.9 ± 20.3
Stroop C	148.9 ± 45.2	165.2 ± 59.2	177.4 ± 63.8	231.1 ± 72.2

[STROOP.12] Stuss, Ely, Hugenholtz, Richard, LaRochelle, Poirier, and Bell, 1985 (Comalli Version)

These authors collected Stroop data on 20 control subjects (13 male, seven female) in Canada as a part of their investigation of the neuropsychological effects of closed head injury. Subjects spoke either English or French. Mean age was 29.2 ± 12.0, mean years of education was 12.5 ± 2.0, and mean WAIS IQ was 106.6 ± 13.4. Subjects were paid $15 for their participation.

The Comalli test stimuli and administration procedures were employed. Means and standard deviations for time in seconds to name colors is reported. (Data from the two other trials are not provided.) Performance on color-naming was significantly depressed in the head injury group relative to controls; groups did not differ in word reading or color interference.

Study strengths

1. Data provided on gender, age, education, IQ, language, and geographic area.
2. Test stimuli and administration procedures are specified.
3. Mean and standard deviation for time to name colors is reported.

Considerations regarding use of the study

1. No information on exclusion criteria.
2. Data were collected in Canada with at least some subjects French-speaking; cultural and linguistic factors may limit usefulness for clinical interpretive purposes in the United States.
3. Data from the word reading and color interference trials are not reported.

Table 6.15. Stroop.12

Color Naming	64.0 ± 12.9

4. Small sample size.
5. Undifferentiated age range (Table 6.15).

[STROOP.13] Connor, Franzen, and Sharp, 1988 (Golden Version)

Stroop data were obtained on 40 college student volunteers in West Virginia (17 male, 23 female) who ranged in age from 18 to 25 with the exception of one 32-year-old.

The Golden version of the Stroop was administered with either standard instructions as detailed in the test manual or standard instructions plus six suggestions ("looking at no more than three words at a time; focusing on only one letter in the word; remembering that the same color never occurs twice consecutively; going at an even steady pace; trying not to become distracted or lose one's place; and not repeating an already-correct answer when correcting a mistake").

Subjects were administered the Stroop at baseline (pretest), following five practice sessions (post-test) and at a 1-week follow-up.

No effect of gender or instruction format was documented. A significant effect of practice was found between the pre- and post-test, but not between the post-test and follow-up.

Data are presented in means and standard deviations for number of items completed for the pre-, post-, and follow-up sessions.

Study strengths

1. Information on the effects of practice, sex, and alternative instructions on Stroop performance is provided.
2. Information on age, gender, and geographic area, with some information on education and recruitment procedures, is reported.
3. Test stimuli and procedures are specified.
4. Data are presented in means and standard deviations for number of items completed.

Table 6.16. Stroop.13

	Pre-Test	Post-Test	Follow-Up
Word	113.52 ± 14.72	123.22 ± 19.28	130.87 ± 17.00
Color	81.22 ± 9.38	93.80 ± 16.85	99.18 ± 14.67
Color-word	49.75 ± 7.53	70.62 ± 15.74	75.07 ± 16.30

Considerations regarding use of the study
1. Relatively small sample size.
2. Undifferentiated age range although it is somewhat restricted.
3. No information on exclusion criteria or IQ.
4. Data are not broken down by sex or education (Table 6.16).

[STROOP.14] Boone, Miller, Lesser, Hill-Gutierrez, and D'Elia, 1990 (Comalli Version)

Data were collected on 61 middle-aged and older individuals ranging in age from 50 to 79 recruited as controls in Southern California through newspaper ads, flyers, and personal contacts as a part of study of the effect of aging on executive abilities. Subjects had no history of psychotic, major affective, or alcohol and other drug dependence disorder and spoke English fluently (a handful of subjects spoke English as a second language). Subjects were excluded if there was a history of physical findings of neurologic disease, such as stroke, Parkinson's disease, or seizure disorder. Also excluded were individuals with laboratory findings showing serious metabolic abnormalities (e.g., low sodium level, elevated glucose level, or thyroid or liver function abnormalities). Eighteen percent of the original sample of 74 were eventually excluded due to the presence of previously unidentified strokes or other significant lesions documented on magnetic resonance imaging (MRI) ($n = 9$), metabolic abnormalities or undiagnosed medical illness ($n = 2$), or evidence from laboratory studies and electroencephalografy (EEG) findings of alcohol abuse and substance intoxication ($n = 2$). The final sample ($n = 61$) included 25 men and 36 women grouped by three age decades: 50–59 ($n = 25$), 60–69 ($n = 21$), and 70–79 ($n = 15$). All but 10 subjects were white: Four were African-American, three were Asian, and three were Hispanic.

Mean educational level was 14.34 ± 2.63 and mean WAIS-R FSIQ was 113.79 ± 13.51.

The Comalli version of the Stroop was administered (i.e., word reading, color naming, and color interference). Mean time in seconds, as well as number of errors, with standard deviations, is presented by age grouping for each card. A significant decline with age was observed for word reading and color naming, with a trend toward a decline with age on color interference.

Study strengths
1. Overall sample size is large although the individual cell sizes are small.
2. Data are presented by age groupings.
3. Good exclusion criteria.
4. Information regarding gender, educational level, IQ, geographic area, ethnicity, fluency in English, and recruitment procedures is provided.
5. Test stimuli and procedures are specified.
6. Means and standard deviations are reported for both time and errors.

Considerations regarding use of the study
1. The sample size within each age group interval is small (see 1 above).
2. High educational and IQ levels of the sample (Table 6.17).

[STROOP.15] Fisher, Freed, and Corkin, 1990 (Golden Version)

The authors collected Stroop data on 36 older controls (typically spouses of patients) from Southern California as a part of investigation of Stroop performance in Alzheimer's disease. Mean age was 72.9 ± 8.3, mean educational level was 14.6 ± 2.7, and mean Blessed Dementia Scale score was 1.5 ± 6.1. The sample included 13 males and 23 females. Subjects had no history (as judged through medical records) of color blindness, cataracts, or glaucoma.

Table 6.17. Stroop.14

	Age Groupings		
	50–59	60–69	70–79
Word Reading			
Time	40.25 ± 4.95	46.05 ± 9.02	44.07 ± 6.39
Errors	0.42 ± 0.72	0.55 ± 1.15	0.40 ± 0.63
Color Naming			
Time	57.75 ± 9.74	63.30 ± 8.25	74.27 ± 17.16
Errors	2.00 ± 2.11	1.55 ± 1.99	2.00 ± 2.27
Color Interference			
Time	120.79 ± 38.07	135.50 ± 29.81	148.67 ± 41.09
Errors	1.75 ± 1.42	2.20 ± 2.12	1.60 ± 1.50

The Golden Stroop Test stimuli and administration procedures were employed. Means and standard deviations are reported for number of items completed on each trial.

Some subjects (five female, three male) had difficulty discriminating between the colors blue and green on the color trial.

Study strengths

1. Data presented in homogenous age grouping.

2. Information is given regarding mean age, mean educational level, gender, mean Blessed Dementia Scale score, geographic area, and recruitment procedures.

3. Information is given on test stimuli and administration procedures.

4. Means and standard deviations reported for number of items completed.

5. Test administration format was described.

Considerations regarding use of the study

1. Relatively small sample size.

2. No information regarding IQ.

3. High educational level of the sample.

4. Unclear exclusion critera (Table 6.18).

[STROOP.16] Boone, Ananth, Philpott, Kaur, and Djenderedjian, 1991 (Comalli Version)

Stroop data were collected on 16 controls as a part of a study on the neuropsychological characteristics of obsessive-compulsive disorder (OCD). Subjects were recruited in Southern California from newspaper advertisements and from siblings (n = 9) of OCD patients. Medical exclusion criteria included history of alcohol or drug abuse, head injury, seizure disorder, cerebral vascular disease or stroke, current or past psychiatric disorder, or any renal, hepatic, or pulmonary disease. Subjects included nine women and seven men, and 19% were left-handed (n = 3). Fourteen were Caucasian and two were Asian and all were fluent in English. Two subjects had a history of learning disability. Mean age was 35.8 ± 13.7, mean educational level was 15.2 ± 2.8, and mean WAIS-R FSIQ was 109.1 ± 10.9.

The Comalli version of the Stroop (i.e., word reading, color-naming, color interference) was administered. Mean and standard deviation for time in seconds to complete the color-interference portion of the test is provided. Controls and patients did not differ in test performance.

Study strengths

1. Good exclusion criteria with the exception that two subjects had histories of learning disability.

2. Information regarding age, education, FSIQ, gender, handedness, fluency in English, ethnicity, recruitment procedures, and geographic area is reported.

Table 6.18. Stroop.15

Word	96.6 ± 15.8
Color	64.9 ± 13.9
Color-word	33.4 ± 10.8
Interference scores	−5.2 ± 8.6

Table 6.19. Stroop.16

Color interference	112.9 ± 22.5

3. Information on test stimuli and administration procedures.

4. Mean time in seconds and standard deviation are provided but only for the color-interference card.

Considerations regarding use of the study
1. Small sample size.
2. Undifferentiated age range.
3. High educational level and two subjects had a history of learning disability.
4. No data reported for word reading and color-naming trials (Table 6.19).

[STROOP.17] Sacks, Clark, Pols, and Geffen, 1991 (Dodrill Version)

Stroop data were obtained on 12 male university student volunteers in Australia, ranging in age from 18 to 32 (averaging 22.4 ± 5 years) as a part of development of five alternate forms of the Dodrill Stroop. All subjects had normal vision (20:20 as tested with a standard Snellen wall chart) and no evidence of color blindness (as assessed through Ishihara charts). Subjects averaged 13.7 ± 2.3 years of education. Mean abbreviated WAIS-R FSIQ, VIQ, and PIQ were 109.1 ± 9.5 (range = 100–124), 108.4 ± 8.7 (range = 100–124), and 106.6 ± 7.1 (range = 97–120), respectively.

The exact procedures used to develop the alternate forms are specified. All subjects were administered all six forms of the test in 1 day with a 50-minute rest period between trials on each form. Order of completion of the six forms was randomized. Subjects were halted at each error and instructed to correct the mistake before proceeding. Means and standard deviations for time in seconds are reported for each form. The forms were judged to be equivalent, although a significant practice

effect was still present between the first and second test administrations. Sets of the six alternate forms are available from the test authors.

Study strengths
1. Data provided on six alternate forms and practice effects.
2. Information reported on education, gender, IQ, vision, age, and geographic area.
3. Test stimuli development and administration procedures are carefully described.
4. Means and standard deviations for time in seconds are reported for each form.

Considerations regarding use of the study
1. Small sample size (n = 12).
2. All-male sample.
3. Data collected in Australia; cultural differences may render the data questionable for clinical interpretive use in the United States.
4. No exclusion criteria (Table 6.20).

[STROOP.18] Daigneault, Braun, and Whitaker, 1992 (Golden Version)

Stroop data were obtained on 128 French-speaking subjects in Canada as a part of a study investigating the effects of aging on prefrontal lobe skills. Subjects were recruited through ads, trade union collaboration, and the help of a large sports center. Exclusion criteria included consumption of more than 24 beers, 5 bottles of wine, or 15 ounces of spirits per week; consumption of cocaine, LSD, or psychostimulants; any neurological of psychiatric consultation, psychoactive medication, head trauma with hospitalization, or major surgery (e.g., cardiac). Subjects were divided into two age groupings: 20 to 35 (mean = 27.71 ± 4.05, n = 70) and 45 to 65 (mean = 56.62 ± 5.29, n = 58). The younger group contained 38 men and 32 women; they were primarily specialized blue-collar workers although some specialized white-collar and unskilled blue-collar

Table 6.20. Stroop.17

Dodrill form	Alternate Forms				
	1	2	3	4	5
72.6 ± 18.2	63.7 ± 13.4	68.8 ± 21.0	68.6 ± 13.3	67.4 ± 18.1	66.0 ± 18.0

professions were represented. The older group contained 30 men and 28 women, and slightly more than half were specialized blue-collar workers but some unskilled blue collar professions, specialized white-collar occupations, and professional occupations were represented. The mean educational level of the younger group was 12.36 ± 2.09 and the mean educational level of the older group was 12.11 ± 3.63.

The Golden (1978) version of the Stroop Test was employed. Mean number of items completed and standard deviations for the color-interference portion of the test are reported. The two age groups differed significantly in test performance, with the younger group outperforming the older group.

Study strengths
1. Good exclusion criteria.
2. Large overall sample size and the two age groupings each have more than 50 subjects.
3. Information regarding educational level, gender, occupations, geographic area, and recruitment procedures.
4. Information on the test stimuli and administration procedures.
5. Means and standard deviations for number of items completed on part C provided.

Considerations regarding use of the study
1. Data were obtained on French-speaking subjects in Canada, and thus it is unclear whether these data are appropriate for clinical interpretive use on English-speaking subjects in the United States.
2. No information regarding IQ (although mean scores on the vocabulary subtest of the French language WAIS analog are reported).
3. No data provided for the first two sections of the Stroop Test.
4. Test administration format may have been altered (i.e., subjects appeared to scan the stimulus cards across rows from left to right) (Table 6.21).

Table 6.21. Stroop.18

	Young Group	Old Group
Color interference	48.80 ± 8.63	37.87 ± 7.67

[STROOP.19] D'Elia, Satz, and Uchiyama, Unpublished Data (Kaplan Version)

These data were collected in 1993 and 1994 during the course of an FAA/EEOC-mandated study to examine neuropsychological functioning of airline pilots. The sample consisted of 197 male, Caucasian, airline pilots aged 40 to 59 employed by major airplane manufacturers in the United States. All pilots had recently passed their yearly comprehensive FAA physical examination. Data are presented in two age groupings: 40–49 ($n = 118$) and 50–59 ($n = 79$). The 40–49-year-old group had an average of 16.1 ± 1.9 years of education, and the 50–59-year-old group had 15.6 ± 2.0 years of education.

The Comalli cards and Kaplan administration procedures (i.e., color-naming, word reading, color interference) were used to obtain Stroop data on the pilots as part of a 55-minute neuropsychological screening battery. Means and standard deviations for time in seconds, errors, and near-miss (i.e., self-corrected) errors are provided.

Study strengths
1. Overall sample size is large and individual cell sizes exceed *n*s of 50.
2. Data are presented by age groupings.
3. Adequate exclusion criteria.
4. Information regarding gender, educational level, recruitment procedures, ethnicity, and occupation, and some information regarding geographic region.
5. Test stimuli and procedures are indicated.
6. Means and standard deviations for time and near-miss (i.e., self-corrected) errors are provided.

Considerations regarding use of the study
1. All-male sample.
2. High educational level of the sample.
3. No information regarding IQ (Table 6.22).

[STROOP.20] Selnes and Miller, Personal Communication (Kaplan Version)

Baseline Stroop data were collected on a sample of 482 HIV-negative gay and bisexual males aged 30–49 with greater-than-high-school

Table 6.22. Stroop.19

	Age Groupings	
	40-49	50-59
Color-Naming		
Time	60.0 ± 10.2	63.9 ± 15.7
Near-misses	0.63 ± 1.0	0.33 ± 0.63
Errors	0.39 ± 0.67	0.39 ± 0.67
Word Reading		
Time	45.8 ± 8.8	47.2 ± 9.1
Near-misses	0.18 ± 0.41	0.28 ± 0.58
Errors	0.26 ± 0.52	0.20 ± 0.49
Color Interference		
Time	105.7 ± 21.4	112.4 ± 22.6
Near-misses	0.72 ± 1.4	0.94 ± 1.7
Errors	0.70 ± 1.1	0.95 ± 1.8

education who served as controls in an ongoing, multicenter epidemiological study of HIV-1 infection known as the Multi-Center AIDS Cohort Study (MACS). Subjects for this report were recruited in Los Angeles. Exclusion criteria included English as second language, history of head trauma with a loss of consciousness lasting more than 1 hour, or a history of drinking, on average, more than 21 drinks per week in the preceding 6 months. Over 90% of the sample was non-Hispanic Caucasian.

The Comalli stimulus card and Kaplan administration procedures (i.e., color-naming, word reading, and color interference) were used to obtain Stroop Test data. Means and standard deviations for time in seconds to complete each card are reported in two-age (30–39, 40–49)-by-three-education (13–15 years, 16 years, >16 years) groupings.

Study strengths

1. Very large sample size and individual cells generally exceed *ns* of 50.
2. Data presented by age and education groupings.
3. Information regarding geographic areas, ethnicity, sexual orientation, gender, and fluency in English.
4. Minimally adequate exclusion criteria.
5. Test stimuli and test administration procedures are specified.

6. Mean time in seconds and standard deviations are reported.

Considerations regarding use of the study

1. All-male sample.
2. Generally highly educated sample.
3. No information regarding IQ (Table 6.23).

[STROOP.21] Boone, In Press (Comalli Version)

The author obtained Stroop data on 155 middle-aged and older individuals (ranging in age from 45 to 84) recruited as described in the Boone et al. (1990) publication; data from the 1990 study were included in the 1998 publication. The mean age of the sample was 63.07 ± 9.29, mean educational level was 14.57 ± 2.55, and mean WAIS-R FSIQ was 115.41 ± 14.11. Fifty-three were male and 102 were female. Medical and psychiatric exclusion criteria are the same as in the 1990 publication with the exception that subjects with significant white-matter hyperintensities documented on MRI were retained in the sample. All subjects considered themselves healthy although 51 subjects had some evidence of vascular illness (defined as cardiovascular disease and/or significant white-matter hyperintensities on MRI) based on self-report or evidence on examination of at least one of the following: current or past history of hypertension ($n = 39$), arrhyth-

Table 6.23. Stroop.20

	Color-Naming	Word Reading	Interference
Age 30–39			
13–15 years education (n = 64)	59.19 ± 11.45	45.59 ± 9.58	110.39 ± 25.15
College degree (n = 93)	53.68 ± 9.32	41.26 ± 6.84	98.14 ± 22.20
>16 years education (n = 95)	52.62 ± 9.64	39.48 ± 6.09	97.59 ± 21.67
Age 40–49			
13–15 years education (n = 49)	56.14 ± 8.36	43.88 ± 7.62	110.33 ± 23.15
College degree (n = 65)	57.15 ± 11.70	43.15 ± 7.94	106.02 ± 24.04
>16 years education (n = 116)	54.96 ± 9.27	41.06 ± 7.22	103.75 ± 23.17

mia (n = 8), large area of white-matter hyperintensities on MRI (e.g., >10 cm^2; n = 7), coronary artery bypass graft (n = 3), angina (n =2), and old myocardial infarction (n =1). Twenty-four subjects were currently on cardiac and/or antihypertensive medications.

The Comalli version of the Stroop was administered. Mean and standard deviations for time in seconds to complete the color-interference portion of the test are provided. A stepwise regression analysis revealed that age and FSIQ were significant contributors to Stroop color-interference performance, accounting for 15% and 13%, respectively, of test score variance; educational level, gender, and vascular status did not account for a significant amount of unique test score variance. Stroop normative data are presented for color-interference time in seconds stratified by IQ and age (< age 65 and ≥ age 65, and average IQ, high average, and ≥ superior IQ).

Study strengths

1. Large overall sample size.
2. Presentation of the data by IQ and age groupings.
3. Comprehensive medical and psychiatric exclusion criteria including MRI brain scans on all subjects.
4. Information regarding educational level, gender, geographic area, recruitment procedures, and fluency in English.
5. Mean times in seconds and standard deviations for color interference reported.
6. Test administration format specified.

Considerations regarding use of the study

1. The individual IQ by age groupings have *n*s ranging from 16 to 37.
2. High IQ and educational level of the sample.
3. No data reported for word reading and color-naming trials (Table 6.24).

Table 6.24. Stroop.21

	Average IQ	High Average IQ	≥Superior IQ
< age 65	132.64 ± 34.51 (n = 33)	128.65 ± 26.87 (n = 23)	110.29 ± 22.37 (n = 35)
≥ age 65	164.65 ± 51.90 (n = 20)	153.75 ± 56.99 (n = 16)	137.08 ± 33.14 (n = 24)

CONCLUSIONS

The Stroop has a lengthy history as an experimental measure in psychological studies and more recently has been adapted for clinical neuropsychological use. However, the plethora of test stimuli and administration formats has been confusing. Compilation of the data sets suggests that the Kaplan version has the largest sample ($n = 1,724$), followed by the Golden ($n = 560+$), Comalli ($n = 317$), Trenerry ($n = 156$), Victoria ($n = 126$), and Dodrill ($n = 62$) versions. However, within the datasets there are problems regarding representation of age groups:

1. There does not appear to be any data on the Victoria version for subjects aged 36 to 49.

2. There does not appear to be any data on the Dodrill version for subjects older than age 40.

3. It is unclear whether there is any Golden version normative data on English-speaking subjects less than age 56.

4. There is a paucity of data on the Comalli version for subjects less than 45 years of age.

5. The Trenerry data were lumped into two large age groupings (18 to 49, 50 to 59) which are of limited clinical use.

Examination of the means across Kaplan and Comalli studies suggests that there is no difference in performance of controls on the two administration versions, raising the possibility that these two normative datasets can be used interchangeably. This would increase the total Kaplan/Comalli sample size to 2,041 and would remedy the lack of data on younger subjects in the Comalli version. Future research is needed to determine whether the Kaplan administration format elicits a more pronounced color-interference effect in clinical groups; it does not appear to have this effect in normals, as observed here.

One difficulty in interpreting Stroop scores has been how to partial out the effect of slowed information processing, as reflected in lowered scores on the first sections of the Stroop, from color-interference performance to obtain a more "pure" measure of executive dysfunction. Some authors have utilized difference scores (Demick & Harkins, 1997; Dodrill, 1978a; Jensen, 1965) although this approach has been questioned (Koss et al., 1984; Trenerry et al., 1989). Koss and colleagues (1984) recommend an analysis of covariance model, and Jensen and Rohwer (1966) report 16 different methods for relating individual Stroop scores. Future research is needed to determine if there is a more effective approach to Stroop interpretation than the typical independent analysis of individual Stroop scores.

7

Auditory Consonant Trigrams

BRIEF HISTORY OF THE TEST

The Auditory Consonant Trigram Test (ACT), also referred to as the Brown-Peterson Consonant Trigram Memory Task or CCC (Stuss, 1987), which is a variant of the Peterson and Peterson technique (Milner, 1970, 1972; Samuels et al., 1972), was originally developed as an experimental verbal memory procedure (Brown, 1958; Peterson & Peterson, 1959). The ACT is sensitive both to deficits in short-term auditory verbal memory (the ability to recall rote verbal information over a distractor; Milner, 1970, 1972; Samuels et al., 1972) and divided attention/working memory (amount of information which can be processed simultaneously; Fleming et al., 1995; Marie et al., 1995; Stuss et al., 1985; Stuss et al., 1987). Individuals with memory impairment associated with left temporal lobe damage have been found to perform poorly on this task (Giovagnoli & Avanzini, 1996; Milner, 1970, 1972; Samuels et al., 1972), but in the absence of a significant verbal memory deficit, poor performance on this measure may also be associated with frontal system dysfunction secondary to closed head injury (Stuss et al., 1985), discrete frontal lobe lesions (Stuss et al., 1992), white-matter hyperintensities (Boone et al., 1992), Korsakoff syndrome (Cermak & Butters, 1972; Leng & Parkin, 1989), schizophrenia (Fleming et al., 1995), and Parkinson's disease (Marie et al., 1995). The impaired test performance of both the memory-dysfunctional patients and patients with frontal system defects may lie in susceptibility to proactive interference; in the former group the impairment may stem from verbal encoding deficits, while in the latter group the difficulty may be due to vulnerability to interfering stimuli which disrupts sustained attention (Stuss et al., 1992). For further information regarding Auditory Consonant Trigrams and its variants, please refer to Lezak (1995, pp. 432–434).

Administration Procedures

The ACT involves the auditory presentation of three consonant trigrams followed by a number. The patient is instructed to subtract 3's from the number for several seconds, after which he/she is asked to recall the letters. The exact administration instructions and test stimuli used by Dr. Stuss and colleagues at Ottawa General Hospital are contained in Appendix 2 and those used by Boone and colleagues at Harbor-UCLA Medical Center are contained in Appendix 3. Some examiners use counting intervals of 3, 9, and 18 seconds (Boone et al., 1990, 1992; Boone, in press; Cermak & Butters, 1972; Corsi, 1969 as reported in Milner, 1972; Samuels et al., 1972), while other investigators have lengthened the subtraction times to 9, 18, and 36 seconds to increase task difficulty and reduce ceiling effects (Stuss et al., 1987).

RELATIONSHIP BETWEEN ACT PERFORMANCE, DEMOGRAPHIC FACTORS, AND VASCULAR STATUS

Relatively few studies are available on the impact of demographic factors and IQ on ACT performance.

A recent examination of the unique contribution of IQ and demographic factors to ACT performance in a large sample of healthy, older subjects found that FSIQ accounted for 17% of unique test score variance while age accounted for a significant but very modest amount (6%) of unique test score variance; gender and educational level did not contribute to test performance (Boone, in press). The remaining literature on the relationship between ACT performance and age has been equivocal, with some investigators failing to detect an association (Boone et al., 1990; Puckett & Lawson, 1989; Stuss et al., 1987), while other studies have documented some deterioration with increasing age (Inman & Parkinson, 1983; Parkin & Walter, 1991; Parkinson et al., 1985; Schonfield et al., 1983). No other literature aside from the Boone (in press) publication could be located on the impact of IQ on ACT scores. A single other study found no contribution of educational level or gender to ACT performance (Stuss et al., 1987).

Of interest, there is some evidence that some medical conditions previously thought to be cognitively benign may lead to decrements in performance on the ACT Test. Specifically, the presence of cerebrovascular risk factors (e.g., hypertension, post-MI (myocardial infarction), cardiovascular disease, arrhythmias, coronary artery bypass graft, angina, old myocardial infarction, white-matter hyperintensities) accounts for 3% of ACT test score variance (Boone, in press), and once a threshold amount of total white-matter hyperintensity volume is detected on MRI (i.e., greater than 10 cm^2), significant declines are detected in ACT performance (Boone et al., 1992). In fact, the ACT test may be one of the most sensitive cognitive tests to the presence of white-matter damage sustained through hyperintensities of probable vascular origin (Boone et al., 1992) or white-matter and/or frontal-limbic-reticular activating system disruption secondary to acceleration–deceleration closed head injury (Stuss et al., 1985).

METHOD FOR EVALUATING THE NORMATIVE REPORTS

Our review of the literature located two ACT normative reports published since 1987 (Stuss et al., 1987; Stuss et al., 1988) as well as data from two studies examining the impact of age, education, IQ, gender, and medical illness on ACT performance (Boone et al., 1990; Boone, in press) and which included unique features such as large sample size (Boone, in press) and reporting of a wide range of ACT scores (Boone et al., 1990).

In order to adequately evaluate the ACT normative reports, six key criterion variables were deemed critical. The first four of these relate to subject variables, and the remaining two dimensions relate to procedural variables.

Minimal criteria for meeting the criterion variables were as follows:

Subject Variables

IQ-Group Intervals

Given the evidence that IQ may account for more unique test score variance than do demographic factors, ACT data should preferably be presented in IQ intervals.

Sample Size

As discussed in previous chapters, a minimum of at least 50 subjects per group interval is optimal.

Reporting of Age

Given the equivocal modest relationship between age and ACT performance, ACT normative data probably do not need to be presented by age-group intervals, but information on the ages of the normative samples should be provided.

Sample Composition Description

Given the evidence that ACT performance may be significantly impacted by medical status (e.g., vascular illness), information regarding medical exclusion criteria is critical. In addition, as discussed previously, information should probably also be provided regarding educational level, gender, psychiatric exclusion criteria, geographic region, ethnicity, occupation, handedness, and recruitment procedures even though there is not yet any data indicating that these factors influence test performance.

Procedural Variables

Description of the Administration Format Used

Given that different test administration formats involving differing lengths of distraction intervals, specific information regarding the delays should be provided.

Data Reporting

Means and standard deviations, and, preferably, ranges, for total score out of 60 are important. In addition, it is advantageous for data to be provided for each of the distraction intervals separately.

SUMMARY OF THE STATUS OF THE NORMS

In terms of subject variables, only one study provides data by IQ level (Boone, in press), although IQ data are reported in a second study (Boone et al., 1990).

Information on age, gender, educational level, geographic area, and recruitment procedures is reported for all studies. In addition, medical, psychiatric, neurologic, and substance abuse exclusion criteria are described and judged to be adequate for all studies. Ethnic composition was described in only one study (Boone et al., 1990), and handedness data were only provided in the investigations conducted by Stuss and colleagues (Stuss et al., 1987, 1988). While all studies exceeded a total sample size of 50, no study reached the criterion of 50 subjects per individual grouping cells.

In terms of procedural variables, information is available regarding the precise administration formats for all studies. Means and standard deviations are reported for total score in all studies, and means and standard deviations for individual distractor delays are provided in all but one study (Boone, in press). Practice effects are investigated in the reports by Stuss and colleagues (Stuss et al., 1987, 1988), and data on qualitative performance variables (perseverations, errors in letter sequence) are provided in the Boone et al. (1990) publication.

Table 7.1 summarizes information provided in the studies described in this chapter.

SUMMARIES OF THE STUDIES

Normative Reports

[ACT.1] Stuss, Stethem, and Poirier, 1987

ACT baseline and 1-week retest data were collected on 60 subjects in Canada recruited through employment agencies who were paid $10 for the two testing sessions. Subjects ranged in age from 16 to 69 with a mean of 39.6 ± 2.62. Years of education ranged from 8 to 20 with a mean of 14.5 ± 2.63. Thirty-three subjects were male and 27 were female. Forty-nine were right-handed. None had a history of significant medical, neurological, or psychiatric disorder; substance abuse; or current psychotropic medication use.

Subjects were tested in their native language (English or French). Each three-consonant combination was presented at a rate of one consonant per second followed by a three-digit number. Subjects were instructed to count backwards by 3's from the number for random delays of 9, 18, and 36 seconds and then required to recall the trigram. Practice trials were employed until the subjects demonstrated understanding of the procedures. Five trials were conducted for each delay interval, with intertrial delays of 2 to 5 seconds. The counting delays were extended from those employed by Cermak and Butters (1972) to minimize ceiling effects. A total score of 15 was possible per each of the three delays. An alternate form was employed on retesting.

Test performance was not impacted by age, educational level, or gender. A practice effect

Table 7.1. ACT.L; Locator Table for the Auditory Consonant Trigrams Test

Study[*]	Age[**]	N	Sample Composition	IQ,[**] Education	Country/ Location
ACT.1 Stuss et al., 1987 page 103	16-19 20-29 30-39 40-49 50-59 60-69	60 10 10 10 10 10 10	Data presented by age, gender, and education groups; 33 male, 27 female; 49 right-handed; nonpsychiatric, nonneurologic, no substance abuse	Educ. 14.5 (2.63)	Canada
ACT.2 Stuss et al., 1988 page 105	16-29 30-49 50-69	90 30 30 30	Data presented by age groups; 44 male, 46 female; 76 righthanded; nonpsychiatric, nonneurologic		Canada
ACT.3 Boone et al., 1990 page 106	50-59 60-69 70-79	61 25 21 15	Data presented by age groups; 25 men, 36 women; all but 10 white; nonpsychiatric, nonneurologic, no substance abuse, no major medical condition	Educ. 14.34 (2.63) IQ 113.8 (13.5)	California
ACT.4 Boone, in press page 107	<65, average IQ High average IQ superior IQ ≥65, average IQ High average IQ superior IQ	155 32 23 37 20 16 23	Data presented by IQ and age groups; 53 male, 102 female; no substance abuse, nonpsychiatric, nonneurologic	Educ. 14.6 (2.6) IQ 115.4 (14.1)	California

[*]The study number corresponds to the number provided in the text of the chapter.

[**]Age column and IQ/education column contain information regarding range and/or mean and standard deviation for the whole sample and/or separate groups, whichever information is provided by the authors.

for the 9 and 18-second delays was observed despite the alternate form.

ACT data are provided by six age groupings (16–19, 20–29, 30–39, 40–49, 50–59, and 60–69) for baseline testing, retesting, and the two testing sessions combined for the three delay intervals separately. Data on sex distribution, handedness, mean age and standard deviation, and mean years of education, standard deviation, range, and frequency of ≤high school and >high school for each age grouping are provided. In addition, data are also presented by gender and educational level (≤high school, >high school), separately.

Study strengths

1. Information regarding age, education, gender, and handedness for the total sample and for individual age groupings.

2. Adequate exclusion criteria.

3. Information on practice effects.

4. Precise description of test administration procedures.

5. Data presented by age groupings, gender groupings, and education groupings.

6. Data presented separately for each distraction interval.

7. Information on geographic area and recruitment procedures.

Table 7.2. ACT.1a; Data Partitioned by Age Group

Delay Interval	Age Group					
	16–19	20–29	30–39	40–49	50–59	60–69
Combined Visits						
9 seconds	12.4	12.6	12.7	11.1	10.9	12.3
	(1.6)	(2.3)	(2.6)	(2.6)	(2.8)	(1.6)
18 seconds	12.0	12.2	12.6	11.0	10.5	11.2
	(2.1)	(2.7)	(2.8)	(2.5)	(3.2)	(1.8)
36 seconds	10.0	9.8	11.3	9.9	8.2	9.9
	(3.0)	(2.8)	(2.8)	(2.8)	(3.6)	(2.1)
First Visit						
9 seconds	11.8	12.2	12.8	11.0	10.9	12.2
	(1.9)	(2.5)	(1.8)	(2.8)	(2.5)	(1.6)
18 seconds	11.8	11.7	12.5	10.0	9.8	10.5
	(2.2)	(2.9)	(3.0)	(2.8)	(3.4)	(1.7)
36 seconds	9.9	8.7	11.0	8.7	8.2	10.0
	(2.3)	(3.3)	(2.5)	(3.4)	(3.1)	(1.8)
Second Visit (1 Week Later)						
9 seconds	13.0	13.0	12.6	11.2	11.0	12.3
	(1.4)	(2.0)	(3.5)	(2.5)	(3.0)	(1.7)
18 seconds	12.2	12.6	12.7	12.0	11.1	11.8
	(2.4)	(2.6)	(2.5)	(2.2)	(2.9)	(2.0)
36 seconds	10.1	10.9	11.5	11.0	8.2	9.8
	(3.6)	(2.3)	(3.0)	(2.1)	(4.1)	(2.4)

8. Means and standard deviations are reported.

Considerations regarding use of the study
1. Small individual cell sizes ($n = 10$).
2. Data collected in Canada with some test administrations conducted in French; cultural and linguistic factors may limit usefulness of data for clinical interpretation purposes in the United States.
3. No information regarding IQ level (Tables 7.2 and 7.3).

[ACT.2] Stuss, Stethem, and Pelchat, 1988

In this publication the authors supplement the data reported in 1987 by expanding the number of subjects, increasing cell sizes by collapsing the data from six to three age groupings (16–29, 30–49, and 50–69), and presenting the combined data from the two testing sessions in boxplots, which has the advantage of visual display of data variability. Each of three age groupings contained baseline and 1-week retest data on 30

subjects, none of whom had a positive psychiatric or neurologic history. Data are presented on sex distribution, handedness, mean age and standard deviation, and mean years of education, standard deviation, and range for each age group separately.

Study strengths
1. Large overall sample size ($n = 90$).
2. Information on practice effects.
3. Adequate exclusion criteria.
4. Information on gender, educational level, and handedness for each age grouping.
5. Presentation of test score variability via box plots.
6. Test administration format is the same as Stuss, Stethem, and Poirier (1987).
7. Means, standard deviations, and ranges are reported.

Considerations regarding use of the study
1. Same as above; although the sample has been increased by 50%, the three age groupings

Table 7.3. ACT.1b; Data Collapsed Across Age Groups Divided According to Sex and Educational Level

Delay Interval	Males	Females	≤ High School	> High School
9 seconds	11.71 (2.65)	12.35 (1.94)	11.46 (2.60)	12.44 (2.06)
18 seconds	11.17 (2.74)	12.04 (2.31)	11.13 (2.55)	11.91 (2.56)
36 seconds	9.20 (3.13)	10.61 (2.57)	9.32 (3.25)	10.26 (2.67)

still only have 30 subjects each (Tables 7.4 and 7.5).

Control Groups in Clinical Studies

[ACT.3] Boone, Miller, Lesser, Hill-Gutierez, and D'Elia, 1990

Data were collected on 61 middle-aged and older individuals ranging in age from 50 to 79 recruited as controls in Southern California through newspaper ads, flyers, and personal contacts as a part of ongoing research on late-life depression and psychosis. Subjects had no history of psychotic, major affective, or alcohol and other drug dependence disorder, and spoke English fluently. (A handful of subjects spoke English as a second language.) Subjects were excluded if there was a history of physical findings of neurologic disease, such as stroke, Parkinson's disease, or seizure disorder. Also excluded were individuals with laboratory findings showing serious metabolic abnormalities (e.g., low sodium level, elevated glucose level, or thyroid or liver function abnormalities). Eighteen percent of the original sample of 74 were eventually excluded due to the presence of previously unidentified strokes or other sig-

nificant lesions documented on MRI ($n = 9$), metabolic abnormalities or undiagnosed medical illness ($n = 2$), or evidence from laboratory studies and EEG findings of alcohol abuse and substance intoxication ($n = 2$). The final sample ($n = 61$) included 25 men and 36 women grouped by three age decades: 50–59 ($n = 25$), 60–69 ($n = 21$), and 70–79 ($n = 15$). All but 10 subjects were white; four were African-American, three were Asian, and three were Hispanic. Mean educational level was 14.34 ± 2.63 and mean WAIS-R FSIQ was 113.79 ± 13.51.

No significant effect of age on ACT performance was documented in comparisons of the three age groups.

Means and standard deviations are presented for ACT total score, as well as for 3-second delay, 9-second delay, and 18-second delay, for each age group separately. Total possible was 60 (15 points for each delay interval as well as 15 points for a five-trial zero-delay condition). Means and standard deviations are also reported for number of perseverations and altered sequences. A perseveration was defined as the reporting of an incorrect letter which was used as an answer on the preceding trial; a total of 57 perseverations were possible. Altered sequence referred to reporting of correct letters but in

Table 7.4. ACT.2a; Demographic Characteristics of the Three Groups

Group	N	Sex M	Sex F	Hand Preference R	Hand Preference L	Age (Years) M	Age (Years) SD	Education (Years) M	Education (Years) SD	Education (Years) Range
1	30	16	14	22	8	22.43	2.67	14.1	1.34	11–18
2	30	14	16	26	4	40.63	2.97	14.9	3.95	5–20
3	30	14	16	28	2	61.77	3.0	13.2	2.38	8–18

Table 7.5. ACT.2b; ACT Performance Across Three Age Groups for the Initial Test and the Retest 1 Week Later

| Delay Interval | Age Group | | | | | |
| | 16–29 | | 30–49 | | 50–69 | |
	Test	Retest	Test	Retest	Test	Retest
9 seconds	12.0	12.6	12.0	12.1	11.5	11.7
	(2.2)	(2.0)	(2.5)	(2.9)	(2.3)	(2.3)
18 seconds	11.4	12.3	10.5	12.0	10.2	10.7
	(2.8)	(2.4)	(3.1)	(2.6)	(2.5)	(2.9)
36 seconds	9.4	10.9	9.9	11.1	8.7	8.6
	(2.7)	(2.9)	(3.0)	(2.4)	(2.9)	(3.5)

the wrong position within the trigram; a total of 20 altered sequences were possible.

Study strengths

1. Information on IQ level, years of education, gender distribution, geographic area, recruitment procedures, ethnicity, and fluency in English.

2. Data reported in terms of total score but also by individual delay intervals; information also provided on perseverations and altered sequences.

3. Comprehensive medical and psychiatric exclusion criteria including MRI brain scans on all subjects.

4. Test administration format is described.

5. Means and standard deviations are reported.

Considerations regarding use of the study

1. Fairly small individual cell sizes (ns of 15 to 25) (Table 7.6).

[ACT.4] Boone, In Press

The author obtained ACT data on 155 middle-aged and older individuals (ranging in age from 45 to 84) recruited as described above; data from the 1990 study are included in the 1998 publication. The mean age of the sample was 63.07 ± 9.29, mean educational level was 14.57 ± 2.55, and mean FSIQ was 115.41 ± 14.11; 53 were male and 102 were female. Medical and psychiatric exclusion criteria are listed above with the exception that subjects with significant white-matter hyperintensities documented on MRI were retained in sample. All subjects considered themselves healthy although 51 subjects had some evidence of vascular illness (defined as cardiovascular disease and/or significant white-matter hyperintensities on MRI) based on self-report or evidence on examination of at least one of the following: current or past history of hypertension ($n = 39$), arrhythmia ($n = 8$), large area of white-matter hyperintensities on MRI (e.g., >10 cm^2; $n = 7$), coronary artery bypass graft ($n = 3$), angina ($n = 2$), and old myocardial infarction ($n = 1$). Twenty-four subjects were currently on cardiac and/or antihypertensive medications.

A stepwise regression analysis revealed that FSIQ, age, and vascular status were significant contributors to total ACT score, accounting for

Table 7.6. ACT.3; Data on ACT Performance for Three Age Groups

| | Age Group | | |
	50–59	60–69	70–79
Total	44.76 (7.36)	48.15 (8.02)	42.50 (7.70)
Perseverative errors	6.36 (3.81)	4.20 (2.78)	5.71 (2.87)
Altered sequence	2.00 (1.50)	1.85 (1.73)	2.71 (2.55)
3 seconds	12.56 (2.02)	12.95 (2.42)	11.21 (3.17)
9 seconds	9.44 (3.79)	10.75 (3.34)	8.93 (2.70)
18 seconds	8.20 (3.56)	9.65 (3.59)	7.50 (3.32)

Table 7.7. ACT.4; Data Presented in Age by WAIS-R IQ Groupings

	Average IQ (90–109)	High Average IQ (110–119)	>Superior IQ (120+)
< age 65	($n = 32$) 45.81 ± 6.05	($n = 23$) 45.91 ± 6.45	($n = 37$) 50.38 ± 8.01
≥ age 65	($n = 20$) 39.95 ± 9.99	($n = 16$) 43.31 ± 9.23	($n = 23$) 49.22 ± 6.02

17%, 6%, and 3% of test score variance, respectively; educational level and gender did not account for a significant amount of unique test score variance. ACT normative data are presented for total ACT score stratified by IQ and age (<age 65 and ≥age 65, and average IQ, high average, and ≥ superior IQ).

Study strengths

1. Large overall sample size.
2. Presentation of data by IQ and age groupings.
3. Comprehensive medical and psychiatric exclusion criteria including MRI brain scans on all subjects.
4. Information regarding educational level, gender, geographic area, recruitment procedures, and fluency in English.
5. Though not stated, test administration procedures are the same as those in Boone et al., 1990.
6. Means and standard deviations are reported.

Considerations regarding use of the study

1. The individual IQ-by-age groupings have *n*s ranging from 16 to 37.
2. Data are presented in terms of total score rather than separately for each distraction interval (Table 7.7).

CONCLUSIONS

The Auditory Consonant Trigram Test has been underutilized as a clinical measure of executive dysfunction despite evidence that it may be particularly sensitive to white-matter disturbance. Given emerging interest in working memory paradigms, the Consonant Trigrams task may experience an increase in popularity. Most working-memory paradigms have been used in experimental studies and normative data are typically not available. The fact that a normative data pool of upward of 240 subjects has been collected for Consonant Trigrams may make it an attractive working-memory procedure for clinical practice.

In addition, the fact that the Auditory Consonant Trigram task does not involve a timed response makes it a desirable executive measure in that test performance is not confounded by declines in mental speed. For tasks such as Trails B, Stroop Color Interference, and word and design generation, poor scores may reflect slowing in information processing speed rather than executive dysfunction per se.

Future research is needed to determine which delay intervals (i.e., 3, 9, and 18 seconds vs. 9, 18, and 36 seconds) are most sensitive and appropriate for clinical use. Also, normative data need to be obtained on populations with less than average IQs.

III
LANGUAGE

8

Boston Naming Test

BRIEF HISTORY OF THE TEST

The Boston Naming Test (BNT) is a test of confrontation naming consisting of simple line-drawn pictures. Its experimental version includes 85 drawings (Kaplan et al., 1978). The modified version of the BNT, published in 1983, includes 60 of the original 85 drawings, arranged in order of ascending difficulty (Kaplan et al., 1983). Subjects are allowed 20 seconds to name each item. Stimulus cues are offered to correct for misperception errors. They are followed by phonemic cues, which provide the first phonemes of the word, facilitating lexical retrieval. The total score on the test is the number of correct responses produced spontaneously and with the aid of stimulus cues. (For detailed administration and scoring instructions see Lezak, 1995; Spreen & Strauss, 1998; and instructions in the test stimulus booklet.)

The authors provided normative data on the 60-item version for children 5.5 to 10.5 years of age, broken down into six age groups based on five subjects in each group; for normal adults between ages 18 and 59 years of age, broken down into two educational groups and five age groups (based on a total of 84 subjects); and for 82 aphasic patients partitioned by aphasia severity level.

Thompson and Heaton (1989) and Heaton et al. (1991) reported high correlation between the 85-item and the 60-item versions ($r = 0.96$). However, the mean percent of correct responses was somewhat lower for the original version (85.1% vs. 87.8%) in their sample of clinical referrals for neuropsychological evaluation.

Studies Using BNT Error Quality Analyses

Several authors have studied the errors made on the BNT by different clinical vs. normal groups (Albert et al., 1988; LaBarge et al., 1992; Nicholas et al., 1985; Smith et al., 1989). Approaches to the classification of naming errors are typically based on the presumed underlying mechanisms: perceptual (analysis of the visual features of the picture), semantic (access of the underlying conceptual representation), and lexical (retrieval of the appropriate name for the stimulus) (Snodgrass, 1984).

Following Borod et al.'s (1980) study pointing to an impaired lexical retrieval mechanism underlying naming difficulties in the normal elderly, Nicholas et al. (1985) explored the integrity of lexical retrieval in normal aging through qualitative analyses of naming errors in the 85-item version of the BNT. The authors identified several error types, which are outlined in Table 8.1.

Using this system in the analysis of BNT errors for a group of 162 healthy subjects aged 30 to 79 years, the authors concluded that confrontation naming requires several stages of information processing: (1) perception of the object; (2) semantic identification; (3) retrieval of the label that corresponds to that semantic

Table 8.1. Types of Naming Errors Identified by Nicholas et al. (1985)°

Coding Category	Example from BNT
No response (comment)	"I have one of those on my porch"
Augmented-correct	"Propeller on an airplane"
Semantically related	"Harness" for yoke
Phonologically related	"Prong" for tongs
Perceptually related	"Flower" for pinwheel
Whole-part, part-whole	"Clock" for pendulum
Off-target utterance (circumlocution)	"Artistic thing for flowers" for trellis

°For the description of each type of error, see Nicholas et al. (1985).

"concept"; (4) encoding the articulatory program; (5) correct articulation of that label or name.

The authors reported a decline in naming ability with age, especially after age 70. Based on the higher frequency of circumlocutory descriptions and semantically related responses in the elderly, the authors sited difficulty with perception and semantic identification as unlikely contributors to the naming difficulty. They concluded that the major age-related difficulty lies in the label (lexical) retrieval stage.

Using the same taxonomy of naming mechanisms, LaBarge et al. (1992) identified 17 types of errors which were classified into three categories: no content, linguistically related, and perceptually related, described in Table 8.2. The authors hypothesized that the linguistic errors reflect a loss in lexical (and potentially semantic) information; no-content errors are representative of a loss in semantic content; and perceptual errors are indicative of a breakdown in the perceptual mechanism.

Based on the analysis of errors produced by 49 elderly with very mild or mild Senile Dementia of the Alzheimer's Type (SDAT), the authors identified loss of lexical information as well as some disruption in specific semantic attributes as processes underlying confrontational naming difficulty in early SDAT. With the progression of the disease, increasing involvement of core semantic structures is implicated.

Hodges et al. (1991) developed a different error classification system, which, in reference to the item "beaver," can be illustrated as follows: category names ("animal"), within-category semantic errors ("skunk"), semantic associates ("dam"), and semantic circumlocutions ("an animal that builds dams").

To further refine the process of error classification along a semantic dimension, Nicholas et al. (1996) proposed a system of rating errors on a five-point scale of semantic relatedness to the target name with 1 being not at all similar in meaning (for single word responses) and poor, incomplete definition or description (for multiword descriptions), and 5 being very similar in meaning (for single word responses) and good, complete definition or description (for multiword responses).

Current Views on the Mechanisms Underlying Confrontation Naming Deficits

There is a general consensus in the literature regarding access to the lexical network as the leading mechanism of naming difficulty in normal aging (Bowles & Poon, 1985; Nicholas et al., 1985). It should be noted that according to some studies, uncomplicated aging is not associated with a decline in naming ability (LaBarge et al., 1986). In contrast, understanding of faulty processes in Alzheimer's disease (AD) still remains highly controversial.

Whereas the majority of the more recent investigations ruled out disruption in the perceptual stage as a primary cause of this breakdown (Bayles & Tomoeda, 1983; Frank et al., 1996; Huff et al., 1986b; LaBarge et al., 1992; Martin and Fedio, 1983; Smith et al., 1989), the relative contributions of lexical vs. semantic dysfunction are highly debated in the literature.

Regarding the semantic deficit hypothesis, disruption in the content and organization of semantic information is implicated as the primary source of naming difficulties in AD (Bayles & Tomoeda, 1983; Flicker et al., 1987; Frank et al., 1996; Henderson et al., 1990;

Table 8.2. Types of Errors Described by LaBarge et al. (1992)

Type of Error	Examples
No Content	
Empty phrase	I don't know
	Can't think of it
No interpretation possible	No response or jargon
Linguistically Related	
Phonological	
Phonologically related	Pelican = pentagon
	Unicorn = hornicorn
	Rhinoceros = nostros
	Sphinx = phoenix
Semantic	
Same category	Latch = hasp
Super- or subordinate	Camel = animal
	Asparagus = vegetable
Function	Funnel = used for pouring
	Compass = makes circles
Attribute	Beaver = eats wood or builds dams
	Volcano = fire
Context	Stethoscope = doctors use it
	Sphinx = found in Egypt
Description	Noose = a rope with a slip knot
Acoustic	
Meaningful sound	Whistle = make a whistling sound or blow noiselessly
	Volcano = make a whooshing sound
Pantomime or Gesture	
Gesture	Comb = gesture to head like combing
	Accordion = swing arms and hands like playing
Perceptually Related (Visually)	
Whole	Whistle = trailer hitch or pacemaker
	Knocker = chandelier
	Igloo = turtle or spider's web
Part	Dart = feather
	Rhinoceros = two big horns
Perspective	Harmonica = windows or apartment
	building or file drawers
Function	Dart = nurse to give shot
	Broom = wash my clothes
Attribute	Beaver = fella who goes underground
	Mask = a bad picture
Context	Wreath = see 'em at wedding
	Whistle = hanging on a tree limb

Hodges et al., 1991; Huff et al., 1986b; Margolin et al., 1990; Martin and Fedio, 1983). A number of studies suggest that this contribution increases as a function of dementia severity (Hodges et al., 1991; Huff et al., 1986b; LaBarge et al., 1992; Shuttleworth & Huber, 1988). As a result, in the early stages of AD, a naming deficit might manifest itself through lexical access difficulties (LaBarge et al., 1992; Neils et al., 1988), which resembles the pattern characteristic for normal aging.

Data challenging the common view of semantic disruption as the cause of naming difficulties in AD was presented by Nebes and his colleagues (Nebes et al., 1984; Nebes, 1989; Nebes & Brady, 1990), who viewed lexical retrieval as the source of naming difficulties. Similarly, Nicholas et al. (1996) pointed to the breakdown in lexical access in AD and referred to the previous findings of semantic breakdown as an artifact of methodologies of the previous studies.

Studies supporting the lexical deficit hypothesis suggest a breakdown in the retrieval stage which is based on the following findings: (1) Incidence of errors in low-frequency words is higher than in high-frequency words: This mechanism is modulated by lexical processing (Kirshner et al., 1984; Skelton-Robinson & Jones, 1984); (2) facilitation of lexical access by phonemic cues (Martin & Fedio, 1983); (3) semantic relatedness of the words produced by the subjects to the target word (Bayles & Tomoeda, 1983; Smith et al., 1989).

In spite of the controversy regarding mechanisms accounting for naming difficulties in AD vs. normal aging, the majority of studies demonstrated utility of the BNT in distinguishing between AD and age-related decline in naming ability (Huff et al., 1986b; Margolin et al., 1990; Storandt & Hill, 1989).

Several studies have explored mechanisms of naming deficits in different types of aphasia. According to Nicholas et al. (1985), aphasic subjects (across all major aphasic groups, except for anomics) have difficulty in the phonological encoding of words. Kohn and Goodglass (1985) support this finding by demonstrating considerable similarity in error types across different aphasic groups in their study. In addition, they provide a more specific analysis of anomic errors associated with different types of aphasia: "Negated responses were associated with Broca's aphasia, whole-part errors (hose for *nozzle*) were associated with frontal anomia, and poor phonemic cuing was associated with Wernicke's aphasia" (p. 266). The authors also reported that anomic aphasics produced the highest frequency of multiword circumlocutions and the lowest number of phonemic errors, which they relate to minimal word production difficulty in anomic aphasia relative to other aphasia syndromes.

In addition to the obvious use of the BNT in assessing word retrieval, Kaplan (1988) observed that analysis of misperception errors allows identification of perceptual fragmentation and inattention to a part of the visual field, which are associated with nondominant hemisphere dysfunction.

Short Versions of the BNT

An attempt to create two shorter equivalent forms of the BNT for repeated testing was undertaken by Huff et al. (1986b). Based on the experimental 85-item version, these authors developed two 42-item versions that proved to be reliable ($r = 0.71$ to 0.81 for controls and $r = 0.97$ for AD patients) and equivalent in difficulty. Both versions were standardized on normal and brain-damaged subjects.

A comparison of different forms of the test was provided by Thompson and Heaton (1989). They administered an 85-item version of the BNT to a clinical group of subjects; data were then rescored according to the criteria for the 60-item and 42-item forms. Although certain differences between forms were found, there were high correlations among different versions of the test (ranging between 0.82 and 0.96) and between BNT scores and other language measures.

Four recently developed 15-item versions of the BNT, one 15-item version used by the Consortium to Establish a Registry for Alzheimer's Disease (CERAD), and three 30-item versions were compared by Mack et al. (1992) and Williams et al. (1989) in patients suffering from Alzheimer's disease and neurologically intact elderly. Scores on each version could be extrapolated to a complete 60-item BNT score.

Franzen et al. (1995) compared different short forms on a sample of 320 individuals with various neuropsychiatric diagnoses. They report adequate internal consistency for all forms and reasonable correlations between forms. Based on their analysis of item difficulty, the authors identified the CERAD version as least desirable.

Farmer (1990) proposed modifications of the administration, response coding, and scoring procedures for the full version of the BNT which were used by the author in assessment of non-brain-damaged adults.

Ponton et al. (1996) described the Ponton-Satz Boston Naming Test, which is an adaptation of the standard version for assessment of

Hispanic patients. It consists of 30 items derived from the original test, which are presented in different order. Some items have several possible correct responses listed on the answer sheet, depending on the country of origin of the examinee.

A French version of BNT was introduced by Colombo and Assal (1992). This paper provides data for 420 normal French-speaking Swiss adults between ages 20 and 89 years.

Performance on a shortened version of the BNT has also been reported for Native Americans (Ferraro & Bercier, 1996). Fillenbaum et al. (1997) report performance of elderly white and African American community residents on the CERAD version of the test.

Psychometric Properties of the BNT

Review of the literature suggests that validation studies for the BNT have focused on its diagnostic and predictive properties in discriminating between normal and clinical groups (Jacobs et al., 1995; Knesevich et al., 1986).

High test–retest reliability over a 1–2-week interval in a group of elderly subjects was documented by Flanagan and Jackson (1997). Mitrushina and Satz (1995) reported test–retest reliability over three annual probes for a sample of neurologically intact elderly ranging between 0.62 and 0.89.

High correlation of BNT performance with verbal fluency was reported by Locascio et al. (1995) with $r = 0.5$ for AD patients and $r = 0.52$ for the normal control subjects. In contrast, a comparison of BNT performance with measures of different aspects of memory suggested that BNT scores are unrelated to learning and memory scores (Albert et al., 1988).

RELATIONSHIP BETWEEN BNT PERFORMANCE AND DEMOGRAPHIC FACTORS

There is abundant evidence of the effect of age on BNT performance, particularly decline in scores and increase in performance variability with advancing age (see above). Several investigators suggest that the most pronounced decline occurs only after age 70 (Albert et al.,

1988; Mitrushina & Satz, 1995; Nicholas et al., 1985). Furthermore, Welch et al. (1996) suggest that individuals with higher than 12 years of education retain intact naming ability into their 80s.

Education was found to be related to BNT scores in several studies. Of note, higher variability in BNT performance was observed in groups with lower educational levels (Borod et al., 1980; Hawkins et al., 1993; Neils et al., 1995; Nicholas et al., 1985; Ross et al., 1995; Thompson & Heaton, 1989; Welch et al., 1996; Worrall et al., 1995). In contrast, Farmer (1990), Ivnik et al. (1996), and LaBarge et al. (1986) did not find any association between BNT performance and educational level.

Albert et al. (1988) and Thompson and Heaton (1989) suggest that verbal intelligence, as measured by WAIS-R Vocabulary score, strongly affects BNT performance. Similarly, Hawkins et al. (1993) found reading vocabulary score to be strongly correlated with BNT performance in a sample of psychiatric and normal subjects. The authors presented BNT performance expectation guidelines based on the Gates-MacGinite Reading Vocabulary Test for use as a complement to the published norms.

Gender was shown in several studies to be unrelated to naming efficiency in normal samples (Ivnik et al., 1996; LaBarge et al., 1986). However, based on the analysis of BNT performance, Ripich et al. (1995) suggest that naming skills for women are poorer than those for men with similar clinical dementia rating (CDR) scores and demographic characteristics in their sample of 60 early AD subjects. Similarly, Welch et al. (1996) reported males outperforming females in a normal elderly sample.

Ethnicity was related to BNT performance in the study by Ross et al. (1995) with higher scores obtained by Caucasian subjects as compared to African-Americans in a group of medical inpatients.

METHOD FOR EVALUATING THE NORMATIVE REPORTS

The normative reports reviewed will be limited to those employing the standard English 60-item version.

In order to adequately evaluate the BNT normative reports, six key criterion variables were deemed critical. The first five of these relate to *subject* variables, and the remaining dimension refers to *procedural* variables.

Minimal requirements for meeting the criterion variables were as follows:

Subject Variables

Age Group Intervals

This criterion refers to grouping of the data into limited age intervals. This requirement is especially relevant for this test, since the effect of age on BNT performance has been unequivocally demonstrated in the literature.

Sample Size

Fifty cases has been considered adequate sample size. Although this criterion is somewhat arbitrary, a large number of studies suggest that data based on small sample sizes is highly influenced by individual differences and does not provide a reliabile estimate of the population mean.

Sample Composition Description

As discussed previously, information regarding medical and psychiatric exclusion crtieria is important; it is unclear if gender, geographic recruitment region, handedness, socioeconomic status or occupation, ethinicity, or recruitment procedures are relevant, so until this is determined, it is best that this information be provided.

Information on Educational Level

Given several studies suggesting a link between BNT performance and education, it is important that the normative studies either provide data by education groupings or at least indicate the educational level of the samples.

Information of Intellectual Level

Given some studies suggesting a relationship between BNT performance and IQ, especially verbal IQ, it is important that the normative studies either provide data by IQ groupings or at least indicate the overall intellectual level of the samples.

Procedural Variables

Data Reporting

In order to facilitate interpretation of the data, group mean and standard deviation should be presented at a minimum. It should be noted, however, that standard deviations should be used with caution in evaluating relative standing of an individual score because BNT scores are not normally distributed.

SUMMARY OF THE STATUS OF THE NORMS

According to a survey of the participants of the 1988 and 1989 Clinical Aphasiology Conference, the BNT was identified as one of the two tests most frequently used to supplement comprehensive aphasia batteries (Jackson & Tompkins, 1991). Similarly, the BNT is used in many studies to explore efficiency of confrontational naming in normal and clinical samples across various demographic groups and diagnostic categories. These studies vary from several perspectives: (1) versions of the BNT utilized: experimental 85-item version, 80-item version, standard 60-item version, as well as a variety of short versions (see above); (2) administration procedures, particularly in respect to provisions for the stimulus cues; (3) aspects of performance reported: total score and/or error analysis (error classification systems also differ between studies), percent of correct responses per item, and recommended cutoff criteria for impaired performance rating.

Russell and Starkey (1993) developed the Halstead-Russell Neuropsychological Evaluation System (HRNES), which includes the BNT among 22 tests. In the context of this system, individual performance is compared to that of 576 brain-damaged subjects and 200 subjects who were initially suspected of having brain damage but had negative neurological findings. Data were partitioned into seven age groups and three educational/IQ levels. This study will not be reviewed in this chapter because the "normal" group consisted of the VA patients who presented with symptomatology requiring neuropsychological evaluation. For

Table 8.3. BNT.L; Locator Table for the BNT

Study[°]	Age[°°]	N	Sample Composition	IQ,[°°] Education	Country/ Location
BNT.1 VanGorp et al., 1986	59–95	78	Ss are normal, independently living elderly (29 M, 49F).	FSIQ 122	California
page 118	59–64	12			
	65–69	20			
	70–74	24			
	75–79	13			
	≥80	9			
BNT.2 Farmer, 1990	20–69	125	Ss are neurologically intact	8-22	California
page 119	43.9		males. Data are presented	14.6	
	(14.3)		for 5 age decades	(2.2)	
	20–29	25			
	30–39	25			
	40–49	25			
	50–59	25			
	60–69	25			
BNT.3 Boone et al., 1995			3 elderly groups are compared:		California
	63.06	110	1. Control (52 M, 58F)	14.84	
page 119	(9.19)			(2.61)	
	60.54	37	2. Mildly depressed (15 M, 22 F)	15.30	
	(9.19)			(2.60)	
	62.22	36	3. Moderately depressed	14.39	
	(7.94)		(20 M, 16 F)	(3.72)	
BNT.4 Mitrushina & & Satz, 1995	57–85	122	Ss are normal, independently living elderly (49 M, 73 F).	14.1 (2.7)	California
page 120	57–65	19	Test-retest data over 3	FSIQ	
	66–70	40	annual probes are provided.	118.2	
	71–75	47		(13.0)	
	76–85	16			
BNT.5 Neils et al., 1995	65–97	323	Neurologically intact volunteers (244 F, 79 M); 167 Ss	6-9 10-12	Northern Kentucky,
page 121	65–74		were living independently,	>12	Cincinnati
	75–84		156 were institutionalized in		
	85–97		extended care facilities. The data is presented in age-by-education-by-living environment matrix		
BNT.6 Ross et al., 1995		123	The sample was comprised of geriatric medical inpatients	11.3 (3.1)	Michigan
page 122	70–74	40	from an urban rehab hospital		
	75–79	40	with a variety of physical		
	≥80	43	diagnoses, some of whom were 2-3 weeks postorthopedic surgery		
BNT.7 Worrall et al., 1995	70.43	136	Ss are independently living, neurologically intact elderly		Australia
page 123	(7.8)		(74.3% F). Interrater reliability		
	55–59	7	data are provided. Error		
	60–64	29	analysis was performed		
	65–69	35			
	70–74	31			
	75-79	14			

continued

Table 8.3. *(Continued)*

Study[*]	Age[**]	N	Sample Composition	IQ,[**] Education	Country/Location
	80-84	13			
	≥85	7			
BNT.8 Ivnik et al., 1996 page 123	56–59 60–64 65–69 70–74 75–79 80–84 85–89 90–94 95+	663	Normal elderly volunteers. The article provides tables for age correction and a regression equation for education correction	Mayo FSIQ 106.2 (14.0)	Minnesota
BNT.9 Welch et al., 1996 page 125	60-93 X̄=74 60–64 65–69 70–74 75–79 ≥80	176	Ss were neurologically intact volunteers (74 M, 102 F) representative of the regional population across most demographic parameters. Data are presented for 5 age groups, age × educ., and age × gender cells. Suggested cutoffs are presented	3-18 X̄=12.28	Middle Tennessee
BNT.10 Tombaugh & Hubley, 1997 page 125	25–88 25–34 35–44 45–54 55–59 60–64 65–69 70–74 75–79 80–88	219 22 28 33 24 19 22 18 24 29	Community dwelling volunteers (46% male) with no known history of neurological or psychiatric illness, head injury or stroke	Education 12.9 (2.3)	Canada

[*]The study number corresponds to the number provided in the text of the chapter.

[**]Age column and IQ/education column contain information regarding range, and/or mean and standard deviation for the whole sample and/or separate groups, whichever information is provided by the authors.

further discussion of the HRNES system see Lezak (1995, pp. 714–715).

Among all the studies available in the literature, we selected for review those investigations based on large, well-defined samples. Only those studies utilizing the 60-item version were reviewed. In all articles reviewed below, the score represents the total number of correctly named drawings (spontaneously or with a stimulus cue) out of 60.

Table 8.3 summarizes information provided in the studies described in this chapter.

SUMMARIES OF THE STUDIES

Normal Reports

[BNT.1] Van Gorp, Satz, Kiersch, and Henry, 1986

The article provides normative data on BNT for 78 normal, independently living elderly residing in Southern California (29 male, 49 female) between the ages 59 and 95 with a mean FSIQ of 122 (range 87 to 150). The subjects were screened for neurological disorders based on their self-report. The data are presented in five

Table 8.4. BNT.1; BNT Data for Five Age Groups

	Age Groups				
	59–64	65–69	70–74	75–79	80+
N	12	20	24	13	9
Education	13.58	14.40	15.25	14.23	15.23
	(2.37)	(2.38)	(3.30)	(3.58)	(4.59)
WAIS-R Verbal IQ	122	123	130	115	118
BNT score	56.75	55.60	54.46	51.69	51.56
	(3.05)	(4.29)	(5.17)	(6.20)	(7.00)
Cutoff	51	47.12	44.12	39.29	37.56

age groupings. The correlation of BNT scores with age was $r = -0.33$, with more variability demonstrated by older groups. The authors provide suggested cutoff criteria for impaired performance which are based on a score falling over two standard deviations below the mean for the respective age group.

Study strengths
 1. Demographic characteristics of the sample are well described in terms of age, education, IQ, gender, and geographic area.
 2. Adequate exclusion criteria were used.
 3. The data are stratified into five age groups.
 4. The authors provide suggested cutoff criteria.
 5. Means and standard deviations are reported.

Considerations regarding use of the study
 1. Standard deviations for the IQ indices describing the whole sample and the individual age groups are not provided.
 2. Sample sizes for age groups are small.
 3. Mean education and intelligence levels are high (Table 8.4).

[BNT.2] Farmer, 1990

The author provides data on the BNT for 125 normal male subjects between the ages 20 and 69 years (M = 43.9, SD = 14.3) recruited in California. Their education ranged from 8 to 22 years (M = 14.6, SD = 2.2). All subjects were native English speakers and had vision and hearing within normal limits. None of the sub-

jects reported a history of brain injury or disease. The BNT was administered according to standard instructions. Data are presented for five age decades with 25 subjects in each age group. Analysis of errors is discussed. According to the results, age was significantly correlated with BNT, but educational level was not.

Study strengths
 1. Demographic characteristics of the sample are described in terms of age, education, gender, geographic area, and fluency in English.
 2. The data are stratified into five age groups.
 3. Minimally adequate exclusion criteria.
 4. Means and standard deviations are reported.

Considerations regarding use of the study
 1. Mean educational level is high.
 2. Individual cell sizes are relatively small.
 3. The sample is all male.
 4. No information regarding IQ level is provided (Table 8.5).

[BNT.3] Boone, Lesser, Miller, Wohl, Berman, Lee, Palmer, and Back, 1995

The authors compared 73 outpatient depressed elderly and 110 controls on a battery of neuropsychological tests. All subjects were fluent English speakers over age 45 residing in Southern California who were recruited through newspaper ads. For the depressed group, at least a 4-week duration of depression was required. The diagnosis was made after adminis-

Table 8.5. BNT.2

Age group	N	Age	Education	BNT
20–29	25	24.08 (2.53)	14.88 (1.67)	56.04 (3.60)
30–39	25	33.92 (3.35)	15.04 (2.32)	57.04 (2.25)
40–49	25	44.60 (2.50)	15.12 (1.94)	57.76 (2.19)
50–59	25	53.56 (2.77)	14.40 (2.26)	58.24 (1.88)
60–69	25	63.68 (2.93)	13.64 (2.50)	58.28 (3.19)
All	125	43.97(14.31)	14.62 (2.19)	57.47 (2.79)

tration of the Structured Clinical Interview (SCID) by an experienced clinician. Based on their Hamilton Depression Scale (HAM-D) scores, the patient group was divided into mildly (≤18) and moderately (≥19) depressed subgroups. Both clinical and control groups underwent physical and neurological examinations and psychiatric interviews. Strict exclusion criteria were utilized.

Study strengths
1. The overall sample sizes are large.
2. A comparison of normal controls with depressed elderly is provided.
3. Information regarding VIQ, age, education, gender, geographic area, recruitment procedures, and fluency in English is reported.
4. Means and standard deviations are reported.
5. Good exclusion criteria.

Considerations regarding use of the study
1. Education and intelligence levels of the samples are high.
2. Undifferentiated age range (Table 8.6).

Table 8.6. BNT.3

	Controls	Mildly Depressed	Moderately Depressed
N	110	37	36
Age	63.06 (9.19)	60.54 (9.19)	62.22 (7.94)
Education	14.84 (2.61)	15.30 (2.60)	14.39 (3.72)
Men (number)	52	15	20
Women (number)	58	22	16
VIQ	115.78 (14.18)	116.08 (14.74)	110.61 (16.03)
BNT	54.97 (6.30)	55.95 (6.01)	53.64 (5.91)

[BNT.4] Mitrushina and Satz, 1995

The article provides BNT data based on a sample of neurologically intact, highly functioning, independently living subjects residing in Southern California who were tested over three longitudinal annual probes. The sample of 156 subjects who participated in the first probe included most of the sample of 78 subjects described by Van Gorp et al. (1986) [BNT.1]. Due to attrition over a period of 3 years, only 122 subjects participated in all three probes. Subjects in this sample (49 M, 73 F) had MMSE scores >24 and ranged in age from 57 to 85 years with a mean age of 70.4 (5.0) years at the first testing probe. Their mean education was 14.1 (2.7) years and the mean FSIQ was 118.2 (13.0). The sample was partitioned into four age groups which did not differ in level of education.

Subjects were screened for a history of neurological or psychiatric disorder. All subjects were native English speakers. The BNT was administered according to standard instructions as a part of a large neuropsychological battery.

Some decline in scores after age 70 was apparent from cross-sectional age-group comparisons. The pattern of correlations with various neuropsychological measures suggests a predominantly verbal mode of information processing in BNT performance on the first probe, as opposed to a visuospatial mode by the third probe.

A comparison of BNT scores across the three probes revealed adequate stability of scores over time, with test–retest correlations ranging from $r = 0.62$ to 0.89.

Study strengths
1. Information regarding age, education, gender, geographic area, IQ, and fluency in English is reported.
2. Adequate exclusion criteria were used.

Table 8.7. BNT.4a; Demographic Characteristics for the Total Sample and for Each Age Group

		Age Groups			
	All	57–65	66–70	71–75	76–85
Education	14.1 (2.7)	14.4 (2.0)	13.7 (1.8)	14.5 (3.1)	14.0 (3.6)
Age	70.4 (5.0)	62.6 (2.5)	68.2 (1.2)	72.9 (1.4)	78.3 (2.5)
WAIS-R FSIQ	118.2 (13.0)	115.0 (12.1)	119.4 (15.2)	119.9 (11.3)	114.4 (12.3)
N	122	19	40	47	16

3. The data are stratified into four age groups.

4. Test–retest data are provided.

5. Overall sample size is large and some cells approach N of 50 while some cell sizes are rather small.

6. Means and standard deviations are reported.

Considerations regarding use of the study

1. Mean education and intelligence levels are high (Tables 8.7 and 8.8).

[BNT.5] Neils, Baris, Carter, Dell'aira, Nordloh, Weiler, and Weisiger, 1995

The study addressed the effects of demographic factors on BNT performance. Subjects were 323 normal elderly (244 F and 79 M) between the ages 65 and 97 residing in northern Kentucky and the greater Cincinnati, Ohio, area; 167 subjects were living independently and 156 subjects were institutionalized in extended care facilities for at least 1 month. All subjects were carefully screened for neurological disorders and had adequate vision, language comprehension, and attention.

Table 8.8. BNT.4b; BNT Data for the Total Sample and for Four Age Groups Over Three Testing Probes

	Time 1	Time 2	Time 3
All	54.5 (5.9)	54.7 (6.2)	54.8 (5.7)
57–65	56.0 (3.3)	56.2 (2.8)	56.0 (2.4)
66–70	56.1 (3.1)	56.0 (2.9)	56.1 (2.9)
71–75	53.7 (7.3)	54.6 (5.3)	54.2 (6.9)
76–85	51.2 (7.3)	51.1 (8.6)	51.4 (7.9)

The administration procedure differed from standard in that the stimulus cues were offered after any error was made—irrespective of whether it was a visual-perceptual error.

The data are presented in an age by education by living environment matrix.

The combination of age, education, and living environment accounted for 32% of the performance variance. The results suggest that scores for low-education and high-education groups are less affected by age and living environment than scores for the subjects with 10–12 years of education. Correlation between BNT scores and education was $r = 0.38$, whereas the correlation of BNT with age was $r = -0.33$.

Study strengths

1. Information regarding age, education, gender, and geographic area is provided. Data across wide ranges of different demographic characteristics are presented.

2. Strict selection criteria were used for neurological disorders and cognitive dysfunction.

3. Overall very large sample size.

4. The data are presented in age by education by living environment matrix.

5. Means and standard deviations are reported.

Considerations regarding use of the study

1. No information regarding intellectual level.

2. Sample sizes in individual cells are small.

3. The administration procedure somewhat differed from standard instructions (Table 8.9).

Table 8.9. BNT.5; BNT Data for the Sample Stratified Into Three Age Groups, Three Educational Levels, and Two Living Environment Settings: Noninstitutionalized/Institutionalized

Age Group	Education Level			All Education Levels
	6–9	10–12	12+	
Noninstitutionalized				
(N = 167)				
65–74	47.58	53.00	53.10	51.83
	(SD = 6.14, n = 12)	(SD = 6.63, n = 22)	(SD = 6.55, n = 20)	(SD = 6.77, n = 54)
75–84	42.79	50.73	48.55	47.54
	(SD = 10.99, n = 19)	(SD = 5.72, n = 22)	(SD = 7.96, n = 20)	(SD = 8.89, n = 61)
85–97	36.00	45.53	49.88	43.75
	(SD = 12.46, n = 17)	(SD = 10.70, n = 19)	(SD = 7.19, n = 16)	(SD = 11.72, n = 52)
Total	41.58	49.95	50.55	
	(SD = 11.36, n = 48)	(SD = 8.29, n = 63)	(SD = 7.40, n = 56)	
Institutionalized				
(N = 156)				
65–74	35.14	46.95	49.54	44.09
	(SD = 6.77, n = 14)	(SD = 8.78, n = 19)	(SD = 6.42, n = 13)	(SD = 9.59, n = 46)
75–64	36.90	39.95	48.30	41.82
	(SD = 11.84, n = 19)	(SD = 10.05, n = 19)	(SD = 6.62, n = 20)	(SD = 10.71, n = 58)
85–97	34.53	38.11	40.20	37.40
	(SD = 9.78, n = 19)	(SD = 7.48, n = 18)	(SD = 7.62, n = 15)	(SD = 8.60, n = 52)
Total	35.56	41.73	46.10	
	(SD = 9.80, n = 52)	(SD = 9.51, n = 56)	(SD = 7.87, n = 48)	

[BNT.6] Ross, Lichtenberg, and Christensen, 1995

This article represents an expansion on the previously reported data in Lichtenberg et al. (1994).

In study 1 the authors provided data for 123 geriatric medical inpatients at an urban rehabilitation hospital in Michigan (60% African-American, 40% Caucasian, 62% female, 38% male). Mean age was 75.87 (7.42), mean education 11.05 (3.38). Rigorous exclusion criteria for neurologic disorders and depression were used. Mean Mattis Dementia Rating Scale (DRS) score for the sample was 132.76 (4.93). Patients who were treated for hypertension, diabetes, and hypothyroidism were included if their conditions were well controlled with medications, and without neurological complication. Some subjects were tested 2 to 3 weeks after orthopedic surgeries and were not on narcotic medications at the time of the assessment.

In study 2 subjects from study 1 were compared as a "normative" group to a cognitively "impaired" group of 151 subjects with Mattis DRS scores below 123 (61% African-American, 39% Caucasian, 30% male, 70% female). Mean age for this group was 79.7, mean education 8.9 years. Subjects from this group presented with a wide variety of physical disorders which are likely to affect cognitive status. Twenty-four percent of these subjects had scores above 10 on the Geriatric Depression Scale.

The results of study 1 indicated significant correlations of BNT scores with age, education and ethnicity (−0.308, 0.375, and 0.326, respectively). The combined effects of demographic variables accounted for 21% of the BNT variance.

In study 2, a discriminant function analysis based on the BNT and demographic data discriminated between cognitively intact and impaired subjects with an accuracy of 72.75% (with a sensitivity of 63% and a specificity of 80%).

The authors underscore the importance of using a demographically appropriate set of normative data and suggest use of their data in urban medical settings.

Study strengths

1. Means and standard deviations are reported.

2. Data are presented by age group.

3. A comparison of BNT performance for clinical and medical control groups is presented.

4. Information regarding age, education, ethnicity, gender and geographic area is reported.

5. Individual cell sizes approach an *N* of 50.

Considerations regarding use of the study

1. "Normal" subjects were geriatric inpatients, many of whom had physical illnesses potentially affecting cognitive status.

2. Standard deviations for the mean age and education for the clinical group are not reported.

3. The age range for the oldest age group is not reported.

4. No information on intellectual level.

5. Low educational level (Table 8.10).

[BNT.7] Worrall, Yiu, Hickson and Barnett, 1995

The authors assessed the validity of the BNT as a part of a large educational project on a sample of 136 independently living older Australians. Subjects were recruited through advertisements. Subjects with reported history of neurological disease or non-native English speakers were excluded. The mean age for the sample was 70.43 (SD=7.8) years and 74.3% were female.

The BNT was administered according to standard instructions, followed by a trial of seven alternative items as potential substitutes for low-frequency original items. In addition to standard scoring, an analysis of errors was conducted according to currently existing systems (e.g., Nicholas et al., 1989).

The results revealed that the mean BNT score was two to five points below that reported for North American samples. Interrater reliabilities for the total score and for error scoring were high (94.89% and 98.17% agreement, respectively). Age, education, visual acuity, and backward digit span were significantly related to BNT scores (*r* ranging between 0.23 and 0.33). The analysis of errors idicated that semantically related errors and "Don't know" responses were most frequent.

The authors emphasized an effect of culture-related word frequency on BNT performance. The proposed alternate items for "beaver" and "pretzel" were "platypus" and "pizza."

Study strengths

1. Minimally adequate exclusion criteria are reported.

2. Data are presented by age group.

3. Authors recommend cutoff scores.

4. Analysis of errors was performed.

5. Information regarding age, gender, geographic area, and recruitment procedures is reported.

Considerations regarding use of the study

1. Education and intellectual level are not reported.

2. Sample sizes for most of the age groups are small.

3. Subjects were recruited in Australia, and it is unclear if these norms are suitable for clinical interpretive purpose in the United States given that this sample scored two to five points below North American samples (Table 8.11).

[BNT.8] Ivnik, Malec, Smith, Tangalos, and Petersen, 1996

The study provides age-specific norms for the BNT test obtained in Mayo's Older Americans Normative Studies (MOANS) projects, which

Table 8.10. BNT.6; Data for a Sample of Geriatric Medical Inpatients From an Urban Rehabilitation Hospital With a Variety of Physical Diagnoses, Some of Whom Were 2–3 Weeks Postorthopedic Surgery

Age	N	Education	DRS Scores	BNT Scores
70–74	40	11.3 (3.1)	133.2 (4.48)	43.1 (11.7)
75–79	40	10.6 (3.3)	133.4 (4.75)	40.1 (10.9)
≥80	43	10.2 (3.2)	131.4 (4.83)	35.8 (11.3)

Table 8.11. BNT.7; Data on BNT Performance for an Australian Sample

Age Groups	N	BNT Mean	BNT SD	BNT Range	Recommended Cutoff
55–59	7	52.57	3.10	47–57	46.37
60–64	29	53.65	5.60	36–60	42.45
65–69	35	54.17	4.47	39–59	45.23
70–74	31	52.29	6.38	34–60	39.53
75–79	14	49.43	8.01	32–60	33.41
80–84	13	47.46	7.54	33–58	32.38
85+	7	47.14	6.12	39–57	34.90

obtain normative data for elderly individuals on different neuropsychological tests. The total sample consisted of 746 cognitively normal volunteers residing in Minnesota, over age 55, and 663 of them participated in the BNT testing. Mean MAYO FSIQ (which differs somewhat from standard WAIS-R FSIQ) for the whole sample was 106.2 (±14.0) and mean Mayo General Memory Index on the WMS-R was 106.2 (±14.2). For a description of their samples the authors refer to their earlier publications.

Age categorization utilized the midpoint interval technique. The raw score distribution for each test at each midpoint age was "normalized" by assigning standard scores with a mean of 10 and SD of 3, based on actual percentile ranks. The authors provided tables of age-corrected norms for each age group (see below). The procedure for clinical application of these data is described in the original article (Ivnik et al., 1996) as follows: "first select the table that corresponds to that person's age. Enter the table with the test's *raw score;* do not use 'corrected' or 'final' scores for tests that might present their own age- or education-adjustments. Select the appropriate column in the table for that test. The corresponding row in the leftmost column in each table provides the MOANS Age-Corrected Scaled Score . . . for your subject's raw score; the corresponding row in the right-most column indicates the percentile range for that same score."

Further, linear regressions should be applied to the normalized, age-corrected MOANS Scaled Scores (A-MSS) derived from the tables, to adjust patient scores for education. Age-and-education-corrected scores for the BNT (A&E-MSS) can be calculated as follows:

$$A\&E-MSS_{BNT} = K + (W_1 \circ A - MSS_{BNT}) - (W_2 \circ \text{Education})$$

where the following indices are specified for the BNT:

K	3.32
W_1	1.07
W_2	0.34

Education should enter the formula as years of formal schooling.

Study strengths

1. Information regarding age, education, IQ, gender, ethnicity, handedness, and geographic area is reported.

2. The data were stratified by age group based on midpoint interval technique.

3. The innovative scoring system was well described. The authors developed new indices of performance.

4. The sample sizes for each group are generally large.

Considerations regarding use of the study

1. The measures proposed by the authors are quite complicated and might be difficult to use in clinical practice.

2. Subjects with prior history of neurological, psychiatric, or chronic medical illnesses were included.

Other comments

1. The theoretical assumptions underlying this normative project have been presented in Ivnik et al. (1992a,b).

2. The authors cautioned that the validity of the MAYO indices depends heavily on the match of demographic features of the individ-

Table 8.12. BNT.8a; Demographic Description of the Sample Used in BNT Testing

	N
Age Groups	
56–59	55
60–64	87
65–69	79
70–74	85
75–79	125
80–84	132
85–89	71
90–94	24
95+	5
Education	
≤7	4
8–11	103
12	218
13–15	163
16–17	115
≥18	60
Sex	
Males	263
Females	400
Race	
Caucasians	662
Blacks	1
Handedness	
Right	607
Left	27
Mixed	29
Total	663

ual to the normative sample presented in this article.

3. Correlation of the BNT with age was −0.46, whereas correlations with education and sex were 0.26 and −0.19, respectively (Tables 8.12 and 8.13).

[BNT.9] Welch, Doineau, Johnson, and King, 1996

The study provides data on BNT performance for 176 normal older adults from Middle Tennessee (74 M, 102 F), ranging in age from 60 to 93, with a mean age of 74 years. Education ranged from third grade to 18 years with a mean of 12.28. The subjects were recruited mostly from senior-citizen organizations and retirement centers to ensure sample representation approximating the general population for the

following parameters: across various occupational levels (skilled, professional, or manual labor), race and living characteristics (urban vs. rural). Strict medical and psychiatric exclusion criteria were utilized. Subjects with well-controlled hypertension or who had adequate corrected vision were included.

The data were presented for five age groups and then further stratified into five age groups by two educational levels, and into five age groups for males and females separately. The table for five age groups includes suggested cutoff scores.

The results indicated that an interaction of age and education is a better predictor of BNT performance than age alone. Performance variability was higher in the older-age and lower-education groups. In the ≥12th-grade educational group, BNT performance remained stable until 80 years, while in the <12 years of education group the decrement was evident at 70 years. Gender differences were also reported, with males outperforming females.

Study strengths
1. Information regarding age, education, gender, ethnicity, occupation, recruitment procedures, and geographic area is reported. The sample is representative of the regional population along most demographic parameters.
2. Strict exclusion criteria were used.
3. Data are presented by age group and by different combinations of demographic variables (education, gender).
4. Authors recommend cutoff scores.
5. Means and standard deviations are reported.

Considerations regarding use of the study
1. Sample sizes for some of the age groups are small.
2. No information regarding IQ is provided (Tables 8.14–8.17).

[BNT.10] Tombaugh and Hubley, 1997

The study provides age- and education-stratified norms for 219 community-dwelling cognitively intact volunteers, who participated in a large study on the effect of aging on acquisition and retention of information. They were recruited through booths at shopping centers, so-

Table 8.13. BNT.8b; Age-Corrected Norms for Each Age Group (A-MSS)°

Scaled Score	Ages					
	56–62	63–65	66–68	69–71	72–74	75–77
2	<41	<39	<39	<38	<25	<25
3	41–42	39–42	39	38	25–32	25–27
4	43–44	43	40–43	39	33–37	28–33
5	45–48	44–46	44–46	40–43	38–41	34–38
6	49–50	47–49	47–48	44–47	42–45	39–42
7	51	50–51	49–51	48–50	46–48	43–46
8	52–53	52	52	51–52	49–50	47–48
9	54	53–54	53–54	53	51–52	49–51
10	55–56	55	55	54–55	53–54	52–53
11	—	56	56	56	55	54–55
12	57	57	57	57	56	56
13	58	58	58	58	57	57
14	—	—	—	—	58	58
15	59	59	—	—	—	—
16	60	60	59–60	59	59	59
17	—	—	—	60	60	60
18	—	—	—	—	—	—
N	171	243	187	197	220	247

Scaled Score	Ages					Percentile Ranges
	78–80	81–83	84–86	87–89	90–97	
2	<25	<25	<25	<25	<22	<1
3	25–27	25	25	25	22	1
4	28–33	26–30	26–29	26–27	23–24	2
5	34–37	31–35	30–33	28–33	25–30	3–5
6	38–40	36–38	34–37	34–36	31–33	6–10
7	41–44	39–42	38–41	37–39	34–36	11–18
8	45–48	43–45	42–43	40–42	37–40	19–28
9	49–50	46–48	44–48	43–46	41–42	29–40
10	51–53	49–52	49–52	47–51	43–48	41–59
11	54	53	53	52	49–50	60–71
12	55	54	54	53–54	51–52	72–81
13	56	55–56	55–56	55–56	53–55	82–89
14	57–58	57	57	57	56	90–94
15	—	58	58	58	57	95–97
16	59	59	59	59	58	98
17	60	60	60	60	59	99
18	—	—	—	—	60	>99
N	309	255	209	138	78	

°The procedure for application of these data is described in the text.

cial organizations, places of employment, psychology classes, and by word-of-mouth. The sample included subjects between 25 and 88 years (M = 59.0, SD = 16.9). Average educational level of the sample was 12.9 (2.3) years; 46% were male. Mean WAIS-R Vocabulary scaled score was 11.6 (2.4). Subjects were screened based on a self-reported history of medical and psychiatric problems, including a list of currently prescribed medications. Persons with a known history of neurological disease, psychiatric illness, head injury, or stroke were excluded. Subjects with MMSE score below 25, and GDS score above 13 were also excluded.

Participants were administered all items for 20 seconds, starting with item one. Specific administration procedures are described by the authors in detail. Standard scoring procedure was used. The authors recorded rates of correct spontaneous responses (SR), number correct after a stimulus cue (SC), and number correct after a phonemic cue (PC). Rates of SR + SC (according to the original scoring procedure) and the sum of all correct responses (SR + SC + PC) are provided.

Study strengths

1. Administration procedures are well outlined.

2. Sample composition is well described in terms of age, education, gender, WAIS-R Vocabulary score, and recruitment procedures.

3. Strict selection criteria were used.

4. The table of means is stratified by age group, by education, and by gender; the table of percentiles is presented in age by education cells.

5. Means, standard deviations and percentiles are reported.

Considerations regarding use of the study

1. Sample sizes for age groupings are relatively small, although overall sample size is quite large.

2. Data were collected in Canada and, therefore, might be of limited use for clinical interpretative purposes in the United States (Tables 8.18 and 8.19).

Table 8.14. BNT.9a; Demographic Description of the Sample Compared to the Population

	Sample (n = 176)	Middle Tennessee (1,101,890)
Living		
Urban	61%	60.9%
Rural	39%	31.9%
Occupation		
Professional	29%	29%
Skilled	28%	32%
Labor	43%	38%
Education		
Median grade completed	12.2%	12.3%
Race		
White	71%	74%
African-American	28%	23%
Other	1%	3%
Age		
60–64	11%	25%
65–69	21%	23%
70–74	23%	18%
75–79	16%	14%
80+	29%	18%

CONCLUSIONS

Review of the literature suggests that confrontation naming ability is affected by many factors that need to be considered in interpreting BNT performance. Inspection of the data sets suggests that educational level is as important, if not more important, than age in BNT performance. This indicates that future normative studies need to present data by education groupings. In addition, all studies except one were limited to older samples.

Table 8.15. BNT.9b; BNT Data for Five Age Groups

Age Group	N	BNT Score	Cutoff
60–64	20	51.6 (5.4)	45
65–69	37	53.4 (4.7)	45
70–74	40	50.1 (8.5)	42
75–79	28	42.9 (12.4)	35
80+	51	44.7 (9.6)	35

Table 8.16. BNT.9c; BNT Data for Five Age Groups by Two Educational Levels

	<12 years			≥12 years		
Age Group	N	M	SD	N	M	SD
60–64	6	49.8	5.4	14	52.4	5.5
65–69	5	49.2	3.6	32	54.0	4.5
70–74	7	38.4	12.3	33	52.6	4.7
75–79	17	36.6	10.9	11	53.4	4.9
80+	20	40.7	11.3	31	47.2	7.5

Table 8.17. BNT.9d; BNT Data for Five Age Groups for Males and Females Separately

	Male			Female		
Age group	N	M	SD	N	M	SD
60–64	10	54	4.3	10	49.2	5.6
65–69	22	54.5	3.7	15	51.7	5.4
70–74	11	52.9	8.8	29	49.0	8.2
75–79	11	46.7	12.0	17	40.4	12.4
80+	31	45.7	9.7	20	43.9	9.7

Table 8.18. BNT.10a; Mean Scores by Age, Education, and Gender

		SR		SR + SC		SR + SC + PC	
	N	M	(SD)	M	(SD)	M	(SD)
Age							
25–34	22	55.9	(2.8)	56.0	(2.9)	58.4	(2.5)
35–44	28	55.5	(3.9)	56.1	(3.6)	58.2	(2.2)
45–54	33	54.8	(4.1)	55.4	(3.6)	58.5	(1.8)
55–59	24	55.2	(3.6)	56.0	(3.1)	58.8	(1.3)
60–64	19	55.6	(3.5)	56.6	(2.9)	58.7	(1.7)
65–69	22	54.9	(3.9)	55.8	(3.5)	58.4	(1.7)
70–74	18	52.5	(4.6)	54.3	(4.4)	57.2	(2.7)
75–79	24	51.7	(5.5)	53.4	(4.6)	57.8	(1.9)
80–88	29	53.1	(4.0)	54.3	(3.8)	58.1	(1.6)
Education (years)							
9–12	123	53.4	(4.4)	54.5	(3.9)	57.8	(2.1)
13–21	96	55.6	(3.7)	56.3	(3.2)	58.8	(1.7)
Gender							
Male	100	54.9	(4.3)	55.9	(3.7)	58.5	(1.8)
Female	119	53.9	(4.1)	54.8	(3.7)	58.0	(2.0)
Total	219	54.3	(4.2)	55.3	(3.7)	58.3	(2.0)

Note: SR = Spontaneous Response; SR + SC = Sum of Spontaneous Response (SR) + Stimulus Cue (SC); SR + SC + PC = Sum of Spontaneous Response (SR) + Stimulus Cue (SC) + Phonemic Cue (PC). *Because scores on the BNT are not normally distributed, standard deviations should not be used to compute normative data.*

Table 8.19. BNT.10b; 60-Item BNT Norms Expressed as Percentiles for Age and Education

	Age					
	25–69		70–88		Total	
Education (years)	9–12	13–21	9–12	13–21		
%tiles	(n = 78)	(n = 70)	(n = 45)	(n = 26)	(n = 219)	
SR						
90	59	60	58	58	59	
75	58	59	56	56	58	
50	55	58	53	54	56	
25	53	55	48	52	53	
10	49	53	45	48	49	
SR + SC						
90	59	60	59	59	60	
75	58	60	58	58	58	
50	56	58	55	56	57	
25	54	56	52	53	54	
10	51	53	47	49	51	
SR + SC + PC						
90	60	60	60	60	60	
75	60	60	59	60	60	
50	59	60	58	59	59	
25	57	59	57	58	58	
10	56	58	54	57	56	
Demographics						
Age	52.1 (12.2)	47.5 (12.4)	78.0 (4.8)	78.0 (4.7)	59.0 (16.9)	
Education	11.3 (0.9)	15.1 (1.9)	11.2 (1.0)	14.9 (1.4)	12.9 (2.3)	
Vocab. (raw)	51.0 (9.0)	57.2 (7.4)	53.3 (9.1)	58.6 (6.9)	54.3 (8.8)	
% Male	41%	41%	56%	54%	46%	

Additional normative studies are needed on younger populations, especially to ascertain if the same relationships betwen BNT scores and educational level are found in younger groups.

BNT performance also is directly affected by one's culturally determined linguistic background and accumulated vocabulary. Therefore, uncritical use of cutoff criteria might result in false-positive misclassification errors. To avoid unsubstantiated determination of a naming impairment, the BNT score needs to be interpreted within the context of a patient's linguistic background and cultural/educational exposure. In addition, qualitative analysis of performance (frequency of "Don't know" responses, misperceptions, tip-of-the-tongue errors, readiness to give up, response latencies, etc.) could contribute to interpretation accuracy.

It should be noted that the distribution of performance scores for the BNT is far from normal. The performance of the majority of subjects falls at the upper range of the score distribution. As a result, this test does not discriminate well at the high-performance level (e.g., the distinction between "well above average" and "superior" performance levels cannot be well defined). On the other hand, this test discriminates well at the lower range of performance. It is sensitive to identifying outliers whose performance falls below the expected range.

The involvement of different information processing mechanisms in confrontational naming has been extensively researched. Due to controversial findings, however, further research in this area would enhance understanding of the processes underlying naming ability and their relation to visual-perceptual/recognition ability. Consequently, the differential mechanisms determining age-related decline in naming ability vs. anomia associated with degenerative brain conditions would be further illuminated.

9

Verbal Fluency Test

BRIEF HISTORY OF THE TEST

There are several types of tasks measuring verbal fluency (VF). Their historical roots stem back to the Thurston Word Fluency Test (TWFT; Thurstone & Thurstone, 1962), which is a component of the Thurstone's Primary Mental Abilities Tests. The major disadvantage of the Thurston's task was the format of the test, which required the examinees to *write* words beginning with the letter S in 5 minutes, followed by writing four-letter words beginning with the letter C in 4 minutes (Heaton et al., 1991; Lezak, 1995; Pendleton et al., 1982). Normative data and *T*-score equivalents for this version of the test, based on a sample of 486 subjects grouped into 10 age categories by six education categories for males and females separately, are provided by Heaton et al. (1991).

Because of the confounds introduced by the writing format of this test, Benton developed an oral version, the Controlled Verbal Fluency Task (CVFT), in which examinees orally generated words beginning with letters F, A, and S, with 60 seconds for each letter (Bechtoldt et al., 1962; Borkowski et al., 1967). This version became part of the Neurosensory Center Examination for Aphasia (Benton, 1967; Spreen & Benton, 1969).

Later, this test was included in the Multilingual Aphasia Examination Battery (Benton & Hamsher, 1978; Benton et al., 1994) under a new name—Controlled Oral Word Association

(COWA)—to eliminate a potentially misleading reference to a fluent/nonfluent aphasia (see Ruff et al., 1996). The COWA test is based on two sets of letters—CFL and PRW. Whereas the former stimuli (FAS) were chosen at random, the selection of the letters for the COWA was based on the analysis of the word difficulty as determined by number of words in English language which begin with that particular letter. As a result, the CFL and PRW versions of the COWA are of equal difficulty and can be used interchangeably.

According to the analysis of letter difficulty (Borkowski et al., 1967), which was based on frequency of associations for 24 different letters, the letters F, A, S, C, P and W were classified as easy, whereas L and R fell in a category of moderately difficult letters. In spite of unequal difficulty levels for letters included in FAS vs. CFL and PRW sets, a study of equivalency between the three letter sets conducted on 106 patients with various neuropsychological dysfunctions yielded correlation coefficients ranging from 0.87 to 0.94 for different samples (Lacy et al., 1996). The authors concluded that these intercorrelations even surpass correlations between CFL and PRW. In spite of such an optimistic view, the norms for the FAS should be used with caution in application to the COWA sets (CFL and PRW) due to different levels of letter difficulty (Ruff et al., 1996).

Other combinations of letters have been used in several studies. For example, Barr and

Brandt (1996) used letters S and P in a study on fluency deficits in dementia, and Ganguli et al. (1993) used the same letters in the study on cognitive impairment in an elderly rural population. Cavalli et al. (1981) used letters P, F, and L in a study on lateralized deficits in linguistic processing. Nielsen et al. (1989) used letters S, N, and F on a large neurologically intact Danish sample.

Other versions of the fluency tests involve generation of words from certain semantic categories (Category Naming), such as animal naming (Barr & Brandt, 1996; Ganguli et al., 1993; Morris et al., 1989; Rosen, 1980; Ylikoski et al., 1993), types of transportation, parts of a car (Weingartner et al., 1984), items found in a supermarket (Barr & Brandt, 1996), fruits and vegetables, things people drink (Randolph et al., 1993), tools, and clothing (Huff et al., 1986b). Fuld (1981) used category naming tasks, such as proper names of people (same sex as the examinee), foods, vegetables, things that make people happy and things that make people sad, as distractor trials for delayed recall of the originally presented stimuli in her Fuld Object-Memory Evaluation (see also Marcopulos et al., 1997). Food, clothing, animals, and things-to-ride categories are included in the McCarthy Scales for Children's Abilities (McCarthy, 1972).

One of the versions of category naming tests is the Set Test (Isaacs & Kennie, 1973), which involves generating items from four successive categories: colors, animals, fruits, and towns. According to this version, examinees are to recall up to 10 items from each category, after which they are instructed to shift to the next category. The score was total number of items recalled for all categories. The versions proposed by Newcombe (1969), used in assessing patients with lateralized missile wounds, involved naming objects, animals, and alternating between naming birds and colors, over 1 minute for each of the three trials. The number of correctly generated items for the first two conditions and correct alternations for the third condition were recorded. Villardita et al. (1985) used a modification of the Set Test in assessment of normal elderly employing the following categories: proper names of persons, foods, and animals over 1-minute trials. The score was the total number of items for all categories.

Animal naming is frequently used in the assessment of demented individuals and has been shown in some studies to be performed at higher levels than word generation tasks (Ober et al. 1986; Rosen, 1980). Similar findings are reported with reference to other semantic category naming tests (e.g., fruits: Ober et al., 1986; Randolph et al., 1993). Rosen explained this distinction from the perspective of different hierarchical organizations for these tasks, with retrieval by letter requiring exploration of more category subsets than retrieval by animal name.

In contrast, Bayles et al. (1989) and Monsch et al. (1994) did not find differences in efficiency of word generation for semantic vs. phonemic tasks. Futhermore, greater impairment of semantic fluency in comparison to phonemic fluency tasks in clinical samples was documented by Barr and Brandt (1996), Butters et al. (1987), Mickanin et al. (1994), Rosser and Hodges (1994), and other authors. This pattern of semantic fluency lower than phonemic fluency is viewed as being mostly due to deterioration of semantic memory in dementia.

Performance on a verbal fluency task relies on efficient organization of verbal retrieval and recall and involves short-term memory (in keeping track of the words have already been said), ability to initiate and maintain word production set, and cognitive flexibility (in rapidly shifting from one word to the next within the selected category) (Cauthen, 1978b; Estes, 1974; Lafleche & Albert, 1995; Martin & Fedio, 1983; Perlmuter et al., 1987), as well as response inhibition capacity (Parks et al., 1992). These processes are commonly viewed as aspects of "executive" functioning, which are subserved by frontotemporal region, particularly left frontal area, as demonstrated in clinical and radiological studies (Benton, 1968; Elfgren et al., 1996; Frith et al., 1995; Miceli et al., 1981; Milner, 1964; Parks et al., 1988; Perret, 1974; Pujol et al., 1996).

Efficiency and rate of verbal production are affected by different types of brain pathology, including brain injuries and different degenerative dementing conditions (Barr & Brandt, 1996; Huff et al., 1986b; Lafleche & Albert,

1995; Locascio et al., 1995; Margolin et al., 1990). Impairment in verbal fluency also accompanies most of the aphasias and some amnesiac conditions, such as Korsakoff's syndrome, which is known to affect the frontal-subcortical system (Miller, 1985).

The analysis of internal consistency for the COWA version (CFL/PRW), reported by Ruff et al. (1996), revealed a high coefficient α ($r = 0.83$) for the three letters, indicating high test homogeneity. Interrater reliability is reported to be near-perfect in several studies (Spreen & Strauss, 1998). Norris et al. (1995) report an interrater reliability of $r = 0.98$. Test–retest reliability for different versions of this test is quite high (see Spreen & Strauss, 1998). Test–retest reliability reported by Ruff et al. (1996) for a 6-month retest with an alternate set of letters yielded reliability coefficient of $r = .74$. A gain of about three words on the retest was interpreted by the authors as a practice effect.

Normative data for children are provided in Spreen and Strauss (1998). Ponton et al. (1996) provide normative data for an FAS version of the test for a sample of 300 Hispanic subjects stratified by gender, age, and education. Furthermore, a Spanish version of this test is available, which is based on different sets of letters (Rey & Benton, 1991).

For test administration instructions and further discussion of the verbal fluency tasks see Lezak (1995) and Spreen and Strauss (1998).

RELATIONSHIP BETWEEN VFT PERFORMANCE AND DEMOGRAPHIC FACTORS

The original normative data for the Controlled Verbal Fluency Task (based on FAS letter set) presented in the Neurosensory Center Examination for Aphasia manual (Spreen & Benton, 1969) was based on a rural sample with low educational background and therefore has limited clinical relevance (Spreen & Strauss, 1991). Norms compiled more recently on demographically advanced samples yield consistently higher scores across different studies. Benton and Hamsher's (1978) manual for the Multilingual Aphasia Examination (based on CFL and PRW letter sets) provides corrections for age, sex, and education, implicating effects of these variables on test performance. (See Lezak 1995, for the correction table and the percentile rank table.)

A decline with age was documented by Furry and Baltes (1973), and Norris et al. (1995). Schaie and Parham (1977) and Schaie and Strother (1968b) reported decline associated with advancing age in cross-sequential comparisons. Benton et al. (1981) reported a decline in verbal fluency only after age 80 based on a sample of 65–84-year-olds. Parkin and Lawrence (1994) identified significant decline with age only in older cohorts with low educational level.

In contrast, Axelrod and Henry (1992), Bolla et al. (1990), Boone (in press), Boone et al. (1990), Cauthen (1978b), Daigneault et al. (1992), Mittenberg et al. (1989), Ruff et al. (1996), Selnes et al. (1991), and Tomer and Levin (1993) did not find age-related differences in VF performance. Relative stability in VF performance with advancing age was also reported by Miller (1984), Perlmuter et al. (1987), and Yeudall et al. (1987). Hultsch et al. (1993) demonstrated that after controlling for self-reported health status and activity levels, age no longer significantly contributed to the variance in word generation.

The discrepancy between different studies can be explained by numerous confounding factors which differentially affect the studies. Schaie (1983) suggested that a requirement for motor response is a factor contributing to age-related decline. Norris et al. (1995) hypothesized that the discrepancy in the findings across different studies regarding effect of age on VF performance might be due to several factors: (1) sampling differences with selection of high IQ participants reducing a correlation that might be observed in a broader sample; (2) the use of clinical samples may mask the unique contribution of age, which is attenuated by the effect of brain damage; (3) cohort effect might influence the results with smallest VF performance differences among middle-aged adults to young-old adults and greater differences across older samples; (4) diversity in the elderly populations subjects are drawn from (community vs. institutionalized elderly) is another factor contributing to discrepant findings.

The effect of gender with superiority of female performance was documented by Bolla et al. (1990), Gaddes and Crockett (1975), Ruff et al. (1996), and Veroff (1980). However, no gender differences in verbal fluency in normal and clinical samples were found by Cauthen (1978b), Ripich et al. (1995), Yeudall et al. (1987), and Boone (in press).

Ivnik et al. (1996) and Norris et al. (1995) found a significant effect of education on VF performance; however, in the studies by Axelrod and Henry (1992), and Bolla et al. (1990) education was not significantly related to efficiency of word generation. Ruff et al. (1996) suggested that gender moderated effect of education.

A positive relationship between verbal intelligence and verbal fluency was documented by Bolla et al., (1990), Boone (in press), Cauthen (1978b, for $\geq$60-year-old subgroup only), Borkowski et al. (1967), and Miller (1984). In contrast, Axelrod and Henry (1992) did not find an effect of verbal intelligence on VF performance. Bolla et al. (1990) and Boone (in press) suggest that effect of education is mediated by verbal intelligence. Bolla et al. (1990) concluded that data based on verbal intelligence rather than on education would be more accurate in differentiating between normal and abnormal performance.

In addition to demographic variables, functional status was found to contribute to the efficiency of VF performance, especially in geriatric samples. An effect of depression on VF performance is well documented (Caine, 1986; Boone et al., 1995; Norris et al., 1995). Effects of levels of physical and mental activity are documented by Craik et al. (1987). Neuropathological changes in the brain associated with cardiovascular disease and cerebrovascular risk factors also contribute to decline in VF efficiency (Breteler et al., 1994; Boone et al., 1993b).

METHOD FOR EVALUATING THE NORMATIVE REPORTS

In order to adequately evaluate the VF normative reports, six key criterion variables were deemed critical. The first four of these relate to

subject variables and the two remaining dimensions refer to *procedural* issues.

Minimal requirements for meeting the criterion variables were as follows:

Subject Variables

Age-Group Intervals

This criterion refers to grouping of the data into limited age intervals. In spite of the controversy in the literature regarding the effect of age on the VF performance, accuracy of data interpretation is facilitated by using a narrow-range age group as a reference sample.

Sample Size

Fifty cases has been considered an adequate sample size. Although this criterion is somewhat arbitrary, a large number of studies suggest that data based on small sample sizes are highly influenced by individual differences and do not provide a reliabile estimate of the population mean.

Grouping by Educational and/or Intellectual Level

Given consistent evidence of effects of educational and intellectual levels on VF performance, normative data should be grouped by or corrected for educational and/or intellectual level.

Sample Composition Description

As discussed previously, information regarding medical and psychiatric exclusion criteria is important; it is unclear if gender, socioeconomic status or occupation, ethnicity, handedness, geographic recruitment region, and recruitment procedures are relevant, so until this is determined, it is best that this information be provided.

Procedural Variables

Description of Administration Procedures

Due to variability in administration procedures (see below), a detailed description of the procedures, including identification of the version of the test administered, is desirable. This would allow one to select the most appropriate norms or to make corrections in interpretation of the data.

Data Reporting

In order to facilitate interpretation of the data, group mean and standard deviation should be presented at minimum.

SUMMARY OF THE STATUS OF THE NORMS

There are a number of studies exploring efficiency of word generation in normal and clinical samples across various demographic groups and diagnostic categories. A considerable variability between studies obscuring their comparability includes the following aspects: time alotted for each category, the type of semantic or phonemic category utilized, relative difficulty of letters within a phonemic category, presence/absence of feedback on intrusion or repetition errors, instructions for item exclusion (inconsistency regarding exclusion of numbers), inconsistent administration of an example with practice trial prior to the first test trial. Some authors do not specify which letters were used in their phonemic categories.

Among all the studies available in the literature, we selected for review those studies based on large, well-defined samples. In the majority of studies reviewed below, the test scores represent a total number of words generated for three letters. Deviations from this format are identified in the context of each table.

Table 9.1 summarizes information provided in the studies described in this chapter.

SUMMARIES OF THE STUDIES

Normative Reports and Control Groups in Clinical Studies

[VF.1] Cauthen, 1978b

The author administered the WAIS (Satz-Mogel short form) and the verbal fluency test as part of a large study in Canada aimed at normative data collection for age and IQ levels on neuropsychological tests. The verbal fluency test consisted of eight letters which were administered in the same order to all subjects—S, G, U, N, F, T, J, P—following the standard procedure (i.e., 1-minute oral production). The sample was divided into two groups: 20–59- and 60–94-year-olds. The younger group consisted of 12 males and 39 females gathered from a variety of sources, with an FSIQ ranging from 100 to 140 (M = 115.6, SD = 8.7). The older group included 28 males and 36 females, living primarily in institutional settings, with the FSIQ ranging from 80 to 140 (M = 111.5, SD = 13.1).

Analysis of the results for the younger group did not indicate any relation between VF performance and FSIQ. Therefore, the VF data were presented for the total sample. In contrast, VF performance differed significantly for the older group across three FSIQ ranges: 80–106, 107–118, 119–140. The authors hypothesized that speed of performance is a determining factor in the relationship between VF scores and IQ (specifically PIQ scale). Further analysis suggested that IQ level did not interact with letter difficulty. No relationship between VF performance and age was evident.

The authors concluded that the use of these norms in the 20–59 group is inappropriate for those with FSIQ below 100.

Study strengths
1. Data are presented in age groupings.
2. Efficiency of word generation for eight letters was compared.
3. Data for the older group were stratified by FSIQ level.
4. Information provided regarding gender and geographic recruitment area.
5. Sample sizes for each age group are adequate but individual cell sizes are small.
6. Test administration procedures were specified.
7. Means and standard deviations are reported.

Considerations regarding use of the study
1. Subjects' level of education was not reported.
2. Younger subjects' FSIQ was high.
3. Exclusion criteria were not specified.

Table 9.1. VF.L; Locator Table for the VF

Study[*]	Age[**]	N	Sample Composition	IQ,[**] Education	Version	Country/ Location
VF.1 Cauthen, 1978b page 135	20–59 ≥60	51 64	Ss included in the younger group were gathered from different sources: 12 M, 39 F. Older Ss lived primarily in institutional settings: 28 M,36 F	FSIQ: 115.6 (8.7) 111.5 (13.1)	Letters S, G, U, N, F, T, J, P	Alberta, Canada
VF.2 Yeudall et al., 1986 page 138	15–40 15–20 21–25 26–30 31–40	225 62 73 48 42	127 M, 98 F volunteers. Data are presented in 4 age groups for M and F separately and combined	Education 14.6 (2.8) FSIQ 118.6 (8.8)	FAS	Alberta, Canada
VF.3 Bolla et al., 1980 page 139	39–89 64.3 (13.5)	199	80 M, 119 F volunteer participants in a study on normal aging. Data were divided by 3 levels of raw WAIS-R Vocabulary scores	8–22 14.7 (3)	FAS	Maryland
VF.4 Boone et al., 1990 page 140	50–59 60–69 70–79	61 25 21 15	Subjects were healthy older adults rigorously screened for health problems. Data are provided by 3 age groups	Education 14.34 (2.63) FSIQ 113.79 (13.51)	FAS	California
VF.5 Selnes et al., 1991 page 141	25–34 35–44 45–54	733 309 290 97	Ss rom MACS study; seronegative homosexual males. Data are presented for 3 age groups and 3 educational levels; mean education = 16 years	<College (229) College (202) >College (302)	FAS, Animals	Baltimore Chicago Los Angeles Pittsburgh
VF.6 Axelrod & Henry, 1992 page 142	50–89 50–59 55.3 (2.5) 60–69 65.2 (2.6) 70–79 74.3 (2.9) 80–89 83.4 (3.0)	80 10 M 10 F 10 M 10 F 10 M 10 F 8 M 12F	Healthy, independently living volunteers	Educ. 15.4 (2.5) 14.4 (2.5) 14.5 (4.2) 14.5 (4.1)	FAS	Michigan
VF.7 Boone et al., 1995 page 142	63.06 (9.19) 60.54 (9.19) 62.22 (7.94)	110 37 36	3 elderly groups are compared: 1. Control 2. Mildly depressed 3. Moderately depressed	14.84 (2.61) 15.30 (2.60) 14.39 (3.72)	FAS	California

continued

Table 9.1. *(Continued)*

Study[*]	Age[**]	N	Sample Composition	IQ,[**] Education	Version	Country/ Location
VF.8 Kozora & Cullum, 1995 page 144	50–89 50–59 60–69 70–79 80–89	174 41 43 47 43	Volunteers screened for major medical and psychiatric disorders	Education: 14.3 (2.3) 14.2 (2.3) 14.3 (3.1) 14.9 (3.3)	FAS, Animals, Supermarket, First names, US States	
VF.9 Norris et al., 1995 page 145	60–86 73.1 (6.1) 62–89 75.3 (7.5) 18–28 19.4 (1.8)	129 54 35 40	3 samples were used: 1. Community elderly living independently 2. Institutionalized elderly with MMSE scores ≥20 3. Undergraduate students Interrater reliability data are provided.	16.7 (2.3) 12.4 (3.7) 13.6 (1.1)	FAS	Texas
VF.10 Ivnik et al., 1996 page 146		743	Normal elderly volunteers. The article provides tables for age correction and a regression equation for education correction	Mayo FSIQ 106.2 (14.0)	COWA	Minnesota
VF.11 Ruff et al., 1996 page 149	16–70 16–24 25–39 40–54 55–70	360 90 90 90 90	Native English speakers: 180 M, 180 F. Data are reported for 3 education groups, M & F separately. Tables for data conversion to *T*-scores and percentile ranks are provided. Test–retest and internal consistency data are reported	Education 7–22 groups: ≤12 13–15 ≥16	COWA	California Michigan Eastern seaboard
VF.12 Crossley et al., 1997 page 149	65–74 75–84 85+	628 (635)	Community-dwelling seniors, cognitively normal	4 educational groups: 0–6 7–9 10–12 13+	FAS Animal naming	Canada
VF.13 Boone, in press page 150	45–84 63.07 (9.29)	155	53 M, 102 F Data are stratified by FSIQ levels: average, high average, superior	Education 14.57 (2.55) FSIQ 115.41 (14.11)	FAS	California

[*]The study number corresponds to the number provided in the text of the chapter.

[**]Age column and IQ/education column contain information regarding range, and/or mean and standard deviation for the whole sample and/or separate groups, whichever information is provided by the authors.

Table 9.2. VF.1; Number of Words Generated by the Two Age Groups for Eight Letters°

| | | | | Age (20 to 59 Years Old) (N = 51) | | | | | |
		S	G	U	N	F	T	J	P
IQ range 100–140	M	16.2	11.7	6.1	9.3	12.9	13.3	8.1	13.4
X̄ FSIQ = 115.6 (8.7)	SD	(4.6)	(3.7)	(2.0)	(2.7)	(3.8)	(3.7)	(3.1)	(3.4)

| | | | | | (60 Years and Older) (N = 64) | | | | | |
IQ range	N		S	G	U	N	F	T	J	P
80–106	21	M	8.8	6.9	3.1	5.5	8.0	7.6	3.7	7.4
		SD	(4.4)	(3.1)	(1.8)	(2.8)	(2.9)	(3.5)	(2.3)	(4.1)
107–118	21	M	10.9	8.9	3.9	6.0	10.1	9.8	4.7	10.0
		SD	(3.9)	(3.3)	(1.7)	(3.0)	(2.7)	(2.7)	(1.8)	(3.3)
119–140	22	M	13.9	10.4	5.5	8.7	12.9	13.0	7.1	13.6
		SD	(4.8)	(3.7)	(2.0)	(3.1)	(4.3)	(3.5)	(2.9)	(4.7)

°Data for the younger group (12 M, 39 F) is presented for the whole sample. Data for the older group (28 M, 36 F, mostly institutionalized elderly) is stratified by the FSIQ level.

4. Subjects from the older group lived in institutional settings; however, the mean FSIQ was quite high. It is unclear from the description of the sample composition why they were institutionalized.

5. Data collected in Canada which may limit its usefulness for clinical interpretive purposes in the United States.

6. Wide age ranges within each age grouping (Table 9.2).

[VF.2] Yeudall, Fromm, Reddon, and Stefanyk, 1986

The authors obtained VF data on 225 Canadian volunteers (127 males, 98 females) recruited from posted advertisements in workplaces and personal solicitations. The participants included meat packers, postal workers, transit employees, and hospital lab technicians, secretaries, ward aides, student interns, student nurses, and summer students. In addition, high school teachers identified for participation average students in grades 10 through 12. Exclusion criteria included evidence of "forensic involvement," head injury, neurological insult, prenatal or birth complications, psychiatric problems, or substance abuse.

Experienced testing technicians gathered VF data and "motivated the subjects to achieve maximum performance," partially through the promise of detailed explanations of their test performance. Stringent exclusion criteria were used.

Data are presented for four age groupings for males and females combined and separately. The data are reported for the FAS and for Written Word Fluency. Norms for the oral version only are reproduced below. No significant effects of gender or age were evident in the data.

Study strengths

1. The sample size is large and individual cells approximate Ns of 50.

2. The sample is stratified into four age groups.

3. Data are presented for males and females separately.

4. Data availability for a 15–20-year-old age group.

5. Adequate medical and psychiatric exclusion criteria.

6. Information regarding handedness, education, IQ, sex, occupation, recruitment procedures, and geographic area is provided.

7. Means and standard deviations are reported.

Table 9.3. VF.2a; Data for the Whole Sample Stratified by Age°

	Age Group				
	15–20	21–25	26–30	31–40	15–40
N	62	73	48	42	225
Age	17.76 (1.96)	22.70 (1.40)	28.06 (1.52)	34.38 (2.46)	24.66 (6.16)
Education	12.16 (1.75)	14.82 (1.88)	15.50 (2.65)	16.50 (3.11)	14.55 (2.78)
WAIS FSIQ	118.14 (8.73)	116.45 (8.57)	120.03 (9.12)	121.87 (8.17)	118.56 (8.81)
F	13.82 (4.36)	14.99 (4.37)	15.65 (4.42)	16.83 (4.04)	15.15 (4.41)
A	12.48 (3.87)	13.33 (4.89)	13.08 (3.41)	14.50 (3.66)	13.26 (4.13)
S	15.87 (4.52)	16.63 (4.97)	16.54 (4.70)	18.10 (4.89)	16.67 (4.80)
Average of 3 trials	14.06 (3.82)	14.98 (4.29)	15.09 (3.34)	16.48 (3.61)	15.03 (3.90)

°The table provides data (total number of words generated for each letter and average for three letters) for four age groups and for the entire sample.

Considerations regarding use of the study

1. Both the written and oral versions of this test were administered but the order of administration is not specified. Issues of practice effect are not addressed.

2. Education and intelligence level for the sample are high.

3. The data were obtained on Canadian subjects which may limit their usefulness for clinical interpretation in the United States (Tables 9.3–9.5).

[VF.3] Bolla, Lindgren, Bonaccorsy, and Bleecker, 1990

The authors examined the effect of demographic factors and influence of different cognitive processes on verbal fluency (FAS) performance in healthy elderly.

The subjects were 199 Caucasian volunteers, 80 men and 119 women, enrolled in the Johns Hopkins Teaching Nursing Home Study of Normal Aging, who were recruited through

Table 9.4. VF.2b; Data for Males Stratified by Age°

	Age Groupings				
	15–20	21–25	26–30	31–40	15–40
N	32	37	32	26	127
Age	17.78 (2.09)	22.57 (1.26)	27.75 (1.57)	34.69 (2.41)	25.15 (6.29)
Education	12.22 (1.96)	15.11 (1.74)	15.78 (2.79)	16.69 (3.55)	14.87 (2.99)
WAIS FSIQ	119.21 (8.36)	118.61 (8.83)	120.30 (8.97)	122.92 (7.06)	119.96 (8.45)
"F"	14.03 (4.48)	14.83 (4.84)	15.84 (4.07)	16.58 (4.31)	15.25 (4.50)
"A"	13.00 (3.91)	13.22 (5.52)	13.03 (3.31)	14.50 (4.13)	13.38 (4.34)
"S"	15.81 (4.79)	16.94 (5.05)	17.44 (5.19)	17.88 (4.41)	16.98 (4.90)
Average of 3 trials	14.28 (3.96)	15.00 (4.73)	15.44 (3.37)	16.32 (3.77)	15.20 (4.04)

°The table provides data (total number of words generated for each letter and average for three letters) for four age groups and for the entire sample.

Table 9.5. VF.2c; Data for Females Stratified by Age°

	Age Groupings				
	15–20	21–25	26–30	31–40	15–40
N	30	36	16	16	98
Age	17.73	22.83	28.69	33.88	24.03
	(1.84)	(1.54)	(1.25)	(2.53)	(5.95)
Education	12.10	14.53	14.94	16.19	14.12
	(1.52)	(1.99)	(2.32)	(2.29)	(2.43)
WAIS FSIQ	116.91	114.29	119.29	120.30	116.79
	(9.15)	(7.86)	(9.78)	(9.73)	(8.99)
"F"	13.60	15.14	15.25	17.25	15.03
	(4.29)	(3.90)	(5.16)	(3.64)	(4.31)
"A"	11.93	13.44	13.19	14.50	13.11
	(3.82)	(4.24)	(3.71)	(2.85)	(3.88)
"S"	15.93	16.31	14.75	18.44	16.29
	(4.31)	(4.94)	(2.91)	(5.72)	(4.68)
Average of 3 trials	13.82	14.96	14.40	16.73	14.81
	(3.71)	(3.86)	(3.27)	(3.43)	(3.73)

°The table provides data (total number of words generated for each letter and average for three letters) for four age groups and for the entire sample.

newspaper advertisements. Subjects' age ranged form 39 to 89 (M = 64.3, SD = 13.5); education ranged from 8 to 22 years with the mean of 14.7 years (SD = 3). Strict exclusion criteria were used.

The FAS version of the verbal fluency test was administered as part of a comprehensive neuropsychological battery. Standard instructions were used. Subjects were instructed to exclude proper nouns. Series of numbers and proper nouns were not scored.

To examine effect of verbal intelligence on the FAS performance, the WAIS-R Vocabulary test scores were used in a regression analysis along with demographic variables. Verbal intelligence and sex accounted for a significant proportion of the variance in FAS performance. Age and education were not related significantly to performance. Therefore, the authors grouped their data by verbal intelligence for males and females separately. Based on their raw WAIS-R Vocabulary scores, subjects were divided into three verbal intelligence groups: average (30–53), high (54–60), and superior (61–68) levels.

Study strengths

1. The sample composition is well described in terms of age, gender, education, verbal IQ, geographic area, and recruitment procedures.

2. The data are presented for three verbal intelligence groups for males and females separately.

3. Adequate exclusion criteria.

4. Test administration procedures are specified.

5. Means and standard deviations are reported.

Considerations regarding use of the study

1. Education and intelligence level for the sample are high.

2. It is unclear whether the subjects were instructed to avoid numbers in the process of word generation.

3. Overall sample is adequate but individual cells are relatively small.

4. Data were collected in Canada and it is unclear if they are appropriate for use in the United States (Table 9.6).

[VF.4] Boone, Miller, Lesser, Hill, and D'Elia, 1990

The authors investigated the effect of aging on frontal lobe functioning. An FAS version of verbal fluency tests was administered among four tests assessing frontal lobe functions.

Subjects were fluent English-speaking, healthy older adults in Southern California rig-

Table 9.6. VF.3; Mean Scores on the FAS for the Sample Divided Into Three Groups Based on the Raw WAIS-R Vocabulary Scores, for Males and Females Separately

	Men on Vocabulary			Women on Vocabulary		
	≤53	54–60	≥61	≤53	54–60	≥61
N	32	25	23	33	39	47
Age	61 (12)	63 (15)	65 (17)	61 (11)	65 (15)	69 (17)
Education	13 (03)	14 (03)	17 (03)	13 (03)	15 (03)	16 (03)
Vocabulary (raw)	47 (05)	57 (02)	65 (02)	45 (06)	52 (02)	65 (02)
FAS	38 (12)	43 (12)	47 (09)	42 (09)	46 (12)	49 (12)

orously screened for health problems. The sample included 61 subjects (25 men and 36 women) grouped by three age decades. Fifty-one subjects were white, four were black, three were Asian, and three were Hispanic. Mean educational level was 14.34 (2.63) and mean FSIQ (Satz-Mogel format) was 113.79 (13.51). Standard administration procedure was utilized with the exception that proper names were allowed; different versions of the same word and number strings were excluded.

The authors concluded that the trend for age differences between the groups did not reach a statistically significant level.

Study strengths
1. The sample is well described in terms of age, education, gender, IQ, fluency in English, ethnicity, and geographic area.
2. Subjects were rigorously screened for health problems.
3. Data are presented for three age decades.
4. Test administration procedures are specified.
5. Means and standard deviations are reported.

Considerations regarding use of the study
1. The sample size for each age group is small.

2. Education and intelligence levels for the samples are high (Table 9.7).

[VF.5] Selnes, Jacobson, Machado, Becker, Wesch, Miller, Visscher and McArthur, 1991

The investigation used subjects from the MACS study. The article presents results of 733 seronegative homosexual and bisexual males for the purpose of establishing normative data for neuropsychological test performance based on a large sample. An FAS version was administered according to standard instructions. The investigators also utilized an animal category task within a 1-minute interval.

Study strengths
1. The overall sample size is large and all individual cells have more than 50 subjects.
2. Normative data are stratified by age and education.
3. Information on ethnicity and handedness is reported.
4. Means, SDs as well as scores for the percentiles 5 and 10 are presented.
5. The paper reports demographic composition for each age and education cell separately.

Considerations regarding use of the study
1. All-male sample.
2. No information on IQ is reported.

Table 9.7. VF.4; FAS Scores for Three Age Groups

	Age		
	50–59	60–69	70–79
N	25	21	15
WAIS-R FSIQ	116.72 (14.95)	111.19 (12.32)	112.53 (12.44)
Education	14.68 (2.80)	13.81 (2.04)	14.53 (3.11)
FAS	43.56 (6.51)	42.33 (14.21)	36.00 (8.93)

Table 9.8. VF.5; Data for the Sample Stratified by Age and Education[*]

Age	N	Mean Age	Education	FAS			Category		
				Mean (SD)	Percentiles		Mean (SD)	Percentiles	
					5th	10th		5th	10th
By Age									
25–34	309	31.0 (2.6)	16.1 (2.2)	45.7 (12.7)	26	30.5	23.4 (5.8)	15	17
35–44	290	39.3 (2.9)	16.4 (2.3)	46.1 (12.6)	26	29	23.4 (5.4)	14	17
45–54	97	48.5 (2.6)	16.7 (2.6)	45.9 (12.3)	25	29	23.3 (4.7)	15	17
By Education									
<College	229	36.1 (7.4)	13.7 (1.2)	41.7 (11.6)	23	26	22.0 (5.3)	13	15
College	202	35.6 (7.2)	16.0 (0.0)	46.2 (12.3)	28	31	23.1 (4.8)	16	17
>College	302	38.4 (7.8)	18.6 (1.3)	49.0 (12.4)	29	32	24.6 (5.7)	16	18

[*]The table presents data for the total number of words generated on FAS test and the number of words from animal category generated within 1 minute.

3. Test administration procedures are not specified.

4. No information on exclusion criteria.

5. High educational level of the sample.

Other comments

1. The majority of sample consisted of Caucasian subjects. Percent of African-American subjects ranged from 3.4 to 4.1 for different age groups. Percent of left-handers ranged from 11.3 to 14.9 (Table 9.8).

[VF.6] Axelrod and Henry, 1992

The authors compared performance of 80 healthy independently living individuals between ages 50 and 89 on tests tapping executive functioning and WAIS-R (Satz-Mogel abbreviation). The subjects were recruited from a university-related project and the community. Strict exclusion criteria were utilized. A FAS version of the VF test was administered according to standard criteria. Items excluded were proper names and variations of the same word. In addition, subjects self-rated their health status on a 1-to-5 scale and reported the number of physicians' appointments in the past 12 months as an objective measure of health status. Verbal intelligence was measured with WAIS-R vocabulary scores. No relationship was found between VF performance and intellectual competence, educational experience, or the general health status.

Study strengths

1. Administration procedures are well outlined.

2. Sample composition is well described in terms of IQ, age, education, gender, and ethnicity.

3. Strict subject selection criteria were used.

4. Data are stratified by age group.

5. Means and standard deviations are reported.

Considerations regarding use of the study

1. The sample sizes for each age group are small.

2. High educational level of the sample (Table 9.9).

[VF.7] Boone, Lesser, Miller, Wohl, Berman, Lee, Palmer, and Back, 1995

The authors compared 73 outpatient depressed elderly and 110 controls on a battery of neuropsychological tests. All subjects were fluent

Table 9.9. VF.6; Demographic Characteristics and Performance on FAS for Four Age Groups

Variables	Age groups			
	50s	60s	70s	80s
Age				
M	55.3	65.2	74.3	83.4
SD	(2.5)	(2.6)	(2.9)	(3.0)
Males	10	10	10	8
Females	10	10	10	12
Blacks	4	4	4	2
Caucasians	16	16	16	18
WAIS-R Vocabulary				
M	10.3	10.3	9.8	10.0
SD	(2.1)	(2.3)	(2.8)	(2.5)
Education (years)				
M	15.4	14.4	14.5	14.5
SD	(2.5)	(3.0)	(4.2)	(4.1)
Health Rating				
M	4.3	4.0	4.0	3.9
SD	(0.7)	(0.9)	(0.9)	(0.8)
Number of Physicians Appointments				
M	2.4	2.7	3.6	3.1
SD	(3.0)	(2.6)	(3.2)	(2.5)
F Words				
M	14.6	14.2	11.8	13.1
SD	(3.8)	(4.7)	(3.2)	(4.1)
A Words				
M	11.5	11.2	10.8	11.5
SD	(4.3)	(3.7)	(4.3)	(5.1)
S Words				
M	14.0	14.2	13.4	13.2
SD	(3.9)	(3.8)	(3.9)	(5.4)
Total FAS Words				
M	41.1	39.6	36.0	37.8
SD	(9.9)	(10.7)	(9.3)	(14.0)

English speakers over age 45 who were recruited through newspaper ads in Southern California. For the depressed group, at least a 4-week duration of depression was required. The diagnosis was made after administration of the structured clinical interview (SCID) by an experienced clinician. Based on their HAM-D scores, the patient group was divided into mildly ($\leq$18) and moderately ($\geq$19) depressed subgroups. Both clinical and control groups underwent physical and neurological examinations and psychiatric interviews. Strict exclusion criteria were utilized including history of psychosis, head injury, neurological disorder, or major medical illness. No patient was on antidepressant medication.

The FAS version of the test was used; proper names were allowed, but different versions of the same word and number strings were excluded.

Study strengths
1. The sample size is large.
2. Composition of the samples is well described in terms of IQ, age, fluency in English, education, gender, recruitment procedures, and geographic area.
3. A comparison of normal controls with depressed elderly is provided.
4. Test administration procedures were specified.
5. Means and standard deviations are reported.
6. Administration procedures are specified.
7. Good exclusion criteria.

Considerations regarding use of the study
1. Education and intelligence levels of the samples are high.
2. Undifferentiated age range (Table 9.10).

[VF.8] Kozora and Cullum, 1995

The authors compared category and letter fluency in normal aging individuals. Subjects were volunteers ($N = 174$) between 50 and 89 years of age, who were recruited through local media announcements as part of an ongoing aging study. Subjects were screened using a semistructured neuromedical interview. None of the subjects selected for the study had a known history of substance use, major psychopathology, uncontrolled hypertension, other major

medical illnesses, learning disability, or neurological disorder, and none was taking medications known to affect CNS functioning. Subjects with the MMSE score below 24 were excluded. The sample was divided into four age groups by decade, which were equated for educational level, gender distribution, and verbal intellectual level (as measured by WAIS-R Vocabulary subtest).

Five different verbal fluency tasks were administered as part of a larger study. Letter fluency was measured using the FAS task, with instructions not to use proper names, numbers, or the same word with different suffixes. Category fluency was measured with four tasks: (1) the supermarket item list from the Dementia Rating Scale (Mattis, 1988), which was administered according to standard instruction, but the total number of items generated in 1 minute was used as the total score; (2) animal naming; (3) state naming, listing USA states; and (4) first name generation, listing both male and female names. Performance within 1 minute was recorded for each task.

Study strengths
1. Administration procedures are well outlined.
2. Sample composition is well described in terms of age, education, gender, and verbal intelligence (based on the Vocabulary score).
3. Strict subject selection criteria were used.
4. Data are stratified by age group.
5. Means and standard deviations are reported.
6. Sample sizes for each age grouping approximate Ns of 50.

Considerations regarding use of the study
1. High educational level of the sample.

Other comments
1. Qualitative aspects of verbal fluency were assessed by calculating the hierarchical structure of words generated on supermarket fluency task, and by examining frequency of perseverative responses and intrusion errors made on each task.
2. The authors concluded that category fluency appears to be disproportionately reduced compared with letter fluency in normal aging,

Table 9.10. VF.7; Demographic Characteristics and Performance on FAS for Three Groups

	Controls	Mildly Depressed	Moderately Depressed
N	110	37	36
Age	63.06	60.54	62.22
	(9.19)	(9.19)	(7.94)
Education	14.84	15.30	14.39
	(2.61)	(2.60)	(3.72)
Men (number)	52	15	20
Women (number)	58	22	16
VIQ	115.78	116.08	110.61
	(14.18)	(14.74)	(16.03)
FAS	40.45	37.41	32.42
	(11.12)	(10.90)	(14.69)

Table 9.11. VF.8a; Mean Demographic and Group Characteristic by Decade

Age Group	50–59 $n = 41$	60–69 $n = 43$	70–79 $n = 47$	80–89 $n = 43$
Male/Female Ratio	21/20	16/27	15/32	16/27
Mean Age	54.5	64.6	74.6	83.8
(SD)	(3.0)	(2.8)	(2.5)	(3.1)
Mean Education	14.3	14.2	14.3	14.9
(SD)	(2.3)	(2.3)	(3.1)	(3.3)
Mean Vocabulary Raw Score	57.15	58.8	60.02	58.79
(SD)	(6.37)	(5.63)	(8.72)	(8.87)

which would be consistent with some degradation of semantic memory systems (Tables 9.11 and 9.12).

[VF.9] Norris, Blankenship-Reuter, Snow-Turek, and Finch, 1995

The study addressed the effect of depression on cognitive deficits in the elderly. The subjects were 54 community elderly, 35 institutionalized elderly, and 40 young adults who were paid or received course credit for their participation and whose first language was English.

The first group included independently living individuals between ages 60 and 86 (M = 73.1, SD = 6.1) who were solicited through ads and personal references. Subjects comprising the second group ranged in age between 62 and 89 years (M = 75.3, SD = 7.5), were living in institutional settings (skilled care and intermediate care facilities), and had MMSE scores ≥20. The third group included undergraduate students from a large southwestern university,

ranging in age between 18 and 28 years (M = 19.4, SD = 1.8).

Subjects were assessed with the FAS version of the VF test. A standard procedure was used. Subjects were instructed to exclude proper names, numbers, and different extensions of the same word. The letter T was used as an example. Two scorers rated all protocols with interrater reliability of $r = .98$. Depression was assessed with the Geriatric Depression Scale (GDS; Yesavage et al., 1983).

A hierarchical regression was used to examine the incremental effects of age, education, depression and functional status on VF performance. Age alone explained 15.8% of the variance in VF scores, while age and education together accounted for 25.2% of the variance. Depression was associated with deflated scores on VF only in functionally independent adults. The role of this finding in differential diagnosis of depression in older adults is underscored by the authors.

Table 9.12. VF.8b; Letter and Category Fluency Scores by Decade

Age Group	50–59 M	(SD)	60–69 M	(SD)	70–79 M	(SD)	80–89 M	(SD)
Letter Total	41.23	(12.10)	45.76	(14.26)	46.49	(10.46)	40.74	(11.19)
Letter F	14.05	(4.55)	15.69	(5.25)	15.98	(3.91)	14.21	(3.69)
Letter A	12.98	(4.08)	14.17	(4.92)	14.40	(4.26)	12.95	(4.44)
Letter S	14.13	(5.19)	15.91	(5.36)	16.11	(4.51)	13.49	(4.40)
Category Total	108.55	(17.08)	105.13	(18.40)	92.53	(16.23)	82.63	(17.36)
Animals	20.95	(4.16)	21.07	(5.08)	18.96	(4.67)	15.81	(4.51)
Supermarket	26.85	(6.75)	25.58	(5.11)	22.60	(5.27)	19.93	(5.41)
First Names	29.21	(5.67)	26.76	(6.74)	23.73	(5.90)	20.47	(5.27)
U.S. States	30.77	(7.24)	31.60	(7.40)	26.67	(5.78)	27.81	(8.05)

Table 9.13. VF.9; Demographic Characteristics and Data on FAS Performance for the Independently Living Elderly (60–86-Year-old), Institutionalized Elderly (62–89-Year-old), and Undergraduate Students (18–28-Year old)

	Group		
Variable	Old (Community)	Old (Institution)	Young
N	54	35	40
Age	73.1	75.3	19.4
	(6.1)	(7.5)	(1.8)
Education	16.7	12.4	13.6
	(2.3)	(3.7)	(1.1)
Depression	3.8	9.7	6.5
	(3.6)	(7.4)	(4.3)
Functional status	8.1	14.0	—°
	(0.3)	(3.1)	
Verbal fluency	36.9	21.5	40.5
	(10.1)	(9.8)	(7.8)
Mini-mental state exam	27.5	24.7	—°
	(2.1)	(3.0)	

° Young participants did not receive these measures due to anticipated ceiling and floor effects.

Study strengths

1. Data for two older groups and a young group were presented.

2. Sample composition was well described in terms of age, native language, recruitment procedures, and education.

3. The sample sizes for each group approach Ns of 50.

4. Test administration procedures were specified.

5. Means and standard deviations are reported.

Considerations regarding use of the study

1. There is a considerable difference in educational level between the two elderly groups, which might partially account for the differences in VF performance.

2. Data are of limited clinical use due to overinclusive age ranges for each group.

3. Subject exclusion criteria were not specified.

4. No data on intellectual level or gender are provided.

5. High educational level of the two control (non-institutional) groups (Table 9.13).

[VF.10] Ivnik, Malec, Smith, Tangalos, and Petersen, 1996

The study provides age-specific norms for the COWA test obtained in Mayo's Older Americans Normative Studies (MOANS) projects, which aim at obtaining normative data for elderly individuals on different neuropsychological tests. The total sample consisted of 746 cognitively normal volunteers over age of 55, and 743 of them participated in COWA testing. Mean MAYO FSIQ (which differs somewhat from standard WAIS-R FSIQ) for the whole sample was 106.2 (±14.0) and mean Mayo General Memory Index on the WMS-R was 106.2 (±14.2). For description of their samples the authors refer to their earlier publications.

Age categorization utilized the midpoint interval technique. The raw score distribution for each test at each midpoint age was "normalized" by assigning standard scores with mean of 10 and SD of 3, based on actual percentile ranks. The authors provided tables of age-corrected norms for each age group (see below). The procedure for clinical application of these data is described in the original article (Ivnik et al., 1996) as follows: "first select the table that corresponds to that person's age. Enter the table with the test's *raw score*; do not use corrected or final scores for tests that might present their own age- or education-adjustments. Select the appropriate column in the table for that test. The corresponding row in the leftmost column in each table provides the MOANS Age-Corrected Scaled Score ... for your subject's raw score; the corresponding row in the right-most column indicates the percentile range for that same score."

Further, linear regressions should be applied to the normalized, age-corrected MOANS Scaled Scores (A-MSS) derived from the tables to adjust the patient's score for education. Age-and-education-corrected scores for the COWA (A&E-MSS) can be calculated as follows:

$$A\&E-MSS_{COWA} = K + (W_1 \cdot A - MSS_{COWA}) - (W_2 \cdot \text{Education})$$

where the following indices are specified for the COWA:

K	3.50
W_1	1.16
W_2	0.40

Education should enter the formula in years of formal schooling.

Study strengths

1. Information regarding age, education, gender, ethnicity, occupation, recruitment procedures, and geographic area is reported.
2. The data were stratified by age group based on midpoint interval technique.
3. The innovative scoring system was well described. The authors developed new indices of performance.
4. The sample sizes for each group are large.

Considerations regarding use of the study

1. The measures proposed by the authors are quite complicated and might be difficult to use in clinical practice.
2. Subjects with prior history of neurological, psychiatric, or chronic medical illnesses were included.
3. It is assumed that the authors used the CFL set of letters based on specification that

MAE COWA test was used. However, due to frequent reporting of FAS as "COWA test," this assumption is only tentative.

Other comments

1. The theoretical assumptions underlying this normative project have been presented in Ivnik et al. (1992a,b).
2. The authors cautioned that validity of the MAYO indices depends heavily on the match of demographic features of the individual to the normative sample presented in this article.
3. Correlation of COWA with age and sex were -0.15 and 0.12, whereas correlation with education was 0.38. The authors underscore effect of education on the test scores (Tables 9.14 and 9.15).

Table 9.14. VF.10a; Demographic Description of the Sample Used in COWA Testing

	N
Age Groups	
56–59	55
60–64	90
65–69	85
70–74	93
75–79	146
80–84	149
85–89	84
90–94	33
95+	8
Education	
≤7	8
8–11	121
12	239
13–15	181
16–17	128
≥18	66
Sex	
Males	286
Females	457
Race	
Caucasians	741
Blacks	2
Handedness	
Right	682
Left	29
Mixed	32
Total	743

Table 9.15. VF.10b; Age-Corrected Norms for Each Age Group (A-MSS)°

Scaled Score	Ages					
	56–62	63–65	66–68	69–71	72–74	75–77
2	<13	<13	<13	<13	<12	<11
3	13–16	13–16	13–16	13–14	12	11
4	17–18	17–18	17	15	13–15	12–13
5	19–20	19–20	18–20	16–19	16–19	14–19
6	21–25	21–24	21–23	20–22	20–22	20–22
7	26–28	25–26	24–25	23–25	23–24	23–24
8	29–31	27–29	26–29	26–28	25–28	25–28
9	32–33	30–32	30–32	29–31	29–31	29–31
10	34–39	33–37	33–37	32–36	32–36	32–36
11	40–42	38–40	38–40	37–39	37–39	37–39
12	43–45	41–44	41–44	40–43	40–43	40–43
13	46–51	45–49	45–49	44–49	44–49	44–49
14	52–56	50–56	50–56	50–56	50–56	50–56
15	57–62	57–62	57–62	57–61	57–61	57–61
16	63–67	63–67	63–67	62–67	62–66	62–64
17	68–71	68–71	68–71	68–71	67–70	65–70
18	>71	>71	>71	>71	>70	>70
N	175	257	201	215	250	282

Scaled Score	Ages					Percentile Ranges
	78–80	81–83	84–86	87–89	90–97	
2	<6	<6	<6	<5	<5	<1
3	6–8	6–8	6	5	5	1
4	9–10	9–10	7–10	6–10	6–10	2
5	11–15	11–15	11–15	11–15	11–15	3–5
6	16–21	16–19	16–18	16–18	16–18	6–10
7	22–23	20–23	19–22	19–22	19–22	11–18
8	24–26	24–25	23–25	23–24	23	19–28
9	27–30	26–30	26–29	25–28	24–26	29–40
10	31–35	31–35	30–35	29–35	27–34	41–59
11	36–39	36–39	36–39	36–39	35–37	60–71
12	40–43	40–43	40–42	40–42	38–41	72–81
13	44–48	44–48	43–48	43–48	42–48	82–89
14	49–52	49–52	49–52	49–52	49–51	90–94
15	53–61	53–60	53–59	53–58	52–56	95–97
16	62–64	61–62	60–62	59–61	57	98
17	65–70	63–70	63–67	62–63	58	99
18	>70	>70	>67	>63	>58	>99
N	309	293	242	165	100	

°The procedure for applications of these data is described in the text.

[VF.11] Ruff, Light, Parker, and Levin, 1996

The authors summarized the history of verbal fluency tasks. Their normative study was based on 360 native English-speaking normal volunteers between 16 and 70 years of age and ranging in education between 7 and 22 years who resided in mostly urban/suburban areas of California, Michigan, and the eastern seaboard. Subjects with positive history of psychiatric hospitalizations, chronic polydrug abuse, or neurological disorders were excluded from the sample.

The COWA (letters CFL and PRW) was administered as a part of a comprehensive neuropsychological battery. The standard aministration procedure was used. The investigators instructed subjects to exclude proper names and same words with different ending. The numbers of correctly generated words and perseverative errors were recorded.

Total numbers of words for the three letters are reported for three educational groups for males and females separately.

Analyses revealed that age did not have a significant effect on word generation. Gender moderated the effect of education and education alone accounted for 8% of total variance. The authors proposed correction factors computed for each cell in a gender-by-education group matrix. A table of percentile ranks and normalized T scores from the 360 subjects is provided.

According to the design of the test, the three letters differ in terms of difficulty. The authors confirmed that the mean production for letters C (14.1, SD = 4.15), F (13.3, SD = 4.10), and L (12.7, SD = 4.0) was significantly different.

The analysis of internal consistency revealed a high coefficient α ($r = 0.83$) for the three letters, indicating high test homogeneity.

Test–retest reliability assessment was based on five or more randomly selected subjects from each cell, resulting in the total of 120 subjects, who were retested after a 6-month delay with the alternate version. The order of versions administered was the same for all subjects. The results yielded an acceptably high test–retest reliability coefficient ($r = 0.74$). However, a gain of about three words on the retest was interpreted by the authors as a practice effect.

The authors pointed out that the raw scores for FAS and COWA versions of the test are not comparable. However, percentiles or standard scores are comparable, based on a comparison with other studies.

Study strengths
1. The sample composition is well described in terms of geographic area, age, education, gender, and IQ.
2. Test instructions are given in detail.
3. The data are presented in education by gender matrix.
4. Correction factor and T-score/percentile equivalents for the raw scores are provided.
5. Exclusion criteria are adequate.
6. The sample size is sufficiently large for the elaborate analyses conducted by the authors. The data cover a wide age span.
7. Means and standard deviations are reported.

Considerations regarding use of the study
1. The raw data for separate age groups are not presented.
2. Data for the retest are not provided.
3. High intellectual (WAIS-R FSIQ: 110–111) and educational (14 years) levels.

Other comments
A raw score for a given individual must be education-adjusted according to Table 9.17. Then the percentile and T-score ranking can be obtained by comparing an education-adjusted score to Table 9.18.

The analysis of errors (repetitions or perseverations) revealed effect of age on the error rate, with 16–24-year-olds perseverating at a much lower rate than 25–79-year-old subjects. Based on their analysis of error rate, the authors proposed the cutoff scores listed in Table 9.19. (Tables 9.16–9.19).

[VF.12] Crossley, D'Arcy, and Rawson, 1997

The authors compared performance on letter and category fluency in a sample of cognitively normal seniors ($N = 635$) and in samples of DAT and vascular dementia patients partici-

Table 9.16. VF.11a; Total Number of Words for the Three Letters for Three Educational Groups for Males and Females Separately for the COWA Version°

Education	Men	Women	Combined Sex
N	180	180	360
≤12	36.9 (9.8)	35.9 (9.6)	36.5 (9.9)
13–15	40.5 (9.4)	39.4(10.1)	40.0 (9.7)
≥16	41.0 (9.3)	46.5(11.2)	43.8(10.6)
All education levels	39.5 (9.8)	40.6(11.2)	40.1(10.5)

°A raw score for a given individual must be education-adjusted according to Table 9.17.

pating in the Canadian Study of Health and Aging. The control sample included community-dwelling individuals who were screened for cognitive impairment using the Modified Mini-Mental State Examination (3MS). All participants were fluent in either English or French. Detailed overview of the study participants, methods, and findings is provided in the *Canadian Study of Health and Aging*, (1994).

Letter fluency was assessed with the FAS task administered in three 60-second trials. Subjects were instructed to avoid proper nouns and the same word with a different suffix. Category fluency was assessed with animal name generation task within 60 second interval.

The data are reported by age group, by gender, and by the educational level.

Study strengths
1. Administration procedures are well outlined.
2. Sample composition is well described in the previous reports.
3. Subject selection criteria are outlined.
4. Data are stratified by age group, by gender, and by education.

Table 9.17. VF.11b; Correction Factors by Gender and Education

Education (in No. of Years)	Men	Women
≤12	+3	+4
13–15	−1	+1
≥16	−1	−7

5. Means and standard deviations are reported.
6. Sample sizes for each demographic grouping are very large.

Considerations regarding use of the study
1. Data were collected in Canada and, therefore, might be of limited use in the United States.
2. It is unknown to what extent having some data collected in French impacted the overall results (Table 9.20).

[VF.13] Boone, In Press

In a follow-up study on Boone et al. (1995), the sample size was increased to 155 subjects: 53 males, 102 females, with an age range of 45 to 84 years (M = 63.07, SD = 9.29). Mean education was 14.57 (2.55) and mean FSIQ was 115.41 (14.11). The same criteria for subject selection and administration procedure were used as described in Boone et al. (1995).

The results identified the FSIQ as the only significant predictor of FAS performance responsible for 15% of test score variance, based on the stepwise regression analysis.

Study strengths
1. The sample size is large.
2. Composition of the samples is well described in terms of fluency in English, gender, age, education, IQ, and geographic area.
3. Adequate exclusion criteria.
4. Test administration procedures are specified.

Table 9.18. VF.11c; Percentile Ranks, Normalized T Scores, and
Interpretation for the Education-Corrected Scores for the COWA Letters

Corrected Score	Percentile	T Score	Interpretation
17 or less	1	26.7	
20	2	29.5	Seriously deficient
21	3	31.2	Deficient
23	4	32.5	
25	5	33.5	Deficient
26	8	35.8	Borderline
27	9	36.6	
28	10	37.2	Borderline
29	13	38.7	Low average
30	16	40.2	
31	19	41.2	
32	21	41.9	
33	27	43.9	Low average
34	30	44.7	Average
35	34	45.9	
36	38	46.9	
37	43	48.2	
38	47	49.2	
39	51	50.3	
40	58	52.0	
41	61	52.8	
42	64	53.6	
43	67	54.4	
44	69	55.0	
45	72	55.8	Average
46	76	57.0	High average
47	78	57.7	
48	80	58.5	
49	82	59.1	
50	85	60.4	
51	87	61.3	
52	89	62.3	High average
53	91	63.4	Superior
54	92	64.1	
55	94	65.5	
56	95	66.5	
58	97	68.9	Superior
60	98	70.6	Very superior
64 and up	99	73.3	

5. Means and standard deviations are reported.

Considerations regarding use of the study
  1. Education and intelligence level for the sample are high.
  2. Data are not presented by age groupings (Table 9.21).

Table 9.19. VF.11d; Cutoff Scores for Interpretation of COWA

Perseverations	Percent of Total Sample	Interpretation
0	56	Intact
1	26	Low average
2	11	Borderline
3	5	Deficient
≥ 4	2	Seriously deficient

Table 9.20. VF.12; Letter and Category Fluency Performance for Cognitively Normal Participants According to Age, Gender, and Educational Level

	Fluency Task					
	FAS (Letter Fluency)			Animal Naming (Category Fluency)		
Group	M	SD	N	M	SD	N
Age Group (years)						
65–74	24.0	12.4	139	14.2	4.3	144
75–84	25.8	11.5	343	14.2	3.8	343
85+	24.0	10.8	146	12.5	3.8	148
Gender						
Male	23.2	12.1	258	14.2	4.2	258
Female	26.2	11.0	370	13.6	3.9	377
Education (years)						
0–6	16.2	6.9	140	12.1	3.1	149
7–9	23.7	9.9	170	13.4	3.8	169
10–12	27.0	10.2	202	14.1	3.9	203
13+	34.2	12.6	115	16.3	4.1	113
Sample	25.0	11.6	628	13.8	4.3	635

CONCLUSIONS

Different versions of the VF task are widely used in clinical practice as measures sensitive to executive dysfunction. Use of the normative data assuring accurate interpretation of the test results is obscured by variability in procedural and reporting aspects of the studies. There is a confusion across studies in identifying the version of the test administered: the CVFT test (FAS) is commonly presented as the COWA test (see introduction to this chapter). This confusion undermines accuracy of interpretation, since due to different levels of letter difficulty, the norms for the FAS should be used with caution in application to the COWA sets (CFL and PRW) and vice versa. Other issues of concern are time alotted for each category, the type of semantic or phonemic category admin-

Table 9.21. VF.13; FAS Performance Partitioned into Three IQLevels

	WAIS-R IQ Level		
	Average	High Average	Superior
N	53	39	59
FAS score	36.45 (9.26)	38.87 (9.22)	44.31 (11.88)

istered, presence/absence of feedback on intrusion or repetition errors, instructions for item exclusion (whether or not numbers were excluded), and administration of an example with practice trial prior to the first recorded trial. These procedural aspects are not consistent across studies. Attention to these aspects of administration and data reporting is recommended for future studies involving the VF tasks.

Other issues of interest to future investigators of this test might include the following: (1) comparative efficiency of word generation for semantic vs. phonemic categories in normal and clinical samples; (2) a comparison of psychometric properties for different types of VF tasks, aiming at the possibility of interchangeable use of the normative data across tasks; (3) effect of demographic variables on test performance across different age ranges, educational/intelligence levels, genders, and clinical diagnoses.

Of concern, nearly every normative study was confined to subjects of high educational and/or IQ levels; there is no FAS normative data for individuals with ≤average IQ and ≤HS education. Because some studies indicate that IQ and/or education are more predictive of VF performance than is age, the lack of normative data for lower IQ and educational groups is a clear problem for clinical practice.

IV

PERCEPTUAL ORGANIZATION: VISUOSPATIAL, AUDITORY, AND TACTILE

10

Rey-Osterrieth Complex Figure

BRIEF HISTORY OF THE TEST

The Rey-Osterrieth Complex Figure (ROCF), also known as the Rey Figure and the Complex Figure Test (CFT), consists of a complex two-dimensional line drawing containing 18 details including crosses, squares, triangles, and a circle arranged around a central rectangle (Fig. 10.1).

The patient is instructed to carefully copy the design with pencil on paper. Rey (1941) asserts that the figure does not require a high level of graphic aptitude; each of the details is simple to reproduce separately and the difficulty of the task is due to the arrangement of the elements. Organizational strategy is documented by having the patient use different-colored pencils when executing the task (Rey & Osterrieth, 1993). Some studies report alternate methods for recording strategy of the reproduction, such as numbering lines on a copy of the ROCF or replicating subject's drawing with indication of directionality of lines, as the subject proceeds with reproduction (Binder, 1982; Kirk & Kelly, 1986; Waber & Holmes, 1986).

Administration Procedures

Rey's (1941) original instructions are as follows: The subject is presented the stimulus figure with the isosceles triangle and circle oriented to the right and is instructed to "make a copy of this design as best as possible" on a plain sheet of paper with a colored pencil. The subject is told that "the copy can be an approximation as far as the proportions are concerned but that care should be taken not to forget any detail." The subject is handed a different colored pencil with which to draw "each time an element is determined;" typically five to six pencils are utilized. The order in which the colored pencils are used is noted on the side of the paper. Time to complete the copy is recorded. The subject is not allowed to change the orientation of the stimulus figure but may reposition the drawing sheet. When the subject stops drawing, he/she is asked if he/she is finished, and the copy sheet and the model are removed from view. After 3 minutes the subject is handed a new sheet of paper and a regular pencil and asked to draw the design from memory.

L. B. Taylor's (1969) instructions are a commonly used variation: "copy this drawing as well as you can. Make sure you do not leave out anything." No time limit is imposed but the length of time required to complete the copy is recorded. Forty minutes later a reproduction of the drawing from memory is requested" (p. 278). In a second publication, L. B. Taylor (1979) provided additional information regarding instructions: "Exposure of the figure for copying is limited to 5 minutes. Then 45 minutes later the patient is asked to reproduce as much of the figure as he can remember" (p. 167). According to Osterrieth (1944), the subjects are not allowed to make erasures.

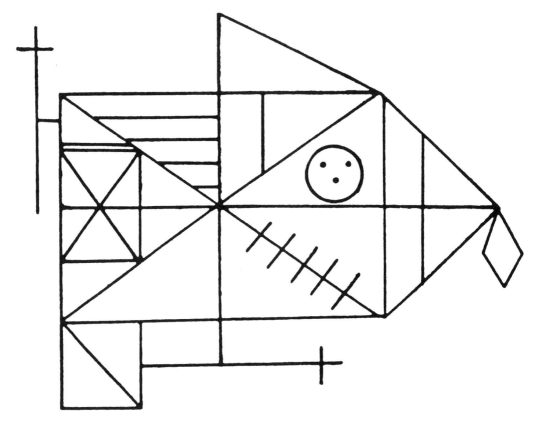

Figure 10.1. Rey-Osterrieth Complex Figure. (Osterrieth, 1944)

Copy and recall administration procedures have varied across investigations. It should be pointed out that according to standard procedure, subjects are asked to recall the figure without being forewarned. Of interest, pilot data collected by Wood et al. (1982) have indicated that there are no differences in Taylor figure scores obtained on 30 minute vs. 60-minute delayed recall in patients or normals.

In some studies, the copy condition is followed by immediate recall. Reported interval for delayed recall varies between 3 minutes and 24 hours. According to recent findings, varying the delay interval between 15 and 60 minutes has minimal effect on the rate of recall (Berry & Carpenter, 1992; Lezak, 1995). The delayed recall, however, is affected by administration of the immediate recall trial or repeated delayed recall trials, which have a facilitating effect on delayed performance (Chiulli et al., 1989; Loring et al., 1990). Loring et al. (1990) reported

an increase in accuracy of 30-minute delayed recall of about six points due to interposing a 30-second recall trial.

The interested reader is also referred to Lezak (1995) and Spreen and Strauss (1998) for additional ROCF administration instructions.

Alternate Version

Repeated administration of the ROCF results in inflation of the retest scores due to the practice effect. According to Spreen and Strauss (1991), the inflation reaches about 10% of the original score on the 1 month retest. The Taylor figure (L. B. Taylor, 1969; Lezak, 1995) was produced as an alternate version of the complex figure to avoid practice effects in repeated testing situations. The assumption of comparability of the two figures stems from the fact that both figures have an equal number of details of assumed equal complexity.

To validate this assumption, several studies compared scores obtained by subjects on Rey-Osterrieth and Taylor figures in normal and clinical populations (Berry et al., 1991; Delaney et al., 1992; Duley et al., 1993; Hamby et al., 1993; Hubley, unpublished honor thesis; Kuehn & Snow, 1992; Peirson & Jansen, 1997; Strauss & Spreen, 1990; Tombaugh & Hubley, 1991; Tombaugh et al., 1990; Tombaugh et al., 1992a). The results indicated that the figures yielded equivalent copy scores. However, recall scores or percentage of the copy score retained on recall condition was much higher for the Taylor figure, irrespective of the delay interval, learning paradigm (incidental or intentional), or scoring system. According to Casey et al. (1991) this might be attributed to the fact that the Taylor figure is more likely than ROCF to be encoded verbally. This finding limits interchangeable use of these figures in test–retest situations.

Scoring Systems

Osterrieth's (1944) scoring system, adapted by Taylor (1959), is most commonly used in scoring the copy and recall reproductions of the ROCF. It is based on the accuracy of a subject's reproduction and assigns zero to two points based on placement and presence of distortion for each of 18 structural elements of the figure. This system replaced scoring criteria proposed by Rey (1941) for scoring copy and 3-minute delayed recall, which was based on a 47-point scale. Translations of Rey's (1941) and Osterrieth's (1944) original articles describing scoring criteria, along with critical commentaries and recommendations for administration, are offered by Corwin and Bylsma (1993).

Scoring criteria published by E. M. Taylor (1959, adapted from Osterrieth, 1944) are reproduced in Figure 10.2 and Table 10.1.

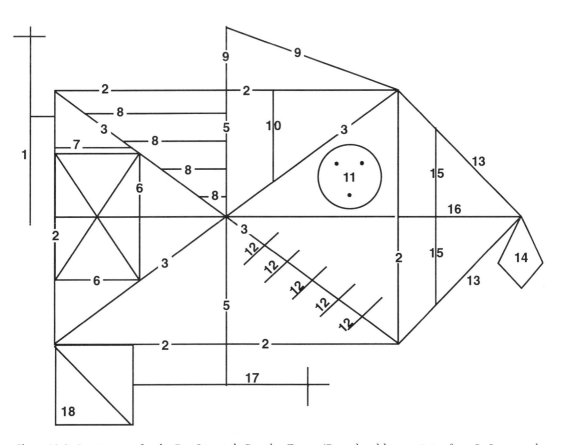

Figure 10.2. Scoring units for the Rey-Osterrieth Complex Figure. (Reproduced by permission from O. Spreen and E. Strauss)

Table 10.1. ROCF.Score1; Scoring Criteria

Units:

1. Cross upper left corner, outside of rectangle;
2. Large rectangle;
3. Diagonal cross;
4. Horizontal midline of 2;
5. Vertical midline;
6. Small rectangle, within 2, to the left;
7. Small segment above 6;
8. Four parallel lines within 2, upper left;
9. Triangle above 2, upper right;
10. Small vertical line within 2, below 9;
11. Circle with three dots within 2;
12. Five parallel lines with 2 crossing 3, lower right;
13. Sides of triangle attached to 2, on the right;
14. Diamond attached to 13;
15. Vertical line within triangle 13, parallel to the right vertical of 2;
16. Horizontal line within 13, continuing 4 to the right;
17. Cross attached to 5, below 2;
18. Square attached to 2, lower left.

Scoring: Consider each of the 18 units separately. Appraise accuracy of each unit and relative position within the whole of the design. Rating for each unit is presented in Table 10.2.

In order to improve quantitative objectivity of scoring and to address organizational aspects of performance, several other scoring systems were proposed:

1. Visser (1973) developed a system which quantifies figure accuracy (based on the presence or omission of certain details) and organization (based on interruption and sequence scores). The method of test administration has been altered to record the sequence of segments reproduced by the patient. Three aspects of performance are scored: (a) omission of a detail or its portion; (b) interruption of a line before being completed; (c) sequence of reproduction. This system was developed for research with brain-damaged patients.

Table 10.2. ROCF.Score2; Rating for Each ROCF Unit

Correct	Placed properly	2 points
	Placed poorly	1 point
Distorted or	Placed properly	1 point
incomplete	Placed poorly	1/2 point
but recognizable		
Absent or not recognizable		0 points
Maximum		36 points

2. Binder (1982) used original Osterrieth scoring criteria to quantify accuracy of the reproduction but developed his own system to quantify organization. Five structural elements of the figure were identified, which were drawn as a single unit by non-brain-damaged subjects in the pilot study: the horizontal midline, vertical midline, two diagonals, and the vertices of the pentagon. The organizational score is based on the number of structural units drawn as a single vs. fragmented units, and on the number of missing units. This system was used to evaluate reproductions of patients with unilateral cerebrovascular brain pathology.

3. Klicpera (1983) used original Osterrieth scoring to assess the accuracy of the reproduction. In addition, he introduced organizational criteria, such as presence of parts of the configuration (main rectangle, internal structural components, external and internal details, intersections, and the segments forming the large rectangle, diagonals, and the perpendiculars); organization (intersections, alignment and arrangement of details); and approach to drawing (sequence of the construction, continuity of lines, segmentation of key parts). Klicpera used this system to explore planning abilities in dyslexic children.

4. Denman (1984) developed an itemized scoring system for the ROCF as a part of the Denman Neuropsychology Memory Scale, which assigns zero to three accuracy points to each of the 24 "designs" of the figure, which are divided into eight sectors. Rapport et al. (1995) developed several measures of hemispatial deficits that may be incorporated in this scoring system.

Tombaugh (unpublished research) developed a similar system for scoring the Taylor complex figure. Both systems consist of a total possible of 72 (69) points and are more detailed than the original 36-point scoring system to provide more objective interpretation.

5. Bennett-Levy (1984) proposed scoring criteria to evaluate strategy in addition to original Osterrieth's accuracy criteria. "Strategy total" included scores for "good continuation" (requiring a line to be drawn as one piece and continued until intersection with another line) and for "symmetry" (reflecting construction of symmetrical units and their components).

6. Waber and Holmes (1985, 1986) developed a scoring system to quantify goodness of organization and style in the context of developmental changes in children. The administration of the ROCF required usage of five colored pencils which were switched after specific time periods had elapsed. The figure was separated into the smallest segments, which were categorized as part of the four major components: base rectangle, main substructure, outer configuration, and internal detail. The presence of intersections and alignment of key components (base rectangle, main substructure, and outer configuration) was scored.

In addition, ratings of organization and style of the reproduction were obtained. Quality of reproduction of 24 organizational features resulted in placement of the protocol in one of the five organizational levels ranging from poor (1) to excellent (5). The rating of the style was based on reproduction of 18 "criterial juncture features," which placed the protocol into part-oriented, intermediate, or configurational categories.

7. Kirk and Kelly (1986) adapted the scoring method for accuracy and error from the system developed by Waber and Holmes (1985). In addition, they developed a system designed to provide an objective basis for recording, classifying, and evaluating starting strategy (configurational vs. piecemeal) and the level of organization (structured vs. nonstructured) in ROCF reproductions by children. Starting strategies were also evaluated from a part/whole perspective. In addition, progression strategies were assessed. This system allows evaluation of the relationship between strategy, accuracy, and errors in ROCF reproductions.

8. A modified scoring system was used by Becker (Becker, 1988; Becker et al., 1988) to evaluate visuoconstructional skills and visual memory in Alzheimer's patients. According to this system, 12 "bits" of the drawing were scored for accuracy and placement (two points) and for accuracy only (one point).

9. Loring et al. (1988, 1990) developed an 11-point method for scoring qualitative errors reflecting accuracy of reproduction of each of 18 original details in recall of the ROCF. Scoring allowed a certain degree of "reproduction tolerance" due to the focus on memory functioning, rather than on constructional ability.

These criteria were applied to reproductions produced by the patients with temporal lobe epilepsy and were found to be effective in discriminating between right and left temporal lobe epilepsies. It should be noted, however, that application of this method to scoring reproductions produced by a sample of college students resulted in over 95% of the sample scoring 36 out of 36 points.

10. Simplified versions of ROCF and Taylor figures were developed by Hubley and colleagues (Hubley, unpublished honors thesis; Tombaugh et al., 1990) to assess elderly and neurologically impaired individuals. Fifty-point itemized scoring systems were developed to score the figures. These systems are similar to the itemized scoring systems developed for the full versions of the figures, with the exception of scoring only 19, rather than 24 (23) "designs" of the figures.

11. Berry et al. (1991) modified the original scoring criteria to improve sensitivity of the score to distortion and displacement of details. Scores for each of the 18 details ranged from 0 to 2 in half-point increments. A score of one-quarter point was also allowed to denote gross distortion or severe displacement of the detail. These criteria were applied to scoring of the ROCF for a sample of elderly subjects. The modified system scores are on the average two points higher than those obtained using the original scoring system; however, the correlations between the two systems are high (ranging between 0.82 and 0.96 for different conditions).

12. Chervinsky (see Chervinsky et al., 1992) developed the "organizational scoring system," which is designed to assess organization of the reproductions and is minimally affected by the reproduction accuracy. According to this system, the subject is offered a different color pencil when it is judged by the examiner that he has completed a "chunk" of the figure. The figure is separated into six sections, consisting of different combinations of conceptual "chunks." A total score reflecting organizational quality of the reproduction is based on the scores assigned for completeness of the conceptual "chunks" (reproduced with the same color pencil) minus penalty scores. (One conceptual detail is reproduced with different color pencils.)

13. Meyers and Meyers' (1992) modified administration procedure of ROCF includes four conditions: copy (recording the time to completion), 3-minute delayed recall (from the time of completing the copy), 30-minute delayed recall (from the time of completing the copy), and a recognition subtest. Scoring of the copy and recall conditions is based on the original system, and is similar to the system presented by Loring et al. (1990). However, the authors introduced a ¼" rule for "misplacement" and an ⅛" rule for drawing errors, which reduce the effect of subjective judgment on scoring.

The recognition subtest is composed of 12 parts of the ROCF presented in their proper size, shape, and orientation, mixed randomly with 12 distractors. The subject is to circle all the parts recognized from the original design. Scoring of the recognition subtest is based on the number of correct, false-positive, and false-negative responses. In their recent study, Meyers and Lange (1994) compared scores on the recognition subtest for different clinical groups and a normal group. The results suggested that this subtest discriminates best between brain-injured and normal subjects or subjects with minor brain injuries.

14. Duley et al. (1993) developed explicit scoring criteria for the ROCF and Taylor figures, which substantially increase interrater reliability of scoring. These criteria define scorable distortions and misplacements and outline clear rules for scoring deviations in drawings for each of 18 elements of the original 36-point scoring system for both figures. This system was used by the authors in a study with subjects infected with HIV.

15. Hamby et al. (1993) developed an organizational quality scoring system for ROCF and Taylor figures. Administration of the figures requires use of colored pens which are switched at equal points in the construction of the figure. The scoring is based on 18 standard elements for each figure. It focuses, however, on the reproduction strategy through determining the order of placement of configural elements (base rectangle or square, horizontal and vertical midlines), the appropriate continuation of lines, and the order of placement of details. The ratings of organizational quality are made on a five-point scale and reflect presence of three types of

mistakes (configural, diagonal, and detail), with higher scores indicating better organization. This system was used by the authors to discriminate between asymptomatic and symptomatic HIV-positive patients.

16. Stern et al. (1994) proposed the Boston Qualitative Scoring System (BQSS), which divides the ROCF into three hierarchical sets of elements: configural elements, clusters, and details. These sets are scored for different combinations of the following features: presence, accuracy, fragmentation, and placement. The reproductions are also evaluated in respect to planning, organization, size distortion, perseveration, confabulation, rotation, neatness, symmetry, and immediate and delayed retention. Quality of these features yield 17 initial scores for each of the three reproductions (copy, immediate recall, and 20-minute delayed recall). In addition, six Summary scores are calculated. Akshoomoff and Stiles (1995a,b) applied this system (with some modifications) to explore strategies used by children in ROCF copy and recall. Cahn et al. (1996) used the BQSS system to examine qualitative features of ROCF performance in ADHD.

A review and critical analysis of different scoring systems are provided in several sources (Chervinsky et al., 1992; Hamby et al., 1993; Lezak, 1995).

In summary, a number of different scoring systems for ROCF and Taylor's figure were proposed which focus on different aspects of reproduction: accuracy, organization, strategy, and style. Due to the variations in scoring systems and differences in operationalization of conceptual aspects of reproduction, results of different studies and normative data reported in these studies should be interpreted with caution.

Reliability

Of some concern in the use of the ROCF is the issue of interrater reliability. Most clinicians use the E. M. Taylor (1959) scoring criteria, and those familiar with the system are aware of the subjective judgment involved in determination of a "distortion." Bennett-Levy (1984) reports that pilot study data have indicated that only by use of very strict or very lenient scoring criteria can adequate interrater reliability be attained. He states that Taylor conveyed to him in a personal communication that he, in fact, employs very strict criteria involving quality of draughtsmanship, as well as presence, distortion, and misplacement of figures. However, Bennett-Levy (1984), Berry and Carpenter (1992), Berry et al. (1991), Boone et al. (1993a), Carr & Lincoln (1988), Delaney et al. (1992), Rapport et al. (1997), and Stern et al. (1994) report respectable interrater reliabilities of between 0.80 and 0.99.

Liberman et al. (1994) assessed interrater and intrarater reliability of the ROCF scoring in a large sample of male boxers. The authors report very high intrarater reliability and good interrater reliability for copy and immediate and delayed recall of the figure.

Tupler et al. (1995) established an excellent inter- and intrarater reliability for total scores (ranging between 0.85 and 0.97) in a sample of 95 memory-impaired elderly subjects. However, corresponding reliabilities for the 18 individual items were highly variable, ranging from 0.14 to 0.96. The authors recommended amplified delineation of relevant decision criteria for scoring of individual items.

Berry et al. (1991) and Rapport et al. (1997) reported adequate internal consistency reliabilities for the standard scoring system. The latter study also reported higher internal consistency for the Denman system in comparison to the standard system.

Data on test–retest reliability of the ROCF over a 1-year period were provided by Berry et al. (1991). Based on performance of a sample of 41 elderly "normal" subjects, they reported low reliability for the copy condition but moderate reliability for immediate and delayed recall.

Similarly, test–retest reliability coefficients for ROCF performance of elderly subjects, reported by Mitrushina and Satz (1991a), were quite low. Assessed over three annual probes, the coefficients ranged from 0.56 to 0.68 for the copy and from 0.57 to 0.77 for the 3-minute delayed recall conditions.

Clinical Utility

ROCF assesses visuoperceptual/constructional skills, spatial organizational skills, and visual memory. It has frequently been found to be sensitive to nondominant hemisphere functioning, and right temporoparietal area integrity in particular (Binder, 1982; Milner, 1975; Taylor, 1969; Wood et al., 1982), although some investigators have failed to document this relationship (King, 1981). Some authors have suggested that right-hemisphere- and left-hemisphere-damaged patients may show different types of ROCF copy and recall failure. On copy, right-hemisphere-damaged patients have been reported to exhibit distortions, while left-hemisphere-damaged patients have been observed to produce the design in a piecemeal and fragmented fashion but still frequently produce an adequate copy (Binder, 1982). On recall, right-hemisphere-damaged patients have been documented to show distortions and loss of the general organization of the figure (based on Taylor version), while left-hemisphere-damaged patients have shown preservation of the four-square quadrant but loss of details (Wood et al., 1982).

Kaplan (1988) emphasized the importance of qualitative interpretation of the drawing strategy in the context of the process analysis of patient's performance. According to Kaplan, both frontal and posterior damage might result in poor reproduction of the ROCF. In case of left frontal pathology, patients retain the outer contour and the major structural lines. In case of a right parietal lesion, the breakdown in contour and organization is expected on the side contralateral to the lesioned hemisphere (i.e., the left side of the design).

Regard and Landis (1994) analyzed clinical findings in 37 patients who produced a happy face ("smiley") instead of the detail involving a circle with three dots. The authors concluded that the "smiley" is rare, but its presence is associated with dysfunction of the anterior part of the right hemisphere.

Seidman et al. (1995, 1997) found that developmental analysis of ROCF identifies organizational difficulties related to ADHD, which is associated with developmentally lower levels of *copy organization* and *recall style.* However, Reader et al. (1994) did not find lower ROCF performance to be associated with attention deficit hyperactivity disorder (ADHD) when using a traditional scoring system. In a study by Waber et al. (1994), long-term survivors of childhood acute leukemia recalled fewer organizing-scheme components on ROCF but more incidental features in comparison to normative expectations. The authors suggest a metacognitive basis for this weakness, rather than visuoperceptual deficit.

The quality of ROCF copy and immediate and delayed recall can also be interpreted from the perspective of cognitive processes involved. Shorr et al. (1992) computed measures of copy accuracy, perceptual clustering, encoding, and savings for 50 neuropsychiatric patients, based on their ROCF performance. The authors concluded that perceptual clustering in the copy condition was a better predictor of memory performance than was copy accuracy.

Quality of ROCF performance of normal elderly (57–85 year-old) was analyzed by Mitrushina et al. (1990). The authors found equally efficient recall of basic structure of the figure across all ages represented in the sample. However, pronounced decline in recall of outer configuration was demonstrated by older subjects. Loss of details (coded verbally) with advancing age lends partial support to the hypothesis of age-related compromise in interaction between verbal and visual codes.

Waber et al. (1989) studied ROCF recall in children in the context of a dual-code cognitive neuropsychological model. Recall was compared after copying the figure vs. after visual inspection for the two experimental groups, respectively. Fifth-graders who did not copy the design prior to recall remembered its organization better and produced it more configurationally than the other group. However, there was no treatment-group difference for eighth-graders. The authors explain these results from the perspective of complementary functioning of the visual system, which favors configurational processing, and the motor system, which relies on sequential or part-oriented processing. Therefore, performance style can be indicative of the relative strength of the visual and motor codes, which can be interpreted in terms of the neuropsychological referents—sequential motor programming being associated with the left cerebral hemisphere and Gestalt pattern perception with the right. In the context of this theory, the results of this experiment sug-

gested that among preadolescent children, motor aspect interfered with efficient encoding of visuospatial information. An explanation based on differential involvement of cerebral hemispheres in information processing was also offered.

Further review of the effect of localization and lateralization of brain dysfunction on ROCF performance is provided in Spreen and Strauss (1998) and Lezak (1995).

RELATIONSHIP BETWEEN ROCF PERFORMANCE AND DEMOGRAPHIC FACTORS

Of importance to the clinician is the frequently reported relationship between ROCF performance and intellectual level in both patients and control subjects. Hemsley (1974) documented a significant correlation between ROCF percent loss on 40-minute delay and WAIS FSIQ ($r = -0.405$). He suggested that "it may be necessary to take IQ into consideration when interpreting scores on the Rey-Osterrieth test" (p. 1134). Wood et al. (1982) report significant correlations between ROCF 40-minute delayed recall and WAIS Block Design scaled scores ($r = 0.628$) with minimal associations with WAIS Vocabulary ($r = 0.258$), Digit Span forward ($r = 0.079$), and Digit Span backward ($r = 0.221$). They argue that ROCF performance is "dominated by variation in intellectual skills unrelated to memory" (p. 181). A majority of other investigators have found significant correlations between IQ variables and ROCF copy and recall performance (Bennett-Levy, 1984; Boone et al., 1993a; King, 1981; Mitrushina et al., 1989; Powell, 1979; Visser, 1980), although some negative findings have been documented (Speers & Ribbler, unpublished manuscript).

A robust relationship has also generally been found for ROCF copy and recall performance with age in patients and control subjects (Ardila & Rosselli, 1989; Ardila et al., 1989; Bennett-Levy, 1984; Boone et al., 1993a; Chiulli et al., 1995; Janowsky & Thomas-Thrapp, 1993; King, 1981; Mitrushina et al., 1995; Mitrushina & Satz, 1991a; Powell, 1979; Rapport et al., 1997; Speers & Ribbler, unpublished manuscript;

Visser, 1980), although some negative findings have been reported (Brooks, 1972; Delaney et al., 1992). King (1981) concluded "the strong effect of age . . . indicates a need for caution in the interpretation of copy and recall data from elderly subjects. It may be that the complexity of the Rey Figure renders it an unsuitable task for the discrimination of brain-damaged from non-brain-damaged elderly subjects. Further data are needed to answer this question" (pp. 642–643).

Tombaugh et al. (1992a) used a multiple-trial, intentional learning procedure to explore recall of ROCF and Taylor figures in 20–80-year-old healthy subjects. In their study, 60–80-year-old subjects scored lower than 20–59-year-old subjects on recall of both figures, which was attributed by the authors to less efficient encoding and retrieval strategies used by older people.

In another study, Tombaugh et al. (1992b) used a similar procedure to explore intentional learning of the Taylor figure in 20–79-year-old neurologically intact subjects. The Taylor figure was presented for observation for 30 seconds, after which subjects were to reproduce it from memory within 2 minutes. The procedure was repeated over four acquisition trials, which were followed by a retention trial 15 minutes later, and concluded with copying the figure from the model within 4 minutes. An itemized scoring system was used (Tombaugh, unpublished research). The results indicated that performance on the Taylor figure is not affected by gender, depression, or education and is not related to performance on the Vocabulary and Block Design subtests of the WAIS-R. Effect of age, however, was evident, with a greater rate of age-related decline on recall than on copy trials. The authors concluded that age has an effect on constructional as well as on memory processes.

Similarly, Mitrushina et al. (1990) did not find differences on the copy condition between 73 young-old (57–70-year-old) and 80 old-old (71–85-year-old) subjects. However, pronounced differences between these two age cohorts were reported on the 3-minute delayed recall condition. Changes in the accuracy and organizational quality of the copy and recall of ROCF as a function of advancing age were also reported by Chervinsky et al. (1992).

Waber and Holmes (1985, 1986) reported maturational changes in children which affect accuracy and organization of the ROCF reproduction in the copy and recall conditions. According to these authors, improvement in accuracy of reproductions is evident up to the age of 9 years, after which accuracy remains relatively stable. In contrast, developmental changes in planning and organization of the reproduction continue into adolescence.

Berry et al. (1991) found a significant relationship of ROCF immediate and 30-minute delayed recall with age and education. Scores on copy condition were not related to age, education, or sex in this study.

In general, no differences in ROCF performance between men and women have been found (Berry et al. 1991; Boone et al., 1993a; Browers et al., 1984). In some studies men outperformed women, but the amount of variance accounted for by this factor generally has been minimal (Ardila & Rosselli, 1989; Ardila et al., 1989; Bennett-Levy, 1984; King, 1981). The relationships between education and ROCF performance have been equivocal, with some reporting a significant relationship (Ardila & Rosselli, 1989; Ardilla et al., 1989; Berry et al., 1991) and others failing to document an association (Boone et al., 1993a; Delaney et al., 1992; Speers & Ribbler, unpublished manuscript).

Some studies addressed the relative importance of, or interaction between, ROCF scores and IQ/demographic factors. Boone et al. (1993a) documented with stepwise regression analyses a significant association between ROCF scores (copy and delay) and age as well as IQ in a healthy middle-aged and elderly population, whereas sex and education were not predictive of ROCF scores. Similarly, Bennett-Levy (1984) reported that age was strongly related to ROCF copy performance in his young-to-middle-aged sample, while copy score and age were significant predictors of recall scores; sex and IQ were not found to contribute to test scores once the other variables had been considered. While the Boone et al. (1993a) report did not find any interaction between age and IQ in their age-restricted sample, their findings considered in conjunction with Bennett-Levy's results may suggest that IQ is a less important factor in ROCF performance during young-to-middle adulthood but only emerges as an important variable in advanced age.

While many studies did not find the relationship between ROCF reproductions and handedness, Weinstein et al. (1990) report an interaction between handedness and academic major in college women. The highest quality of reproductions (in both copy and recall conditions) was seen in left-handed math/science majors, while the poorest quality was demonstrated by familial right-handed non–math/science majors. The authors attributed this difference to an increased ability to coordinate the use of left- and right-hemisphere processing in high-performing groups.

Ardila et al. (1989) found an interaction between education and age, and education and sex, on ROCF copy scores in their Spanish-speaking sample, with age and sex effects observed primarily in subjects with no formal education. However, in a larger sample of subjects limited to age 55 and older, classified into 0 to 5 years, 6 to 12, and greater than 12 years of education, while main effects for age, education, and sex on ROCF scores were also documented, no interaction between age, education, and sex was found (Ardila & Rosselli, 1989).

In another study, Rosselli and Ardila (1991) reported effects of age, educational level, and sex on the scores for both the copy and the immediate reproduction of the figure.

The discrepancy in the Ardila et al. (1989) and Boone et al. (1993a) reports regarding the importance of education for ROCF performance is probably related to differences in the educational levels sampled. The Boone et al. (1993a) population included only four subjects who had completed less than 12 years of education. It may be that educational level is a predictor of ROCF scores only at low education levels but that once an educational "threshold" is reached, such as completion of high school, education no longer influences ROCF performance.

METHOD FOR EVALUATING THE NORMATIVE REPORTS

In order to adequately evaluate the ROCF normative reports, eight key criterion variables were deemed critical. The first six of these relate to subject variables, and the remaining two dimensions relate to procedural variables.

Minimal requirements for meeting the criterion variables were as follows:

Subject Variables

Age Group Intervals

Given the significant relationship between age and ROCF performance, ROCF normative data should preferably be presented in age intervals.

Sample Size

As discussed in previous chapters, a minimum of at least 50 subjects per age group interval is optimal.

Sample Composition Description

As discussed previously, information regarding medical and psychiatric exclusion criteria, geographic region, ethnicity, occupation, handedness, and recruitment procedures is important.

Reporting of IQ Levels

Given the consistent significant relationship between IQ and ROCF performance, IQ information for the normative samples is critical.

Reporting of Education Levels

Given the probable relationship between education, especially low educational levels, and ROCF performance, information regarding education should be provided.

Reporting of Gender

Given a possible relationship between sex and ROCF performance in favor of males, information regarding sex composition of the sample should be reported.

Procedural Variables

Description of the Scoring System Used

A clear statement of the method used for scoring the ROCF is important because numerous scoring systems are available. In addition, given the rather subjective nature of some of the scoring procedures, information regarding interrater reliability is desirable.

Data Reporting

Means and standard deviations, and preferably, ranges, for copy and recall scores are important. Percent forgetting or percent retention could substitute for a recall score mean.

SUMMARY OF THE STATUS OF THE NORMS

In terms of subject variables, not all the studies provided data according to age intervals, although all datasets did indicate mean ages of the samples. Only a few studies provided data for elderly subjects. Several studies reported IQs or IQ estimates. However, only one publication provided data by IQ intervals. Mean educational level was indicated in many studies, but only a few publications reported data by educational level, or in age-by-education cells. Information on gender composition of the samples was documented in many studies and several publications provided data for males and females separately.

Several datasets had total sample sizes greater than 50; however, medical and psychiatric exclusion criteria were judged to be adequate in only a few studies. Information on geographic recruitment area was present in all datasets. Ethnicity, handedness, and occupation were less commonly reported.

In regard to procedural variables, all studies reported either mean raw scores or mean percent retention, and almost all reports provided standard deviations. Several studies presented copy scores only or recall performance only. Although documentation of copy strategy through use of colored pencils is commonly employed, only a few investigators reported qualitative information on the strategy features of ROCF copy or delay. Similarly, only a few reports indicated that ROCF performance was timed and only a few of these reported the data on performance time. Number and types of errors for copy and recall were described in a few studies.

The length of time elapsed before delayed recall varied widely: immediate recall, 3-minute delay, 30-minute delay, 40-minute delay, and 24-hour delay. In only some studies were the precise scoring systems described.

Only a few studies reported interrater reliability data for ROCF scores and internal consistency indices.

In addition to the studies reviewed in this chapter, normative data for Canadian children and adults between ages 6 and 70+ are provided by Spreen and Strauss (1998).

Among all the studies available in the literature, we selected for review those studies based on large, well-defined samples, or studies that offer some aspects of information that are not routinely reported. A majority of authors provide data based on the Osterrieth-Taylor scoring system. Any deviations from this standard reporting are specified in the context of each table.

Table 10.3 summarizes information provided in the studies described in this chapter.

SUMMARIES OF THE STUDIES

Normative Reports

[ROCF.1] Powell, 1979

The authors report data on 64 Londoners as a part of an examination of the relationship between ROCF performance and IQ and verbal memory performance. The 64 "normal" subjects were a part of a sample of 150 right-handed patients referred for neurological screening but who were "confirmed as having no brain damage on the usual physical tests such as the EMI scan" (p. 336). Twenty-one of the 64 subjects were female, and mean age was 41.0 (SD = 14.05). Mean verbal and performance IQs prorated from scores on the Comprehension, Similarities, Vocabulary, Block Design, and Object Assembly subtests were 107.70 (SD = 16.80) and 83.70 (SD = 21.55), respectively.

Mean and standard deviation for percent retention of the figure following a 40-minute delay as compared to original copy score are reported. Significant correlations were noted in the sample as a whole between ROCF percent retention score and Block Design score (r = 0.51), Object Assembly score (r = 0.50), Digit Span (r = 0.28), Comprehension (r = 0.39), Similarities (r = 0.32), Vocabulary (r = 0.27), Performance IQ (r = 0.38), Verbal IQ (r =

Table 10.3. ROCF.L; Locator Table for ROCF

Study[*]	Age[**]	N	Sample Composition	IQ,[**] Education	Country/ Location
ROCF.1 Powell, 1979 page 167	41.0 (14.05)	64	R-handed patients referred for neurological screening, but brain damage was ruled out	VIQ 107.70 (16.80) PIQ 83.70 (21.55)	London
ROCF.2 King, 1981 page 170	39.6 (21.4) <30 30–60 >60	71	Control group: healthy volunteers or patients with non-neurological or psychiatric conditions; Divided into three age subgroups	Education 11.4 (2.9) FSIQ 104.5 (18.1)	Canada
ROCF.3 Huhtaniemi et al., 1983 page 171	19–29 22	25	Male college students with good and poor attentional abilities (as determined by their performance on CPT) were compared.	College students	Maryland
ROCF.4 Bennett-Levy, 1984 page 171	29.3 (9.3) 17–49	107	Volunteers: 76 M, 31 F. No history of head injury or epilepsy	IQ 104.9 (7.6)	England
ROCF.5 Speers & Ribbler, unpublished manuscript page 173	35.00 (10.79) 23–70	40	20 M, 20 F normal volunteers. Modified ROCF was administered	Education 16.15(2.77) 10–22 Q.T.IQ 107.93(8.73) 87–123	CA
ROCF.6 Ardila et al., 1989 page 174	16–25 26–35 36–45 46–55 56–65	200	Normal Spanish speaking R-handed subjects. The data are stratified into 5 age ranges, by gender, and by education	Education: Illiterate vs. ≥ 10	Columbia
ROCF.7 Van Gorp et al., 1990 page 174	57–85 57–65 66–70 71–75 76–85	156 28 45 57 26	Healthy elderly Ss without history of neurologic or psychiatric disorder; 62 M, 94 F. Four age groups	Education 14.1(2.9) FSIQ 117.21 (12.59)	S. CA
ROCF.8 Berry et al., 1991 page 175	50–79 65 (2.9)	107	55 M, 52 F, elderly Caucasian Ss without cardiac, neurologic or psychiatric disease, or psychoactive medication. Rey and Taylor figures were administered. Test-retest data for 1 year interval are provided for 41 Ss.	Education 15(2.9)	Kentucky
ROCF.9 Tombaugh & Hubley, 1991 page 176		64 67	Study 1 compared performance on ROCF & Taylor figures. Itemized scoring systems were used. Study 2 addressed similar issues with the addition of implementing 2 scoring systems —itemized and Osterrieth-Taylor	3rd year undergraduate students	Canada

continued

Table 10.3. (*Continued*)

Study[*]	Age[°°]	N	Sample Composition	IQ,[°°] Education	Country/ Location
ROCF.10 Berry & Carpenter, 1992 page 178	68 (8.5)	31 M 29 F	Ss were healthy older volunteers with no history of neurological or psychiatric illness. Ss were divided into 4 equal groups, each of which was exposed to different delay period (15, 30, 45, and 60 min.)	Education 15(3.1)	USA
ROCF.11 Delaney et al., 1992 page 179	22–67 45.8	42	Study compared performance of normal adults on ROCF and Taylor figures in test-retest paradigm with intervals of 1-month between the two tests	6–16 12.8	7 VA Medical Center facilities: CT, CA, FL, VA, MA, MN, Ontario, Canada
ROCF.12 Kuehn & Snow, 1992 page 180	46.7	38	Study compared scores on copy, recall and percent recall for ROCF and Taylor figures in a sample of patients referred for evaluation of possible brain damage. Group 1 was presented with ROCF first Group 2 was presented with Taylor figure first	Education 10.9 FSIQ 94.7 Education 13.5 FSIQ 93.4	Canada
ROCF.13 Boone et al., 1993a page 181	45–59 60–69 70–83	91	Fluent English-speaking, healthy older adults; 34 M, 57 F. Three age groupings and four IQ levels	Education 14.5(2.5) FSIQ 115.9(13.0) 90–109 110–119 120–129 130–139	S. CA
ROCF.14 Chiulli et al., 1995 page 181	70–93 70–74 75–79 80–91	153 46 58 49	Ss are healthy elderly without any serious medical illnesses and not taking medications; 3 age groups	Education 15.3(2.4) 15.0(3.6) 13.9(3.0)	
ROCF.15 Meyers & Meyers, 1995 page 182	Group means: 21.2 to 23.8	30 Ss in each of 4 groups	Undergraduate students randomly assigned to 4 experimental groups. Modified scoring procedure was used	Education 12.2–12.6	Iowa
ROCF.16 Rapport et al., 1997 page 183	18-84 55.01 (14.31)	318	Ss were veterans referred to a V.A. hospital assessment service. Majority of Ss were inpatients; 312 M, 6 F. Standard and Denman scoring systems were compared	Education 12.62(2.77)	

[*]The study number corresponds to the number provided in the text of the chapter.

[°°]Age column and IQ/education column contain information regarding range, and/or mean and standard deviation for the whole sample and/or separate groups, whichever information is provided by the authors.

0.30), and age ($r = -0.33$). Powell concludes that ROCF performance is more associated with performance IQ than verbal IQ. He cautions that the ROCF "must be viewed in the light of the patient's intelligence . . . [and] in relation to the patient's age, since older people score lower" (p. 339). Powell describes how the clinician can derive an expected memory score based on IQ from a regression equation which can be used to determine if the patient's actual memory score is worse than expected.

Study strengths

1. Reporting of IQ data, age, sex distribution, geographic recruitment area, and handedness.

2. Relatively large sample size.

3. Means and standard deviations are reported.

Considerations regarding use of the study

1. While no objective evidence of brain dysfunction was found on lab tests, the patients were apparently suspected to have dysfunction—hence the referral for neuropsychological testing. Probably a sizable percent had some type of subtle brain dysfunction not detected by the standard diagnostic laboratory measures. The significantly lower performance IQ corroborates that this group is probably not "normal."

2. Undifferentiated age range.

3. Lack of data regarding education.

4. Lack of data regarding copy scores or raw recall scores.

5. The data were collected in England and may have limited value for use in this country.

6. No information on scoring system or interrater reliability (Table 10.4).

[ROCF.2] King, 1981

The authors obtained ROCF data on 71 Canadian controls as a part of a study on the effects of lateralized nonfocal brain dysfunction and age on the ROCF and the relationship between ROCF and Wechsler Memory Scale–Visual Reproduction performance in a sample of 185 subjects. The controls consisted of healthy volunteers or patients with "non-neurological or psychiatric conditions." Mean age, years of education, and WAIS FSIQ were 39.6 (SD = 21.4)), 11.4 (SD = 2.9), and 104.5 (SD = 18.1), respectively.

Subjects copied the ROCF and drew it from memory following a 40-minute delay during which time verbal tasks were administered. Copy and recall scores were obtained using the E. M. Taylor guidelines. A percent recall score was also calculated by multiplying the ratio of recall to copy score by 100.

Means and standard deviations for copy, recall, and percent recall are reported for three age groups: <30 ($n = 36$), 30 to 60 ($n = 17$), and >60 ($n = 18$). Significant correlations were obtained between ROCF scores (copy, recall, and percent recall) and age and IQ in the patients and controls as a whole. In addition, for the whole sample, males were found to perform significantly better than females on recall and percent recall; however, the amount of variance accounted for was negligible.

Study strengths

1. Data presented by age groupings.

2. Information regarding IQ, education, and geographic recruitment area.

3. Specification of scoring system.

4. Means and standard deviations are reported.

Table 10.4. ROCF.1; Percent Retention of the Figure Following a 40-Minute Delay as Compared to Original Copy Score

			WAIS		
N	Age	Sex (M/F)	VIQ	PIQ	% Retention
64	41.0 (14.05)	43/21	107.70 (16.80)	83.70 (21.55)	56.79 (22.25)

Table 10.5. ROCF.2; Means and Standard Deviations for Copy, Recall, and Percent Recall for the Total Sample and Three Age Groups

| | | | | | ROCF | | |
| | | | | | | 40-Minute | |
	N	Age	Education	WAIS FSIQ	Copy	Recall	% Recall
Total	71	39.6	11.4	104.5	31.1	16.4	52.3
		(21.4)	(2.9)	(18.1)	(4.5)	(7.1)	(20.4)
	36	<30			33.0	20.0	60.4
					(2.8)	(6.4)	(18.1)
	17	30–60			30.5	13.4	44.5
					(4.7)	(6.0)	(19.9)
	18	>60			27.8	12.2	44.3
					(5.4)	(5.9)	(19.9)

Considerations regarding use of the study

1. An unspecified number of subjects were medical or psychiatric patients.

2. The data were collected in Canada and their usefulness for an American sample is unclear.

3. No information on interrater reliability.

4. Below average educational level.

5. No information regarding gender distribution.

6. There is an apparent error in the data presentation table; the recall score for controls less than 30 years reads 0.0. (Our calculations suggest it should read 20.0).

7. The sample sizes for the individual age groupings are small (Table 10.5).

[ROCF.3] Huhtaniemi, Haier, Fedio and Buchsbaum, 1983

Four hundred male college students were screened on a measure of vigilance, the Continuous Performance Test (CPT). Two groups were identified for further study: (1) a Good Attention Group (upper 5% of the CPT score distribution, $N = 13$) and (2) a Poor Attention Group (lower 5% of the CPT score distribution, $N = 12$). Subjects ranged in age from 19 to 29 years with a mean age of 22 years.

Subjects copied the ROCF and reproduced the figure from memory 3 minutes later. The standard scoring system was used.

The authors concluded that attentional dysfunction is associated with performance deficits similar to those seen in patients with bilateral and diffuse cortical damage.

Study strengths

1. A nonclinical sample of subjects with good and poor attentional abilities was studied.

2. Specification of scoring system used.

3. Information on gender, age, and education.

4. Restricted age range.

5. Means and standard deviations are reported.

Considerations regarding use of the study

1. All subjects were male.

2. Demographic variables for each group are not provided.

3. High intellectual level of the subjects.

4. No exclusion criteria.

5. No information on interrater reliability.

6. Small sample size (Table 10.6).

[ROCF.4] Bennett-Levy, 1984

The authors collected ROCF data on 107 English volunteers as a part of a project to develop a quantified technique of scoring copy strategy and assessing the relationship between copy strategy and recall. Forty-five subjects were hospitalized patients tested prior to nonemer-

Table 10.6. ROCF.3; Copy and 3-Minute Delayed Recall Scores for the Two Groups of Subjects

	WAIS-FSIQ	ROCF Copy	ROCF Recall
Good attention	122	30.23	24.92
	(5.2)	(4.62)	(5.62)
Poor attention	107	28.92	22.67
	(12.0)	(5.04)	(6.81)

gency surgery; 62 subjects were auto-assembly line workers. Seventy-six were male and 31 were female. Exclusion criteria included history of head injury or epilepsy. Mean age was 29.3 (SD = 9.3; range = 17–49) and mean estimated IQ based on the Schonell Graded Word Reading Test and the New Adult Reading Test was 104.9 (SD = 7.6).

Subjects were instructed to "Copy the figure as accurately (emphasized) as [possible]. . . . While the subject copied the figure, the experimenter made a note of every line drawn in sequence. . . . When the subject indicated that s/he had finished the copy, the figure and the drawing were removed from sight; 40 minutes later, the experimenter said to the subject: 'You remember that drawing you copied for me. I would now like you to recall as much of it as you possibly can.' When the subject first indicated that s/he could recall no more, the experimenter said: 'Give yourself a little more time. I always say to people to give themselves some more time.' In a number of cases, this procedure resulted in one further detail being recalled. When the subject indicated that s/he had finished, this was accepted" (p. 110).

Bennett-Levy developed precise scoring criteria for the copy and recall of the figure based on Osterrieth's (1944) and E. M. Taylor's (1959) outline. He noted that his scoring system is "almost certainly more stringent than those customarily used by clinical psychologists." He opted for a strict scoring criteria to reduce the presence of ceiling effects on the copy trial; a majority of the protocols would have achieved the maximum possible score if more lenient criteria had been used. Bennett-Levy developed a more lenient scoring system in addition to his strict criteria for the recall trials, reasoning that memory scores should not be penalized due to sloppiness or imprecision of the reproduction when it was clear that the details were in fact accurately remembered. Interrater reliabilities of 0.96 and 0.98, respectively, for the "strict" and "lax" scoring systems were obtained on 25 randomly selected recall protocols. Bennett-Levy also developed scores describing "good continuation" (when a straight line is drawn as one piece until its final intersect with an-

other line), "symmetry" (successive construction of symmetrical units), and "strategy total" (sum of good continuation and symmetry scores).

Means and standard deviations for copy score, strict and lax recall, copy time, symmetry, good continuation, and strategy total are reported for males and females separately and for the sample as a whole. Multiple regression analyses revealed that strategy, copy time, and age were the primary determinants of copy scores, while strategy, copy score, and age were the principal predictors of recall. IQ and sex were significantly associated with copy and recall performance but did not provide a unique contribution to prediction once the other variables were considered. Bennett-Levy provides a regression equation to allow prediction of "lax" recall from strategy total and age. He suggests that a large discrepancy (i.e., more than 2 standard errors) between predicted and observed recall scores in favor of predicted score would argue for the presence of a significant memory impairment. He further cautions that failure to consider strategy and age and reliance solely on normative recall scores might lead to an inaccurate interpretation of memory impairment.

Study strengths

1. Careful specification of a scoring system including quantification of drawing strategy, and information on interrater reliability.
2. Specification of a regression equation which can provide a predicted recall score to be used for comparison with actual test scores.
3. Relatively large overall sample size.
4. Information on IQ, sex, age, occupation, and geographic recruitment area.
5. Presentation of data by sex.
6. Information on time to complete the drawing.
7. Means and standard deviations are reported.

Considerations regarding use of the study

1. Utilization of a unique scoring system which is much more complicated than the Taylor system and which is not in wide usage.

Table 10.7. ROCF.4; Means and Standard Deviations for Copy Score, Strict and Lax Recall, Copy Time, Symmetry, Good Continuation, and Strategy Total for the Sample as a Whole and for Males and Females Separately

N	Age	IQ	Symmetry	Good Continuity	Strat Total	Copy Score	Strict Recall	Lax Recall	Copy Time
107	29.3	104.9	10.1	13.2	23.4	28.1	16.3	20.9	158.0
	(9.3)	(7.6)	(3.2)	(3.1)	(5.0)	(4.2)	(5.2)	(5.8)	(51.5)
76 M	29.3	104.0	10.5	13.7	24.2	28.6	17.1	21.9	159.1
	(9.4)	(7.9)	(3.1)	(3.1)	(4.8)	(3.9)	(5.3)	(5.6)	(52.8)
31 F	29.2	106.9	8.9	12.2	21.1	26.9	14.5	18.3	153.6
	(9.1)	(6.2)	(3.2)	(2.8)	(5.0)	(4.7)	(4.7)	(5.7)	(47.8)

2. Use of hospitalized orthopedic patients for nearly half of the subject sample.

3. Undifferentiated age range.

4. Minimal exclusion criteria.

5. No information on educational level.

6. The data were collected in England and their usefulness for an American sample is unclear (Table 10.7).

[ROCF.5]. Speers and Ribbler, unpublished manuscript

The authors report data on 40 (20 male and 20 female) normal subjects tested as a part of a study on rates of loss for newly learned information over a 24-hour delay. Subjects were recruited from staff and visitors at a rehabilitation hospital in California. Those with abnormal neurological histories were excluded as well as those with signs of language, motor, or visual disability. Mean age was 35.00 (SD = 10.79; range = 23 to 70) and mean years of education was 16.15 (SD = 2.77; range = 10 to 22). IQ estimates obtained through the Quick Test revealed a mean IQ of 107.93 (SD = 8.73; range = 87 to 123).

The Rey Figure was modified to include an additional detail in the left lower quadrant. Subjects copied the design and then drew it from memory immediately and at delays 30 minutes and 24 hours later. They were not informed that they would be requested to recall the figure again after the immediate recall attempt. The subjects were kept occupied during the 30-minute delay interval with a questionnaire and IQ test items; the 24-hour delay period was unstructured. Time to copy the figure averaged 3 minutes 26 seconds.

The authors developed a scoring system involving a zero-, one-, and two-point rating scale for 50 separate scoring units, which resulted in a total possible score of 100. Approximately 12% of the information could not be retrieved on immediate recall, with additional 1% losses noted on 30-minute and 24-hour delayed recall. No mean scores or standard deviations are reported, but rates of forgetting over the three delay periods are plotted in a graph format, and the modal reproduction of the figure at copy, immediate, and 30-minute and 24-hour delays are pictured. The investigators cite significant negative correlations between amount of information loss and age ($r = -0.39$) but found no significant relationship between IQ ($r = -0.12$) or education ($r = 0.09$) and retention of the figure.

Study strengths

1. Presentation of data regarding three different recall intervals (although earlier recall trials no doubt influenced later recall trials to some unknown extent and therefore the data on 30-minute and 24-hour delays should not be used as a comparison reference for subjects who were not administered the earlier recall trials).

2. Reporting of IQ estimates, age, sex distribution, educational level, and geographic recruitment area.

3. Adequate exclusion criteria.

Considerations regarding use of the study

1. Modification of the stimulus figure.

2. Utilization of a unique scoring system not in common usage.

Table 10.8. ROCF.5; Scores for the Copy Condition Based on the Author's Unique Scoring System, and Percent Recalled on Three Recall Conditions°

| N | Age | Education | Quick Test IQ | Copy | ROCF % retention | | |
					Immediate	30 Minutes	24 Hours
40	35.00	16.15	107.93	99	87	84	84
	(10.79)	(2.77)	(8.73)				
	(23–70)	(10–22)	(87–123)				

°IQ was estimated with the Quick Test.

3. Lack of mean scores and standard deviations for the recall conditions.

4. Undifferentiated age range.

5. High mean educational level.

6. No data on interrater reliability.

7. Sample size is relatively small. (Table 10.8).

[ROCF.6] Ardila, Rosselli, and Rosas, 1989

The authors obtained ROCF data on 200 "normal," Spanish-speaking, right-handed Colombians as part of their assessment of neuropsychological functioning in illiterates. Inclusion criteria for the illiterate subjects were as follows: (1) total illiteracy, (2) illiteracy due to lack of opportunity to attend school, (3) no current or past neurologic or psychiatric history, or sensory or motor impairment, (4) adequate performance in activities of daily living. All were of low income, and occupations included factory or construction workers, maids, cooks, or homemakers.

High-education subjects were recruited to match the illiterates on age and sex. Subjects, aged 16 to 25, were students and had at least 10 years of education; subjects over age 25 had at least 17 years of formal education. No exclusion criteria are reported.

The E. M. Taylor (1959, as reported in Lezak, 1983) scoring criteria were employed. Copy and immediate recall data were obtained although only the means for ROCF copy in sex-by-age-by-education cells are reported; the age intervals employed were 16–25, 26–35, 36–45, 46–55, and 56–65, and each cell had 10 subjects. Significant education, sex, and age main effects were documented for copy and immediate recall performance, with better performance associated with males, younger age, and higher education. In addition, significant inter-actions on copy score were noted for education and age, with lower scores primarily observed in the illiterate rather than the educated subjects over age 55. Similarly, a significant education and sex interaction was documented, with men outperforming women only in the illiterate group. No significant interactions were observed for recall performance.

Study strengths

1. Provide data on a Spanish-speaking population.

2. Provide data on ROCF performance in illiterates.

3. Large overall sample size.

4. Report data in age-by-education-by-sex cells.

5. Specification of scoring system.

6. Information regarding sex, occupation, handedness, and geographic recruitment area.

Considerations regarding use of the study

1. Small sample size in the individual cells.

2. ROCF scores for immediate recall are not presented.

3. No standard deviations are reported.

4. No information on interrater reliability.

5. No information on exclusion criteria in the educated subjects.

6. No IQ data available.

7. The data were collected in Colombia and their usefulness for an American sample is unclear (Table 10.9).

[ROCF.7] Van Gorp, Satz, and Mitrushina, 1990

The authors have collected data on 156 healthy elderly adults, aged 57 to 85, living independently in retirement community in Southern California as a part of their investigation of neu-

Table 10.9. ROCF.6; Scores on the Copy Condition for Illiterates and Those Who Completed at Least 10 Years of Education

Age	Illiterate		Educated	
	Men	Women	Men	Women
16–25	21.7	19.7	35.5	35.1
26–35	25.2	16.7	35.6	35.3
36–45	25.3	13.1	34.3	34.1
46–55	22.6	14.5	34.9	35.2
56–65	12.0	10.6	34.7	34.8

ropsychological processes in normal aging. Exclusion criteria included history of neurologic or psychiatric disorder or substance abuse. Thirty-nine percent ($n = 62$) of the sample were male and 61% ($n = 94$) were female. Mean years of education were 14.1 (± 2.9), and mean WAIS-R (Satz-Mogel format) FSIQ, VIQ, and PIQ were 117.21 (± 12.59), 118.77 (± 13.27), and 110.74 (± 13.07), respectively.

Mean scores and standard deviations are provided based on the Taylor (1959) scoring system for the copy and 3-minute delayed recall of the ROCF for four age intervals: 57–65 ($n = 28$), 66–70 ($n = 45$), 71–75 ($n = 57$), and 76–85 ($n = 26$). Mean VIQs for each age interval ranged from 114.8 to 122.9, and mean PIQs ranged from 101.0 to 115.1. No differences in VIQ, PIQ, or education were found between older and younger subjects (<70 vs. >70).

Study strengths
1. Relatively large sample size and some of the individual age groupings approximate Ns of 50.

2. Organization of the data into relatively small age intervals.
3. Adequate exclusion criteria.
4. Specification of scoring system.
5. Reporting of information on IQ, education, sex, and geographic recruitment area.
6. Means and standard deviations are reported.

Considerations regarding use of the study
1. The very high intelligence and educational level of the sample.
2. No information regarding interrater reliability (Table 10.10).

[ROCF.8] Berry, Allen, and Schmitt, 1991

The authors collected ROCF data on 107 (55 male, 52 female) elderly Caucasian subjects from Kentucky, aged 50 to 79, as a part of their evaluation of the psychometric properties of the ROCF and Taylor figures. Mean age was 65 (± 8.6), and subjects were recruited from newspaper ads, flyers at senior-citizen centers, and a volunteer subject pool. Exclusion criteria included history of cardiac, neurologic, or psychiatric disease, or use of psychoactive medication, and all subjects underwent a physical exam by a physician and an EEG evaluation by a neurologist. Ten recruits were excluded due to the discovery of previously undetected diseases.

Subjects were provided with blank sheets of $8\frac{1}{2}'' \times 11''$ paper and were told to draw the complex figure as best they could. Without being forewarned, the subjects were instructed to draw the design from memory immediately after copy and 30 minutes later. The period between immediate and delayed recall was occu-

Table 10.10. ROCF.7; Scores for Copy and 3-Minute Delayed Recall Conditions per Age Group

N	Age	VIQ	PIQ	Copy	3-Minute Recall
28	57–65	117.2 (11.3)	109.2 (11.6)	32.50 (4.7)	14.45 (5.3)
45	66–70	114.8 (17.0)	111.5 (16.8)	32.93 (3.4)	14.13 (7.8)
57	71–75	122.9 (11.4)	115.1 (11.9)	31.73 (3.4)	11.13 (6.7)
26	76–85	110.6 (11.3)	101.0 (8.8)	30.14 (5.6)	8.41 (5.9)

pied with verbal testing. The scoring system was based on the E. M. Taylor protocol, with the following exceptions: (1) distorted but properly placed details, or correctly reproduced but misplaced details, received 1.5 points (rather than 1 point as in the Taylor system), and (2) severely misplaced but correctly drawn details, or severely distorted but correctly placed details received 1.25 points (rather than one point as in the Taylor system). Significant correlations were noted between the revised and Taylor systems (copy, $r = 0.82$; immediate, $r = 0.93$; delay, $r = .96$); scores for the revised system averaged two points higher. Interrater reliability quotients for the revised scoring system on 87 of the protocols were 0.80, 0.93, and 0.96 for the copy, immediate, and delayed recall trials, respectively, and the most experienced rater's scores were used for data analysis.

In a subgroup of 54 subjects, alternate form equivalence was assessed by administering either the ROCF or Taylor figures in a morning testing session; in the afternoon, the version not given in the morning was administered. Interrater reliability for 37 Taylor protocols was comparable to that documented with the ROCF (copy, $r = 0.84$, immediate, $r = 0.97$, delay, $r = 0.93$), and the more experienced rater's scorings were used for data analysis.

Test–retest reliability was evaluated in a subset of 41 subjects who were retested 1 year after original testing. The authors conclude the ROCF copy scores were not reliable, with moderate reliability noted on immediate and delayed recall. However, examination of mean scores suggests that there does not appear to be a clinically significant change in scores over 1 year (e.g., means differed by 0.3 to one point).

Means and standard deviations are reported for copy, immediate recall, and 30-minute delayed recall for the ROCF and Taylor figures for 54 subjects, as well as for baseline and 1-year follow-up ROCF scores in the subset of 41 subjects. Data on internal consistency, construct validity, and criterion-related validity are also reported. Significant correlations between ROCF scores and age and education were documented for immediate and delayed recall, but not for copy scores; sex was not significantly related to any ROCF scores.

Study strengths
1. Relatively large sample size.
2. Information regarding age, education, sex, ethnicity, recruitment procedures, and geographic area.
3. Information regarding interrater reliability.
4. Well specified exclusion criteria.
5. Specification of a scoring system.
6. Data on the Taylor figure, as well as comprehensive psychometric information for the ROCF.
7. Means and standard deviations are reported.

Considerations regarding use of the study
1. Undifferentiated age range spanning three decades.
2. Even though the total sample size is large ($n = 107$), it appeared that the reported means and standard deviations were based on sample sizes of either 54 or 41, but that the information on mean age and education was derived from the whole sample.
3. Idiosyncratic scoring system.
4. High mean educational level.
5. No information regarding IQ.
6. The baseline data on the subset of 41 subjects on whom the 1-year retest data were obtained had mean copy and recall scores five points below the sample of 54 subjects, suggesting that the subset was not randomly chosen and was not representative of the larger sample (Table 10.11).

[ROCF.9] Tombaugh and Hubley, 1991

The goal of the paper was to assess comparability of scores obtained on the Rey and Taylor figures in copy and recall conditions. Four studies were reported in this article.

Study 1 used an incidental learning paradigm, in which the subjects were not informed that recall will follow the copy condition. Subjects were 64 undergraduate students enrolled in a third-year psychology course who were randomly assigned to copy a ROCF or Taylor figure. Subjects reported no history of head injury producing loss of consciousness, neurologic dysfunction, or current use of psychoactive medication. Subjects were allowed 5.5 minutes to copy the complex figure, after which they were instructed to reproduce it from memory.

Table 10.11. ROCF.8; Means and Standard Deviations for Copy, Immediate Recall, and 30-Minute Delayed Recall for the ROCF and Taylor Figures for 54 Subjects, as Well as for Baseline and 1-Year Follow-up ROCF Scores in the Subset of 41 Subjects°

N	Age	Education	ROCF (n = 54)			Taylor (n = 54)		
			Copy	Immediate	Delay	Copy	Immediate	Delay
107	65	15	33.2	23.4	22.5	32.9	24.8	23.3
	(8.6)	(2.9)	(2.1)	(6.1)	(6.0)	(2.3)	(6.3)	(7.1)

	ROCF					
	Baseline (n = 41)			1 Year (n = 41)		
	Copy	Immediate	Delay	Copy	Immediate	Delay
	32.6	17.8	17.2	31.6	17.5	17.9
	(2.4)	(5.1)	(5.1)	(2.8)	(5.1)	(5.0)

°A modified scoring system was used in this study.

After a 4-minute delay filled with a nonpictorial task, the second recall condition was offered. Twenty minutes later, following completion of verbal learning tasks, subjects were administered the third recall condition. A 2-minute time limit was imposed on all recall trials.

Itemized scoring systems allowing a total of 72 points were used for scoring of both figures (Denman, 1984, system for ROCF; and Tombaugh, unpublished research, system for Taylor figure).

The authors concluded that the degree of accuracy on the copy condition was comparable for the two figures. However, all recall trials yielded significantly higher scores for the Taylor figure (Table 10.12).

Study 2 used another sample to replicate the above results and to explore the effect of scoring system on the comparability of the scores for the two figures.

Subjects were 67 undergraduate students enrolled in a third-year psychology course who were randomly assigned to copy the ROCF or Taylor figure. The procedure was similar to that used in study 1, with the exception of omission of the 4-minute delayed trial and inclusion of a 1-month delayed trial (which is based on the data for 52 subjects). In addition, the time required for copy and reproduction of each figure was recorded. The reproductions were scored according to the itemized system and the original Osterrieth-Taylor system.

Results were consistent with study 1 in that both figures were comparable on the copy, but not on the recall conditions, irrespective of scoring system. No forgetting was demonstrated between immediate and 20-min delayed recall trial; however, substantial decline in scores, equivalent for both figures, was seen over the 1-month interval (Table 10.13).

Study 3 utilized a modified size of the base rectangle of the ROCF to equate it to the base square of the Taylor figure (the total area of both figures = 64 cm^2). Itemized scoring systems were used. Results indicated that differences in recall scores cannot be attributed to differences in size of the structural components of the two figures.

Table 10.12. ROCF.9a; Scores for the Copy and Three Recall Conditions Based on the Itemized Scoring Systems for ROCF and Taylor Figures

Figure	N	Copy	Immediate Recall	4-Minute Delay	20-Minute Delay
ROCF	31	69.8	44.1	46.4	48.7
		(2.1)	(13.2)	(13.4)	(12.7)
Taylor	33	69.6	52.1	54.2	55.5
		(1.5)	(11.6)	(10.5)	(10.0)

Table 10.13. ROCF.9b; Scores for Copy and Three Recall Conditions for the ROCF and Taylor Figures Based on Two Scoring Systems

Figure	N	Copy	Immediate Recall	20-Minute Delay	30-Day Delay
Itemized Scoring System					
ROCF	33	69.0	46.9	50.3	29.5
		(1.8)	(11.0)	(12.2)	(12.1)
Taylor	34	69.6	56.4	59.4	39.2
		(1.5)	(11.6)	(10.5)	(10.0)
Osterrieth-Taylor Scoring System					
ROCF	33	34.9	23.5	25.5	14.6
		(1.2)	(5.1)	(6.0)	(6.1)
Taylor	34	35.1	28.6	30.3	19.8
		(1.4)	(5.9)	(5.3)	(8.1)

Study 4 modified administration of the figures to explore the effect of intentional learning and difference in time of exposure on recall efficiency. Seventy-two students enrolled in a first-year psychology course were instructed to study figures for a specified interval of time (15, 30, and 60 seconds) in order to reproduce them from memory after the exposure. Six learning trials were utilized followed by 20-minute delayed recall trial and a copy trial. A maximum of 2 minutes was allowed for all memory trials and 4 minutes for the copy trial. Itemized scoring systems were used. The results suggested that difference in performance was most pronounced with the 60-second presentation interval. The authors inferred that reported differences in recall efficiency of the two figures reflect lower degree of learning of ROCF in comparison to Taylor figure.

Study strengths
1. The authors systematically explore effect of different variables on performance on two figures.
2. Sample sizes are sufficient for these homogeneous samples.
3. Minimally adequate exclusion criteria.
4. Means and standard deviations are reported.

Considerations regarding use of the study
1. Age range and demographic characteristics of the samples are not reported; age range is probably sufficiently narrow.

2. Itemized scoring systems are not sufficiently described, and no information is reported on interrater reliability.
3. High educational level (third year of college) (Tables 10.12 and 10.13).

[ROCF.10] Berry and Carpenter, 1992

The article reports the rate of recall of ROCF over four different delay periods (15, 30, 45, or 60 minutes) in older persons in Kentucky. A sample of 60 subjects was divided into groups of 15, which were equivalent in age, sex, and education. All subjects were volunteers who were in good health with no active illness, no history of neurological or psychiatric illness, and no current use of psychoactive medication. Mini-Mental Status Examination scores were >24, with a mean of 28.5 (SD = 1.7). The sample consisted of 31 males and 29 females. All subjects were white, and 10% of the sample were left-handed.

All subjects were administered copy and immediate recall trials with no time limits, which were followed by one of the four delay durations. Timing of the delay started from the completion of the copy trial. During the delay periods, subjects were administered other neuropsychological tests of a verbal nature. Each protocol was scored for accuracy by two independent raters using the system described by Berry et al. (1991). Interrater reliability for the three trials was as follows: copy $r = .95$; immediate recall $r = .98$; delayed recall $r = .99$. Scores for data analyses represent average of the final scores assigned by two raters for each protocol.

The results revealed no significant effect of delay period on recall. Scores on immediate and delayed-recall trials were similar. The authors inferred that most forgetting occurs very quickly, as a result of an "overloading" of working memory.

Study strengths
1. Sample composition is well described in terms of age, ethnicity, sex, educational level, handedness, and geographic location.
2. Adequate exclusion criteria were used.
3. Interrater reliability and scoring system are reported.
4. Means and standard deviations are reported.
5. Age range is probably sufficiently narrow.

Considerations regarding use of the study
1. While overall sample is adequate, individual sample sizes are small.
2. High educational level.
3. No IQ information is reported (Table 10.14).

[ROCF.11] Delaney, Prevey, Cramer and Mattson, 1992

This study addressed comparability of the ROCF and Taylor Figure in a non-patient sample and is based on the control sample data collected as part of a large study carried out in various locations of the United States on the effect of anticonvulsant medications on memory functioning. Subjects were free of neurological and psychiatric disorders or current drug history.

Their age ranged from 22 to 67 years and education from 6 to 16 years.

The ROCF and Taylor figures were administered in the same order to all subjects, which is consistent with the order used in clinical practice. The time interval between administration of the two figures was approximately 1 month.

Three conditions were administered for both figures: copy, immediate recall, and 20-minute delayed recall, filled with nonvisuospatial tasks. The reproductions were scored according to the standard criteria.

Study strengths
1. Information on interrater reliability.
2. Information regarding age, education, and geographic area.
3. Information on alternate form.
4. Sample size approximates an N of 50.
5. Minimally adequate exclusion criteria.
6. Means and standard deviations are reported.

Considerations regarding use of the study
1. The data were not broken down by age.
2. No information regarding IQ or gender.

Other comments
1. Interrater reliability based on scoring of 10 samples by two experienced neuropsychologists was 0.91.
2. Correlations with age (-0.11 to -0.26) and education (-0.01 to 0.20) were relatively low.
3. The authors concluded that performance on the copy condition for both figures was nearly identical; however, subjects performed sig-

Table 10.14. ROCF.10; Scores for the Copy and Two Recall Conditions for Each Experimental Group (Based on the Length of Delay Interval)

Delay Period	Age	Education	Copy	Immediate Recall	Delayed Recall
15	67.3	15.1	30.8	19.3	19.2
	(7.8)	(2.6)	(3.4)	(3.9)	(3.2)
30	69.2	15.2	31.0	19.1	18.4
	(9.9)	(3.6)	(4.3)	(7.6)	(8.1)
45	67.5	15.2	32.5	22.6	22.1
	(8.5)	(2.7)	(2.7)	(6.3)	(5.5)
60	67.4	15.3	33.4	20.1	18.9
	(8.4)	(3.4)	(2.4)	(7.5)	(6.9)

Table 10.15. ROCF.11; Scores for the Copy and Immediate and 20-Minute Delayed Recall Conditions for the ROCF and Taylor Figures

	N	Age	Education	ROCF	TCF
Copy	42	45.8	12.8	33.8 (2.1)	33.6 (2.2)
Immediate recall				21.0 (7.8)	26.1 (6.4)
20 seconds delayed recall				20.8 (8.0)	25.7 (7.2)

nificantly better on the Taylor figure on both recall conditions (Table 10.15).

[ROCF.12] Kuehn and Snow, 1992

The study explored comparability of the ROCF and Taylor figure in a clinical sample. Subjects were 38 patients in Canada referred for neuropsychological assessment to assess presence of various forms of brain damage. Patients unable to execute drawing of a Greek cross or those who were administered either figure previously were excluded from the study. Mean age of the sample was 46.7 years.

The procedure consisted of copying each figure with a lead pencil with 40-minute delayed recall (without forewarning). Approximately 3 hours elapsed between administration of the two figures, during which time tests involving drawings or visual memory were not administered. Two figures were presented in a counterbalanced order.

The standard scoring systems were used for both figures. Percent recall was calculated.

The authors concluded that performance on both figures is equivalent considering copy and recall scores. Percent recall scores, however, were higher for the Taylor figure, especially when it was administered first.

Study strengths
1. Scoring system was specified.
2. Information on gender, age, education, IQ, and geographic areas provided.
3. Information on alternate form.
4. Means and standard deviations are reported.

Considerations regarding use of the study
1. Data were not broken down by age group. Age range was not specified.
2. The two groups were not comparable in education but were comparable in IQ.
3. Brain-damaged population; no exclusion criteria.
4. No information on interrater reliability.
5. Small sample size.

Table 10.16. ROCF.12; The Table Provides Scores for the Copy Condition, 40-Minute Delayed Recall and Percent Recall for the Rey and Taylor Figures

	Group[*]	N	Gender	Education	FSIQ	ROCF	Taylor
Copy	1	19	12M 7F	10.9	94.7	31.5 (4.0)	32.7 (3.4)
	2	19	7M 12F	13.5	93.4	31.0 (6.5)	30.5 (7.4)
Absolute recall	1					11.2 (5.2)	9.2 (7.5)
	2					9.2 (6.3)	14.2 (6.9)
Percent recall	1					35.2 (14.6)	29.5 (22.1)
	2					28.0 (16.8)	46.0 (17.0)

[*]Group 1: ROCF administered first; group 2: Taylor administered first.

6. Data were collected in Canada and as such may be problematic for use in the U.S (Table 10.16).

[ROCF.13] Boone, Lesser, Hill-Gutierrez, Berman, and D'Elia, 1993a

The investigators collected data on 91 fluent English-speaking, healthy, older adults recruited in Southern California through newspaper ads, flyers, and personal contacts as a part of their investigation of the effects of age, IQ, education, and sex on ROCF performance. Exclusion criteria included current or past history of major psychiatric disorder or alcohol or other substance abuse, neurological illness, and significant medical illness which could affect central nervous system function (e.g., uncontrolled hypertension or diabetes). In addition, potential subjects were rejected if they were found to have abnormal findings on neurological examination, metabolic disturbances detected with laboratory tests, or abnormal findings on EEG or MRI. The final sample included 34 males and 57 females. Seventy-one subjects were Caucasian, 10 were African-American, five were Asian, and five were Hispanic. Mean educational level for the sample was 14.5 ($\pm$2.5) years and mean WAIS-R FSIQ (Satz-Mogel format) was 115.9 ($\pm$13.0).

Subjects were instructed to copy the figure onto a blank paper "as carefully as you can without tracing." Performance was not timed and subjects were allowed to make erasures. Following a 3-minute verbal fluency task and without forewarning, the subjects were instructed to draw what they could remember of the figure onto a second sheet of blank paper. The E. M. Taylor scoring system was employed.

Means and standard deviations are reported for copy scores and percent retention for three age groupings (45–59, 60–69, and 70–83) and four FSIQ levels (90–109, 110–119, 120–129, and 130–139). Interrater reliability between two experienced neuropsychologists was 0.82 for copy and 0.93 for delay. In regression analyses, a relatively small but significant percent of the variance in ROCF performance was associated with age and FSIQ; sex and education were not predictive of ROCF scores. In addition, ROCF copy score was not associated with delay score or percent retention. Significantly

poorer ROCF scores did not emerge until age 70 and older, and individuals of average IQ showed a trend toward poorer performance on ROCF delay relative to subjects falling into very superior intelligence range. No interaction effects between age and FSIQ were observed. The number and types of errors committed on copy and recall are summarized.

Study strengths
1. Comprehensive exclusion criteria.
2. Presentation of data by age and IQ groupings.
3. Specification of scoring system and information on interrater reliability.
4. Information regarding education, sex, geographic recruitment area, ethnicity, and recruitment procedures.
5. Information regarding error number and type for copy and delay.
6. Large overall sample size although individual cells all fall short of 50.
7. Means and standard deviations are reported.

Considerations regarding use of the study
1. High intellectual and educational level.

Other comments
1. For the subjects older than age 74, age-corrected FSIQs were based on Ryan et al. (1990b) tables (Table 10.17).

[ROCF.14] Chiulli, Haaland, LaRue, and Garry, 1995

The study explores rates of decline in ROCF performance after age 70. The subjects were 153 healthy elderly subjects living independently between the ages of 70 and 93 who participated in the New Mexico Aging Process Study, which explored nutrition and aging. Persons taking prescription medications or with serious medical illnesses were excluded. The sample was broken down into three age groups.

The ROCF was administered as part of a brief battery of psychological tests. Standard administration and scoring procedures were used. A copy condition was followed by immediate and 30-minute delayed recall. If the reproduction started with the drawing of the large rectangle, the approach was categorized as configural. All other approaches were determined

Table 10.17. ROCF.13; Means and Standard Deviations for Copy and Three Minute Delayed Recall Scores, and Percent Retention for Three Age Groupings and Four FSIQ Levels

N	Age	Education	FSIQ	Copy	3-Minute Recall	% Retention
38	45–59	14.6 (2.6)	114.7 (14.2)	34.2 (1.8)	18.9 (6.1)	55.0 (17.1)
31	60–69	14.4 (2.1)	114.5 (12.8)	33.8 (2.8)	17.3 (5.2)	51.7 (13.8)
22	70–83	14.5 (2.9)	119.4 (10.6)	31.3 (4.7)	13.8 (5.0)	43.8 (14.8)

N	FSIQ	Age	Education	Copy	3-Minute Recall	% Retention
32	90–109	60.3 (9.8)	13.4 (2.2)	32.6 (4.5)	15.2 (4.9)	46.3 (13.3)
23	110–119	62.1 (9.0)	14.2 (2.2)	33.5 (2.0)	16.7 (5.6)	49.6 (16.1)
21	120–129	63.0 (9.3)	15.1 (2.4)	33.7 (2.2)	18.9 (5.4)	56.0 (14.8)
15	130–139	62.9 (10.4)	16.4 (2.4)	34.3 (2.3)	19.4 (7.6)	56.0 (20.2)

to be nonconfigural. All protocols were checked by a second 'blind' evaluator.

The results revealed a significant main effect for age group. Accuracy was greatest in the copy condition, but did not differ between the immediate and delayed recall conditions. The most pronounced decline in performance was demonstrated between the first and the second group, which did not differ considerably from the third group performance. No gender effects were evident. The number of subjects using configural approach did not differ significantly for the three age groups.

Study strengths

1. The data for elderly sample are provided broken down into three age groups.

2. Relatively large sample size and individual cells approximate *N*s of 50.

3. Specification of administration system.

4. Exclusion criteria are specified.

5. Reporting of information on education, sex, and geographic recruitment area.

6. The study assessed strategy utilized in approach to drawings.

7. Means and standard deviations are reported.

Considerations regarding use of the study

1. Generalizability of the data are low due to high educational level of the sample.

2. Data were checked by a "blind" evaluator, but no information on interrater reliability is provided.

3. No information on IQ (Table 10.18).

[ROCF.15] Meyers and Meyers, 1995

The study explores effect of different administration procedures on the rate of recall of the ROCF. Subjects were undergraduate students from a college in Iowa and had no prior history of head injury, drug abuse, learning disability, or psychiatric illness. Subjects were randomly assigned to one of four groups, each of which received different combinations of trials (30 subjects in each group). There was no significant difference between the groups on age, sex, or education.

Reproductions were scored according to the system developed by Meyers and Meyers (1992), which is based on the standard scoring system with addition of ¼″ rule for misplacement and ⅛″ rule for drawing errors. In addition, the authors used a recognition trial (Meyers & Lange, 1994).

Study strengths

1. Scoring system is described.

2. Sample composition and demographic characteristics are described, as well as geographic area.

Table 10.18. ROCF.14; Means and Standard Deviations for Accuracy of Performance on Three ROCF Conditions*

| | Age Group | | |
	70–74	75–79	80–91
N	46	58	49
Age	72.7	—	82.4
	(1.1)		(3.0)
Education	15.3	15.0	13.9
	(2.4)	(3.6)	(3.0)
Gender (% Women)	52%	59%	49%
Copy			
Accuracy	32.6	31.0	29.8
	(2.8)	(4.0)	(4.6)
Approach	39%	36%	35%
Immediate recall			
Accuracy	17.2	14.2	12.9
	(6.2)	(6.6)	(6.4)
Approach	55%	41%	40%
30-Minute delayed recall			
Accuracy	16.9	14.2	12.4
	(6.3)	(6.2)	(6.0)
Approach	55%	52%	41%

*Data on proportion of subjects adopting a configural approach are provided for each age group.

3. Overall sample size is large (*N* = 120), although individual groupings fall short of an *N* of 50.

4. Adequate exclusion criteria.

5. Means and standard deviations are reported.

6. Age grouping is suitably restricted.

Considerations regarding use of the study

1. No information regarding interrater reliability or IQ.

Other comments

1. The authors suggest use of a 3-minute recall instead of immediate recall due to its higher correlation with the 30-minute recall (Table 10.19).

[ROCF.16] Rapport, Charter, Dutra, Farchione, and Kingsley, 1997

The study addressed interrater and internal consistency reliabilities of the standard (as described in Lezak, 1995) and Denman scoring systems for the ROCF. Subjects were 318 veterans (312 males and six females), ranging in age between 18 and 84 years, who were referred to a V.A. hospital assessment service. The majority of subjects were inpatients. Mean age was 55.01 years (SD = 14.31) and mean education was 12.62 years (SD = 2.77). Three independent raters scored copy and immediate recall reproductions using standard and Denman criteria.

Interrater reliabilities are presented for the entire sample and for three referral sources separately: neurology, psychiatry, and rehabilitation medicine. The authors concluded that internal consistency and interrater reliabilities for both scoring systems were high. Coefficient α reliabilities were also high indicating psychometrically sound interitem congruity for both scoring systems.

Age was found to be modestly related to performance on the copy condition and strongly related to recall. Education was modestly associated with copy and weakly associated with recall performance.

Table 10.19. ROCF.15; Scores for the Copy Condition and Different Combinations of Three Recall Conditions/Recognition Trial for Each Experimental Group,[*] (N = 30 for each group)

	Age	Education	Gender	Copy	Immediate Recall	3-Minute Delay	30-Minute Delay	Recognition
Group 1	23.6	12.2	10 M	34.7	26.7		26.6	21.9
	(7.4)	(0.6)	20 F	(1.7)	(4.6)		(4.4)	(1.3)
Group 2	21.2	12.4	17 M	35.5		27.6	27.7	21.6
	(4.2)	(0.7)	13 F	(0.9)		(4.0)	(3.9)	(1.3)
Group 3	23.8	12.6	11 M	35.2	26.6	27.2	27.4	21.5
	(5.4)	(0.8)	19 F	(1.0)	(4.3)	(3.6)	(3.6)	(1.5)
Group 4	21.6	12.6	18 M	35.5			25.3	20.9
	(4.4)	(0.9)	12 F	(0.6)			(3.7)	(1.6)

[*]Scoring was based on a modified procedure (see text).

Study strengths

1. A large sample size.
2. Data on psychometric properties of the ROCF are provided.
3. Two scoring systems were compared.
4. Information on gender, age, education, and recruitment procedures.
5. Means and standard deviations are reported.

Considerations regarding use of the study

1. Subjects were V.A. inpatients from different wards, including neurology. Selection criteria and subjects' diagnoses are not specified. The data on test scores are of limited use with general population due to likely health confounds of the sample.
2. The sample was not broken down into age groups.
3. No information on IQ.
4. Mostly male population (Table 10.20).

Table 10.20. ROCF.16; Total Scores and Individual Item Scores for the Copy and Immediate Recall Reproductions Scored According to Denman and Standard Systems

	Denman Copy	Denman Recall	Standard Copy	Standard Recall
Total Score				
M	51.79	23.52	26.01	11.94
SD	15.57	15.35	7.89	7.64
Individual Items				
M	2.16	0.98	1.44	0.66
SD	0.33	0.44	0.17	0.30

CONCLUSIONS

A great number of studies exploring the psychometric properties of the ROCF and its clinical utility attest to its popularity among clinicians and investigators alike. However, a tremendous variability in administration and scoring of the ROCF obscures comparability of the results of these studies. To improve consistency across different studies, the procedures for administration and scoring need to be highlighted in detail.

It should be noted that the distribution of scores for ROCF copy condition deviates considerably from normal distribution. A majority of subjects are capable of copying the figure without major distortions. Therefore, a label of "superior" performance given to a subject achieving a high ROCF score is meaningless. On the other hand, the test is highly sensitive to deficits in visuospatial information processing, and achieving low performance score falling in the outlying range has important clinical significance.

In addition to the numerical expression of a subject's performance, the value of qualitative interpretation and the delineation of subject's strategy/type of errors was emphasized in several studies reviewed above. In this context, the two avenues of research on ROCF, namely, studies on clinical utility and on cognitive processes involved in figure drawing, are mutually enriching.

Recommendations for future research on ROCF include careful analysis of the effects of demographic factors on subjects' performance.

The well-documented effects of age and intelligence (and, possibly, education) need to be considered in subject selection and data presentation format. A large number of studies on the learning/processing strategies in children and on the clinical sensitivity of the test to different neurological conditions in adults are available in the literature, but only a few studies are dedicated to cognitive/clinical issues related to older age groups.

The psychometric properties of different scoring systems need to be further assessed. Data on interrater reliability, internal consistency, and test–retest reliability are scarce. From the review of existing studies it appears that different scoring systems are differentially applicable to specific clinical and research situations.

11

HOOPER VISUAL ORGANIZATION TEST

BRIEF HISTORY OF THE TEST

The Hooper Visual Organization Test (HVOT) consists of 30 line drawings of familiar objects which have been fragmented into pieces. The task requires the examinee to mentally reintegrate and name the objects, which are arranged in order of increasing difficulty. The response format can be oral or written, depending on whether the individual administration or the booklet format is used. The score is the number of correctly identified items, with half-points available for some of the items. Wetzel and Murphy (1991) suggest a discontinuation rule of five consecutive errors, based on a rating change of only 1% using this strategy.

The test was first published in 1958 and was revised in 1983. The test manual for the revised edition provides conversion tables to correct raw scores for age and educational level. Corrected or uncorrected raw scores can be converted to T scores according to the tables provided in the manual, with higher T scores representing a greater likelihood of neurological dysfunction. It should be noted that the standardization data reported in the manual are based on Mason and Ganzler's (1964) all male sample of 231 patients, personnel, and volunteer workers from a Veterans Administration hospital. The sample was stratified into nine age cohorts: 25–29, 30–34, 35–39, 40–44, 45–49, 50–54, 55–59, 60–64, 65–69 years old.

In addition to using T-score tables, determi-

nation of impaired vs. normal performance can be made using the cutoff criteria. The cutoff scores recommended by the authors vary depending on test administration setting. In a clinical diagnostic setting, a cutoff score of ≤24 is suggested in determining whether further assessment is needed. On the other hand, if the test is used as part of a screening battery administered to all patients admitted to a facility with a low incidence of organic brain pathology, a cutoff of 20 is recommended to minimize the rate of false-positive errors. Boyd (1981) argued that "no single cutoff score can be recommended for use in all clinical situations. Factors such as the subject's age, educational level, intelligence, and whether the situation requires minimization of false positives or false negatives, must all be weighed in interpreting test results" (p. 19). While the cutoff score suggested by Hooper was judged by Boyd (1981) to be optimal for evaluating chronically ill institutionalized patients, it appeared to be too low for less incapacitated patient populations.

Hooper also developed a qualitative system of response analysis involving four categories: isolate, perseverative, bizarre, and neologistic responses. Lezak (1995) underscores the benefits of qualitative analysis of errors, pointing to the localizing significance of fragmentation tendencies. Nadler et al. (1996) concur that qualitative analysis of errors improves the differentiation between the effects of right vs. left hemisphere dysfunction on HVOT performance.

The HVOT was developed as a screening instrument for organic brain dysfunction. However, the issue of the test's sensitivity to general vs. lateralized dysfunction remains controversial. The test authors suggest that the HVOT "is sensitive to general impairments, not specific visuopractic functions" (Hooper, 1983, p. 6). This view is supported by Boyd (1981, 1982a), Wang (1977), and Wetzel and Murphy (1991). However, HVOT's sensitivity to lateralized dysfunction is demonstrated in several studies. Lewis et al. (1997) report that the HVOT performance is vulnerable to acute lesions in the right anterior quadrant of the brain. In contrast, Fitz et al. (1992), Rathbun and Smith (1982), and Woodward (1982) demonstrate the HVOT's sensitivity to localized dysfunction specifically, of the nondominant parietal lobe. In fact, a heated debate over general vs. specific sensitivity of the HVOT is reflected in a series of articles published in response to Boyd's (1981) article (Boyd, 1982a,b; Rathbun & Smith, 1982; Woodward, 1982).

The above issue is directly related to assumptions regarding which cognitive functions are measured by the HVOT. Two components of information processing involved in HVOT responses are mental reintegration and naming of the objects for each test item. If visual perception and synthesis are the primary mechanisms involved in item analysis, then nondominant hemisphere contribution prevails. If test performance also imposes considerable naming demands, then both dominant and nondominant hemispheres contribute substantially to test performance. Studies exploring the relative contribution of these cognitive processes to HVOT performance are largely equivocal. Lezak (1995) and Spreen and Strauss (1991, 1998) suggest caution in interpreting HVOT failures as a manifestation of visuospatial deficit due to the contribution of the naming component.

In contrast, Ricker and Axelrod (1995) found that perceptual organization accounted for 44% of HVOT performance variance; however, confrontation naming ability was not significantly related to test performance. Similarly, in a study designed to replicate and extend the above research, Paolo et al. (1996) observed the HVOT to be a measure of perceptual organization, whereas performance on the test was not sig-

nificantly impacted by poor naming ability. Similarly, Seidel (1994) found the HVOT to be a measure of general visual-perceptual-constructional abilities in a pediatric population, and Johnstone and Wilhelm (1997) concluded that HVOT measures global visuospatial intelligence and shares 12% to 23% of common variance with WAIS-R PIQ subtests.

Data on reliability and validity of the HVOT are provided in Gerson (1974), Franzen et al. (1989), Lezak (1995), and Spreen and Strauss (1998). Item analysis for use of the HVOT with Indian subjects was performed by Verma et al. (1993).

Normative data for children 5–11 years are provided by Seidel (1994) and for 5–13 years by Kirk (1992).

RELATIONSHIP BETWEEN HVOT PERFORMANCE AND DEMOGRAPHIC FACTORS

Age and intelligence level are consistently shown to be related to HVOT performance. Tamkin and Jacobsen (1984) report an effect of age and IQ on HVOT performance in their sample of 211 male, veteran, psychiatric inpatients. Similarly, Wentworth-Rohr et al. (1974) found a positive relationship between HVOT scores and intelligence level as well as a negative age/HVOT relationship beginning in the late 30s. Age-related changes in HVOT performance are also documented by Farver and Farver (1982) and by Tamkin and Hyer (1984). Hilgert and Treloar (1985) documented an effect of age and IQ level, but no sex differences in elementary school children. An effect of IQ is also reported by Gerson (1974).

Education and sex have been shown to be unrelated to HVOT scores in a study by Wentworth-Rohr et al., 1974. Kirk (1992) reported, however, based on her analysis of HVOT performance of 434 normal children between ages 5 and 13, that boys attained adult performance by age 12, whereas girls participating in this study did not reach the adult level. Based on these data, Kirk documents an effect of age and gender on HVOT performance.

An interaction between age and education in a sample of cognitively intact elderly was reported by Richardson and Marottoli (1996). Nabors et al. (1997) found HVOT scores to be significantly related to age and education in a total sample, which combined cognitively intact and impaired elderly urban medical patients, whereas performance was not significantly related to these demographic variables for the cognitively intact group considered separately.

For further information regarding the HVOT, see Lezak (1995, pp. 409–411) and Spreen and Strauss (1998).

METHOD FOR EVALUATING THE NORMATIVE REPORTS

In order to adequately evaluate the HVOT normative reports, six key criterion variables were deemed critical. The first five of these relate to *subject* variables, and the remaining dimension refers to *procedural* issues.

Minimal criteria for meeting the criterion variables were as follows:

Subject Variables

Sample Size

As discussed in previous chapters, a minimum of at least 50 subjects per grouping interval is optimal.

Sample Composition Description

Information regarding medical and psychiatric exclusion criteria is important; it is unclear if education, geographic recruitment region, socioeconomic status or occupation, ethnicity, handedness, and recruitment procedures are

relevant, so until this is determined, it is best that this information be provided.

Age Group Intervals

Given the association between age and HVOT performance, information regarding age of the normative sample is critical and preferably normative data should be presented by age intervals.

Reporting of IQ Levels

Given the relationship between HVOT performance and IQ, information regarding intellectual level should be provided and preferably normative data should be presented by IQ levels.

Reporting of Gender Distribution

Information regarding sex distribution of the samples should be reported.

Procedural Variables

Data Reporting

Means and standard deviations for the total number of correct responses should be reported.

SUMMARY OF THE STATUS OF THE NORMS

There are several studies providing data for HVOT performance in psychiatric or neurological patients. Among the articles reporting data for normal samples, several studies only used selected HVOT items. A study which can be used to supplement normative data provided in the test manual by extending data toward older age groups is summarized in Table 11.1.

Table 11.1. HVOT.L; Locator Table for the HVOT

Study[*]	Age[**]	N	Sample Composition	IQ,[**] Education	Country/ Location
HVOT.1 Richardson & Marottoli, 1996 page 189	81.5 (3.3) 76–80 81–91	101	All autonomously living elderly Ss, current drivers; 53 M, 48 F. Data are provided for younger-old and older-old by two educational levels	Education 11.0(3.7) <12 ≥12	New Haven, CT

[*]The study number corresponds to the number provided in the text of the chapter.

[**]Age column and IQ/education column contain information regarding range and/or mean and standard deviation for the whole sample and/or separate groups, whichever information is provided by the authors.

SUMMARIES OF THE STUDIES

Normative Report

[HVOT.1] Richardson and Marottoli, 1996

The authors report data for 101 autonomously living, mostly Caucasian elderly subjects who comprise a subsample of a cohort of participants in "Project Safety", a study on driving performance conducted in New Haven, Connecticut. Individuals with a history of neurologic disease, excessive use of alcohol, or those at risk for dementia (based on the MMSE scores), were excluded.

The sample consisted of 53 males and 48 females with a mean age of 81.47 (±3.30) and mean education of 11.02 (±3.68) years. The HVOT was administered and scored according to the standard instructions provided in the test manual.

The data were divided into two age groups of younger-old (76–80) and older-old (81–91), by two education groups. The results indicated that the mean performance for subjects with less than 12 years of education was stable across younger-old (76–80) and older-old (81–91) age groups, and was considerably lower than for their more educated counterparts; however, performance for the younger-old age group with <12 years of education was superior to that of the older-old with comparable education.

Study strengths
1. Data for a relatively large sample of elderly subjects are presented.
2. Sample composition is well described in terms of gender, education, geographic area, and ethnicity.

Table 11.3. HVOT.1b; Means and Standard Deviations for the HVOT Scores for Two Age Groups by Two Education Groups (in Years of Schooling)

	Age			
	76–80		81–91	
Education	<12	≥12	<12	≥12
N	26	24	18	33
HVOT	17.90	21.69	17.62	19.71
	(4.01)	(4.02)	(6.17)	(2.97)

3. Exclusion criteria are described.
4. The data are classified into age-by-education groupings.
5. Means and standard deviations are reported.

Considerations regarding use of the study
1. No information on intelligence level is provided.
2. Sample sizes for each age-by-education cell are relatively small (Tables 11.2 and 11.3).

CONCLUSIONS

The HVOT has been used clinically as a measure of visual perception and organization. However, the effect of naming impairment on HVOT performance still remains controversial. The clinical utility of this test would be enhanced with the availability of normative data for a large sample of neurologically intact subjects of both genders across a wide age span, partitioned by age group and intelligence level.

Table 11.2. HVOT.1a; Demographic Characteristics of the Sample

	Total Sample	Younger-Old	Older-Old
N	101	50	51
Age	81.47 (3.30)	78.80 (1.07)	84.08 (2.56)
Education	11.02 (3.68)	10.44 (3.86)	11.59 (3.45)
MMSE	26.97 (2.55)	26.56 (3.03)	27.37 (1.92)
% female	47.5%	46.0%	49.0%
% white	90.1%	82.0%	98.0%
% black	9.9%	18.0%	2.0%

12

The Seashore Rhythm Test

BRIEF HISTORY OF THE TEST

The Seashore Rhythm Test (SRT) is a subtest of the Seashore Test of Musical Talent (Seashore et al., 1960) incorporated by Halstead in his original neuropsychological battery and subsequently employed by Reitan in his expansion of the Halstead Battery (Reitan & Wolfson, 1993). Subjects are played an audiotape or phonograph recording of 30 pairs of rhythmnic sequences of five to seven beats in length. The test consists of three parts (A, B, and C) each with 10 items. Subjects are instructed to note on a score sheet whether the pairs are the same or different by marking "s" or "d" in the appropriate space. This test requires sustained attention, rhythm discrimination, and immediate auditory memory (Yeudall et al., 1987). The SRT is described as a "nonverbal auditory discrimination test" by Young and Delay (1993). Specific instructions are provided in Reitan's (1979) *Manual for Administration of Neuropsychological Test Batteries for Adults and Children*.

The SRT has been reported to be sensitive to right hemisphere functioning (Jarvis & Barth, 1984; Russell, 1974) and right temporal lobe functioning in particular (Golden et al. 1981b; Lezak, 1983). However, empirical studies have failed to support this hypothesis (Boone & Rausch, 1989; Karzmark et al., 1985; Milner, 1962; Reitan, 1964; Reitan & Wolfson, 1989; Steinmeyer, 1986). Reitan and Wolfson (1989) suggest that the SRT is a "general indicator of

brain functions," performed more poorly by patients with brain injury than control subjects.

Two forms of the test are available. Form B appears to be of greater difficulty than Form A (Moore & Hannay, 1982). Examination of the internal consistency of Form A has yielded reliability coefficients of 0.64 to 0.75 (Bornstein, 1983b; Charter et al., 1987; Moses, 1985; Seashore et al., 1960).

Scoring and interpretation of SRT scores has traditionally involved conversion to rank scores and use of cutoff scores. Reitan (1979) instructed that SRT raw scores should be converted to rank scores, but there does not appear to be any benefit to this procedure, and all reports reviewed in this chapter provide mean number correct or errors rather than rank scores except for one study (Pauker, 1980). Reitan (1979; Reitan & Wolfson, 1985) recommends a cutoff of a rank score greater than 5[1] (which corresponds to a raw correct score less than or equal to 25), although given the significant association between SRT performance and age, education, and IQ, a single cutoff score would not appear to be appropriate. Bornstein (1986a) found that using a cutoff of greater than or equal to 25 correct, 35.3% of a large normal sample of subjects between ages 18 and 69 were misclassified in the abnormal range. Bornstein

[1] Reitan attributes this cutoff to Halstead (1947), but we could not document this in our examination of Halstead's publication. Halstead suggests a cutoff of greater than 35 errors for the Seashore Battery as a whole.

et al. (1987b), Ernst (1988), and Bak and Greene (1980) using the same cutoff, found that 44%, 37%, and 40%, respectively, of a healthy elderly sample were misclassified as brain damaged. Similarly, Dodrill (1987) documented a 27.5% misclassification rate in a young control sample. Bornstein and colleagues (1987b) note that a 95% correct classification rate was obtained when a cutoff of greater than or equal to 20 was used (but 61% of brain damaged subjects were then misclassified with this cutoff). The authors emphasize that cutoff scores may be useful but only if considered in the context of other neuropsychological information obtained in a test battery and if age, education, and other appropriate adjustments are made.

An alternative approach to scoring the SRT utilizing the Signal Detection Theory (SDT) was proposed by Young and Delay (1993). The set of instructions included statements specifying the proportion of the test stimuli that would be identical or different. The standard scores and SDT d' scores reflected age difference (young vs. old nonclinical groups), and level of signal probabilities. The authors inferred that use of SDT allows exploration of decision-making process and response bias, in addition to sensory sensitivity.

Clinical utility of the SRT was questioned by Sherer et al. (1991) based on the literature review and their own empirical studies. They argue against a premise that the SRT is a sensitive measure of alertness and sustained attention and that it has lateralizing significance. The authors concluded that the SRT as well as the SSPT are "most appropriately interpreted as being general indicators of cerebral integrity" (p. 749); however, the unique diagnostic contribution of these tests was questioned.

Findings by Charter (1994) raise further concerns regarding clinical significance of the SRT scores. The author examined frequency of random responding for three tests from the Halstead-Reitan Battery using a formula approximating binomial distribution for a large sample, based on observed score and a probability of guessing. To illustrate use of this formula, Charter utilizes the Seashore Rhythm Test as an example. Frequency of random responses for the 90%, 95%, and 99% confidence intervals presented in this article are summarized below:

90%		95%		99%	
Low	High	Low	High	Low	High
11	19	10	20	8	22

The article includes the percentage of SRT scores falling within the random range for different studies reviewed by the author. Based on this review, Charter infers that 39% of the normative subjects' scores fell within the random range of responding, which raises questions regarding the utility of the SRT.

In a more recent article, Charter and Webster (1997) present results of the item analysis and internal consistency reliability study of the SRT. The results confirm their earlier findings regarding a large number of scores falling in the range of random responding. The reliabilities for the scores from all three series were quite low—less than 0.7. In addition, the results of the item analysis revealed that only about half of all items are good discriminators, and the majority of the items are too easy. The authors suggest limited use of this test "only as part of a neuropsychological battery, and/or when it contributes to a composite score, such as the Impairment Index . . . , the General Neuropsychological Deficit Scale . . . , and the Brain Intactness Quotient" (p. 172).

On the other hand, a moderately strong relationship between SRT scores and ADLs (as measured by the Scale of Competence in Independent Living Skills, SCILS) in a sample of geriatric patients was reported by Searight et al. (1989). The authors report correlation coefficients between the SRT scores and measures of 16 activities of daily living ranging between 0.26 and 0.57. Correlation between the SRT and the Total SCILS score was moderately high (0.56).

RELATIONSHIP BETWEEN SRT PERFORMANCE AND DEMOGRAPHIC FACTORS

The literature to date generally suggests that SRT performance in normal individuals is associated with age, education, and IQ. Specifically, younger age (Bornstein, 1985; Heaton et al., 1986, 1991; Pauker, 1980; Vega & Parsons, 1967; Yeudall et al., 1987; Young & Delay, 1993), higher education (Bornstein, 1985; Bornstein & Suga, 1988; Finlayson et al., 1977; Heaton et al., 1986, 1991; Vega & Parsons, 1967), and higher IQ (Dodrill, 1987; Matarazzo et al., 1974; Yeudall et al., 1987) have been tied to better SRT performance, although the amount of variance explained by each of these variables never exceeded 15%. Wiens and Matarazzo (1977) argue that IQ scores within the top half of the population (greater than or equal to 105) do not "materially influence performance on the Halstead-Reitan neuropsychological measures" (p. 119). Of particular interest, Moore and Hannay (1982) found that different patterns of VIQ and PIQ scores are differentially related to SRT performance; subjects with higher VIQ than PIQ scores or VIQ scores equal to PIQ scores obtained significantly higher SRT scores than subjects in whom PIQ exceeded VIQ by 10 to 19 points.

Some authors have failed to document a relationship between SRT performance and age and education (Bak & Greene, 1980; Reed & Reitan, 1963; Reitan & Wolfson, 1989), although subject selection criteria were problematic in at least one of these publications. For example, Reed and Reitan (1963) compared SRT performance of younger subjects, the majority of whom were hospitalized with non-neurological conditions, with older subjects, the majority of whom were nonhospitalized "normals"; it is now known that non-neurological medical conditions are frequently associated with mild cognitive decline.

As might be expected, age and education are less related to SRT performance in brain-injured populations (Vega & Parsons, 1967), although Prigatano and Parsons (1976) did note a significant positive correlation between SRT scores and education in brain-injured subjects. Prigatano and Parsons (1976) argue that SRT performance is relatively independent of age in a brain-injured population, but their conclusions must be viewed with caution given the young mean age of their sample. (The majority of the primarily head-injured population ranged in age from 16 to 29.)

The majority of investigators have not found sex to be related to SRT scores (Bornstein, 1985; Dodrill, 1979; Fromm-Auch & Yeudall, 1983; Heaton et al., 1991; Reitan & Wolfson, 1989; Yeudall et al., 1987). Only the Young and Delay (1993) study reports small but significant gender differences in favor of male performance, which, according to the authors, might be a function of education, IQ differences, or altered scoring procedure utilizing Signal Detection Theory.

A recent article by Arnold et al. (1994) documents a significant effect of acculturation on SRT performance for a sample of Mexican-American subjects, with more acculturated subjects performing better on the test.

METHOD FOR EVALUATING THE NORMATIVE REPORTS

Our review of the literature located nine SRT normative reports published since 1965 (Bornstein, 1985; Bornstein & Suga, 1988; Dodrill, 1987; Ernst, 1988; Fromm-Auch & Yeudall, 1983; Harley et al., 1980; Heaton et al., 1991; Pauker, 1980; Yeudall et al., 1987) as well as two interpretive guides for the Halstead-Reitan Battery (Gilandas et al., 1984; Reitan & Wolfson, 1985) and the original norms published with the Seashore Measures of Musical Talents (Seashore et al., 1960). Numerous studies have also reported control subject data, and we have included discussion of 10 of those investigations which involved some unique feature, such as large sample size (greater than or equal to 100), data collected on non-English-speaking subjects, retest data, elderly population, etc. (Alekoumbides et al., 1987; Anthony et al., 1980; Bak & Greene, 1980; Bornstein et al., 1987a; Heaton et al., 1986; Karzmark et al., 1985; Klove & Lochen, 1974: Moore & Hannay, 1982; Russell, 1987; Wiens & Matarazzo, 1977).

Of note, Russell and Starkey (1993) developed the Halstead-Russell Neuropsychological Evaluation System (HRNES), which includes SRT among 22 tests. In the context of this system, individual performance is compared to that of 576 brain-damaged subjects and 200 subjects who were initially suspected of having brain damage but had negative neurological findings. Data were partitioned into seven age groups and three educational/IQ levels. This study will not be reviewed in this chapter because the "normal" group consisted of the V.A.

patients who presented with symptomatology requiring neuropsychological evaluation. For further discussion of the HRNES system see Lezak, 1995 (pp. 714–715).

Interestingly, few relevant manuscripts have emerged since the 1980s, perhaps due either to the publication of Heaton et al.'s (1991) comprehensive normative tables or to the escalating use in research and clinical practice of flexible neuropsychological test protocols which include newer tasks rather than traditional fixed neuropsychological batteries.

In order to adequately evaluate the SRT normative reports, six key criterion variables were deemed critical. The first five of these relate to *subject* variables, and the one remaining dimension refers to *procedural* issues.

Minimal requirements for meeting the criterion variables were as follows:

Subject Variables

Sample Size

As discussed in previous chapters, a minimum of at least 50 subjects per grouping interval is optimal.

Sample Composition Description

As discussed previously, information regarding medical and psychiatric exclusion criteria is important; it is unclear if geographic region, ethnicity, occupation, handedness, recruitment procedures, or sex is relevant, so until this is determined, it is best that this information is provided.

Age-Group Intervals

Given the association between age and SRT performance, information regarding age of the normative sample is critical, and preferably normative data should be presented by age intervals.

Reporting of IQ Levels

Given the relationship between SRT performance and IQ, information regarding intellectual level should be provided. In addition, due to the unique association between VIQ/PIQ discrepancies and SRT scores, information regarding these specific IQ dimensions preferably should be included.

Reporting of Education Levels

Given the association between education level and SRT scores, information regarding highest educational level completed should be reported.

Procedural Variables

Data Reporting

Means and standard deviations, and preferably ranges, for total correct or total errors on the SRT should be reported.

SUMMARY OF THE STATUS OF THE NORMS

In terms of subject variables, the majority of the studies provided data according to limited age intervals (Bak & Greene, 1980; Bornstein, 1985; Ernst, 1988; Fromm-Auch & Yeudall, 1983; Heaton et al., 1991; Moore & Hannay, 1982; Pauker, 1980; Wiens & Matarrazo, 1977; Yeudall et al., 1987). In addition, 12 datasets reported information on mean IQ (Alekoumbides et al., 1987; Anthony et al., 1980; Bak & Greene, 1980; Bornstein et al., 1987a; Dodrill, 1987; Fromm-Auch & Yeudall, 1983; Heaton et al., 1991; Klove & Lochen, in Klove, 1974; Russell, 1987; Vega & Parsons, 1967; Wiens & Matarrazo, 1977; Yeudall et al., 1987), although only two studies grouped data by IQ levels (Moore & Hannay, 1982; Pauker, 1980). All but two studies reported information on educational levels (Bornstein et al., 1987a; Pauker, 1980); but in only three datasets were test scores grouped by educational levels (Bornstein, 1985; Bornstein & Suga, 1988; Heaton et al., 1991) and data from one study were limited to college students (Moore & Hannay, 1982). Only two studies consistently provided at least 50 subjects for each age, IQ, and/or education grouping (Ernst, 1988; Seashore et al., 1960), although some studies approximated this number, e.g., ≥40 (Bornstein & Suga, 1988; Yeudall et al., 1987) or had at least some cells which met this criterion (Bornstein, 1985; Dodrill, 1987; Fromm-Auch & Yeudall, 1983; Pauker, 1980). All datasets provided some description of sample characteristics, but medical and psychiatric exclusion criteria were judged to be adequate in only nine studies (Anthony et al., 1980; Bornstein et al., 1987a; Bornstein & Suga, 1988; Ernst, 1988; Dodrill, 1987; Fromm-Auch & Yeudall, 1983; Heaton et al., 1991; Karzmark et al., 1985; Pauker, 1980; Yeudall et al., 1987). Four reports cite information on occupation (Alekoumbides et al., 1987; Dodrill, 1987; Ernst, 1988; Yeudall et al., 1987), six studies provide handedness data (Bornstein, 1985; Dodrill, 1987; Ernst, 1988; Fromm-Auch & Yeudall, 1983; Moore & Hannay, 1982; Yeudall et al., 1987), and five datasets describe the ethnic composition of the samples (Alekoumbides et al., 1987; Dodrill, 1987; Ernst, 1988; Russell, 1987; Vega & Parsons, 1967). Information regarding geographical recruitment areas was availble for all but one investigations (Bornstein et al., 1987a).

In regard to procedural variables, all studies except three provided either SRT mean correct or errors and standard deviations. Pauker reported mean rank scores and standard deviations, and Klove and Lochen, in Klove (1974) and Heaton et al. (1986) do not include a standard deviation with their reported mean. Fromm-Auch and Yeudall (1983) and Harley et al. (1980) are the only authors to publish test score ranges. Some publications also include information on IQ equivalent scores (Dodrill, 1987), T scores (Harley et al., 1980; Heaton et al., 1991), and computational methods for obtaining standard scores corrected for age and education (Alekoumbides et al., 1987).

Table 12.1 summarizes information provided in the studies described in this chapter.

SUMMARIES OF THE STUDIES

Given that the use of the SRT has typically been within the context of the Halstead-Reitan Battery, the Reitan interpretation recommendations will be reported first, followed by a summary of the other interpretation formats, and then the normative publications presented in order of recency of publication. The chapter will conclude with a review of SRT control data reported in various clinical studies. Halstead's 1947 publication will not be reviewed since he used a total error score for all six subtests of the Seashore Measures of Musical Talents and did not provide separate information on the Rhythm Test.

Interpretive Guide

[SRT.1] Reitan and Wolfson, 1985

The authors cite SRT data published by Reitan in 1955 on 50 (35 male and 15 female) controls in Indiana. Twelve were "normal" while the remainder were either hospitalized with paraplegia ($n = 13$) or various psychiatric disorders (depression = 17, acute anxiety state = 6, obsessive-compulsive neurosis = 2). On neurological exam, none showed evidence of cerebral damage or dysfunction, and histories were negative for head injuries or brain diseases. Mean age was 32.36 ± 10.78, and mean years of education was 11.58 ± 2.85.

Mean standard deviation for number correct is reported. In addition, score severity ranges reflecting "perfectly normal," "normal," "mildly impaired," and "seriously impaired" performance are provided. The authors also report cutoff scores for "normal range" and "brain-damaged range" to be used in computing the Halstead Impairment Index. Of interest, they report that Halstead's original cutoff score for the SRT was a ranked score of 6 (5 or less reflected normal performance; 6 or more was abnormal); however, our examination of Halstead's (1947) publication indicates that he provided a single cutoff error score for the entire Seashore test battery (>35 errors) (p. 174), but no cutoff score specific to the Rhythm Test.

Considerations regarding use of the study
The authors argue that only general normative score ranges are necessary rather than exact percentile ranks because "other methods of inference are used to supplement normative data in clinical interpretation of results for individual subjects" (p. 97). However, given the reported association between SRT scores and age, education, and IQ, this approach to interpretation utilizing the same set of single cutoff scores and severity ranges for all patients will lead to excessive false positive errors in identifying the presence of cognitive dysfunction

Table 12.1. SRT.L; Locator Table for the SRT

Study[°]	Age[°°]	N	Sample Composition	IQ,[°°] Education	Country/ Location
SRT.1 Reitan & Wolfson, 1985 page 194	32.36 (10.78)	50	35 M, 15 F, 12 were normal, while the remainder were hospitalized with paraplegia or various psychiatric disorders. Cutoffs for impairment severity ranges were offered.	Education 11.58(2.85)	Indiana
SRT.2 Seashore et al., 1960 page 197		4,024	Ss were students recruited from high schools and colleges	Education 9-16	Numerous locations across country
SRT.3 Harley et al., 1980 page 198	55–79	193	V.A. hospitalized patients. T-score equivalents are reported	IQ>80	Wisconsin
	55–59	56		Education 8.8	
	60–64	45			
	65–69	35			
	70–74	37			
	75–79	20			
SRT.4 Pauker, 1980 page 199	19–71	363	152 M, 211 F volunteers. Rank scores are provided for 3 age groups by 4 IQ levels	IQ levels:	Toronto Canada
	19–34			89–102	
	35–52			103–112	
	53–71			113–122	
				123–143	
SRT.5 Fromm-Auch & Yeudall, 1983 page 200	15–64 25.4 (8.2)	193	111 M, 82 F. Participants described as nonpsychiatric and non-neurological. 83% are R-handed. Ss classified in 5 age groupings	Education 8–26 14.8(3.0) FSIQ 119.1(8.8)	Canada
	15–17	32			
	18–23	75			
	24–32	57			
	33–40	18			
	41–64	10			
SRT.6 Bornstein, 1985 page 201	18–69 43.3 (17.1)	365	178 M, 187 F. 91.5 % were R-handed. Data are stratified by 3 age groups, 2 education levels for males and females separately	Education 5–20 12.3(2.7) <HS ≥HS	Canada
	20–39				
	40–59				
	60–69				
SRT.7 Dodrill, 1987 page 202	27.73 (11.04)	120	60 M, 60 F volunteers. Data for various intelligence levels are presented	Education 12.28(2.18) FSIQ 100(14.3)	Washington
SRT.8 Yeudall et al., 1987 page 202	15–40	225	Volunteers, four age groupings. 127 M, 98 F	Education 14.55 (2.78) FSIQ 112.25 (10.25)	Canada
	15–20	62			
	21–25	73			
	26–30	48			
	31–40	42			

continued

Table 12.1. (*Continued*)

Study[°]	Age[°°]	N	Sample Composition	IQ,[°°] Education	Country/ Location
SRT.9 Bornstein & Suga, 1988 page 204	55–70 62.7 (4.3)	134	Healthy elderly volunteers. No history of neurological or psychiatric disease. Sample divided into 3 groups based on education	Education 5–10 ($n = 46$) 11–12 ($n = 44$) >12 ($n = 44$)	Canada
		49 M 85 F			
SRT.10 Ernst, 1988 page 204	65–75	85	39 M, 46 F. All but one were R-handed. Ss free of neuro-logical or psychiatric illness	Education 10.4(3.1) 4–20	Brisbane, Australia
SRT.11 Heaton et al., 1991 page 205	42.1 (16.8) groups: 20–34 35–39 40–44 45–49 50–54 55–59 60–64 65–69 70–74 75–80	486	Volunteers: urban and rural. Data collected over 15 years through multi-center collabo-rative efforts. Strict exclusion criteria. 65% M. Data are presented in *T*-score equivalents for M and F separately in 10 age groupings by 6 educational groupings	Education 13.6(3.5) FSIQ 113.8(12.3) groups 6–8 9–11 12 13–15 16–17 18+	California, Washington, Texas, Oklahoma, Wisconsin, Illinois, Michigan, New York, Virginia, Massachusetts, Canada
SRT.12 Klove & Lochen, (1n Klove, 1974) page 206	31.6 32.1	22 22	Controls: American and Norwegians	Education 11.1 12.2 FSIQ 109.3 111.9	Wisconsin, Norway
SRT.13 Wiens & Matarazzo 1977 page 206	23.6 24.8	48	All male, neurologically normal. Divided into 2 groups. Random sample of 29 were retested 14–24 weeks later	Education 13.7 14.0 FSIQ 117.5 118.3	Oregon
SRT.14 Anthony et al., 1980 page 207	38.88 (15.80)	100	Normal volunteers. Ss had no history of medical or psychiatric problems, head traumas, brain disease, or substance abuse	Education 13.33(2.56) FSIQ 113.5(10.8)	Colorado
SRT.15 Bak & Greene, 1980 page 207	50–62 55.6 (4.44)	15	R-handed Ss. Equally divided into 2 age groupings. Ss fluent in English and had no history of CNS disorders. 9 Ss in 1st group were female. 10 Ss in 2nd group were female	Education 13.7(1.91) 14.9(2.99)	Texas
	67–86 74.9 (6.04)	15			
SRT.16 Moore & Hannay, 1982 page 208	20.83 (2.25) 20.17 (1.57) 20.40 (1.89)	90	College students. Data are presented for 3 VIQ/PIQ discrepancy groups for forms A and B; 62 M, 28 F		Alabama

continued

Table 12.1. (*Continued*)

Study[*]	Age[**]	N	Sample Composition	IQ,[**] Education	Country/ Location
SRT.17 Karzmark et al., 1985 page 209	37.58 (15.70)	112	Paid normal controls with no history of brain trauma, alcohol or drug abuse, or psychiatric disorder	Education 13.27(2.94)	Colorado
SRT.18 Heaton et al., 1986 page 210	15–81 39.3 (17.5) <40 40-59 ≥60	553 319 134 100	356 M, 197 F normal controls. Data are presented for 3 age groups and 3 education groups. % classification as normal is presented	Education 0–20 13.3 (3.4) <12 (n = 132) 12–15 (n = 249) ≥16 (n = 172)	Colorado, California, Wisconsin
SRT.19 Alekoumbides et al., 1987 page 210	19–82 46.85 (17.17)	114	Medical and psychiatric inpatients and outpatients from V.A. hospitals. Regression equation for computation of age- and education-corrected scores is provided	Education 1–20 11.43(3.20) FSIQ 105.9 (13.5)	S. California
SRT.20 Bornstein et al., 1987a page 211	17-52 32.3 (10.3)	23	Volunteers, 9 M, 14 F. No neurological or psychiatric illness. Test-retest data for a 3-week interval are provided	VIQ 105.8 (10.8) PIQ 105.0 (10.5)	
SRT.21 Russell, 1987 page 212	46.19 (12.86)	155	Controls from VA hospitals. 148 M, 7 F. Ss with suspected neurological disorders were excluded	Education 12.29(3.00) FSIQ 111.9	Cincinnati, Miami

[*]The study number corresponds to the number provided in the text of the chapter.

[**]Age column and IQ/education column contain information regarding range, and/or mean and standard deviation for the whole sample and/or separate groups, whichever information is provided by the authors.

and should no longer be endorsed. The methods used to determine the score ranges and cut-offs are not described and warrant concern given that the mean error score for controls (5.20 ± 3.45) reported by Reitan in 1955 and summarized in this 1985 publication falls at the cutoff between normal and mildly impaired. Normative data reported in this publication are presented in Table 12.2.

An alternate classification of scores into severity ranges is proposed by *Gilandas et al.* (1984, p. 97). The authors suggest that "clinically significant" performance on the SRT corresponds to scores less than 26 out of 30 for both children and adults. "Borderline impairment" refers to scores between 21 and 25, "mild impairment" is reflected by scores between 16 and 20, and "severe impairment" is represented by scores less than 16.

Normative Studies

[SRT.2] Seashore, Lewis, and Saetveit, 1960

The study provides SRT data on 4,024 students in grades 9 through 16 collected in high schools in Illinois, Michigan, Minnesota, Montana, New York, Ohio, Pennsylvania, and Washington, and the University of Maine, Union College of Schenectady, New York, and Casper Junior College in Wyoming. The mean and standard deviation for SRT number correct as well as percentile equivalents for all possible raw scores are provided. No other information is given regarding subject characteristics.

Study strengths
1. Very large sample size.
2. Presentation of percentile equivalents for raw scores.

Table 12.2. SRT.1; a) Number of Errors, b) Severity Ranges Based on the Number of Correct Responses

a)		Mean				
SRT No. errors		5.20 (3.45)				

b)						
Normal	Perfectly Normal	28–30		Impaired	Mildly	20–24
	Normal	25–27			Seriously	0–19

3. Data were collected in several communities and states.

4. Information on educational level.

Considerations regarding use of the study

1. Data were collected nearly 40 years ago, raising the issue of possible cohort effects.

2. No exclusion criteria are reported, although the large size of the sample and the fact that the subjects were healthy enough to be currently enrolled in school renders this less of an issue.

3. Nothing is known of IQ level, ethnicity, sex ratio, handedness, or age.

4. An educational range of 9 to 16 is probably too wide to be clinically useful.

N	No. correct
4024	26.5 (2.8)

[SRT.3] Harley, Leuthold, Matthews, and Bergs, 1980

The authors collected SRT data on 193 V.A.-hospitalized patients in Wisconsin, ranging in age from 55 to 79. Exclusion criteria included Full Scale IQ less than 80, active psychosis, unequivocal neurological disease or brain damage, and serious visual or auditory acuity problems. Patients with diagnosis of chronic brain syndrome *were* included. Patient diagnoses were as follows: chronic brain syndrome unrelated to alcoholism (28%), psychosis (55%), alcoholic (37%), neurotic (9%), and personality disorder (4%). Mean educational level was 8.8 years. The sample was divided into five age groupings: 55–59 (n = 56), 60–64 (n = 45), 65–69 (n = 35), 70–74 (n = 37), and 75–79 (n = 20). Mean educational level and percent of sample included in each of the diagnostic classifications are reported for each age grouping. The authors also provided test data on a subgroup of 160 subjects equated for percent diagnosed with alcoholism across the five age groupings. The "alcohol-equated sample" was developed "to minimize the influence that cognitive or motor/sensory differences uniquely attributable to alcohol abuse might have upon group test performance levels" (p. 2). This subsample remained heterogeneous regarding representation of the other diagnostic categories.

Means, standard deviations, ranges, and T-score equivalents for raw scores are reported for SRT number correct for each age interval for the whole sample and for the alcohol-equated sample. We reproduce selected data due to space considerations.

Study strengths

1. Large sample size and many individual cells approximate Ns of 50.

2. Reporting of IQ data, geographic area, age, and education.

3. Data presented in age groupings.

4. Means and standard deviations are reported.

Considerations regarding use of the study

1. The presence of substantial neurologic (chronic brain syndrome), substance abuse, and major psychiatric disorders in the sample.

2. Low educational level, although IQ levels are average.

3. No information regarding sex, although given that data were obtained in a V.A. setting, the sample is likely all, or nearly all, male.

Table 12.3. SRT.3; Means, Standard Deviations, and Ranges for SRT Number Correct for Five Age Intervals for the Whole Sample and for the Alcohol-Equated Sample

Age	N	WAIS			Educ	SRT No. Correct
		FSIQ	VIQ	PIQ		
Total sample						
55–59	56	98.57 (11.43) 80–129	99.39 (12.92) 77–131	97.00 (10.65) 72–129	10.1	22.48 (5.19) 11–30
60–64	45	98.58 (9.93) 80–121	101.27 (11.42) 78–123	95.00 (9.82) 78–116	9.8	23.13 (3.91) 15–30
65–69	35	97.51 (11.18) 80–130	100.37 (12.51) 80–135	93.66 (10.20) 68–120	8.7	22.46 (4.70) 12–29
70–74	37	100.41 (9.92) 82–125	102.95 (11.81) 80–133	97.24 (10.08) 75–114	8.8	19.03 (4.77) 12–28
75–79	20	101.75 (10.18) 81–119	101.40 (11.40) 77–117	102.15 (9.95) 83–119	6.5	21.22 (3.46) 16–30
Alcohol–equated sample						
55–59	47	99.00 (11.73) 80–129	100.00 (13.02) 77–131	98.00 (11.13) 72–129	10.1	22.09 (5.40) 11–30
60–64	33	96.00 (9.43) 80–117	99.00 (11.33) 78–123	93.00 (9.30) 78–112	9.3	22.97 (4.10) 15–29
65–69	23	99.00 (12.06) 80–130	102.00 (13.06) 80–135	95.00 (11.52) 68–120	8.8	22.57 (5.08) 17–28
70–74	37	100.00 (9.92) 82–125	103.00 (11.81) 80–133	97.00 (10.08) 75–114	8.8	19.03 (4.77) 12–28
75–79	20	102.00 (10.18) 81–119	101.00 (11.40) 77–117	102.00 (9.95) 83–119	6.5	21.22 (3.46) 16–30

Other comments

The scores for the two oldest age groups are identical in the whole sample and alcohol-equated group because these two groups did not have overrepresentation of alcoholics, so they did not need to be adjusted (Table 12.3).

[SRT.4] Pauker, 1980

The authors obtained SRT scores on 363 Toronto citizens fluent in English recruited through announcements and notices. Subjects ranged in age from 19 to 71 years and included 152 men and 211 women. Exclusion criteria included significant physical disability, sensory deficit, current medical illness, use of medication that might affect test performance, history of actual or suspected brain disorder, and alcoholism; MMPI profiles "could not suggest severe disturbance" or include more than three clinical scales with T scores greater than or equal to 70 or an F scale score greater than 80.

The SRT was administered according to Reitan's guidelines. Means and standard deviations for SRT *rank* scores are reported for the sample as a whole and for three age groupings (19–34, 35–52, 53–71) by four WAIS IQ levels (89–102, 103–112, 113–122, 123–143). Individual cell sample sizes ranged from 4 to 60. Age by IQ categories were determined "in a compromise between what would be desirable and what the obtained sample characteristics and size dictated" (p. 1). No differences in SRT performance between men and women were documented.

Study strengths

1. Large sample size, although individual cell sizes are substantially less than 50.
2. Presentation of the data for age by IQ groupings.
3. Adequate medical and psychiatric exclusion criteria.
4. Information regarding language, recruitment procedures, gender, and geographic area.
5. Means and standard deviations are reported.

Considerations regarding use of the study

1. Reporting of SRT rank scores rather than mean number correct or number errors; this unduly complicates scoring to no apparent benefit.

2. No information regarding education.
3. Subjects were recruited in Canada which possibly limits use of these data for clinical interpretation purposes in the United States.
4. The age by IQ cell representing subjects aged 53 to 71 with IQs of 89 to 102 contained only four subjects; Pauker comments that this category "should not be considered to be of any more than interest value" (p. 2).
5. IQ levels below the average range are not represented (Table 12.4).

[SRT.5] Fromm-Auch and Yeudall, 1983

The authors obtained SRT data on 193 Canadian subjects (111 male, 82 female) recruited through posted advertisements and personal contacts. Participants are described as "nonpsychiatric" and "nonneurological." Eighty-three percent of the sample were right-handed and mean age was 25.4 (SD = 8.2, range = 15 to 64). Mean years of education were 14.8 (SD = 3.0, range = 8 to 25) and included technical and university training. Mean WAIS FSIQ, VIQ, and PIQ were 119.1 (SD = 8.8, range = 98 to 142), 119.8 (SD = 9.9, range = 95 to 143), and 115.6 (SD = 9.8, range 89 to 146), respectively. Of note, no subject obtained a FSIQ which was lower than the average range.

Means, standard deviations, and ranges for

Table 12.4. SRT.4; Means and Standard Deviations for SRT *Rank* Scores for the Sample as a Whole, and for Three Age Groupings by Four WAIS IQ Levels

	Age			
WAIS FSIQ	19–34	35–52	53–71	19–71
123–143	1.57	1.76	2.70	1.95
	(1.35)	(1.69)	(2.41)	(1.84)
	n = 28	n = 25	n = 20	n = 73
113–122	2.40	2.96	4.63	3.04
	(2.37)	(2.34)	(2.75)	(2.55)
	n = 60	n = 56	n = 27	n = 143
103–112	3.15	3.21	5.40	3.50
	(2.71)	(2.80)	(2.95)	(2.86)
	n = 53	n = 34	n = 15	n = 102
89–102	4.05	5.15	7.25	4.82
	(3.02)	(3.42)	(2.22)	(3.23)
	n = 21	n = 20	n = 4	n = 45
89–143	2.72	3.13	4.38	3.17
	(2.54)	(2.71)	(2.91)	(2.73)
	n = 162	n = 135	n = 66	n = 363

total SRT errors are reported for five age group-ings: 15–17, 18–23, 24–32, 33–40, and 41–64, with sample sizes ranging from 10 to 75. The two oldest age groupings both had sample sizes less than 20. No sex differences were document-ed and male and female data were collapsed.

Study strengths
  1. The large overall sample size and some in-dividual cells approximate Ns of 50.
  2. Presentation of the data by age groupings. However, essentially no differences in perfor-mance were noted between the 18–23-year-olds, the 24–32-year-olds and the 33–40-year olds, suggesting that use of a single age group-ing for 18 to 40 would have been appropriate.
  3. Information regarding mean IQ, age, ed-ucational levels, gender, handedness, recruit-ment procedures, and geographic area.
  4. Some psychiatric and neurological exclu-sion criteria.
  5. Means and standard deviations are re-ported.

Considerations regarding use of the study
  1. The high intellectual and educational lev-el of the sample.
  2. An age grouping of 41 to 64 with an N of 10 would not appear to be particularly useful.
  3. Subjects were recruited in Canada which may limit the usefulness of these data for clini-cal interpretation purposes in the United States (Table 12.5).

[SRT.6] Bornstein, 1985

The author collected data on 365 Canadian in-dividuals (178 males and 187 females) recruit-ed through posted notices on college campuses and unemployment offices, newspaper ads, and senior citizen groups. Subjects were paid for their participation. Participants ranged in age from 18 to 69 (mean = 43.3 ± 17.1) and had completed between 5 and 20 years of education (mean = 12.3 ± 2.7). Ninety-one and a half percent of the sample were right-handed. No other demographic data or exclusion criteria are reported.
  Means and standard deviations for total cor-rect on the SRT are reported for three age groupings (20–39, 40–59, and 60–69), two ed-ucational levels (less than high school, greater

Table 12.5. SRT.5; Means, Standard Deviations, and Ranges for Total SRT Errors for Five Age Groupings

Age	N	SRT
15–17	32	2.1 (1.4) Range = 0–5
18–23	75	2.5 (2.1) Range = 0–9
24–32	57	2.4 (1.9) Range = 0–9
33–40	18	2.3 (2.1) Range = 0–8
41–64	10	3.9 (2.1) Range = 1–6

than or equal to high school) and sex, resulting in a total of 12 separate groups. Individual group sample sizes ranged from 13 to 86. Sig-nificant correlations were obtained between SRT scores and age ($r = -0.17$) and education ($r = 0.33$), suggesting that better performance was associated with younger age and more years of education. No significant differences be-tween males and females were documented.

Study strengths
  1. Very large overall sample size and several individual cells approximate Ns of 50.
  2. Stratification of the data by age, sex, and educational level.
  3. This dataset is unique in that it reports data for subjects with less than a high school ed-ucation.
  4. Information on handedness, recruitment procedures, and geographic area.
  5. Means and standard deviations are re-ported.

Considerations regarding use of the study
  1. Individual sample sizes of some cells were small (e.g., 13, 16, 17).
  2. The lack of any reported exclusion crite-ria.
  3. The data were collected on Canadian cit-izens which may limit generalizability for use in the United States.

Table 12.6. SRT.6; Means and Standard Deviations for the Total Number of Correct Responses on the SRT for Three Age Groupings, Two Educational Levels (Less Than High School [HS], Greater Than or Equal to High School), and for Males and Females Separately

| | Education Groups | | | |
| | Males | | Females | |
Age Groups	<HS	≥HS	<HS	≥HS
20–39	25.8	26.7	25.1	27.0
	(4.0)	(2.6)	(3.6)	(2.5)
	n = 21	n = 86	n = 13	n = 50
40–59	23.8	25.9	23.9	26.5
	(3.7)	(2.8)	(3.4)	(2.5)
	n = 13	n = 17	n = 22	n = 42
60–69	25.8	26.9	23.8	25.6
	(3.4)	(2.8)	(2.7)	(2.5)
	n = 16	n = 23	n = 21	n = 34

4. The lack of IQ data. The concern over the lack of IQ data is somewhat mitigated by the fact that the mean educational level was not unduly elevated (12.3 years), which might suggest that mean intellectual levels were within the average range.

5. Inexplicably, males aged 60 to 69 outperformed males aged 40–59, and the 60–69-year-olds performed virtually identically to males aged 20 to 39. This data runs counter to the correlational evidence of poorer SRT performance with age and should be used with caution (Table 12.6).

[SRT.7] Dodrill, 1987

The author collected SRT data on 120 subjects in Washington during the years 1975–1976 (n = 81) and 1986–1987 (n = 39). Half of the sample was female and 10% were minorities (six black, three native American, two Asian American, one unknown). Eighteen were left-handed, and occupational status included 45 students, 37 employed, 26 unemployed, 11 homemakers, and one retiree. Subjects were recruited from various sources, including schools, churches, employment agencies, and community service agencies, and were either paid for their participation or offered an interpretation of their abilities. Exclusion criteria included history of "neurologically relevant dis-

ease (such as meningitis or encephalitis)," alcoholism, birth complications "of likely neurological significance," oxygen deprivation, peripheral nervous system injury, psychotic or psychotic-like disorders, or head injury associated with unconsciousness, skull fracture, persisting neurological signs, or diagnosis of concussion or contusion. Of note, one-third of potential participants failed to meet the above medical and psychiatric criteria, resulting in a final sample of 120. Mean age was 27.73 (±11.04) and mean years of education was 12.28 (±2.18). The subjects tested in the 1970s were administered the WAIS and the subjects assessed in the 1980s were administered the WAIS-R; WAIS scores were converted to WAIS-R equivalents by subtracting seven points from the VIQ, PIQ, and FSIQ. Mean FSIQ, VIQ, and PIQ scores were 100.00(±14.35), 100.92 (±14.73), and 98.25 (±13.39), respectively. IQ scores ranged from 60 to 138 and reflected an exactly normal distribution.

SRT mean total scores and standard deviations are reported as well as IQ-equivalent scores for various levels of intelligence. Slightly more than one-quarter (27.5%) of a subgroup of the sample were misclassified as brain damaged using Reitan's cutoff of 25.

Study strengths
1. Large sample size.
2. Comprehensive exclusion criteria.
3. Information regarding education, IQ, occupation, sex ratio, age, handedness, ethnicity, recruitment procedures, and geographic area.
4. IQ-equivalent scores provided.
5. Data for different IQ levels provided.
6. Means and standard deviations are reported.

Considerations regarding use of the study
1. Undifferentiated age range (Table 12.7).

[SRT.8] Yeudall, Reddon, Gill, and Stefanyk, 1987

The authors obtained SRT data on 225 Canadian subjects recruited from posted advertisements in workplaces and personal solicitations. The participants included meat packers, postal workers, transit employees, hospital lab technicians, secretaries, ward aides, student in-

Table 12.7. SRT.7; Mean Number of Correct Responses and Standard Deviations for the Total Sample and for Various Levels of Intelligence

Data for the Total Sample:

| N | Age | Education | WAIS-R | | | SRT |
			FSIQ	VIQ	PIQ	
120	27.73	12.28	100.00	100.92	98.25	26.64
	(11.04)	(2.18)	(14.35)	(14.73)	(13.39)	(2.53)

Data broken down by FSIQ levels:

N	FSIQ	SRT	FSIQ	SRT
7	130	29	>89	26–30
18	125	29	80–89	23–25
34	120	28	70–79	19–22
64	115	28	<70	<19
93	110	27		
101	105	27		
75	100	26		
60	95	26		
48	90	26		
33	85	26		
19	80	25		
10	75	24		
	70	23		

terns, student nurses, and summer students. In addition, high school teachers identified for participation average students in grades 10 through 12. Exclusion criteria included evidence of "forensic involvement," head injury, neurological insult, prenatal or birth complications, psychiatric problems, or substance abuse.

Experienced testing technicians gathered SRT data and "motivated the subjects to achieve maximum performance" partially through the promise of detailed explanations of their test performance.

Means and standard deviations for number of SRT errors are presented for four age groupings (15 to 20, 21 to 25, 26 to 30, and 31 to 40) for males and females combined and separate. Information regarding percent right-handers, mean years of education, and mean WAIS/WAIS-R FSIQ, VIQ, and PIQ are reported for each age grouping and age-by-sex grouping. For the sample as a whole, 88% were right-handed and had completed an average of 14.55 (SD = 2.78) years of schooling. The mean FSIQ, VIQ, and PIQ were 112.25 (SD = 10.25),

112.60 (SD = 10.86), and 108.13 (SD = 10.63), respectively.

No significant correlations were found between age or education and SRT performance. A significant correlation emerged for VIQ ($r = -0.14$) but accounted for only 2% of the variance in test scores. Age and sex effects on means were not significant, although variance effects for age emerged, leading the authors to recommend use of age norms, which we report below.

Study strengths

1. Large sample size and individual cells approximate Ns of 50.

2. Grouping of data by age.

3. Data availability for a 15–20-year-old age group.

4. Adequate medical and psychiatric exclusion criteria.

5. Information regarding handedness, education, IQ, sex, occupation, recruitment procedures, and geographic area.

6. Means and standard deviations are reported.

Table 12.8. SRT.8; Means and Standard Deviations for Number
of SRT Errors per Four Age Groupings and for the Whole Sample
(for Males and Females Combined)

	Age Grouping				
	15–20 ($n = 62$)	21–25 ($n = 73$)	26–30 ($n = 48$)	31–40 ($n = 42$)	15–40 ($n = 225$)
SRT No. errors	2.23 (1.61)	2.58 (2.29)	2.13 (1.58)	2.57 (2.11)	2.38 (1.94)
% righthanded	79.03	86.30	89.58	90.48	85.78
Education	12.16 (1.75)	14.82 (1.88)	15.50 (2.65)	16.50 (3.11)	14.55 (2.78)
VIQ	111.18 (10.92)	110.48 (10.43)	114.10 (11.45)	117.76 (9.32)	112.60 (10.86)
PIQ	108.30 (10.47)	105.88 (11.20)	110.28 (8.72)	109.72 (11.45)	108.13 (10.63)
FSIQ	111.75 (10.16)	109.79 (9.97)	113.95 (10.61)	116.09 (9.51)	112.25 (10.25)

Considerations regarding use of the study

1. The sample was atypical in terms of its high average intellectual level and high level of education.

2. The data were obtained on Canadian subjects which may limit its usefulness for clinical interpretation in the United States due to possible subtle cultural differences (Table 12.8).

[SRT.9] Bornstein and Suga, 1988

In a more recent publication, the authors report SRT data on 134 healthy elderly Canadian volunteers, aged 55 to 70, according to three educational levels: 5–10 years ($n = 46$), 11–12 years ($n = 44$), and greater than 12 years ($n = 44$). Nearly two-thirds of the sample were female ($n = 85$). The average age for the sample was 62.7 (± 4.3), and the mean ages of the three educational groups were comparable (62.3, 62.9, and 63.0, respectively). Exclusion criteria included history of neurological or psychiatric disease.

Significant group differences in SRT performance were obtained across the three education groups, which was due to the group with 5–10 years of education performing significantly more poorly than the groups with 12 years or greater. Mean correct and standard deviation on the SRT are reported for the three education groups.

Study strengths

1. Large sample size and individual cells approximate Ns of 50.

2. Reporting of data by three education groups; the study is unique in terms of representation of subjects with less than 12 years of education.

3. Information regarding sex, age, and geographic area.

4. Means and standard deviations are reported.

5. Minimally adequate exclusion criteria.

Considerations regarding use of the study

1. No information regarding IQ or ethnicity or SES data.

2. Greater than 12 years education too large a category.

3. Data collected in Canada which may limit generalizability for use in the United States (Table 12.9).

[SRT.10] Ernst, 1988

The author collected SRT data on 85 Brisbane (Australian) uncompensated volunteers, aged 65 to 75, recruited from the Queensland State electoral roll. All but one participant were Caucasian, and all but one were right-handed. Thirty-nine were males and 46 were females. The sample was derived from 518 names random-

Table 12.9. SRT.9; Mean Number of Correct Responses and Standard Deviations for Three Education Groups and for the Total Sample

	Years of Education			
	5–10	11–12	>12	Total
SRT	24.0	25.6	26.5	25.4
	(3.6)	(3.2)	(2.1)	(3.2)
Education	8.5	11.7	15.0	11.7
				(2.9)

ly selected based on date of birth and residence. These potential subjects were sent information regarding the project and a health questionnaire and asked to participate. Individuals with histories of substance abuse, head trauma, stroke, psychiatric hospitalization, or epilepsy were excluded. A large minority of the subjects (42%) had a history of at least one treated and/or well-controlled chronic illness (10 heart disease, 17 hypertension, five asthma, two emphysema, 10 hypo- or hyperthyroidism, two diabetes). A majority of subjects were currently using prescribed medications (55%) for the above chronic diseases or as a hypertensive preventative. Mean educational level was 10.4 ($\pm$3.1) with a range of 4 to 20 years, which was comparable to the modal educational level for that age range according to the Australian Bureau of Statistics. A wide range of occupations was represented, including unskilled laborers, homemakers, business persons, and teachers.

The SRT was administered according to Reitan's 1959 procedures. Mean number correct and standard deviations are reported. Thirty-seven percent of the sample were misclassified as impaired using Reitan's (1959) cutoff score of 24. Education was found to be significantly related to SRT scores ($r = -0.22$) while no effect of sex, chronic disease, medication or their interaction was found for SRT performance.

Study strengths
1. Relatively large sample size for constricted age range.
2. Reporting of ethnic characteristics, sex, education, handedness, recruitment procedures, and geographic area.

3. Means and standard deviations are reported.

Considerations regarding use of the study
1. Data collected in Australia which may limit their usefulness for clinical interpretation in the United States.
2. Below average educational level.
3. No information regarding IQ.
4. Approximately half of the subjects had at least one chronic illness, and over half were taking prescribed medications.

	Mean	Standard Deviation
SRT No. correct	25.4	3.5

[SRT.11] Heaton, Grant, and Matthews, 1991

The authors provide normative data on the SRT from 486 (378 in the base sample and 108 in the validation sample) urban and rural subjects recruited in several states (California, Washington, Colorado, Texas, Oklahoma, Wisconsin, Illinois, Michigan, New York, Virginia, and Massachusetts) and Canada. Data were collected over a 15-year period through multicenter collaborative efforts; the authors trained the test administrators and supervised data collection. Exclusion criteria included history of learning disability, neurologic disease, illnesses affecting brain function, significant head trauma, significant psychiatric disturbance (e.g., schizophrenia), and alcohol or other substance abuse. Mean age for the total sample was 42.06 $\pm$ 16.8, and mean educational level was 13.6 $\pm$ 3.5. Sixty-five percent of the sample were males. The majority of the subjects ($N = 486$) were administered the WAIS; mean FSIQ, VIQ, and PIQ were 113.8 $\pm$ 12.3, 113.9 $\pm$ 13.8, and 111.9 $\pm$ 11.6, respectively.

The SRT was administered according to procedures outlined by Reitan and Wolfson (1985). Subjects were generally paid for their participation, and were judged to have provided their best efforts on the tasks. Fourteen percent of score variance was accounted for by age, while 15% was attributable to educational level; a total of 22% of test score variance was accounted for by age and education. Sex did not account for any unique variance in performance. The normative data, which are not reproduced here, are presented in comprehensive tables in *T*-score equivalents for test-scaled scores for males and females separately in 10 age groupings (20–34, 35–39, 40–44, 45–49, 50–54, 55–59, 60–64, 65–69, 70–74, 75–80) by six educational groupings (6–8 years, 9–11 years, 12 years, 13–15 years, 16–17 years, 18+ years). Mean score correct on the SRT for the sample as a whole was 26.1 ± 3.2.

Study strengths
1. Large sample size.
2. *T* scores corrected for age, education, and sex.
3. Comprehensive exclusion criteria.
4. Information regarding IQ and geographic recruitment area.

Considerations regarding use of the study
1. Above average mean intellectual level (which is probably less of an issue given that these are WAIS rather than WAIS-R IQ data).

Other comments
1. The interested reader is referred to 1996 critique of Heaton et al. (1991) norms, and Heaton et al.'s (1996) response to this critique.

Control Groups in Clinical Studies

[SRT.12] Klove and Lochen (in Klove, 1974)

The authors obtained SRT data on 22 American controls from Wisconsin and 22 Norwegian controls as a part of a validation study of the ability of the Halstead-Reitan Battery to detect brain damage. The mean number correct on the SRT is reported for each group. The mean age, educational level, and IQ for the American subjects were 31.6, 11.1, and 109.3, respectively. The mean age, educational level, and IQ for the Norwegian subjects were 32.1, 12.2, and 111.9, respectively.

Study strengths
1. This publication is unique in providing SRT data on a Norwegian population.
2. Information regarding educational level, IQ, age, and geographic recruitment area is reported.

Considerations regarding use of the study
1. The small sample size.
2. Undifferentiated age ranges.
3. No test score standard deviations reported.
4. Lack of specification of exclusion criteria.
5. No information on gender.
6. Low educational level of the United States sample, although IQ is average (Table 12.10).

[SRT.13] Wiens and Matarazzo, 1977

The authors collected SRT data on 48 male applicants to a patrolman program in Portland, Oregon, as a part of an investigation of the WAIS and MMPI correlates of the Halstead-Reitan Battery. All subjects passed a medical exam and were judged to be neurologically normal. Subjects were divided into two equal groups which were comparable in age (23.6 vs. 24.8), education (13.7 vs. 14.0), and WAIS FSIQ (117.5 vs. 118.3). SRT mean number correct and standard deviation were provided for each group. A random subsample of 29 of the applicants was readministered the SRT 14 to 24 weeks following the original administration. Means and standard deviations for SRT number correct for both the original testing and retest are reported. Four of the 29 subjects obtained scores lower than Reitan's suggested cutoff of 26 correct. A single significant correlation was obtained between SRT scores and FSIQ in the second control group; no significant correlations were obtained between SRT performance and VIQ or PIQ.

Table 12.10. SRT.12; Means for SRT Number Correct, IQ, Education, and Age for the Two Cultural Groups Separately

	N	Age	Educ	IQ	SRT No. correct
Americans	22	31.6	11.1	109.3	25.7
Norwegians	22	32.1	12.2	111.9	24.7

Study strengths
1. Information on test/retest performance.
2. Relatively large sample size for the small age range.
3. Adequate medical exclusion criteria.
4. Information provided regarding educational level, IQ, sex, and geographic recruitment area.
5. Means and standard deviations are reported.

Considerations regarding use of the study
1. High IQ level.
2. High educational level.
3. All male sample (Table 12.11)

[SRT.14] Anthony, Heaton, and Lehman, 1980

The authors amassed SRT data on 100 normal volunteers from Colorado as a part of a cross-validation of two computerized interpretive programs for the Halstead-Reitan Battery. Subjects had no history of medical or psychiatric problems, head trauma, brain disease, or substance abuse. In addition, for 85% of the controls, normal EEGs and neurological exams were obtained; in the remaining 15% of the subjects it appears that this information was not available. Mean age was 38.88 (SD = 15.80) and mean years of education was 13.33 (SD = 2.56). Mean WAIS VIQ and PIQ were 113.24 (SD = 11.59) and 112.26 (SD = 10.88), respectively. SRT data are presented in terms of mean number correct and standard deviation.

Study strengths
1. Large sample size.
2. Adequate exclusion criteria.
3. Information regarding education, IQ, age and geographic recruitment area is provided.
4. Means and standard deviations are reported.

Considerations regarding use of the study
1. The large undifferentiated age groupings.
2. The IQ range is high average.
3. No information regarding gender (Table 12.12).

[SRT.15] Bak and Greene, 1980

The authors gathered SRT data on 30 right-handed Texan subjects as a part of an investigation of the effect of age on performance on the Halstead-Reitan Battery and the Wechsler Memory Scale. The participants were equally divided into two age groupings: 50 to 62 and 67 to 86. Subjects were fluent in English and denied history of CNS disorders, uncorrected sensory deficits or illnesses, or "incapacities" which might affect test results; subjects in poor health were excluded. The mean age of the two groups was 55.6 (SD = 4.44) and 74.9 (SD = 6.04), respectively. Subjects in the first group were born between the years 1916 and 1929, and subjects in the second group were born between 1892 and 1912. Nine individuals in the first group were female, and 10 subjects in the second group were female. Four WAIS subtests were administered (Information, Arithmetic, Block Design, Digit Symbol); the mean scores

Table 12.11. SRT.13; Means and Standard Deviations for SRT Number of Correct Responses for the Original Testing for the Two Equal Groups°

N	Age	Education	WAIS			SRT	Retest
			FSIQ	VIQ	PIQ		
24	23.6 (21–27)	13.7 (12–16)	117.5 (8.3) (105–139)	117.4 (8.4)	115.4 (10.5)	27.5 (2.3)	
24	24.8 (21–28)	14.0 (12–16)	118.3 (6.8) (108–131)	116.4 (6.9)	118.2 (8.6)	27.1 (1.8)	
29	24 (21–28)	14 (12–16)	118	116	118	27.24 (1.94)	27.76 (1.48)

°For 29 subjects test-retest data are reported (14–24 weeks).

Table 12.12. SRT.14; Mean Number of Correct Responses and Standard Deviations

| N | Age | Education | WAIS | | | SRT |
			FSIQ	VIQ	PIQ	
100	38.88	13.33	113.54	113.24	112.26	26.96
	(15.80)	(2.56)	(10.83)	(11.59)	(10.88)	(2.70)

on these measures suggested that IQ levels were within the high average range or higher. Mean educational levels for the two groups were 13.7 ± 1.91 and 14.9 ± 2.99, respectively.

Means and standard deviations for SRT number correct are presented for the two groups. No significant differences in performance were documented between the two groups.

Study strengths

1. It provides data on a very elderly age group not found in other published normative data.

2. Adequate exclusion criteria.

3. Information regarding education, IQ, sex, handedness, fluency in English, and geographic recruitment area is provided.

4. Means and standard deviations are reported.

Considerations regarding use of the study

1. The high IQ level.

2. High educational level.

3. The older age grouping spans nearly two decades and may be too broad for optimal clinical interpretative use.

4. Small sample sizes (Table 12.13).

[SRT.16] Moore and Hannay, 1982

The authors published SRT data on 90 Alabama college students in an examination of the relationship between SRT performance and WAIS VIQ/PIQ discrepancies. Course extra credit was awarded for participation in the project. Subjects were strongly right-handed (use of right hand on at least nine of 10 hand activities on the Neurosurgery Center Handedness Questionnaire) and had no left-handed parents or siblings. Students with histories of CNS dysfunction, 3 or more years of formal musical training, and music lessons within the previous year were excluded. Subjects were divided into three groups (equal in terms of age) based on WAIS test scores: VIQ minus PIQ ≥10 but <20, PIQ minus VIQ ≥10 but <20, and VIQ and PIQ within five points of each other. The means and standard deviations for FSIQ, VIQ, and PIQ for the three groups are summarized in Table 12.14.

The three groups included 20, 20, and 22 males, respectively, and had a mean age of 20.83 (SD = 2.25), 20.17 (1.57), and 20.40 (1.89), respectively. All subjects were administered both form A and form B; half of the subjects in each group were presented with form A first and the other half received form B first.

Table 12.13. SRT.15; Mean Number of Correct Responses and Standard Deviations for the Two Age Groups

| N | Age | Education | WAIS° | | | | SRT |
			Information	Arithmetic	Block Design	Digit Symbol	
15	50–62						
	55.6	13.7	20.13	11.87	34.33	54.67	25.27
	(4.44)	(1.91)	(3.38)	(1.92)	(6.79)	(12.19)	(2.68)
15	67–86						
	74.9	14.9	21.07	13.60	28.07	39.47	24.60
	(6.04)	(2.99)	(3.84)	(2.97)	(5.36)	(12.11)	(3.31)

°WAIS raw scores.

Table 12.14. SRT.16a; Sample Composition Based on the WAIS VIQ/PIQ Discrepancy

	FSIQ		VIQ		PIQ	
	M	SD	M	SD	M	SD
High VIQ	113.37	(6.22)	118.60	(6.62)	104.26	(5.53)
High PIQ	114.97	(8.06)	108.83	(7.93)	120.96	(7.36)
Equal VIQ/PIQ	114.27	(7.67)	112.96	(7.81)	114.00	(6.87)

Means and standard deviations for SRT number correct and percent correct are reported for each VIQ/PIQ discrepancy group for forms A and B. The high PIQ group scored significantly below the high VIQ and equal VIQ/PIQ groups; 30% of the high PIQ group scored within the brain damaged range (≥ 5 errors) vs. none of the high VIQ and 7% of the equal VIQ/PIQ groups. The authors suggest that the superior performance of high VIQ and equal groups could be related to the use of a left-hemisphere strategy of sequential analysis (suitable for the short rhythmic sequences found on the SRT) vs. holistic analysis (Moore & Hannay, 1981).

Study strengths
1. The information on VIQ/PIQ discrepancy.
2. Large sample size for a restricted age range.
3. Data on form B.
4. Information regarding handedness, sex, musical training, age, educational background, geographic area, and recruitment procedures.
5. Means and standard deviations are reported.

Considerations regarding use of the study
1. Above average intellectual level.
2. Exclusion criteria are minimal.

(Because of the unique pattern of SRT performance associated with variations in VIQ/PIQ performance, these data would be the best normative set for use with patients who match the age and IQ characteristics of this sample. The authors conclude: "for college students or perhaps all people with average to superior intelligence . . . IQ discrepancy may be important in interpreting lowered performance on the Seashore Rhythm Test" (Moore & Hannay, 1981, p.824) (Table 12.15).

[SRT.17] Karzmark, Heaton, Lehman, and Crouch, 1985

The authors gathered SRT data on 112 paid normal controls from Colorado as a part of an investigation of the sensitivity of the SRT to right vs. left hemisphere lesions. Exclusion criteria included history of brain disease or trauma, alcohol or other drug abuse, and psychiatric disorder. The mean age of the group was 37.58 (SD = 15.70) and mean years of education was

Table 12.15. SRT.16b; The Table Provides Means and Standard Deviations for Number Correct and Percent Correct for Each VIQ/PIQ Discrepancy Group for SRT Forms A and B

	SRT A		SRT B	
IQ Discrepancy Group	Number Correct	Percent Correct	Number Correct	Percent Correct
High VIQ	28.47	94.89	23.70	79.00
	(1.28)	(4.19)	(2.90)	(9.51)
High PIQ	26.80	89.33	24.63	82.11
	(1.83)	(5.99)	(2.36)	(7.72)
Equal VIQ/PIQ	27.67	92.22	23.70	79.00
	(1.42)	(4.66)	(2.33)	(7.66)

13.27 (SD = 2.94). The authors provide the mean and standard deviation for number correct on the SRT. The SRT was sensitive to the presence of brain damage in the patient sample but was not useful in providing localizing information regarding which hemisphere was dysfunctional.

Study strengths
1. Large sample size.
2. Medical exclusion requirements are adequate.
3. Information on education, geographic area, age, and education.
4. Means and standard deviations are reported.

Considerations regarding use of the study
1. Lack of presentation of the data in smaller age groupings.
2. No information is provided regarding IQ level, ethnicity, sex ratio, or handedness.

N	Age	Education	SRT No. Correct
112	37.58 (15.70)	13.27 (2.94)	26.83 (2.86)

[SRT.18] Heaton, Grant, and Matthews, 1986

The authors obtained SRT data on 553 normal controls in Colorado, California, and Wisconsin as a part of an investigation into the effects of age, education, and sex on Halstead-Reitan Battery performance. Nearly two-thirds of the sample was male (males = 356, females = 197). Exclusion criteria included history of neurologic illness, significant head trauma, and substance abuse. Subjects ranged in age from 15 to 81 (mean = 39.3 ± 17.5), and mean years of education was 13.3 (±3.4) with a range of 0 to 20 years. The sample was divided into three age categories (less than 40, 40–59, and greater than or equal to 60 years) with 319, 134, and 100 subjects, respectively, and was classified into three education categories (less than 12 years, 12 to 15 years, and greater than or equal to 16 years) with *N*s of 132, 249, and 172, respectively.

Testing was conducted by trained technicians and all participants were judged to have expended their best effort on the task; SRT

mean number correct and percent of subjects classified as normal by Russell et al. (1970) criteria are reported for the six subgroups. Approximately 15% of test score variance was accounted for by age and approximately 10% of test score variance was associated with education level. Significant group differences in SRT scores were found across the three age groups and across the three education groups; no significant age-by-education interaction was documented. No significant differences in performance were found between males and females.

Study strenghts
1. Large size of overall sample and individual cells.
2. Information regarding sex, geographic area, age, and education.
3. Data grouped by age and also by educational level.
4. Minimally adequate exclusion criteria.

Considerations regarding use of the study
1. No reporting of SRT score standard deviations.
2. Mean scores for individual WAIS subtest scaled scores reported but not overall IQ scores (Table 12.16)

[SRT.19] Alekoumbides, Charter, Adkins, and Seacat, 1987

The authors report data on 114 medical and psychiatric inpatients and outpatients without cerebral lesions or histories of alcoholism or cerebral contusion from V.A. hospitals in Southern California as part of their development of standardized scores corrected for age and education for the Halstead-Reitan battery. Among the 41 psychiatric patients, nine were diagnosed as psychotic and 32 were neurotic. In addition to psychiatry services, patients were also drawn from medicine (*n* = 57), neurology (*n* = 22), spinal cord injury (*n* = 9), and surgery (*n* = 6) units. Mean age was 46.85 ± 17.17 (ranging from 19 to 82), and mean years of education was 11.43 ± 3.20 (ranging from 1 to 20). Frequency distributions for age and years of education are provided. Mean WAIS FSIQ, VIQ, and PIQ were within the average range (105.89 ± 13.47, 107.03 ± 14.38, and 103.31 ± 13.02,

Table 12.16. SRT.18; SRT Mean Number of Correct Responses and Percent of Subjects Classified as Normal by Russell et al. (1970) Criteria for the Six Subgroups[°]

N	Age	Education	SRT No. Correct	% Normal	WAIS SS Mean
319	<40		26.9	84.3	11.9
134	40-59		26.1	75.4	11.2
100	≥60		23.8	52.0	9.7
132		<12	24.6	61.2	9.5
249		12–15	26.4	77.5	11.2
172		≥16	27.0	85.5	12.9

[°]Mean scaled scores for the WAIS subtests are also reported.

respectively); means and standard deviations for individual age-corrected subtest scores are also reported. All subjects except one were male; the majority were Caucasian (93%), with 7% African-American. The mean score on a measure of occupational attainment was 11.29.

No differences were found in test performance between the two psychiatric groups and the nonpsychiatric group and the data were collapsed. Mean SRT correct and standard deviation are reported. In addition, regression equation information to allow correction of raw scores for age and education is included.

Study strengths
1. Large sample size.
2. Information regarding age, IQ, education, ethnicity, sex, occupational attainment, and geographic area.
3. Regression equation data for computation of age- and education-corrected scores.
4. Means and standard deviations are reported.

Considerations regarding use of the study
1. Data were collected on medical and psychiatric patients.

2. Undifferentiated age range (mitigated by the regression equation information).
3. Somewhat low educational level although IQ is average.
4. Nearly all male sample (Table 12.17).

Raw scores were corrected by the following equation:

$$Xc = X - b1X1 - b2X2 + C$$

where Xc is the corrected score, X is the uncorrected score, $X1$ is the age, $X2$ is the education, $b1$ and $b2$ are the weights of age and education, respectively, and C is a constant:

B1	B2	C
−0.036	0.244	1.123

[SRT.20] Bornstein, Baker, and Douglass, 1987a

The authors collected SRT test/retest data on 23 volunteers (14 women, nine men) who ranged in age from 17 to 52 (mean = 32.3 ± 10.3), as a part of an examination of the short-term retest reliability of the Halstead-Reitan

Table 12.17. SRT.19; Sample Composition and the Number of Correct SRT Responses

N	Age	Education	WAIS FSIQ	VIQ	PIQ	SRT No. correct
114	46.85 (17.17)	11.43 (3.20)	105.89 (13.47)	107.03 (14.38)	103.31 (13.02)	24.72 (3.47)

Table 12.18. SRT.20; Means and Standard Deviations for SRT Number of Correct Responses for Two Testing Sessions° (3 Weeks Apart)

N	Age	VIQ	PIQ	Test	Retest	Raw Score Change	Median Raw Score Change	% Change
23	32.3	105.8	105.0	27.7	27.6	0	0	0
	(10.3)	(10.8)	(10.5)	(2.1)	(2.1)	(1.5)		
	17–52	88–128	85–121					

°Raw score change and standard deviation, median raw score change, and mean percent of change are also reported.

Battery. Exclusion criteria consisted of a positive history of neurological or psychiatric illness. Mean verbal IQ was 105.8 ± 10.8 (range = 88 to 128) and mean performance IQ was 105.0 ± 10.5 (range = 85 to 121).

Subjects were administered the Halstead-Reitan Battery in standard order both on initial testing and again 3 weeks later. Means, standard deviations, and ranges for SRT number correct for both testing sessions are provided, as well as raw score change and standard deviation, median raw score change, and mean percent of change. No significant correlations between mean change and age ($r = 0.18$) or education ($r = -0.12$) or between mean percent of change and age ($r = 0.20$) or education ($r = -0.09$) were documented.

Study strengths
1. Information on short-term (3-week) retest data.
2. Information on IQ level, age, and gender.
3. Minimally adequate exclusion criteria.
4. Means and standard deviations are reported.

Considerations regarding use of the study
1. Undifferentiated age range.
2. No information regarding education.
3. Relatively small sample size (Table 12.18).

[SRT.21] Russell, 1987

The author obtained SRT data on 155 controls during the years 1968 to 1982 in V.A. hospitals in Cincinnati and Miami for his development of a reference scale method for neuropsychological test batteries. The 148 male and seven female subjects were suspected of having neurological disorders but had "negative neurological findings." No other exclusion criteria are described. Mean age was 46.19 ± 12.86, and mean years of education was 12.29 ± 3.00. All but eight of the participants were Caucasian; the remainder were African-American. Mean WAIS FSIQ, VIQ, and PIQ were 111.9, 112.3, and 109.9, respectively.

Mean SRT errors and standard deviation are provided.

Study strengths
1. Large sample size.
2. Information regarding IQ, education, ethnicity, sex, age, and geographic area.
3. Means and standard deviations are reported.

Considerations regarding use of the study
1. Undifferentiated age range.
2. Insufficient exclusion criteria.
3. High mean intellectual level.
4. Mostly male sample (Table 12.19).

Table 12.19. SRT.21; Sample Composition and the Number of SRT Errors

N	Age	Education	WAIS			SRT Errors
			FSIQ	VIQ	PIQ	
155	46.19	12.29	111.9	112.3	109.9	3.95
	(12.86)	(3.00)				(3.02)

CONCLUSIONS

The above review suggests that the SRT has received relatively wide scrutiny. In spite of the diversity in demographic characteristics of the samples, the mean level of performance (in No. of correct responses or, conversely, in No. of errors) is quite consistent across different studies. A comparison of data reported in this chapter suggests that variability in SRT performance is determined by age, education, IQ level, and VIQ/PIQ discrepancy. Therefore, an adjustment of the cutoff score to account for differences in these demographic and cognitive variables would improve psychometric properties of this test.

Considerable controversy exists regarding utility of the SRT in detection of brain dysfunction ranging from its localizing/lateralizing effectiveness to its general diagnostic classification accuracy. Future studies exploring incremental validity of the SRT with different clinical and control groups would be of utmost importance in establishing the utility of this test in neuropsychological assessment.

13

Speech Sounds Perception Test

BRIEF HISTORY OF THE TEST

The Speech Sounds Perception Test (SSPT) was incorporated by Halstead (1947) in his original neuropsychological battery and subsequently employed by Ralph Reitan in his expansion of the Halstead Battery (Reitan & Wolfson, 1993). Subjects are played an audiotape of 60 spoken single-syllable "nonsense" words divided into six series of 10 items all containing the long "e" vowel sound. They are given a score sheet with four multiple-choice options for each of the 60 "words" which differ in beginning and/or ending consonant sounds and instructed to underline the option which matches the "word" heard on the audiotape. This test requires sustained attention, immediate auditory memory, and phoneme discrimination, but also intact spelling and reading ability. The task attempts to measure the ability to discriminate between spoken phonemes, but, unfortunately, individuals with intact auditory discrimination ability may fail this measure due to the response format. In our experience if an individual has reading and/or spelling deficits, he/she is likely to perform poorly on this task because these problems cause them to have difficulties in choosing the correct multiple choice item. In addition, Schear et al. (1988), based on their investigation of the effect of simulated hearing loss on the SSPT, caution that decreased hearing in the elderly may artificially lower SSPT performance. Finally, the integrity

of the test is further compromised by Bolter et al.'s (1984) finding that it is possible to deduce the correct answers on the SSPT according to the manner of construction of the multiple choices; an adolescent of average IQ was able to consistently choose the correct answers without actually attending to the auditory stimuli.

The SSPT has traditionally been used by neuropsychologists as a measure of left hemisphere and/or left temporal lobe dysfunction (Golden et al., 1981b; Jarvis & Barth, 1984; Lezak, 1983), but this assumption has not been supported empirically (Doehring & Reitan, 1961; Reitan, 1964; Goldstein & Shelly, 1972). Bornstein & Leason (1984) suggest that error type rather than total score may provide useful information regarding lesion lateralization. They documented that right-hemisphere-damaged patients committed significantly more beginning errors while left-hemisphere-damaged patients made significantly more ending errors. They recommend that use of a cutoff of greater than 70% ending errors and less than 29% beginning errors may be helpful in identifying patients with left hemisphere dysfunction.

Specific administration and scoring instructions are provided in Reitan's (1979) *Manual for Administration of Neuropsychological Test Batteries for Adults and Children.* Ryan et al. (1982) report that a shortened version of the test consisting of the first 30 items may be substituted for administration of the entire test with no loss in diagnostic accuracy. Bornstein (1982a) documented a split-half reliability on the SSPT of between 0.74 and 0.87 in patient samples, with reliability increasing with greater levels of overall cognitive impairment (e.g., lower IQ, higher Impairment Index). The greatest number of errors were committed on series B and A and the fewest were documented on E and D. Significantly more errors occurred on the first half of the test. The formula of score correct on series A + series B + series C + 2 effectively predicted total test score although Bornstein recommended against the use of an abbreviated format. In a subsequent publication, Bornstein et al. (1984) found that the pattern of errors across the six series could not be attributed to order of presentation or learning but rather appeared to be due to differences in item difficulty related to phonetic similarity of the correct choices to real words.

Reddon et al. (1989) report that the nonrandom organization of response choices leads to response bias that can confound interpretations derived from test scores. They developed a revised, randomized form but they do not recommend its clinical use due to the absence of normative data. They suggest that the original form be used with caution, or that other, more modern speech perception tests be substituted.

Clinical utility of the SSPT was further questioned by Sherer et al. (1991) based on a literature review and their own empirical studies. They argue against the premise that the SSPT is a sensitive measure of alertness and concentration and that it specifically targets left hemisphere dysfunction. The authors concluded that SSPT and SRT are "most appropriately interpreted as being general indicators of cerebral integrity" (p. 749); however, a unique diagnostic contribution of these tests was questioned.

A more positive view of SSPT utility was offered by Charter (1994), who examined the frequency of random responding for three tests from the Halstead-Reitan Battery using a formula approximating binomial distribution for a large sample, based on observed score and a probability of guessing. Frequency of random responses on the SSPT for the 90%, 95%, and 99% confidence intervals presented in this article are summarized:

90%		95%		99%	
Low	High	Low	High	Low	High
40	51	39	52	38	55

Charter's review of the different articles did not reveal any studies reporting normative subjects' scores falling in the random range for the SSPT.

A moderately high relationship between SSPT scores and activities of daily living (as measured by the Scale of Competence in Independent Living Skills; SCILS) in a sample of geriatric patients was reported by Searight et al. (1989). The authors report correlation coefficients between the SSPT scores and measures of 16 activities of daily living ranging between 0.24 and 0.53. Correlation between the SSPT and the total SCILS score was 0.44.

Scoring and interpretation of SSPT scores has traditionally involved use of cutoff scores. Reitan and Wolfson (1985) recommend a cutoff of 10 errors. They report that Halstead's 1947 cutoff was between seven and eight errors (seven and fewer errors as normal and eight or greater as abnormal). However, our examination of Halstead's text suggests that Halstead's cutoff was actually 20 errors (1947, p. 147). Regardless, given the significant association between SSPT performance and age, education, and IQ, a single cutoff would not appear to be appropriate. Ernst (1988) found that using a cutoff of eight errors, 37% of a healthy elderly sample were misclassified as brain damaged. Bak and Greene (1980) report that their elderly sample aged 67–86 averaged 7.13 ± 4.26 errors "indicating that a large portion of these subjects would be classified as dysfunctional based on these non-age-corrected cutoff scores" (p. 397). Similarly, Dodrill (1987) reported a 19.2% misclassification rate using a cutoff of seven errors in a young control sample. Bornstein and colleagues (1987b) emphasized that cutoff scores may be useful but only if considered in the context of other neuropsychological information obtained in a test battery, and if age, education, and other appropriate adjustments are made. Bak and Greene (1980) recommended that if a cutoff approach is to be used with older individuals, new cutoffs need to be developed, but they question whether useful cutoffs can be identified given the increased variability in performance in the elderly.

RELATIONSHIP BETWEEN SSPT PERFORMANCE AND DEMOGRAPHIC FACTORS

The available literature indicates that SSPT performance in normal individuals is associated with age (Heaton et al., 1986, 1991), education (Ernst, 1988; Heaton, Grant, & Matthews, 1986, 1991), VIQ (Reitan & Wolfson, 1985; Yeudall et al., 1987), and PIQ (Yeudall et al., 1987), with high intellectual and educational level and younger age associated with better SSPT scores. However, some investigators have failed to document these relationships, possibly due to methodological factors. Bak and Greene (1980) did not find any relationship between age and SSPT performance, but their sample was limited to 30 subjects above age 50. Reed and Reitan (1962) could not document an association between older age and poorer SSPT scores, but their young sample included a majority of patients hospitalized with non-brain-related diseases while the majority of the older subjects were nonhospitalized normals. Fromm-Auch and Yeudall (1983) did not find a relationship between age and SSPT scores but their sample included very few subjects above age 40, and they concluded that their data cannot adequately address this issue. Yeudall et al. (1987) failed to find a significant association between SSPT performance and age or education, but this sample was limited to subjects aged 40 and less. Wiens and Matarazzo (1977) failed to document significant correlations between SSPT scores and FSIQ, VIQ, or PIQ, but the IQ range was restricted to the average level and higher. No FSIQ was below 105. No studies have revealed any significant differences in SSPT test scores between men and women (Dodrill, 1979; Fromm-Auch & Yeudall, 1983; Heaton et al., 1991; Yeudall et al., 1987).

Relationships between SSPT scores and age, education, and IQ have been found for patient groups, although the associations decline with increasing severity of brain disturbance. Seidenberg et al. (1984) found education to be a predictor of SSPT performance (accounting for 13% of the test score variance) in their sample of seizure patients; age was not a significant predictor but the age range was limited to 52 and less. Finlayson et al. (1977) noted a significant relationship between education and SSPT performance in hospitalized psychiatric and non-neurological medical patients and a brain-damaged sample. In the hospitalized sample, poorer SSPT performance was documented in subjects with less than 10 years of formal education relative to high-school- and university-educated subjects, while in the brain-damaged sample, lower SSPT scores were found in the subjects with less than 10 years of education vs. those wih 15 or more years of college. Vega and Parsons (1967) observed the presence of a significant positive correlation between SSPT scores and education, and a significant negative correlation between SSPT scores and age in a medically or psychiatrically hospitalized population, but failed to find significant relationships between SSPT scores and these variables in a brain-damaged sample. Prigatano and Parsons (1976) found no association between age or education and SSPT performance in their brain-damaged sample but reported a relationship between age, but not education, and SSPT scores in psychiatric and medical–surgical patients. Seidenberg et al. (1984) reported no association between SSPT performance and sex, handedness, or socioeconomic status.

METHOD FOR EVALUATING THE NORMATIVE REPORTS

Our review of the literature located seven SSPT normative reports published since 1965 (Dodrill, 1987; Ernst, 1988; Fromm-Auch & Yeudall, 1983; Harley et al., 1980; Heaton et al., 1991; Pauker, 1980; Yeudall et al., 1987), as well as Halstead's (1947) original data and three interpretative guides for the Halstead-Reitan Battery (Gilandas et al., 1984; Reitan & Wolfson, 1985; Golden et al., 1981b). Numerous studies have also reported control subject data and we have included discussion of seven of those investigations which involved some unique feature, such as large sample size (greater than or equal to 100), retest data, and elderly population (Alekoumbides et al., 1987; Anthony et al., 1980; Bak & Greene, 1980; Bornstein et al., 1987; Heaton et al., 1986; Russell, 1987; Wiens & Matarazzo, 1977).

Russell and Starkey (1993) developed the Halstead-Russell Neuropsychological Evaluation System (HRNES), which includes the SSPT among 22 tests. In the context of this system, individual performance is compared to that of 576 brain-damaged subjects and 200 subjects who were initially suspected of having brain damage but had negative neurological findings. Data were partitioned into seven age groups and three educational/IQ levels. This study will not be reviewed in this chapter because the "normal" group consisted of the V.A. patients who presented with symptomatology requiring neuropsychological evaluation. For further discussion of the HRNES system see Lezak, 1995 (pp. 714–715).

Of note, few relevant manuscripts have emerged since the 1980s, perhaps due either to the publication of Heaton et al.'s (1991) comprehensive normative tables or to the escalating use in research and clinical practice of flexible neuropsychological test protocols which include newer tasks rather than traditional fixed neuropsychological batteries.

In order to adequately evaluate the SSPT normative reports, six key criterion variables were deemed critical. The first five of these relate to *subject* variables, and the one remaining dimension refers to *procedural* issues.

Minimal requirements for meeting the criterion variables were as follows:

Subject Variables

Sample Size

As discussed in previous chapters, a minimum of at least 50 subjects per grouping interval is optimal.

Sample Composition Description

As discussed previously, information regarding medical and psychiatric exclusion criteria is important; it is unclear if gender, geographic region, ethnicity, occupation, handedness, or recruitment procedures are relevant, so until this is determined, it is best that this information is provided.

Age Group Intervals

Given the apparent association between age and SSPT performance, information regarding age of the normative sample is critical and preferably normative data should be presented by age intervals.

Reporting of IQ Levels

Given the relationship between SSPT performance and IQ, information regarding intellectual level should be provided.

Reporting of Education Levels

Given the association between education level and SSPT scores, information regarding highest educational level completed should be reported.

Procedural Variables

Data Reporting

Means and standard deviations, and preferably ranges, for total errors on the SSPT should be reported.

SUMMARY OF THE STATUS OF THE NORMS

In terms of subject variables, only seven studies provided SSPT data by age groupings (Bak & Greene, 1980; Fromm-Auch & Yeudall, 1983; Harley et al., 1980; Heaton et al., 1986, 1991; Pauker, 1980; Yeudall et al., 1987), and two studies limited their total sample to a suitably restricted age range (Ernst, 1988; Wiens & Matarazzo, 1977). Twelve of the publications reported information on IQ levels for their samples as a whole and/or for individual age groupings (Alekoumbides et al., 1987; Anthony et al., 1980; Bak & Greene, 1980; Bornstein et al., 1987a; Dodrill, 1987; Fromm-Auch & Yeudall, 1983; Harley et al., 1980; Halstead, 1947; Heaton et al., 1991; Russell, 1987; Wiens & Mattarrazzo, 1977; Yeudall et al., 1987), although only one publication actually presented SSPT data by IQ levels (Pauker, 1980); he provided these data in age by IQ cells. Similarly, 10 reports indicated the mean educational levels of their sample as a whole and/or mean educational levels for age groupings (Alekoumbides et al., 1987; Bak & Greene, 1980; Dodrill, 1987; Ernst, 1988; Fromm-Auch & Yeudall, 1983; Halstead, 1947; Harley et al., 1980; Russell, 1987; Wiens & Matarazzo, 1977; Yeudall et al., 1987), although only two studies presented data by educational level (Heaton et al., 1986, 1991).

The majority of the studies involved large total sample sizes, but only three publications consistently achieved individual age groupings of at least 50 subjects (Ernst, 1988; Heaton et al., 1986; Pauker, 1980), although several studies had one or more age groupings (or age by IQ groupings) which met this criterion (Fromm-Auch & Yeudall, 1983; Harley et al., 1980; Pauker, 1980; Yeudall et al., 1987).

Medical and psychiatric exclusion criteria were judged to be excellent in seven reports (Anthony et al., 1980; Dodrill, 1987; Ernst, 1988; Heaton et al., 1991; Pauker, 1980; Wiens & Matarazzo, 1977; Yeudall et al., 1987) and minimally adequate in four others (Bak & Greene, 1980; Bornstein et al., 1987a; Fromm-Auch & Yeudall, 1983; Heaton et al., 1986). Of particular concern, four publications actually included psychiatric, neurologic, medical, and/or alcoholic patients or subjects suspected of having neurological disorders but with negative neurological findings (Alekoumbides et al., 1987; Halstead, 1947; Harley et al., 1980; Russell, 1987).

Indications of geographic recruitment area were available in the majority of studies (Alekoumbides et al., 1987; Bak & Greene, 1980; Ernst, 1988; Fromm-Auch & Yeudall, 1983; Harley et al., 1980; Heaton et al., 1986, 1991; Reitan & Wolfson, 1985; Russell, 1987; Wiens & Matarazzo, 1977; Yeudall et al., 1987). Four publications reported data collected outside of the United States; one study reported SSPT norms on an Australian population (Ernst, 1988) while three reports sampled a Canadian population (Fromm-Auch & Yeudall, 1983; Pauker, 1980; Yeudall et al., 1987). Sex distribution was reported in all studies but two (Anthony et al., 1980; Harley et al., 1980), although since the Harley et al. data were collected in a V.A. setting, it can probably be assumed the sample was primarily male. Yeudall et al. (1987) provide SSPT data in age-by-sex cells. Information regarding handedness (Dodrill, 1987;

Ernst, 1988; Fromm-Auch & Yeudall, 1983; Yeudall et al., 1987), ethnicity (Alekoumbides et al., 1987; Dodrill, 1987; Ernst, 1988; Halstead, 1947; Russell, 1987), and occupation (Alekoumbides et al., 1987; Dodrill, 1987; Ernst, 1988; Fromm-Auch & Yeudall, 1983; Halstead, 1947; Yeudall et al., 1987) was less commonly provided.

In terms of procedural variables, mean errors or number correct is reported in all publications, with standard deviations indicated in all but two reports (Halstead, 1947; Heaton et al., 1986). Test score ranges are provided in four datasets (Bornstein et al., 1987a; Fromm-Auch & Yeudall, 1983; Halstead, 1947; Harley et al., 1980), and some reports also presented information on IQ-equivalent scores (Dodrill, 1987), computation methods for obtaining standardized scores corrected for age and education (Alekoumbides et al., 1987), and T scores (Harley et al., 1980; Heaton et al., 1991).

Table 13.1 summarizes information provided in the studies described in this chapter.

SUMMARIES OF THE STUDIES

Given that the use of the SSPT has typically been within the context of the Halstead-Reitan Battery, the Halstead and Reitan data and interpretation recommendations will be reported first, followed by a summary of the other interpretation formats, and then the normative publications, presented in ascending chronological order. The chapter will conclude with a review of SSPT control data reported in various clinical studies.

Interpretive Guides

[SSPT.1] Halstead, 1947

The author obtained data on 28 control subjects apparently from the Chicago area, half of whom had psychiatric diagnoses. The 14 subjects without psychiatric diagnoses were nine male and five female civilians ranging in age from 15 to 50 (mean = 25.9), without a history of brain injury. The eight subjects who carried diagnoses of mild psychoneurosis were male soldiers ranging in age from 22 to 38 (mean =

Table 13.1. SSPT.L; Locator Table for the SSPT

Study°	Age°°	N	Sample Composition	IQ°° Education	Country/ Location
SSPT.1 Halstead, 1947 page 218	15–50	28	14 Ss without psychiatric diagnosis, 14 Ss with psychiatric diagnosis	Education 7-18 years IQ 70–140	Chicago
SSPT.2 Reitan & Wolfson, 1985 (Reitan, 1955) page 221	32.3 (10.78)	50	12 normal, 38 hospitalized with psychiatric disorders	Education 11.58 (2.85)	Indiana
SSPT.3 Harley et al., 1980 page 222	55–79 55–59 60–64 65–69 70–74 75–79	193 56 45 35 37 20	V.A. hospitalized patients; 5 age groups T-score equivalents are reported	FSIQ>80 Education 8.8 years	Wisconsin
SSPT.4 Pauker, 1980 page 222	19–71 19–34 35–52 53–71	363	152 M, 211 F volunteers fluent in English. Data are presented in age by IQ groupings	4 IQ levels	Toronto, Canada
SSPT.5 Fromm-Auch & Yeudall, 1983 page 224	15–64 25.4 (8.2) 15–17 18–23 24–32 33–40 41–64	193 32 76 57 18 10	111 M, 82 F volunteers 83% R-handed; 5 age groups	Education 8-25 years 14.8 (3.0) FSIQ,VIQ, PIQ: 119.1 (8.8) 119.8 (9.9) 115.6 (9.8)	Canada
SSPT.6 Dodrill, 1987 page 225	27.73 (11.04)	120	60 M, 60 F volunteers 10% minorities 18 L-handed. No neurologically relevant diseases, alcoholism, birth complications, psychoses, head injury	Education 12.28(2.18) FSIQ, VIQ, PIQ: 100.00(14.35) 100.29(14.73) 98.25(13.39)	Washington
SSPT.7 Yeudall et al., 1987 page 225	15–40 15–20 21–25 26–30 31–40	225	Volunteers: no neurological insult, prenatal/birth complications, psychiatric problems or substance abuse. 4 age groups, 88% R-handed; 127 M, 98 F	Education 14.55 (2.78) FSIQ 112.25 (10.25)	Canada
SSPT.8 Ernst, 1988 page 226	65–75	85	Volunteers: all but 1 Caucasian, all but 1 R-handed, 39 M, 46 F. No history of substance abuse, head trauma, stroke, psychiatric hospitalization, epilepsy	Education 10.4(3.1) 4-20 years	Brisbane, Australia
SSPT.9 Heaton et al., 1991 page 227	42.1 (16.8) Groups: 20–34 35–39 40–44	486	Volunteers: urban and rural Data collected over 15 years through multi-center collaborative efforts. Strict exclusion criteria. 65% M. Data are presented	Education 13.6(3.5) FSIQ 113.8(12.3) Groups 6–8	California, Washington, Texas, Oklahoma, Wisconsin, Illinois,

continued

Table 13.1. *(Continued)*

Study[*]	Age[**]	N	Sample Composition	IQ[**] Education	Country/ Location
(SSPT.9 Heaton et al., 1991 continued)	45–49 50–54 55–59 60–64 65–69 70–74 75–80		in T-score equivalents for M and F separately in 10 age groupings by 6 educational groupings	9–11 12 13-15 16-17 18+	Michigan, New York, Virginia, Massachusetts, Canada
SSPT.10 Wiens & Matarazzo, 1977 page 228	23.6 vs. 24.8	48	All male participants: neurologically normal control group, divided in 2 equal groups. Test-retest data are provided	Education 13.7 vs. 14.0 FSIQ 117.5 vs. 118.3	Portland, Oregon
SSPT.11 Anthony et al., 1980 page 228	38.88 (15.80)	100	Normal volunteers: No history of medical or psychiatric problems, head trauma, brain disease or substance abuse	Education 13.33 (2.56) FSIQ 113.5 (10.8)	Colorado
SSPT.12 Bak & Greene, 1980 page 229	50–62 67–86	15 15	Volunteers: R-handed, 2 age groupings, fluent in English, no CNS disorders, sensory deficits, illnesses, or incapacities. 1st group—9 F 2nd group—10 F	Education 13.7 (1.9) 14.9 (3.0)	Texas
SSPT.13 Heaton, et al., 1986 page 230	15–81 39.3 (17.5) <40 40–59 ≥60	553 319 134 100	Normal controls 356 M, 197 F No neurological illness, head trauma, substance abuse. Data are presented for 3 age groups and 3 education groups	Education 13.3 (3.4) 0–20 years <12 (n = 132) 12–15 (n = 249) ≥16 (n = 172)	Colorado, California, Wisconsin
SSPT.14 Alekoumbides et al., 1987 page 230	46.85 (17.17) 19–82	113	Outpatients w/o cerebral lesions or histories of cerebral contusions from V.A. hospitals. The study provides a regression equation for computation of age-and-education-corrected scores	Education 11.43 (3.20) 1–20 years FSIQ 105.9 (13.5)	Southern California
SSPT.15 Bornstein et al., 1987a page 231	17–52 32.3 (10.3)	23	Volunteers 9 M, 14 F No neurological or psychiatric illness. Data on 3-week retest are provided	VIQ 105.8 (10.8) PIQ 105.0 (19.5)	
SSPT.16 Russell, 1987 page 232	46.19 (12.86)	155	Controls in V.A. hospitals 148 M, 7 F suspected of having neurological disorders	Education 12.29 (3.00) FSIQ 111.9	Cincinnati, Miami

[*]The study number corresponds to the number provided in the text of the chapter.

[**]Age column and IQ/education column contain information regarding range and/or mean and standard deviation for the whole sample and/or separate groups, which ever information is provided by the authors.

29.6); some had had combat experience, but none had a history of head injury. The last six subjects ranged in age from 27 to 39 and included a depressed military prisoner facing execution, a severely depressed female with suicidal and homicidal impulses tested prior to lobotomy, and a suicidal/homicidal female and a suicidal male tested pre- and *post*lobotomy. Educational level ranged from 7 to 18 years, and the following occupations were represented: artist, entertainer, farmer, housewife, semiskilled and unskilled laborers, professional, secretary, teacher, technician, trade, and student. Ethnic background included American, Balkan, English, French, German, Irish, Polish, Scandinavian, and Scottish. IQ levels ranged from 70 to 140.

The mean SSPT errors for the total group and each control "subgroup" are reported as well as the individual error score for each subject. The SSPT criterion score used in calculating the Impairment Index was greater than 20 errors out of 60.

Study strengths
1. Information provided regarding geographic area, IQ, age, education, occupation, ethnicity, and gender.

Considerations regarding use of the study
1. Small sample size including use of two subjects twice.
2. Inclusion of subjects with psychiatric diagnoses and postlobotomy.
3. No reporting of standard deviations.
4. Undifferentiated age range (Table 13.2).

[SSPT.2] Reitan and Wolfson, 1985
The authors cite SSPT data published by Reitan in 1955 on 50 (35 male and 15 female) controls in Indiana. Twelve were "normal" while the remainder were either hospitalized with paraplegia ($n = 13$) or had various psychiatric

disorders (depression = 17, acute anxiety state = 6, obsessive-compulsive neurosis = 2). On neurological exam, none showed evidence of cerebral damage or dysfunction, and histories were negative for head injuries or brain diseases. Mean age was 32.3 ± 10.78 and mean years of education was 11.58 ± 2.85.

Mean and standard deviation for number errors are reported. In addition, score severity ranges reflecting "perfectly normal," "normal," "mildly impaired," and "seriously impaired" performance are provided. The authors also list cutoff scores for "normal" and "brain-damaged range" to be used in computing the Halstead Impairment Index. Of interest, they report that Halstead's original cutoff score was 8 (seven or less errors reflected normal performance; eight or more errors was abnormal); however, our examination of Halstead's (1947) publication, as reported above, indicates that his cutoff was greater than 20 errors (p. 174). Reitan and Wolfson suggest that a cutoff score of 8 is too stringent given their experience that normal individuals make up to 10 errors on the test. They report a significant negative correlation between SSPT errors and verbal IQ ($r = -0.73$).

Considerations regarding use of the study
The authors argue that only general normative score ranges are necessary rather than exact percentile ranks because "other methods of inference are used to supplement normative data in clinical interpretations of results for individual subjects" (p. 97). However, given the reported association between SSPT scores and education, age, and IQ, this approach to interpretation utilizing the same set of single cutoff scores and severity ranges for all patients will lead to excessive false-positive errors in identifying the presence of cognitive dysfunction and should no longer be endorsed (Table 13.3).

It should be noted that *Gilandas et al. (1984, p. 95)* suggest use of a cutoff score of six errors for the short form of the SSPT to classify abnormal performance. *Golden et al. (1981b)* use the SSPT to provide information regarding lesion lateralization, reporting that more than 20 errors "is almost always associated with a left hemisphere injury" (p. 19).

Table 13.2. SSPT.1

	N	SSPT Errors	Range
Total	28	10.36	3–20
Civilian	14	8.0	3–15
Military	8	14.5	8–20
Miscellaneous	6	7.0	3–12

Table 13.3. SSPT.2; Severity Ranges (Based on the Number of Errors)

Normal	Perfectly Normal	0–6	Impaired	Mildly	11–15	Mean	7.08
	Normal	7–10		Seriously	≥16		(5.31)

Normative Studies

[SSPT.3] Harley, Leuthold, Matthews, and Bergs, 1980

The authors collected SSPT data on 193 V.A.-hospitalized patients in Wisconsin ranging in age from 55 to 79. Exclusion criteria included full-scale IQ less than 80, active psychosis, unequivocal neurological disease or brain damage, and serious visual or auditory acuity problems. Patient diagnoses were as follows: chronic brain syndrome unrelated to alcoholism (28%), psychosis (55%), alcoholism (37%), neurosis (9%), and personality disorder (4%). Mean educational level was 8.8 years. The sample was divided into five age groupings: 55 to 59 ($n = 56$), 60 to 64 ($n = 45$), 65 to 69 ($n = 35$), 70 to 74 ($n = 37$), and 75 to 79 ($n = 20$). Mean educational level and percent of sample included in each of the diagnostic classifications are reported for each age grouping. The authors also provide test data on a subgroup of 160 subjects equated for percent diagnosed with alcoholism across the five age groupings. The "alcohol-equated sample" was developed "to minimize the influence that cognitive or motor/sensory differences uniquely attributable to alcohol abuse might have upon group test performace levels " (p. 2). This sample remained heterogeneous regarding representation of the other diagnostic categories.

Means, standard deviations, ranges, and T-score equivalents for raw scores are reported for SSPT number errors for each age interval for the whole sample and for the alcohol-equated sample. We reproduced selected data due to space considerations.

Study strengths
1. Large sample size and many individual cells approximate Ns of 50.

2. Reporting of IQ data, geographic area, and education.
3. Data presented in age groupings.
4. Means and standard deviations are reported.

Considerations regarding use of the study
1. The presence of substantial neurologic disease (chronic brain syndrome), substance abuse, and major psychiatric disorders in the sample.
2. Low educational level, although IQ levels are average.
3. No information regarding sex although given that data were obtained in a V.A. setting, the sample is likely all, or nearly all, males.

Other comments
The scores for the two oldest age groups are identical in the whole sample and alcohol-equated group because these two groups did not have overrepresentation of alcoholics, so they did not need to be adjusted (Table 13.4).

[SSPT.4] Pauker, 1980

The author obtained SSPT scores on 363 Toronto citizens fluent in English recruited through announcements and notices. Subjects ranged in age from 19 to 71 and included 152 men and 211 women. Exclusion criteria included significant physical disability, sensory deficit, current medical illness, use of medication that might affect test performance, history of actual or suspected brain disorder, and alcoholism. The MMPI profiles "could not suggest severe disturbance" or include more than three clinical scales with T scores greater than or equal to 70 or an F-scale score greater than 80.

The SSPT was administered according to Reitan's guidelines. Means and standard devia-

Table 13.4. SSPT.3; Means, Standard Deviations, and Ranges for SSPT Number of Errors for Five Age Intervals for the Whole Sample and for the Alcohol-Equated Sample

Age	N	WAIS			Education	SSPT
		FSIQ	VIQ	PIQ		
Total Sample		.				
55–59	56	98.57	99.39	97.00	10.1	10.57
		(11.43)	(12.92)	(10.65)		(7.00)
		80–129	77–131	72–129		3–32
60–64	45	98.58	101.27	95.00	9.8	10.33
		(9.93)	(11.42)	(9.82)		(5.01)
		80–121	78–123	78–116		3–23
65–69	35	97.51	100.37	93.66	8.7	15.69
		(11.18)	(12.51)	(10.20)		(6.86)
		80–130	80–135	68–120		5–31
70–74	37	100.41	102.95	97.24	8.8	14.97
		(9.92)	(11.81)	(10.08)		(7.38)
		82–125	80–133	75–114		5.36
75–79	20	101.75	101.40	102.15	6.5	14.00
		(10.18)	(11.40)	(9.95)		(6.54)
		81–119	77–117	83–119		6–31
Alcohol–Equated Sample						
55–59	47	99.00	100.00	98.00	10.1	11.00
		(11.73)	(13.02)	(11.13)		(7.32)
		80–129	77–131	72–129		3–32
60–64	33	96.00	99.00	93.00	9.3	11.12
		(9.43)	(11.33)	(9.30)		(5.14)
		80–117	78–123	78–112		3–23
65–69	23	99.00	102.00	95.00	8.8	16.13
		(12.06)	(13.06)	(11.52)		(6.52)
		80–130	80–135	68–120		7–31
70–74	37	100.00	103.00	97.00	8.8	14.97
		(9.92)	(11.81)	(10.08)		(7.38)
		82–125	80–133	75–114		5–36
75–79	20	102.00	101.00	102.00	6.5	14.00
		(10.18)	(11.40)	(9.95)		(6.54)
		81–119	77–117	83–119		6–31

tions for SSPT total errors are reported for the sample as a whole and for three age groupings (19–34, 35–52, 53–71) by four IQ levels (89–102, 103–112, 113–122, 123–143). Individual cell sample sizes ranged from four to 60. Age-by-IQ categories were determined "in a compromise between what would be desirable and what the obtained sample characteristics and size dictated" (p.1). Men committed more errors than the women (5.96 vs. 5.07), but the data on men and women were combined because the scores were so close.

Study strengths

1. Large overall sample size, although individual cell sizes are substantially less than 50.

2. Presentation of the data in age by IQ groupings.

3. Adequate medical and psychiatric exclusion criteria.

4. Information on sex, recruitment procedures, language, and geographic area.

5. Means and standard deviations are reported.

Considerations regarding use of the study

1. No information regarding education.

2. Subjects were recruited in Canada which may limit the usefulness of these data for clinical interpretation purposes in the United States.

3. The age-by-IQ cell representing subjects aged 53 to 71 with IQs of 89 to 102 contained only four subjects; Pauker comments that this category "should not be considered to be of any more than interest value" (p. 2).

4. IQ levels below the average range not represented (Table 13.5).

[SSPT.5] Fromm-Auch and Yeudall, 1983

The authors obtained SSPT data on 193 Canadian subjects (111 male, 82 female) recruited through posted advertisements and personal contacts. Participants are described as "nonpsychiatric" and "non-neurological." Eighty-three percent of the sample were right-handed and mean age was 25.4 (SD = 8.2, range = 15 to 64). Mean years of education were 14.8 (3.0, range = 8 to 25) and included technical and university training. Mean WAIS FSIQ, VIQ, and PIQ were 119.1 (SD = 8.8, range =98 to 142), 119.8 (SD = 9.9, range = 95 to 143), and 115.6 (SD = 9.8, range = 89 to 146), respectively. Of note, no subject obtained a FSIQ which was lower than the average range.

Means, standard deviations, and ranges for total SSPT errors are reported for five age groupings—15–17, 18–23, 24–32, 33–40, and 41–64—with sample size ranging from 10 to 76. The two oldest age groupings both had sample sizes less than 20. No sex differences were documented and male and female data were collapsed.

Study strengths

1. The large overall sample size and some individual cells approximate *N*s of 50.

2. Presentation of the data by age groupings.

3. Information regarding mean IQ, educational levels, age, handedness, occupation, gender, recruitment procedures, and geographic area.

4. Some psychiatric and neurological exclusion criteria.

5. Means and standard deviations are reported.

Considerations regarding use of the study

1. The high intellectual and educational level of the sample.

2. An age grouping of 41 to 64 with an *N* of 10 would not appear to be particularly useful.

3. Subjects were recruited in Canada which may limit the usefulness of these data for clinical interpretation in the United States (Table 13.6).

Table 13.5. SSPT.4; Means and Standard Deviations for SSPT Total Errors for the Total Sample and for Three Age Groupings by Four IQ Levels

WAIS FSIQ	Age			
	19–34	35–52	53–71	19–71
123–143	3.96	4.84	5.85	4.78
	(1.64)	(2.10)	(3.23)	(2.41)
	n = 28	n = 25	n = 20	n = 73
113–122	4.65	4.86	6.41	5.06
	(2.31)	(2.13)	(2.90)	(2.44)
	n = 60	n = 56	n = 27	n = 143
103–112	5.09	6.15	6.80	5.70
	(2.80)	(3.27)	(3.36)	(3.09)
	n = 53	n = 34	n = 15	n = 102
89–102	6.05	6.80	11.25	6.84
	(2.33)	(3.02)	(5.56)	(3.25)
	n = 21	n = 20	n = 4	n = 45
89–143	4.86	5.47	6.62	5.41
	(2.44)	(2.68)	(3.44)	(2.80)
	n = 162	n = 135	n = 66	n = 363

Table 13.6. SSPT.5; Means, Standard Deviations, and Ranges for Total Number of SSPT Errors for Five Age Groupings

Age	N	SSPT
15–17	32	4.6 (2.4) range = 1–13
18–23	76	4.2 (2.0) range = 1–10
24–32	57	4.1 (2.2) range = 1–10
33–40	18	3.6 (2.0) range = 1–8
41–64	10	4.4 (1.8) range = 1–7

[SSPT.6] Dodrill, 1987

The author collected SSPT data on 120 subjects in Washington during 1975–1976 ($n = 81$) and 1986–1987 ($n = 39$). Half of the sample was female and 10% were minorities (six black, three native American, two Asian American, one unknown). Eighteen were left-handed and occupational status included 45 students, 37 employed, 26 unemployed, 11 homemakers, and one retiree. Subjects were recruited from various sources including schools, churches, employment agencies, and community service agencies and either were paid for their participation or offered an interpretation of their abilities. Exclusion criteria included history of "neurologically relevant disease (such as meningitis or encephalitis)," alcoholism, birth complications "of likely neurological significance," oxygen deprivation, peripheral nervous system injury, psychotic or psychotic-like disorders, or head injury associated with unconsciousness, skull fracture, persisting neurological signs, or diagnosis of concussion or contusion. Of note, one-third of potential participants failed to meet the above medical and psychiatric criteria, leaving a final sample of 120.

Mean age for the sample was 27.73 (± 11.04) and mean years of education was 12.28 (± 2.18). The subjects tested in the 1970s were administered the WAIS and the subjects assessed in the 1980s were administered the WAIS-R; WAIS scores were converted to WAIS-R equivalents by subtracting seven points from the VIQ, PIQ, and FSIQ. Mean FSIQ, VIQ, and PIQ scores for the sample were 100.00 (± 14.35), 100.29 (± 14.73), and 98.25 (± 13.39), respectively. IQ scores ranged from 60 to 138 and reflected an exactly normal distribution. SSPT mean error scores and standard deviations are reported as well as IQ-equivalent scores for various levels of intelligence. Nineteen percent of the sample were misclassified as brain damaged using a cutoff of seven or more errors.

Study strengths
1. Large sample size.
2. Comprehensive exclusion criteria.
3. Information regarding education, IQ, occupation, sex ratio, age, handedness, ethnicity, recruitment procedures, and geographic area.
4. IQ equivalent scores provided.
5. Data for different IQ levels provided.
6. Means and standard deviations are reported.

Considerations regarding use of the study
1. Undifferentiated age range.
2. The number of errors associated with an IQ of 130 is greater than that corresponding to IQs of 110 and 125 (Table 13.7).

[SSPT.7] Yeudall, Reddon, Gill, and Stefanyk, 1987

The authors obtained SSPT data on 225 Canadian subjects recruited from posted advertisements in workplaces and personal solicitations. The participants included meat packers, postal workers, transit employees, and hospital employees: lab technicians, secretaries, ward aides, student interns, student nurses, and summer students. In addition, high school teachers identified for participation average students in grades 10 through 12. Exclusion criteria included evidence of "forensic involvement," head injury, neurological insult, prenatal or birth complications, psychiatric problems, or substance abuse.

Experienced testing technicians gathered SSPT data and "motivated the subjects to achieve maximum performance" partially through the

Table 13.7. SSPT.6; SSPT Mean Error Scores for the Whole Sample and for Various Levels of Intelligence

N	Age	Education	WAIS-R			SSPT
			FSIQ	VIQ	PIQ	
120	27.73	12.28	100.00	100.92	98.25	5.02
	(11.04)	(2.18)	(14.35)	(14.73)	(13.39)	(4.16)

N	FSIQ	SSPT	N	FSIQ	SSPT	FSIQ	SSPT
7	130	5	33	85	6	>89	0–6
18	125	4	19	80	8	80–89	7–8
34	120	4	10	75	11	70–79	9–17
64	115	4		70	14	<70	>17
93	110	4					
101	105	5					
75	100	5					
60	95	5					
48	90	5					

promise of detailed explanations of their test performance.

Means and standard deviatons for number of SSPT errors are presented for four age groupings (15 to 20, 21 to 25, 26 to 30, and 31 to 40) for males and females combined and separate. Information regarding percent right-handers, mean years of education, and mean WAIS/ WAIS-R FSIQ, VIQ, and PIQ are reported for each age grouping and age-by-sex grouping. Eighty-eight percent were right-handed, and the sample as a whole had completed an average of 14.55 ± 2.78 years of schooling. The mean FSIQ, VIQ, and PIQ were 112.25 ± 10.25, 112.60 ± 10.86, and 108.13 ± 10.63, respectively.

No significant correlations were found between age or education and SSPT performance. A significant correlation emerged between SSPT scores and VIQ and PIQ, but only in the male subjects ($r = -0.25$ and -0.22, respectively). Age and sex effects on means were not significant nor were there any variance differences with age.

Study strengths

1. Large sample size and individual cells approximate Ns of 50.

2. Grouping of data by age.

3. Data availability for a 15-to-20-year-old age group.

4. Adequate medical and psychiatric exclusion criteria.

5. Information regarding handedness, education, IQ, occupation, sex, recruitment procedures, and geographic area.

6. Means and standard deviations are reported.

Considerations regarding use of the study

1. The sample is atypical in terms of its high average intellectual level and high level of education. The groups differ in educational level, but given that IQ levels are highly similar across groups, the educational discrepancy is probably not an issue.

2. The data were obtained on Canadian subjects which may limit their usefulness for clinical interpretation in the United States due to possible subtle cultural differences (Table 13.8).

[SSPT.8] Ernst, 1988

The author collected SSPT data on 85 Brisbane (Australian) uncompensated volunteers aged 65 to 75 recruited from the Queensland State electoral roll. All but one participant were Caucasian and all but one were right-handed. Thirty-nine were males and 46 were females. The sample was derived from 518 names randomly selected based on data of birth and residence. These potential subjects were sent information regarding the project and a health questionnaire and asked to participate. Individuals with histories of substance abuse, head trauma, stroke, psychiatric hosspitalization, or epilepsy were

Table 13.8. SSPT.7; Number of SSPT Errors for the Total Sample and for Four Age Groupings

	Age Grouping				
	15–20 (n = 62)	21–25 (n = 73)	26–30 (n = 48)	31–40 (n = 42)	15–40 (n = 225)
SSPT No. errors	4.31 (2.10)	4.11 (2.17)	3.94 (2.18)	3.69 (1.99)	4.05 (2.12)
% right-handed	79.03	86.30	89.58	90.48	85.78
Education	12.16 (1.75)	14.82 (1.88)	15.50 (2.65)	16.50 (3.11)	14.55 (2.78)
VIQ	111.18 (10.92)	110.48 (10.43)	114.10 (11.45)	117.76 (9.32)	112.60 (10.86)
PIQ	108.30 (10.47)	105.88 (11.20)	110.28 (8.72)	109.72 (11.45)	108.13 (10.63)
FSIQ	111.75 (10.16)	109.79 (9.97)	113.95 (10.61)	116.09 (9.51)	112.25 (10.25)

excluded. A large minority of the subjects (42%) had a history of at least one treated and/or well-controlled chronic illness (10 heart disease, 17 hypertension, five asthma, two emphysema, 10 hypo- or hyperthyroidism, two diabetes). A majority of subjects were currently using prescribed medications (55%) for the above chronic diseases or as a hypertensive preventative. Mean educational level was 10.4 ± 3.1 with a range of 4 to 20 years, which was comparable to the modal educational level for that age range according to the Australian Bureau of Statistics. A wide range of occupations was represented including unskilled laborers, homemakers, business persons, and teachers.

The SSPT was administered according to Reitan's 1959 procedures. Mean number of errors and standard deviation are reported. Thirty-seven percent of the sample were misclassified as impaired using Reitan's (1979, 1985) cutoff of eight errors. Education was found to be significantly related to SSPT scores ($r = 0.33$), while no effect of sex, chronic disease, medication, or their interaction was found for SSPT performance.

Study strengths
1. Relatively large sample size for constricted age range.
2. Reporting of ethnic characteristics, sex, education, handedness, recruitment procedures, and geographic area.

3. Means and standard deviations are reported.

Considerations regarding use of the study
1. Data were collected in Australia which may limit their usefulness for clinical interpretation in the United States.
2. Below average educational level.
3. No information regarding IQ.
4. Approximately half of the subjects had at least one chronic illness and over half were taking prescribed medications.

	Mean
SSPT No. errors	7.2 (4.3)

[SSPT.9] Heaton, Grant, and Matthews, 1991

The authors provide normative data on the SSPT from 486 (378 in the base sample and 108 in the validation sample) urban and rural subjects recruited in several states (California, Washington, Colorado, Texas, Oklahoma, Wisconsin, Illinois, Michigan, New York, Virginia, and Massachusetts) and Canada. Data were collected over a 15-year period through multicenter collaborative efforts; the authors trained the test administrators and supervised data collection. Exclusion criteria included history of learning disability, neurologic disease, illnesses affecting brain function, significant head trauma, significant psychiatric disturbance (e.g., schizophrenia), and alcohol or other substance abuse. Mean age for the total sample was 42.06 ± 16.8, and mean educational level was 13.6 ± 3.5. Sixty-five percent of the sample were males. The majority of the subjects (N = 486) were administered the WAIS; mean FSIQ, VIQ, and PIQ were 113.8 ± 12.3, 113.9 ± 13.8, and 111.9 ± 11.6, respectively.

The SSPT was administered according to procedures outlined by Reitan and Wolfson (1985). Subjects were generally paid for their participation and were judged to have provided their best efforts on the tasks. Seventeen percent of score variance was accounted for by age, while 21% was attributable to educational level; sex accounted for a negligible amount of unique variance in performance (1%). A total of 28% of test score variance was accounted for by demographic variables. The normative data, which are not reproduced here, are presented in comprehensive tables in T-score equivalents for test-scaled scores for males and females separately in 10 age groupings (20–34, 35–39, 40–44, 45–49, 50–54, 55–59, 60–64, 65–69, 70–74, 75–80) by six educational groupings (6–8 years, 9–11 years, 12 years, 13–15 years, 16–17 years, 18+ years). Mean errors on the SSPT for the sample as a whole was 5.2 ± 4.7.

Study strengths
1. Large sample size.
2. *T* scores corrected for age, education, and sex.
3. Comprehensive exclusion criteria.
4. Information regarding IQ and geographic recruitment area.

Considerations regarding use of the study
1. Above average mean intellectual level (which is probably less of an issue given that these are WAIS rather than WAIS-R IQ data).

Other comments
1. The interested reader is referred to 1996 critique of Heaton et al. (1991) norms, and Heaton et al.'s (1996) response to this critique.

Control Groups in Clinical Studies

[SSPT.10] Wiens and Matarazzo, 1977

The authors collected SSPT data on 48 male applicants to a patrolman program in Portland, Oregon, as a part of an investigation of the WAIS and MMPI correlates of the Halstead-Reitan Battery. All subjects passed a medical exam and were judged to be neurologically normal. Subjects were divided into two equal groups which were comparable in age (23.6 vs. 24.8), education (13.7 vs. 14.0), and WAIS FSIQ (117.5 vs. 118.3). SSPT mean errors and standard deviation are provided for each group. A random subsample of 29 of the applicants was readministered the SSPT 14 to 24 weeks (median of 20 weeks) following the original administration. Means and standard deviations for SSPT errors for both the original testing and retest are reported. One of the 29 subjects obtained a score lower than Reitan's suggested cutoff of eight or more errors. No significant correlations were obtained between SSPT scores and VIQ, PIQ, or FSIQ.

Study strengths
1. Information on test/retest performance.
2. Relatively large sample size for the small age range.
3. Adequate medical exclusion criteria.
4. Information regarding education, IQ, sex, and geographic recruitment area.
5. Means and standard deviations are reported.

Considerations regarding use of the study
1. High IQ level.
2. High educational level.
3. All subjects were male (Table 13.9).

[SSPT.11] Anthony, Heaton, and Lehman, 1980

The authors amassed SSPT data on 100 normal volunteers from Colorado as a part of a cross-validation of two computerized interpretive programs for the Halstead-Reitan Battery. Subjects had no history of medical or psychiatric problems, head trauma, brain disease, or substance abuse. In addition, for 85% of the controls, normal EEG and neurological exams were obtained; in the remaining 15% of the subjects it appears

Table 13.9. SSPT.10; Mean Number of SSPT Errors and Standard Deviations for Two Equal Groups°

| N | Age | Education | WAIS | | | SSPT | Retest |
			FSIQ	VIQ	PIQ		
24	23.6	13.7	117.5	117.4	115.4	4.2	
	(21–27)	(12–16)	(8.3)	(8.4)	(10.5)	(2.6)	
			(105–139)				
24	24.8	14.0	118.3	116.4	118.2	3.9	
	(21–28)	(12–16)	(6.8)	(6.9)	(8.6)	(2.2)	
			(108–131)				
29	24	14	118	116	118	3.8	3.3
	(21–28)	(12–16)				(1.74)	(1.93)

°Test–retest data for 29 subjects are also reported (14–24 weeks).

that this information was not available. Mean age was 38.88 (SD = 15.80) and mean years of education were 13.33 (SD = 2.56). Mean WAIS FSIQ, VIQ, and PIQ were 113.54 ($\pm$10.83), 113.24 ($\pm$11.59), and 112.26 ($\pm$10.88), respectively. SSPT data are presented in terms of mean number errors and standard deviation.

Study strengths
1. Large sample size.
2. Adequate exclusion criteria.
3. Information regarding education, age, and geographic area.
4. Means and standard deviations are reported.

Considerations regarding use of the study
1. The large undifferentiated age grouping.
2. The IQ range is high average.
3. No information is available regarding sex ratio (Table 13.10).

[SSPT.12] Bak and Greene, 1980

The authors gathered SSPT data on 30 right-handed Texan subjects as a part of an investigation of the effect of age on performance on the Halstead-Reitan Battery and the Wechsler Memory Scale. The participants were equally divided into two age groupings: 50 to 62 and 67 to 86. Subjects were fluent in English and denied history of CNS disorders, uncorrected sensory deficits, or illnesses or "incapacities" which might affect test results; subjects in poor health were excluded. The mean age of the two groups was 55.6 (SD = 4.44) and 74.9 (SD = 6.04), respectively. Subjects in the first group were born between the years 1916 and 1929, and subjects in the second group were born between 1892 and 1912. Nine individuals in the first group were female, and 10 subjects in the second group were female. Four WAIS subtests were administered (Information, Arithmetic, Block Design, Digit Symbol); the mean scores on these measures suggested that IQ levels were within the high average range or higher.

Means and standard deviations for SSPT errors are presented for the two groups. No significant differences in performance were documented between the two groups.

Study strengths
1. It provides data on a very elderly age group not typically found in other published normative data.

Table 13.10. SSPT.11

| N | Age | Education | WAIS | | | SSPT Errors |
			FSIQ	VIQ	PIQ	
100	38.88	13.33	113.54	113.24	112.26	5.75
	(15.80)	(2.56)	(10.83)	(11.59)	(10.88)	(3.46)

Table 13.11. SSPT.12; Means and Standard Deviations for the Number of SSPT Errors for Two Age Groups

N	Age	Education	SSPT Errors
15	50–62		
	55.6	13.7	4.93
	(4.44)	(1.91)	(2.81)
15	67–86		
	74.9	14.9	7.13
	(6.04)	(2.99)	(4.26)

2. Adequate exclusion criteria.

3. Information regarding sex, geographic recruitment area, handedness, fluency in English, IQ, and education.

4. Means and standard deviations are reported.

Considerations regarding use of the study

1. High IQ level.

2. High educational level.

3. The older age grouping spans nearly two decades and may be too broad for optimal clinical interpretative use.

4. Small sample sizes (Table 13.11).

[SSPT.13] Heaton, Grant, and Matthews, 1986

The authors obtained SSPT data on 553 normal controls in Colorado, California, and Wisconsin as a part of an investigation into the effects of age, education, and sex on Halstead-Reitan Battery performance. Nearly two-thirds of the sample were male (males = 356, females = 197). Exclusion criteria included history of neurologic illness, significant head trauma, and substance abuse. Subjects ranged in age from 15 to 81 (mean = 39.3 ± 17.5), and mean years of education was 13.3 (±3.4) with a range of 0 to 20 years. The sample was divided into three age categories (less than 40, 40–59, and greater than or equal to 60 years) with Ns of 319, 134, and 100, respectively, and were classified into three education categories (less than 12 years, 12 to 15 years, and greater than or equal to 16 years) with Ns of 132, 249, and 172, respectively.

Testing was conducted by trained technicians and all participants were judged to have expended their best effort on the task. SSPT mean errors and percent of subjects classified as normal by Russell et al. (1970) criteria are reported for the six subgroups. Approximately 10% of test score variance was accounted for by age and approximately 17% of test score variance was associated with educational level. Significant group differences in SSPT scores were found across the three age groups, and across the three education groups, and a significant age-by-education interaction was documented. No significant differences in performance were found between males and females.

Study strengths

1. Large size of overall sample and individual cells.

2. Information regarding sex, geographic area, age, education, and some IQ data.

3. Data grouped by age and education level.

4. Minimally adequate exclusion criteria.

Considerations regarding use of the study

1. No reporting of SSPT score standard deviations.

2. Mean scores for individual WAIS subtest scaled scores reported but not overall IQ scores (Table 13.12).

[SSPT.14] Alekoumbides, Charter, Adkins, and Seacat 1987

The authors report data on 113 outpatients without cerebral lesions or histories of alcoholism or cerebral contusion from V.A. hospitals in Southern California as a part of their development of standardized scores corrected for age and education for the Halstead-Reitan Battery. Among the 41 psychiatric patients, nine were diagnosed as psychotic and 32 were neurotic. In addition to psychiatry services, patients were also drawn from medicine (n = 57), neurology (n = 22), spinal cord injury (n = 9), and surgery (n = 6) units. Mean age was 46.85 ± 17.17 (ranging from 19 to 82), and mean years of education was 11.43 ± 3.20 (ranging from 1 to 20). Frequency distributions for age and years of education are provided. Mean WAIS FSIQ, VIQ, and PIQ were within the average range (105.89 ± 13.47, 107.03 ± 14.38, and 103.31 ± 13.02, respectively); means and standard deviations for individual age-corrected subtest scores were also reported. All subjects

Table 13.12. SSPT.13; SSPT Mean Number of Errors and Percent of Subjects Classified as Normal by Russell et al. (1970) Criteria for the Six Subgroups°

N	Age	Education	SSPT No. error	% Normal	WAIS SS Mean
319	<40		4.3	89.6	11.9
134	40–59		5.0	82.1	11.2
100	≥60		8.4	55.0	9.7
132		<12	7.3	66.7	9.5
249		12–15	5.3	80.7	11.2
172		≥16	3.5	94.2	12.9

°Mean scaled scores for the WAIS subtests are also reported.

except one were male; the majority were Caucasian (93%), with 7% African-American. The mean score on a measure of occupational attainment was 11.29.

No differences were found in test performance between the two psychiatric groups and the nonpsychiatric group; therefore the data were collapsed. Mean SSPT errors and standard deviation were reported. In addition, regression equation information to allow correction of raw scores for age and education was included.

Study strengths

1. Large sample size.
2. Information regarding IQ, age, education, ethnicity, sex, occupational attainment, and geographic area.
3. Regression equation data for computation of age- and-education-corrected scores.
4. Means and standard deviations are reported.

Considerations regarding use of the study

1. Data were collected on medical and psychiatric patients.
2. Undifferentiated age range (mitigated by the regression equation information).
3. Nearly all male sample (Table 13.13).

The regression equation is described as follows: "Raw scores were corrected by the equation $Xc = X - b1X1 - b2X2 + C$, where Xc is the corrected score, X is the uncorrected score, X1 is the age, X2 is the education, b1 and b2 are the weights of age and education respectively, and C is a constant" (p. 16):

$b1$	$b2$	C
0.196	−0.399	4.622

[SSPT.15] Bornstein, Baker, and Douglass, 1987a

The authors collected SSPT test/retest data on 23 volunteers (14 women, nine men) who ranged in age from 17 to 52 (mean = 32.3 ± 10.3), as a part of an examination of the short-term retest reliability of the Halstead-Reitan Battery. Exclusion criteria consisted of a positive history of neurological or psychiatric illness. Mean verbal IQ was 105.8 ± 10.8 (range = 88 to 128), and mean performance IQ was 105.0 ± 19.5 (range = 85 to 121).

Subjects were administered the Halstead-Reitan Battery in standard order both on initial testing and again 3 weeks later. Means, standard deviations, and ranges for SSPT number correct for both testing sessions are provided,

Table 13.13. SSPT.14

N	Age	Education	WAIS FSIQ	VIQ	PIQ	SSPT Errors
113	46.85	11.43	105.89	107.03	103.31	10.64
	(17.17)	(3.20)	(13.47)	(14.38)	(13.02)	(6.90)

Table 13.14. SSPT.15; Means, Standard Deviations, and Ranges for SSPT Number of Correct Responses for Two Testing Sessions° (3 weeks apart)

N	Age	VIQ	PIQ	Test	Retest	Raw Score Change	Median Raw Score Change	% of Change
23	32.3	105.8	105.0	55.0	56.0	1.1	2	4
	(10.3)	(10.8)	(10.5)	(3.5)	(2.3)	(2.2)		
	17–52	88–128	85–121	51–58	53–59			

°The raw score change and standard deviation, median raw score change, and mean percent of change are also reported.

as well as raw score change and standard deviation, median raw score change, and mean percent of change. No significant correlations between mean change and age ($r = 0.12$) or education ($r = 0.28$) or between mean percent of change and age ($r = 0.35$) or education ($r = 0.09$) were documented.

Study strengths
   1. Information on short-term (3-week) retest data.
   2. Information on IQ level, sex, and age.
   3. Minimally adequate exclusion criteria.
   4. Means and standard deviations are reported.

Considerations regarding use of the study
   1. Undifferentiated age range.
   2. No information regarding education.
   3. Small sample sizes (Table 13.14).

[SSPT.16] Russell, 1987

The author obtained SSPT data on 155 controls during the years 1968 to 1982 in V.A. hospitals in Cincinnati and Miami for his development of a reference scale method for neuropsychological test batteries. The 148 male and seven female subjects were suspected of having neurological disorders, but had "negative neurological findings." No other exclusion criteria are described. Mean age was 46.19 ± 12.86, and mean years

of education was 12.29 ± 3.00. All but eight of the participants were Caucasian; the remainder were African-American. Mean WAIS FSIQ, VIQ, and PIQ were 111.9, 112.3, and 109.9, respectively.

Mean SSPT errors and standard deviation are provided.

Study strengths
   1. Large sample size.
   2. Information regarding IQ, education, ethnicity, age, sex, and geographic area.
   3. Means and standard deviations are reported.

Considerations regarding use of the study
   1. Undifferentiated age range.
   2. Insufficient exclusion criteria.
   3. High mean intellectual level.
   4. Mostly male sample (Table 13.15).

CONCLUSIONS

The above review suggests that the SSPT has been extensively studied by clinicians and researchers. In spite of some controversy regarding utility of this test, a number of studies support its usefulness in assessment of brain functioning. The question still remains, however, whether this test has lateralizing signifi-

Table 13.15. SSPT.16

N	Age	Education	WAIS			SSPT Errors
			FSIQ	VIQ	PIQ	
155	46.19	12.29	111.9	112.3	109.9	7.89
	(12.86)	(3.00)				(4.44)

cance. The empirical data suggest that a single cutoff score does not provide sufficient information to establish a pattern of lateralized dysfunction. An association between error type and lateralization of dysfunction proposed by Bornstein and Leason (1984) appears to be a promising avenue in exploring this issue.

Another factor undermining the SSPT utility is the effect of peripheral problems (such as loss of hearing acuity) and reading/spelling problems on test performance. The contribution of these factors needs to be further explored. Development of strategies to concurrently assess and correct for these problems would minimize their effect on the interpretation of the SSPT.

Empirical reports suggest considerable effects of age, education, and intelligence level on SSPT performance. This frequently results in a large proportion of a normative sample being misclassified as impaired. Heaton et al. (1991) made a considerable contribution to improvement of test specificity and accuracy of SSPT interpretation through development of a correction factor taking into account these demographic characteristics. However, further attention to this issue is of critical importance.

14

Tactual Performance Test

BRIEF HISTORY OF THE TEST

The Tactual Performance Test (TPT) is based on the Sequin-Goddard Formboard. It was incorporated by Halstead (1947) in his original neuropsychological battery and subsequently employed by Reitan (1979) in his expansion of the Halstead Battery. Subjects are blindfolded and ten blocks of differing shapes and a matching 10-hole formboard are placed in front of them. They are instructed to insert the blocks in the board as quickly as they can with their dominant hand only. Following this trial, they are required to place the blocks with their nondominant hand, and then both hands together. The blocks and formboard are removed, followed by the blindfold, and the subjects are asked to draw the formboard and as many of the block shapes as they can remember in their relative location. Specific instructions are provided in Reitan's (1979) *Manual for Administration of Neuropsychological Test Batteries for Adults and Children,* Reitan and Wolfson's (1985) *The Halstead-Reitan Neuropsychological Test Battery,* and Swiercinsky's (1978) *Manual for the Adult Neuropsychological Evaluation.* Thompson and Parsons (1985) summarize the literature through 1983 on the status of the TPT in terms of test construction, effect of subject variables on TPT performance, interpretation of TPT scores regarding lateralization and localization, and test performance in specific patient populations; the interested reader is referred to this publication.

The TPT involves several different abilities including tactile perceptual skills, propriospatial ability, tactile/spatial memory, and visual constructional skills. We are not sure precisely which brain areas are involved in TPT performance; deficits in TPT performance have been associated with frontal lesions (Halstead, 1947; Shure & Halstead, 1958), posterior dysfunction (Reitan, 1964), and right hemisphere disturbance (Reitan, 1964; Schreiber et al., 1976). Some reports have indicated that increased right-hand time is associated with left hemisphere damage, and increased left-hand time is tied to right hemisphere dysfunction (Dodrill, 1978a; Reitan, 1964), but no consistent lateralization findings have been documented for the memory and localization scores (Heilbronner et al., 1991; Thompson & Parsons, 1985).

TPT performance has typically been reported in terms of time to complete the task with the preferred hand, nonpreferred hand, both hands, and total time, as well as number of blocks correctly recalled and located. Reitan (1979) recommends Halstead's (1947) cutoff of 15.6 minutes for total time, five or less blocks recalled, and four or less blocks located. However, given the significant association of TPT scores with age and IQ, and possibly, education and sex, a single cutoff would not appear to be appropriate, particularly in older subjects, as documented by the following reports. Price et al. (1980) found that using Halstead's (1947) cutoffs for total time, memory, and localization,

89.8%, 12.2%, and 77.6%, respectively, of a healthy, elderly sample with a mean age of 71.9 were misclassified as brain damaged. Similarly, Ernst (1987) documented in his sample of 65–75-year-olds a misclassification rate of 77%, 36%, and 89% for total, memory, and localization scores, respectively. Bak and Greene (1980) reported that 40% of their healthy sample aged 50 to 62 were misclassified on total time. The mean scores of this group fell below the cutoffs for memory and localization, and the mean scores of an older group (67–86) did not surpass the cutoff for any of the TPT measures. Cauthen (1978a), studying a broader age range, documented a 22%, 15%, and 53% misidentification rate for total time, memory, and localization in his 20–60-year olds; only 2% of the 20-year-olds were misclassified on total time, while 63% of the 50–60-year-olds were miscategorized. Dodrill (1987) documented a 21.7%, 5%, and 39.2% misclassification rate for total time, memory, and localization, respectively, in a young control sample. Chavez et al. (1982) note that the mean localization score (4.87) of their male college students fell below the Reitan cutoff of 5. Bornstein and colleagues (1987b) emphasize that cutoff scores may be useful, but only if considered in the context of other neuropsychological information obtained in a test battery, and if age, education, and other appropriate adjustments are made.

Reitan and Wolfson (1985) and others (Golden et al., 1981b; Jarvis & Barth, 1984) have suggested that nondominant hand performance should be 30% faster than dominant hand performance, although several investigators have documented that a sizable percentage of normals show superior dominant hand performance (Cauthen, 1978a; Thompson & Heaton, 1991) and that this percentage increases with age (Goldstein & Braun, 1974; Price et al., 1980; Thompson et al., 1987).

Criticisms have emerged regarding the lack of standardization of some aspects of TPT administration which could substantially influence the obtained test scores. Snow (1987) notes that Reitan recommends discontinuation of a time trial at 15 minutes if the patient is discouraged and is not close to finishing the task, but continuing if the patient is near completion, while other clinicians (e.g., Russell et al., 1970)

routinely stop at 10 minutes. Snow (1987) points out that differing amounts of exposure time to the blocks could influence memory and localization scores. Snow (1987) also observes that no precise scoring criteria have been developed for the memory and localization scores; for example, some clinicians allow a four- or five-point star, while others give credit for a six-point star. Investigations of interrater reliability have revealed moderate agreement for memory scores (71–76.3%) and poor correspondence for localization scores (56.7–63.8%; Martin & Greene, in Snow, 1987). Chavez et al. (1982) note that some clinicians follow a consistent order in placing the blocks before blindfolded subjects while other examiners randomly arrange the blocks. Chavez and colleagues (1982) report that the order of block presentation did not affect the time trials with their normal college student population but that a standardized block presentation format was associated with higher memory scores, and a trend was noted toward higher localization scores. Kupke (1983) observed better total time scores in his college sample with use of a portable version of the TPT rather than the standard equipment.

In addition to the above concerns regarding TPT administration and interpretation, Lezak (1995) points out that the TPT is very frustrating and stressful for patients due to its length and difficulty, and she questions its practical utility. Also, because moderately to severely impaired individuals fail the test so completely, little information can be gleaned regarding extent of impairment in these subjects (Russell, 1985). In an attempt to shorten and simplify the test, Lezak (1995) has recommended substituting the six-block child's TPT (TPT-6) for the 10-block adult version. Russell (1985) reported that the TPT-6 scores were highly correlated with the 10-block TPT and that the TPT-6 successfully discriminated controls from brain-damaged subjects. Also, test administration was shortened by two-thirds. Clark and Klonoff (1988) examined the internal consistency, test–retest reliability, and construct validity of the TPT-6 and concluded that it was reliable and had construct validity characteristics comparable to those of the 10-block TPT. Unfortunately, although these reports regarding the utility of substituting six-block TPT for the 10-block version in adults are promising, the only "normative" data on the six-block TPT in adults are Clark and Klonoff's (1988) 79 coronary bypass surgery patients and Russsell's (1985) 19 "controls" referred for suspected but unconfirmed brain dysfunction.

In spite of the above-mentioned liabilities, the TPT enjoys popularity in clinical assessment. A number of studies report its sensitivity to brain dysfunction. It was found to be one of the HRB tests which are most useful in assessment of brain impairment (total time and location scores; Mutchnick et al., 1991), most strongly associated with daily living skills in geriatric patients (memory scores; Searight et al., 1989), and most sensitive to learning disabilities (total time and localization scores; Davis et al., 1989). Further discussion of TPT interpretation is provided by Bradford (1992).

RELATIONSHIP BETWEEN TPT PERFORMANCE AND DEMOGRAPHIC FACTORS

Age has been consistently found to be related to TPT performance in normal individuals (Bak & Greene, 1980; Cauthen, 1978a; Fromm-Auch & Yeudall, 1983; Heaton et al., 1986, 1991; Reed & Reitan, 1962, 1963b; Reitan, 1955d; Yeudall et al., 1987), and brain-damaged (Fitzhugh et al., 1964; Prigatano & Parsons, 1976; Reed & Reitan, 1962; Vega & Parsons, 1967), medical (Alekoumbides et al., 1987; Reed & Reitan, 1963b), and psychiatric patients (Alekoumbides et al., 1987; Ernst et al., 1987; Prigatano & Parsons, 1976), with older age associated with poorer scores. To our knowledge, no published study has failed to document a correlation between TPT and age.

Higher IQ also appears to be associated with better TPT performance in various patient groups, including psychiatric (Warner et al., 1987) and mentally retarded subjects (Matthews, 1974). IQ levels have also been found to be associated with TPT scores in normals (Cauthen, 1978a; Wiens & Matarrazzo, 1977), with PIQ showing more of a correlation than VIQ (Wiens & Matarrazzo, 1977; Yeudall et al., 1987).

The data on the relationship of education and sex with TPT indices has been more equivocal; taken as a whole, the available literature does not demonstrate a convincing relationship between these variables and TPT performance. Yeudall et al. (1987), Ernst (1987), and Finlayson et al. (1977) failed to detect a relationship between educational level and TPT scores in normals, while Heaton et al. (1986, 1991) observed significant differences across educational levels only for the memory score. No association has been detected between education and TPT performance in brain-damaged patients (Finlayson et al., 1977; Prigatano & Parsons, 1976; Vega & Parsons, 1967; Warner et al., 1987), although Vega and Parsons observed an effect of education on memory and timed scores in a medical patient sample, and Alekoumbides et al. (1987) apparently detected a relationship between education and TPT scores in a medical and psychiatric sample.

Most publications suggest that there is no difference between males and females on TPT performance in normal subjects (Dodrill, 1979; Filskov & Catanese, 1986; Fromm-Auch & Yeudall, 1983; King et al., 1978; Pauker, 1980; Thompson et al., 1987; Yeudall et al., 1987) and in patients (Dodrill, 1979). On the other hand, Heaton et al. (1986) reported that males outperformed females on total time, although the amount of variance in test scores accounted for by sex was minimal (Heaton et al., 1991). Ernst (1987) documented better male performance on memory, localization and all time scores except dominant hand. Conversely, other reports have suggested that women score better than men on memory (Fabian et al., 1981), localization (Chavez et al., 1982), or both scores (Gordon & O'Dell, 1983), although Gordon and O'Dell (1983) comment that the sex differences they observed were not of "practical significance."

In the two studies addressing the relationship between lateral preference and test performance, no difference in test scores between right- and left-handers were documented (Gregory & Paul, 1980; Thompson et al., 1987).

A recent article by Arnold et al. (1994) documents a significant effect of acculturation (higher performance being associated with higher acculturation level) on TPT dominant hand, nondominant hand, and total time, with no effect of acculturation on localization and memory scores.

METHOD FOR EVALUATING
THE NORMATIVE REPORTS

Our review of the literature located nine TPT normative reports for adults published since 1965 (Cauthen, 1978a; Dodrill, 1987; Ernst, 1987; Fromm-Auch & Yeudall, 1983; Harley et al., 1980; Heaton et al., 1991; Pauker, 1980; Schear, 1986; Yeudall et al., 1987), as well as the original Halstead (1947) and Reitan (1955b, 1959) normative data and three interpretive guides for the Halstead-Reitan Battery (Golden et al., 1981b; Reitan & Wolfson, 1985; Russell et al., 1970). Hundreds of other studies have also reported control subject data, and we have included discussion of 12 of those investigations which involved some unique feature, such as large sample size (≥100), retest data, elderly population, non-English-speaking sample, and use of a shorter version of the test (Alekoumbides et al., 1987; Anthony et al., 1980; Bak & Greene, 1980; Bornstein et al., 1987a; Clark & Klonoff, 1988; El-Sheikh et al., 1987; Heaton et al., 1986; Klove & Lochen, in Klove, 1974; Russell, 1985; Thompson & Heaton, 1991; Weins & Matarazzo, 1977; Matarazzo et al., 1974). (We also found a study in which military personnel were administered the TPT during various field maneuvers of differing intensity to evaluate the effect of environmental stress on TPT performance [Arima, 1965]. However, given the questionable relevance of this information for the typical neuropsychological testing session, we decided not to review this publication.)

Russell and Starkey (1993) developed the Halstead-Russell Neuropsychological Evaluation System (HRNES), which includes 22 tests. In the context of this system, individual performance is compared to that of 576 brain-damaged subjects and 200 subjects who were initially suspected of having brain damage but had negative neurological findings. Data were partitioned into seven age groups and three educational/IQ levels. This study will not be reviewed in this chapter because the "normal" group consisted of the V.A. patients who presented with symptomatology requiring neuropsychological evaluation. For further discussion of the HRNES system see Lezak (1995, pp. 714–715).

Of note, few relevant manuscripts have emerged since the 1980s, perhaps due either to the publication of Heaton et al.'s (1991) comprehensive normative tables, or to the escalating use in research and clinical practice of flexible neuropsychological test protocols which include newer tasks rather than traditional fixed neuropsychological batteries.

In order to adequately evaluate the TPT normative reports, seven key criterion variables were deemed critical. The first six of these related to *subject* variables, and the remaining dimension refers to *procedural* issues.

Minimal requirements for meeting the criterion variables were as follows:

Subject Variables

Sample Size

As discussed in previous chapters, a minimum of at least 50 subjects per grouping interval is optimal.

Sample Composition Description

As discussed previously, information regarding medical and psychiatric exclusion criteria is important; it is unclear if geographic recruitment region, socioeconomic status or occupation, ethnicity, handedness, and recruitment procedures are relevant, so until this is determined, it is best that this information be provided.

Age-Group Intervals

Given the association between age and TPT performance, information regarding age of the normative sample is critical and normative data should be presented by age intervals.

Reporting of IQ Levels

Given the relationship between TPT performance and IQ, data should be presented by IQ intervals, or at least information regarding intellectual levels should be provided.

Reporting of Education Levels

Given a possible, although minor, association between education level and TPT scores, it is preferable that information regarding highest educational level completed be reported.

Reporting of Gender Distribution

Given a possible, although minor, association between gender and TPT scores, it is preferable that information regarding sex be reported.

Procedural Variables

Data Reporting

Means and standard deviations, and preferably ranges, for time in seconds or minutes on the TPT for the dominant and nondominant hand separately and together, and total across all three trials should be reported, as well as means and standard deviations for memory and localization scores.

SUMMARY OF THE STATUS
OF THE NORMS

All but eight datasets had total sample sizes larger than 100 (Bak & Greene, 1980; Bornstein et al., 1987a; Clark & Klonoff, 1988; El-Sheikh et al., 1987; Halstead, 1947; Klove & Lochen, in Klove, 1974; Reitan, 1955b, 1959; Wiens & Matarazzo, 1977). Only three publications consistently had at least 50 subjects in individual subject groupings (Ernst, 1987; Heaton et al., 1986; Schear, 1984), although some reports had some subgroups which met this criterion (Fromm-Auch & Yeudall, 1983; Harley et al., 1980; Pauker, 1980; Yeudall et al., 1987).

Approximately half of the studies summarized in this chapter present TPT data according to circumscribed age ranges (Bak & Greene, 1980; Cauthen, 1978a; Ernst, 1987; Fromm-Auch & Yeudall, 1983; Harley et al., 1980; Heaton et al., 1986, 1991; Pauker, 1980; Schear, 1984; Weins & Matarazzo, 1977; Yeudall et al., 1987). Information on IQ levels is reported in all but five studies (El-Sheikh et al., 1987; Ernst, 1987; Heaton et al., 1986; Klove & Lochen, in Klove, 1974; Russell, 1985), and two reports presented TPT data for age-by-IQ groupings (Cauthen, 1978a; Pauker, 1980). Similarly, education level was also indicated in all but three studies (Bornstein et al., 1987a; Cauthen, 1978a; Pauker, 1980), and Heaton et al. (1986, 1991) organized data by educational levels. Information on gender composition of the samples was available in all but four reports (Anthony et al., 1980; Harley et al., 1980; Klove & Lochen, in Klove, 1974; Thompson & Heaton, 1991); five datasets included only male (Clark & Klonoff, 1988; Schear, 1984; Weins & Matarazzo, 1977) or nearly all male (Alekoumbides et al., 1987; Russell, 1985) populations. Ernst (1987) et al. (1991) presented data separately for male and females.

Information on other subject variables was provided less frequently; data on handedness was indicated in eight studies (Bak & Greene, 1980; Cauthen, 1978a; Clark & Klonoff, 1988; Dodrill, 1987; Fromm-Auch & Yeudall, 1983; Russell, 1985; Schear, 1984; Yeudall et al., 1987), occupation or socioeconomic status was described in five reports (Alekoumbides et al., 1987; Dodrill, 1987; Halstead, 1947; Weins & Matarazzo, 1977; Yeudall et al., 1987), and information regarding ethnicity was presented in four datasets (Alekoumbides et al., 1987; Dodrill, 1987; Halstead, 1947; Russell, 1985). Exclusion criteria were judged to be adequate in only 10 publications (Anthony et al., 1980; Bak & Greene, 1980; Bornstein et al., 1987a; Dodrill, 1987; Fromm-Auch & Yeudall, 1983; Heaton et al., 1991; Pauker, 1980; Thompson & Heaton, 1991; Weins & Matarazzo, 1977; Yeudall et al., 1987). Geographic recruitment areas were specified in all but two publications (Bornstein et al., 1987a; Dodrill, 1987). Fourteen datasets were obtained in the United States (Alekoumbides et al., 1987; Anthony et al., 1980; Bak & Greene, 1980; Halstead, 1947; Harley et al., 1980; Heaton et al., 1986, 1991; Klove & Lochen, in Klove, 1974; Reitan, 1955b, 1959; Russell, 1985; Schear, 1986; Thompson & Heaton, 1991; Weins & Matarazzo, 1977), five in Canada (Cauthen, 1978a; Clark & Klonoff, 1988; Fromm-Auch & Yeudall, 1983; Pauker, 1980; Yeudall et al., 1987), one in Norway (Klove & Lochen, in Klove, 1974), one in Egypt (El-Sheikh et al., 1987), and one in Australia (Ernst, 1987).

Total mean time in seconds or minutes and standard deviations to complete the task across the three time trials as well as means and standard deviations for memory and localization were reported in 18 datasets (Alekoumbides et al., 1987; Anthony et al., 1980; Bak & Greene, 1980; Bornstein et al., 1987a; Cauthen, 1978a; Dodrill, 1987; El-Sheikh et al., 1987; Ernst, 1987; Fromm-Auch & Yeudall, 1983; Harley et al., 1980; Heaton et al., 1986, 1991; Klove & Lochen, in Klove, 1974; Pauker, 1980; Russell, 1985; Schear, 1984; Thompson & Heaton, 1991; Weins & Matarazzo, 1977; Yeudall et al., 1987). Twelve reports provided data for the preferred and nonpreferred hands separately and together (Alekoumbides et al., 1987; Bak & Greene, 1980; Cauthen, 1978a; El-Sheikh et al, 1987; Ernst, 1987; Fromm-Auch & Yeudall, 1983; Heaton et al., 1991; Russell, 1985; Schear, 1984; Thompson & Heaton, 1991; Weins & Matarazzo, 1977; Yeudall et al., 1987). Three studies reported score ranges (Fromm-Auch & Yeudall, 1983; Halstead, 1947; Harley et al., 1980).

Several publications reported supplementary TPT scores such as T-score equivalents (Harley et al., 1980), T scores corrected for age, education, and sex (Heaton et al., 1991), IQ-equivalent scores (Dodrill, 1987), test–retest data (Bornstein et al., 1987a; El-Sheikh et al., 1987; Matarazzo et al., 1974), and data for a six-block version (Clark & Klonoff, 1988; Russell, 1985). In addition, Harley et al. (1980) provide percentage of patients correctly placing blocks, and Harley et al. (1980), Ernst (1987), and Schear (1984) report means and standard deviations for number of blocks correctly placed by each hand, both hands, and total. Alekoumbides et al. (1987) present mean and standard deviation for number of blocks placed per minute and Harley et al. (1980) report mean time and standard deviation to place each block for the three trials.

Table 14.1 summarizes information provided in the studies described in this chapter.

SUMMARIES OF THE STUDIES

Given that the use of the TPT has typically been within the context of the Halstead-Reitan battery, the Halstead (1947) and Reitan (1955b, 1959) data and interpretation formats and then the normative publications are presented in ascending chronological order. The chapter will conclude with a review of TPT control data in various clinical studies.

Original Studies

[TPT.1] Halstead, 1947

The author obtained data on 28 control subjects in Chicago, half of whom had psychiatric diagnoses. The 14 subjects without psychiatric diagnoses were nine male and five female civilians ranging in age from 15 to 50 (Mean = 25.9), without history of brain injury. The eight subjects who carried diagnoses of mild psychoneurosis were male soldiers ranging in age from 22 to 38 (Mean = 29.6); some had had combat experience but none had a history of head injury. The last six subjects ranged in age from 27 to 39 and included a depressed military prisoner facing execution, a severely depressed female with suicidal and homicidal impulses tested prior to lobotomy, and a suicidal/homicidal female and a suicidal male tested pre- and *post*lobotomy. Educational level ranged from 7 to 18 years, and the following occupations were represented: artist, entertainer, farmer, housewife, semiskilled and unskilled laborers, professional, secretary, teacher, technician, trade, and student. Ethnic background included American, Balkan, English, French, German, Irish, Polish, Scandinavian, and Scottish. IQ levels ranged from 70 to 140.

Mean total time for the three trials and mean scores for memory and localization are reported for the total group and each control "subgroup," as well as the individual scores for each subject. The TPT criterion scores used in calculating the Impairment Index were greater than 15.6 minutes for total time, less than six blocks recalled, and less than five blocks located.

Study strengths

1. Information provided regarding IQ, education, occupation, age, gender, ethnicity, and geographic recruitment area.

Considerations regarding use of the study

1. Small sample size including use of two subjects twice.

2. Inclusion of subjects with psychiatric diagnoses and postlobotomy.

3. No reporting of standard deviations.

4. Undifferentiated age range (Table 14.2).

Table 14.1. TPT.L; Locator Table for the TPT

Study[*]	Age[**]	N	Sample Composition	IQ,[**] Education	Country/ Location
TPT.1 Halstead, 1947 page 239	15–50	28	14 Ss without psychiatric diagnosis, no history of brain injury. 14 Ss with psychiatric diagnosis	Education 7–18 IQ 70–140	Chicago
TPT.2 Reitan, 1955b, 1959 page 243	32.36 (10.78)	50	35 M, 15 F volunteers. Ss hospitalized with paraplegia and neurosis were included	Education 11.58(2.85) FSIQ 112.6(14.3)	Indiana
TPT.3 Reitan & Wolfson, 1985 page 243			No information is provided regarding the normative sample. Cutoffs for "severity ranges" (perfectly normal, normal, mildly impaired, seriously impaired) are presented		
TPT.4 Cauthen, 1978a page 244	20–60 20–29 30–39 40–49 50–60	117	35 M, 82 F Ss recruited from hospital volunteers and service clubs. All but 3 Ss were R-handed. Data are represented in age × IQ cells	WAIS IQ 91–111 112–122 123–139	Canada
TPT.5 Harley et. al., 1980 page 245	55–79 55–59 60–64 65–69 70–74 75–79	193 56 45 35 37 20	V.A. hospitalized patients. *T*-score equivalents are reported	Education 8.8 IQ>80	Wisconsin
TPT.6 Pauker, 1980 page 246	19–71 19–34 35–52 53–71	363	Volunteers fluent in English. 152 M, 211 F. Ss had no physical disability, sensory deficit, current medical illness, brain disorder or alcoholism. Data are presented in age × IQ cells	WAIS IQ 89–102 103–112 113–122 123–143	Toronto, Canada
TPT.7 Fromm-Auch & Yeudall, 1983 page 247	15–64 25.4 (8.2) 15–17 18–23 24–32 33–40 41–64	190 32 74 56 18 10	111 M, 82 F. Participants described as nonpsychiatric and non- neurological. 83% are R-handed. Ss classified in 5 age groupings	Education 8-26 years 14.8 (3.0) FSIQ 119.1 (8.8)	Canada
TPT.8 Schear, 1984 page 249	20–69 20–29 30–39 40–49 50–59 60–69	560 111 112 111 155 67	Neuropsychiatric sample. 35% had evidence of various signs of organic brain syndromes, alcohol encaphalopathy, epilepsy, etc. 49% exhibited nonorganic psychotic disorders, schizophrenia, alcoholism, etc. 5 age decades are represented	Education 2–22	Kansas
TPT.9 Dodrill, 1987 page 249	27.73 (11.04)	120	60 M, 60 F volunteers. Data for various intelligence levels are presented	Education 12.28(2.18) FSIQ 100(14.4)	Washington

continued

Table 14.1. (*Continued*)

Study[°]	Age[°°]	N	Sample Composition	IQ,[°°] Education	Country/ Location
TPT.10 Yeudall et. al., 1987 page 251	15–40 15–20 21–25 26–30 31–40	225	Volunteers classfied in four age groupings; 88% were R-handed; 127 M, 98 F	Education 14.55 (2.78) FSIQ 112.25 (10.25)	Canada
TPT.11 Ernst, 1987 page 252	65–75 69.6 (2.7)	110	51 M, 59 F volunteers	Education 10.3	Brisbane, Australia
TPT.12 Heaton et al., 1991 page 253	42.1 (16.8) groups: 20–34 35–39 40–44 45–49 50–54 55–59 60–64 65–69 70–74 75–80	486	Volunteers: urban and rural. Data collected over 15 years through multi-center collaborative efforts. Strict exclusion criteria. 65% M. Data are presented in T-score equivalents for M and F separately in 10 age groupings by 6 educational groupings	Education 13.6 (3.5) FSIQ 113.8 (12.3) Educ groups 6–8 9–11 12 13–15 16–17 18+	California Washington, Texas, Oklahoma Wisconsin, Illinois, Michigan, New York, Virginia, Massachusetts, Canada
TPT.13 Klove & Lochen (in Klove, 1974) page 254	31.6 32.1	22 22	American and Norwegian controls. No exclusion criteria reported	Education 11.1 12.2 FSIQ 109.3 111.9	Wisconsin, Norway
TPT.14 Wiens & Matarazzo, 1977 page 255	23.6 21–27 24.8 21–28	48	All males, neurologically normal. Divided into two groups. Random sample of 29 were retested 14 to 24 weeks later	Education 13.7 14.0 FSIQ 117.5 105–139 118.3 108–131	Portland, Oregon
TPT.15 Anthony et. al., 1980 page 256	38.88 (15.80)	100	Normal volunteers, no history of medical or psychiatric problems, head injury, brain disease or substance abuse	Education 13.33 (2.56) FSIQ 113.5 (10.8)	Colorado
TPT.16 Bak & Greene, 1980 page 256	50–62 55.6 (4.44) 67–86 74.9 (6.04)	15 15	Participants were equally divided in two age groupings: Ss were fluent in English and denied histories of neurological problems. 1st group had 9 F, 2nd group had 10 F	Education 13.7 (1.91) 14.9(2.99)	Texas
TPT. 17 Russell, 1985 page 257	43.5 (13.6)	19	Caucasian control Ss admitted to a neurology ward for suspected neurological condition, but showed no evidence of brain damage. All but 2 Ss were male. 6-block version used 17 M, 2 F	Education 14.8 (6.4)	Miami

continued

Table 14.1. (*Continued*)

Study[*]	Age[**]	N	Sample Composition	IQ,[**] Education	Country/ Location
TPT.18 Heaton et al., 1986 page 258	15–81 39.3 (17.5) <40 40–59 ≥60	553 319 134 100	356 M, 197 F. Exclusion criteria included history of neurologic illness, significant head trauma, and substance abuse. Sample was divided into 3 age groups and 2 education group. % classification as normal provided	Education 0–20 13.3 (3.4) <12 (132) 12-15(249) ≥16(172)	Colorado, California, Wisconsin
TPT.19 Alekoumbides et al. 1987 page 259	19–82 46.85 (17.17)	111	Ss were all medical and psychiatric V.A. inpatients & outpatients without cerebral lesion or histories of alcoholism or cerebral contusions. All Ss except for one were male	Education 1–20 11.43 (3.20) FSIQ 105.9 (13.5)	S. California
TPT.20 Bornstein et al., 1987a page 260	17–52 32.3 (10.3)	23	Volunteers: 9 M, 14 F. No history of neurological or psychiatric illness. Test–retest data for a 3-week interval are provided	Verbal IQ 88-128 105.8(10.8) Performance IQ 85-121 105.0(10.5)	
TPT.21 El-Sheikh et al., 1987 page 260	17–24 20.6 (1.4)	32	Ss were undergraduate and graduate students with no history of brain damage. Test–retest data are provided.		Cairo, Egypt
TPT.22 Clark & Klonoff, 1988 page 261	35-68 55.5 (8.0)	79	Ss were all male, R-handed, coronary bypass surgery patients. Test–retest data, 6-block version was used	WAIS-R FSIQ 77-137 105.9(12.2)	Canada
TPT.23 Thompson & Heaton, 1991 page 262	39.43 (17.76)	489	Healthy Ss	Education 13.19(3.46) FSIQ 113.09(12.07)	California, Colorado, Ohio, Michigan

[*]The study number corresponds to the number provided in the text of the chapter.

[**]Age column and IQ/education column contains information regarding range and/or mean and standard deviation for the whole sample and/or separate groups, whichever information is provided by the authors.

Table 14.2. TPT.1; Mean Total Time for the Three Trials, and Mean Scores for Memory and Localization for the Total Group and for Each Subgroup

| | N | TPT | | |
		Total	Memory	Localization
Total	30[*]	10.8	8.2	5.7
Civilian	14	9.5 (5.2–19.6)	8.4 (6–10)	6.1 (2–10)
Military	10	12.0 (6.3–15.9)	7.8 (6–9)	5.6 (1–8)
Miscellaneous	6	11.7 (5.9–13.3)	8.2 (7–10)	4.9 (1–7)

[*]Two Ss were tested twice.

[TPT.2] Reitan, 1955b, 1959

The author obtained TPT scores on 50 subjects in Indiana who had apparently been referred for neuropsychological testing and "who had received neurological examinations before testing and showed no signs or symptoms of cerebral damage or dysfunction. . . . None . . . had positive anamnestic findings" (p. 29), but subjects hospitalized with paraplegia and neurosis were included. The sample included 35 men and 15 women, and mean age and educational level were 32.36 ± 10.78 and 11.58 ± 2.85, respectively. Mean WAIS VIQ, PIQ, and FSIQ were 110.82 ± 14.46, 112.18 ± 14.23, and 112.64 ± 14.28, respectively.

Study strengths
1. Information regarding IQ, education, sex, age, and geographic recruitment area is provided.
2. Adequate sample size.
3. Means and standard deviations are reported.

Considerations regarding use of the study
1. Undifferentiated age range.
2. Insufficient medical and psychiatric exclusion criteria; the sample included subjects hospitalized with spinal cord injuries and psychiatric disorders (Table 14.3).

Interpretive Guides

[TPT.3] Reitan and Wolfson, 1985

The authors suggest that nondominant hand performance should be about one-third faster than dominant hand time, and performance on the third trial (both hands) should be one-third faster than nondominant hand performance. They provide general guidelines for TPT score interpretation in the form of "severity ranges": "perfectly normal (or better than average)," "normal," "mildly impaired," and "seriously im-paired." They list the test total completion time in minutes and number of blocks recalled and located which correspond to each severity range. No other information is provided such as score means or standard deviations, or any data regarding the normative sample on which these guidelines were developed.

Considerations regarding use of the study
The authors argue that these norms were meant as "general guidelines" and that "exact percentile ranks corresponding with each possible score are hardly necessary because the other methods of inference are used to supplement normative data in clinical interpretation of results of individual subjects" (p. 97). However, we maintain that more precise scores as well as separate normative data for different age, IQ, and educational levels are necessary to avoid false-positive errors in diagnosis.

It is not clear how cutoffs were developed (not reproduced here); they do not match the cutoffs recommended by Halstead (1947).

Of note, *Golden et al., 1981b* (pp. 20–21) recommend that if nondominant hand performance is 40% better than dominant hand performance, a dominant hemisphere lesion should be inferred, and if the nonpreferred hand score is less than 25% better than the preferred hand score, a nondominant hemisphere lesion should be hypothesized.

Russell et al., 1970 (pp. 42–44), in constructing their neuropsychological key approach, devised six rating equivalents of TPT raw scores based primarily on "rules of thumb" recommended by P. M. Rennick and apparently derived from a small group of patients. Russell (1984) subsequently modified the ratings as reflected in Table 14.4.

Russell et al. (1970) suggest that left hemisphere damage is indicated if the right-hand score is worse than the left-hand score by two rating points, and vice versa.

Table 14.3. TPT.2; Mean Total Time for the Three Trials and Mean Scores for Memory and Localization

| N | Age | Education | WAIS | | | Total | Memory | Localization |
			VIQ	PIQ	FSIQ			
50	32.36 (10.78)	11.58 (2.85)	110.82 (14.46)	112.18 (14.23)	112.64 (14.28)	12.59 (5.20)	7.65 (1.41)	5.29 (2.12)

Normative Studies

[TPT.4] Cauthen, 1978a

The author obtained TPT data on 117 subjects recruited from hospital volunteers and service clubs in Canada. Those with "evidence of organic dysfunction" associated with head injuries, illnesses, and symptoms of organic dysfunction were excluded (although the author indicates that five subjects "were judged to have performed in a manner consistent with central nervous system dysfunction" on the TPT and "apparently were suffering from such dysfunction)." The sample included 35 male and 82 female Caucasian urban residents. All but three subjects were right-handed, and given that there were no apparent differences in performance between right- and left-handers, the three left-handers were included in the sample.

Mean time in minutes and standard deviation are reported for preferred hand, nonpreferred hand, both hands, and total, as well as means and standard deviations for memory and localization. The TPT data are presented in four age (20–29, 30–39, 40–49, and 50–60)-by-three-WAIS IQ (91–111, 112–122, 123–139) groupings, with individual cell sizes ranging from five to 18. Significant differences across age groups were documented on all TPT scores, and significant differences across IQ groups were documented for time for both hands, total time, and memory and localization. Using Halstead's (1947) cutoffs of 15.7 minutes for total time, five and below for memory, and four and below for localization, 22% of the sample were misclassified as impaired for total time, 15% were misclassified for memory, and 53% were misidentified as impaired for localization. The authors conclude that "the inclusion of over half the normals in the dysfunctional range

of performance on location indicates that the cutoff point requires adjustment" (p. 458). They also observed that the percent exceeding the cutoff for total time increased dramatically across age groups (e.g., 2% for the 20–29-year-olds, up to 63% for the 50–60-year-olds). The authors provide revised cutoff scores for each age decade for total time, memory, and localization; when all three cutoffs were employed, between 29% and 37% of subjects in each age group fell below the cutoffs for at least one score. Subjects decreased their nondominant hand performance by an average of 1.3 ± 1.9 minutes, but 19% failed to show faster nondominant hand performance.

Study strengths
1. Large overall sample size.
2. Presentation of data in age by IQ groupings.
3. Information regarding handedness, ethnicity, sex, and geographic recruitment area.
4. Means and standard deviations are reported.

Considerations regarding use of the study
1. Small individual cell sizes.
2. No information regarding educational level.
3. Minimal exclusion criteria.
4. No data on individuals with less than average IQs.
5. The IQ groupings are somewhat odd and no information is provided regarding how they were derived.
6. The mean total time for the 30–39-year-olds with average IQs is in error.
7. Several unusual variations occurred in the data which are probably due to the small individual cell sizes. For example, the 30–39-year-

Table 14.4. TPT.Russell

| | Rating Equivalents of Raw Scores | | | | | | |
	0	1	2	3	4	5	6
Dominant	≤3.9	4–7.9	8–9.9	10–12.9	13–15.9	16–19	20,X
Nondominant	≤2.9	3–5.4	5.5–6.7	6.8–9.7	9.8–13.9	14–18	19–20,X
Both	≤1.7	1.8–3.3	3.4–3.9	4–5.7	5.8–9.5	9.6–18	19–20,X
Total	≤8.9	9–16.6	16.7–20.5	20.6–28.5	28.6–39.7	40–56	57–60
Memory	9–10	6–8	4–5	2–3	1	0	6 = TPT tot
Localization	7–10	5–6	3–4	1–2	0	M = 0	6 = TPT tot

olds of average to high average IQ had mean scores on preferred hand time which were higher than the 40–49-year-olds of the same IQ level. Also of concern, the 50–60-year-olds in the highest IQ range scored more poorly than those of lower IQ levels on nonpreferred hand time and memory and localization scores.

8. Data were collected in Canada raising questions regarding its generailizability for clinical interpretive use in the United States (Table 14.5).

[TPT.5] Harley, Leuthold, Matthews, and Bergs, 1980

The authors collected TPT data on 193 V.A.-hospitalized patients in Wisconsin ranging in age from 55 to 79. Exclusion criteria included FSIQ less than 80, active psychosis, unequivocal neurological disease or brain damage, and serious visual or auditory acuity problems. Patients with diagnosis of chronic brain syndrome

were included. Patient diagnoses were as follows: chronic brain syndrome unrelated to alcoholism (28%), psychosis (55%), or alcoholic (37%), neurotic (9%), or personality disorder (4%). Mean educational level was 8.8 years. The sample was divided into five age groupings: 55–59 ($n = 56$), 60–64 ($n = 45$), 65–69 ($n = 35$), 70–74 ($n = 37$), and 75–79 ($n = 20$). Mean educational level and percent of sample included in each diagnostic classification are reported for each age grouping. The authors also provide test data on a subgroup of 160 subjects equated for percent diagnosed with alcoholism across five age groupings. The "alcohol-equated sample" was developed "to minimize the influence that cognitive or motor/sensory differences uniquely attributable to alcohol abuse might have upon group test performance levels" (p. 2). This subsample remained heterogeneous regarding representation of the other diagnostic categories.

Table 14.5. TPT.4; Mean Times in Minutes and Standard Deviations for Preferred Hand, Nonpreferred Hand, Both Hands, and Total, as Well as Means and Standard Deviations for Memory and Localization[°]

N	Age	IQ	Preferred	Nonpreferred	Both	Total	Memory	Localization
18	20–29	91–111	5.1 (1.4)	4.3 (1.3)	3.0 (1.2)	12.4 (3.2)	6.8 (1.4)	3.8 (2.1)
11		112–122	4.3 (0.9)	3.6 (1.4)	2.2 (0.9)	10.1 (2.0)	8.1 (1.6)	5.5 (2.1)
14		123–139	4.7 (1.2)	3.0 (1.1)	1.8 (0.7)	9.6 (2.1)	8.2 (0.9)	6.4 (1.6)
5	30–39	91–111	7.4 (2.5)	4.0 (2.3)	2.5 (0.9)	3.9 (5.3)	5.8 (1.8)	4.2 (0.8)
17		112–122	6.4 (2.8)	4.4 (2.5)	2.5 (1.5)	13.2 (5.9)	7.8 (1.1)	5.5 (2.0)
6		123–139	4.5 (1.1)	3.4 (0.9)	1.9 (0.3)	9.5 (2.3)	8.5 (1.0)	5.2 (3.2)
9	40–49	91–111	6.9 (2.2)	5.5 (1.8)	2.9 (0.8)	15.3 (3.5)	6.1 (1.3)	3.3 (1.9)
8		112–122	5.4 (1.9)	4.6 (1.7)	3.0 (2.1)	12.9 (5.2)	7.6 (1.1)	4.1 (2.2)
10		123–139	5.7 (1.8)	4.0 (1.5)	1.6 (.4)	11.4 (3.4)	6.7 (1.5)	4.5 (2.1)
7	50–60	91–111	8.5 (2.6)	6.2 (1.8)	3.9 (2.1)	18.6 (3.3)	5.3 (1.4)	2.1 (1.1)
4		112–122	7.1 (3.1)	5.3 (2.8)	3.4 (2.0)	16.0 (7.0)	6.5 (3.1)	3.8 (3.1)
8		123–139	6.3 (1.9)	7.4 (3.1)	3.5 (1.2)	17.2 (5.0)	5.5 (1.1)	2.8 (1.8)

[°]The data are presented in four age by three WAIS IQ groupings.

T-score equivalents for raw scores and mean time in minutes per block are reported for dominant, nondominant hands, both hands, and total time per block for the three trials combined by age groupings. In addition, total number of blocks correctly placed; number of blocks correctly placed by the dominant hand, nondominant hand, and both hands; time per block for three trials combined; and percentage of patients correctly placing blocks are provided by age groupings for the total and alcohol-equated samples. We reproduce only the mean, standard deviation, and range for the four time scores.

Study strengths
1. Large sample size in many individual cells, approximate *N*s of 50.
2. Reporting of data on IQ, educational level, and geographic recruitment area.
3. Data presented in age groupings.
4. Means and standard deviations are reported.

Considerations regarding use of the study
1. The presence of substantial neurologic (chronic brain syndrome), substance abuse, and major psychiatric disorders in the sample.
2. Low educational level, although IQ levels are average.
3. No information regarding sex, although given that data were obtained in a VA setting, the sample is likely all, or nearly all, male.

Other comments
The scores for the two oldest age groups are identical in the whole sample and alcohol-equated group because these two groups did not have overrepresentation of alcoholics, so they did not need to be adjusted (Table 14.6).

[TPT.6] Pauker, 1980

The author obtained TPT scores on 363 Toronto citizens fluent in English recruited through announcements and notices. Subjects ranged in age from 19 to 71 and included 152 men and 211 women. Exclusion criteria consisted of significant physical disability, sensory deficit, current medical illness, use of medication that might affect test performance, history of actual or suspected brain disorder,

and alcoholism. MMPI profiles "could not suggest severe disturbance" or include more than three clinical scales with *T* scores greater than or equal to 70 or an F-scale score greater than 80.

The TPT was administered according to Reitan's guidelines. Means and standard deviations for total time in seconds and memory and localization scores are reported for the sample as a whole and by three age groupings (19–34, 35–52, 53–71) by four WAIS IQ levels (89–102, 103–112, 113–122, 123–143). Individual cell sample sizes ranged from four to 60. Age-by-IQ categories were determined "in a compromise between what would be desirable and what the obtained sample characteristics and size dictated" (p. 1). No differences in TPT performance between men and women were documented.

Study strengths
1. Large sample size, although individual cell sizes are substantially less than 50.
2. Presentation of the data in age by IQ groupings.
3. Adequate medical and psychiatric exclusion criteria.
4. Information regarding sex, recruitment procedures, language, and geographic recruitment area.
5. Means and standard deviations are reported.

Considerations regarding use of the study
1. No information regarding education.
2. Individual times for each hand separately and together are not reported.
3. Subjects were recruited in Canada, raising questions regarding usefulness for clinical interpretive purpose in the United States.
4. The age-by-IQ cell representing subjects aged 53 to 71 with IQs of 89 to 102 contained only four subjects; Pauker comments that this category "should not be considered to be of any more than interest value" (p. 2).
5. At least one 53–71-year-old subject in the 123–143 IQ range scored particularly poorly on the total time and localization scores, causing the means to be artificially low and the standard deviations to be excessively large for this age-by-IQ cell.

Table 14.6. TPT.5; Means and Standard Deviations for Time in Minutes per Block for Dominant and Nondominant Hands, Both Hands as Well as Total Time per Block for the Three Trials Combined, by Age Groupings

N	Age	WAIS FSIQ	Education	Dominant	Nondominant	Both	Total
Total Sample							
56	55–59	98.57 (11.43) 80–129	10.1	2.53 (2.42)	2.30 (2.54)	1.83 (2.70)	2.21 (3.31)
45	60–64	98.58 (9.93) 80–121	9.8	2.27 (1.73)	1.94 (1.35)	1.77 (1.93)	2.70 (3.81)
35	65–69	97.51 (11.18) 80–130	8.7	3.56 (3.26)	2.37 (1.67)	2.38 (2.16)	2.17 (1.86)
37	70–74	100.41 (9.92) 82–125	8.8	3.68 (3.24)	4.24 (3.77)	2.43 (2.59)	3.25 (3.41)
20	75–79	101.75 (10.18) 81–119	6.5	4.30 (2.64)	2.15 (2.51)	2.06 (1.43)	2.63 (1.42)
Alcohol-Equated Sample							
47	55–59	99.00 (11.73) 80–129	10.1	2.72 (2.58)	2.47 (2.72)	1.99 (2.89)	2.40 (3.57)
33	60–64	96.00 (9.43) 80–117	9.3	2.41 (1.81)	2.10 (1.41)	2.03 (2.00)	2.94 (3.92)
23	65–69	99.00 (12.06) 80–130	8.8	3.45 (3.16)	1.93 (1.29)	2.10 (2.14)	1.72 (1.47)
37	70–74	100.00 (9.92) 82–125	8.8	3.68 (3.24)	4.24 (3.77)	2.43 (2.59)	3.25 (3.41)
20	75–79	102.00 (10.18) 81–119	6.5	4.30 (2.64)	3.15 (2.51)	2.06 (1.43)	2.63 (1.42)

6. IQ levels below the average range not represented (Table 14.7).

[TPT.7] Fromm-Auch and Yeudall, 1983

The authors obtained TPT data on 193 Canadian subjects (111 male, 82 female) recruited through posted advertisements and personal contacts. Participants are described as "nonpsychiatric" and "non-neurological." Eighty-three percent of the sample were right-handed and mean age was 25.4 ± 8.2 (range = 15 to 64). Mean years of education were 14.8 ± 3.0 (range = 8–26) and included technical and university training. Mean WAIS FSIQ, VIQ, and PIQ

were 119.1 ± 8.8 (range = 98 to 142), 119.8 ± 9.9 (range = 95 to 143), and 115.6 ± 9.8 (range = 89 to 146), respectively. Of note, no subject obtained a FSIQ which was lower than the average range. Subjects were classified into five age groupings: 15–17 (n = 32), 18–23 (n = 74), 24–32 (n = 56), 33–40 (n = 18), and 41–64 (n = 10). Total N for this test = 190.

Mean time in minutes, standard deviation, and range are reported for preferred hand, nonpreferred hand, both hands combined, and total time for each age grouping. Similarly, mean correct blocks, standard deviation, and range are summarized on localization and

Table 14.7. TPT.6; Means and Standard Deviations for Total Time in Seconds, as Well as Memory and Localization Scores for the Sample as a Whole and for Three Age Groupings by Four WAIS IQ Levels

	WAIS IQ				
	89–102	103–112	113–122	123–143	89–143
Age					
19–34	*n* = 21	*n* = 53	*n* = 60	*n* = 28	*n* = 162
Total	932.57	830.79	692.95	616.71	755.93
	(294.57)	(298.21)	(267.62)	(174.93)	(285.73)
Memory	7.10	7.70	8.33	8.61	8.01
	(1.48)	(1.41)	(1.13)	(1.07)	(1.35)
Localization	4.71	4.66	5.68	6.36	5.34
	(2.19)	(2.46)	(2.39)	(2.09)	(2.41)
35–52	*n* = 20	*n* = 34	*n* = 56	*n* = 25	*n* = 135
Total	1139.80	961.79	888.11	788.64	925.53
	(257.07)	(320.49)	(288.75)	(344.50)	(318.45)
Memory	6.30	6.74	7.43	8.16	7.22
	(1.66)	(1.56)	(1.31)	(1.43)	(1.56)
Localization	2.40	3.38	4.05	4.08	3.64
	(1.60)	(2.16)	(2.12)	(2.31)	(2.16)
53–71	*n* = 4	*n* = 15	*n* = 27	*n* = 20	*n* = 66
Total	1591.25	1342.60	1108.70	1189.90	1215.71
	(417.50)	(346.88)	(317.15)	(409.95)	(375.07)
Memory	5.00	5.33	6.22	6.55	6.05
	(0.82)	(1.63)	(1.48)	(1.73)	(1.62)
Localization	0.75	2.07	3.07	2.00	2.38
	(0.96)	(1.71)	(1.66)	(2.25)	(1.92)
19–71	*n* = 45	*n* = 102	*n* = 143	*n* = 73	*n* = 363
Total	1083.22	949.73	847.87	823.63	902.60
	(340.02)	(355.55)	(322.77)	(386.83)	(356.10)
Memory	6.56	7.03	7.58	7.89	7.36
	(1.62)	(1.70)	(1.48)	(1.62)	(1.64)
Localization	3.33	3.85	4.55	4.38	4.17
	(2.30)	(2.43)	(2.38)	(2.81)	(2.50)

memory trials. The authors note that none of their subjects required more than 15 minutes to place the blocks with preferred, nonpreferred, and both hands. No sex differences were documented and male and female data were collapsed.

Study strengths
1. Large overall sample and some individual cells approximate *N*s of 50.
2. Presentation of the data by age grouping.
3. Information regarding mean IQ and edu-

cational levels, handedness, sex, recruitment procedures, and geographic recruitment area.
4. Some psychiatric and neurological exclusion criteria.
5. Means and standard deviations are reported.

Considerations regarding use of the study
1. The high intellectual and educational level of the sample.
2. An age grouping of 41 to 64 with 10 subjects would not appear to be particularly useful.

3. Subjects were recruited in Canada, raising questions regarding the usefulness of the data for clinical interpretive purpose in the United States.

4. At least one subject in the 18–23-year-old group scored particularly poorly on the time scores, causing the means to be artificially low and the standard deviations to be excessively large for this age grouping (Table 14.8).

[TPT.8] Schear, 1984

The author reports "norms" for the TPT from a Kansas neuropsychiatric sample consisting of 560 right-handed males with no "peripheral injuries or defects" which could adversely affect test performance. The sample reflected a large number of diagnostic categories; 35% had evidence of various signs of brain damage (organic brain syndromes, alcohol encephalopathy, epilepsy, etc.) and 49% exhibited psychiatric disturbance (nonorganic psychotic disorders, schizophrenia, alcoholism, etc.).

A maximum of 10 minutes was allowed for each of the three TPT timed trials. Means, standard deviations, and ranges are provided for years of education, and time in minutes for right hand, left hand, both hands, and total for five age decades: 20–29 ($n = 111$), 30–39 ($n = 112$), 40–49 ($n = 111$), 50–59 ($n = 155$), and 60–69 ($n = 67$). Means, standard deviations,

and ranges are also reported for memory and localization, and number of blocks placed with the right hand, left hand, both hands, and total.

Study strengths
1. Large sample size and individual cells exceeded Ns of 50.
2. Presentation of the data by age decades.
3. Information regarding education, sex, handedness, and geographic recruitment area.
4. Data regarding mean number of blocks placed.
5. Means and standard deviations are reported.

Considerations regarding use of the study
1. Insufficient exclusion criteria; subjects were diagnosed with organic, psychiatric, and/or medical illnesses.
2. All male sample.
3. No information on IQ (Tables 14.9 and 14.10).

[TPT.9] Dodrill, 1987

The author collected TPT data on 120 subjects in Washington during the years 1975–1976 ($n = 81$) and 1986–1987 ($n = 39$). Half of the sample was female and 10% were minorities (six African-American, three native American,

Table 14.8. TPT.7; Mean Time in Minutes, Standard Deviations, and Range for Preferred Hand, Nonpreferred Hand, Both Hands Combined, and Total Time for Each Age Grouping°

N	Age	TPT Preferred	Nonpreferred	Both	Total	Localization	Memory
32	15–17	4.6	3.3	1.7	9.5	6.8	8.9
		(1.2)	(1.2)	(0.5)	(2.1)	(2.5)	(1.0)
		2.6–6.8	1.1–6.4	0.8–3.3	4.7–14.1	1–10	6–10
74	18–23	5.1	3.5	2.1	10.6	5.7	8.2
		(2.2)	(1.6)	(1.3)	(4.5)	(2.1)	(1.3)
		1.9–13.5	1.1–10.8	0.4–9.3	4.2–29.1	1–10	4–10
56	24–32	4.5	3.1	1.8	9.4	5.5	8.3
		(1.8)	(1.1)	(.8)	(3.0)	(1.8)	(1.1)
		1.7–9.5	1.5–7.1	.5–4.6	3.8–18.8	2–9	6–10
18	33–40	4.9	3.7	2.3	10.9	5.6	8.6
		(1.7)	(1.0)	(.8)	(2.9)	(2.2)	(1.1)
		1.9–9.0	2.2–5.9	1.4–4.4	5.9–19.4	1–9	6–10
10	41–64	5.6	4.2	2.5	12.2	4.9	7.7
		(1.5)	(1.6)	(1.2)	(3.6)	(1.8)	(1.3)
		4.0–9.0	2.4–8.1	1.4–5.5	8.3–20.6	2–7	6–9

°Mean correct blocks, standard deviation and range are reported for localization and memory trials.

Table 14.9. TPT.8a; Means, Standard Deviations, and Ranges for Time in Minutes Required for Completion and Number of Blocks for the Right Hand, Left Hand, and Both Hands for Five Age Decades

N	Age	Education	Right Minutes	Right Blocks	Left Minutes	Left Blocks	Both Minutes	Both Blocks
111	20–29	11.72	6.98	8.95	5.39	9.36	3.63	9.85
		(1.50)	(2.30)	(2.14)	(2.62)	(1.78)	(2.29)	(1.08)
		6–16	1.8–10	1–10	1.3–10	2–10	0.7–10	1–10
112	30–39	12.11	7.04	8.66	6.30	8.81	4.51	9.53
		(2.21)	(2.43)	(2.49)	(2.75)	(2.39)	(2.80)	(1.52)
		6–18	2.4–10	0–10	1.6–10	0–10	0.9–10	1–10
111	40–49	11.71	7.69	7.81	6.96	8.41	5.07	9.32
		(2.75)	(2.37)	(3.11)	(2.50)	(2.89)	(2.74)	(2.05)
		5–21	2.2–10	0–10	2.4–10	0–10	1–10	1–10
156	50–59	11.16	8.70	7.35	8.20	7.45	6.51	8.40
		(3.61)	(1.85)	(3.03)	(2.21)	(3.24)	(2.92)	(2.86)
		2–22	3.3–10	0–10	2.3–10	0–10	1.2–10	0–10
67	60–69	11.13	8.75	6.85	8.35	6.39	7.36	7.54
		(3.60)	(1.81)	(3.25)	(2.24)	(3.51)	(3.00)	(3.06)
		3–20	3.5–10	0–10	2.6–10	0–10	2.1–10	0–10

two Asian American, one unknown). Eighteen were left-handed. There were 45 students, 11 homemakers, and one retiree; 37 were employed, 26 were unemployed. Subjects were recruited from various sources including schools, churches, employment agencies, and community service agencies. They were either paid for their participation or offered an interpretation of their abilities. Exclusion criteria included history of "neurologically relevant disease (such as meningitis or encephalitis)," alcoholism, birth complications "of likely neurological significance," oxygen deprivation, peripheral nervous system injury, psychotic or psychotic-like disorders, or head injury associated with uncon-sciousness, skull fracture, persisting neurological signs, or diagnosis of concussion or contusion. Of note, one-third of potential participants failed to meet the above medical and psychiatric criteria, resulting in a final sample of 120. Mean age was 27.73 ± 11.04 and mean years of education was 12.28 ± 2.18. The subjects tested in the 1970s were administered the WAIS and the subjects assessed in the 1980s were administered the WAIS-R; WAIS scores were converted to WAIS-R equivalents by subtracting seven

points from the VIQ, PIQ, and FSIQ. Mean FSIQ, VIQ, and PIQ scores were 100.00 ± 14.35, 100.92 ± 14.73, and 98.25 ± 13.39, respectively. IQ scores ranged from 60 to 138 and reflected a normal distribution.

Mean time in minutes and standard deviation are reported for TPT total time, as well as mean and standard deviation for memory and localization. In addition, IQ-equivalent scores for various levels of intelligence are presented. Using Halstead's (1947) cutoff of 15.6 or less minutes for total time, and score of six or greater and five or greater for memory and localization respectively, 21.7%, 5.0%, and 39.2% of a subgroup of the sample were misclassified as brain damaged.

Study strengths
1. Large sample size.
2. Comprehensive exclusion criteria (although the appropriateness of including mentally retarded individuals could be questioned).
3. Information regarding education, IQ, age, occupation, sex ratio, handedness, ethnicity, recruitment procedures, and geographic area.
4. IQ-equivalent scores provided.
5. Data for different IQ levels provided.

Table 14.10. TPT.8b; Means, Standard Deviations, and Ranges for Time in Minutes and the Number of Blocks°

N	Age	Total Minutes	Blocks	Memory	Localization
111	20–29	16.01	28.15	7.14	3.43
		(6.57)	(4.34)	(1.99)	(2.79)
		3.8–30	4–30	2–10	0–10
112	30–39	17.86	27.00	6.40	2.54
		(7.25)	(5.29)	(1.85)	(2.20)
		6.5–30	4–30	0–10	0–8
111	40–49	19.73	25.54	6.02	1.94
		(6.58)	(7.09)	(2.01)	(2.01)
		5.6–30	2–30	2–10	0–9
156	50–59	23.41	23.18	5.49	1.47
		(6.24)	(8.28)	(1.92)	(1.73)
		8.4–30	0–30	1–10	0–7
67	60–69	24.46	20.78	4.96	1.45
		(6.56)	(9.05)	(1.96)	(1.46)
		8.6–30	0–30	1–9	0–5

°The data is also reported for memory and localization.

6. Means and standard deviations are reported.

Considerations regarding use of the study
1. Undifferentiated age range.
2. Individual times for each hand separately and together are not reported.
3. On the IQ-equivalent scores, the two highest IQ groups have lower scores on localization than 100–120 IQ groups (Table 14.11).

[TPT.10] Yeudall, Reddon, Gill, and Stefanyk, 1987

The authors obtained TPT data on 225 Canadian subjects recruited from posted advertisements in workplaces and from personal solicitations. The participants included meat packers, postal workers, transit employers, hospital lab technicians, secretaries, ward aides, student interns, student nurses, and summer students. In addition, high school teachers identified for participation average students in grades 10 through 12. Exclusion criteria included evidence of "forensic involvement", head injury, neurological insult, prenatal or birth complications, psychiatric problems, or substance abuse. Subjects were classified into four age groupings

devised to ensure group homogeneity: 15–20, 21–25, 26–30, and 31–40. Information regarding percent right-handers, mean years of education, and mean WAIS/WAIS-R VIQ, and PIQ are reported for each age grouping for males and females separately and combined. For the sample as a whole, 88% were right-handed and had completed an average of 14.55 ± 2.78 years of schooling. The mean FSIQ, VIQ, and PIQ were 112.25 ± 10.25, 112.60 ± 10.86, and 108.13 ± 10.63, respectively.

TPT data were gathered by experienced testing technicians who "motivated the subjects to achieve maximum performance" partially through the promise of detailed explanations of their test performance.

Means and standard deviations for time in seconds to execute the task with the preferred and nonpreferred hands separately and together are presented, as well as means and standard deviations for memory and localization scores, for each age grouping, and each age by sex grouping.

No significant relationships were found between TPT scores and sex or educational level. Significant age effects were noted for the time, memory, and localization scores, and significant

Table 14.11. TPT.9; Mean Time in Minutes for TPT Total Time and Mean Scores for Memory and Localization for the Total Sample and for Various Levels of Intelligence

N	Age	Education	WAIS-R			Total Time	Memory	Localization
			FSIQ	VIQ	PIQ			
120	27.73	12.28	100.00	100.92	98.25	13.65	7.86	4.97
	(11.04)	(2.18)	(14.35)	(14.73)	(13.39)	(7.21)	(1.26)	(2.36)

N	FSIQ	Total Time	Memory	Localization
7	130	10.8	8	5
18	125	10.9	8	5
34	120	10.9	8	6
64	115	10.8	8	6
93	110	11.6	8	6
101	105	12.1	8	6
75	100	12.4	8	6
60	95	12.9	8	5
48	90	14.2	8	5
33	85	17.7	7	4
19	80	21.0	7	4
10	75	26.5	7	3
	70		6	3

correlations were documented between all scores and PIQ, particularly in males; an association between TPT memory scores and VIQ was also noted. Because no significant differences were found between men and women, only the combined sample data are reproduced below.

Study strengths

1. Large sample size and individual cells approximate Ns of 50.

2. Grouping data by age.

3. Data availability for a 15–20-year-old age group.

4. Adequate medical and psychiatric exclusion criteria.

5. Information regarding handedness, education, IQ, sex, occupation, geographic recruitment area, and recruitment procedures.

6. Means and standard deviations are reported.

Considerations regarding use of the study

1. The sample was atypical in terms of its high average intellectual level and high level of education.

2. The data were obtained on Canadian subjects, which may limit its usefulness for clinical interpretation in the United States due to possible subtle cultural differences.

3. Examination of the data reveals odd, unpredicted variability, with the 21–25-year-olds performing more poorly on the time scores than the 26–30-year-olds (Table 14.12).

[TPT.11] Ernst, 1987

The author obtained TPT data on 110 primarily Caucasian (99%) residents of Brisbane, Australia, aged 65 to 75. Fifty-nine were female and 51 were male, and mean educational level was 10.3 years; men and women did not differ in years of education. Subjects were recruited primarily through random selection from the Queensland State electoral roll ($n = 97$), with the remainder ($n = 13$) solicited through senior citizen centers. Exclusion criteria included history of significant head trauma or neurologic disease. Nearly one-half of the sample were diagnosed with at least one of chronic disease (hypertension = 33, heart disease = 9, thyroid dysfunction = 7, asthma = 5, emphysema = 2, diabetes = 1) for which they were receiving treatment and which was described as well controlled. Sixty-six of the subjects were receiving medications, primarily for the diseases listed above.

Test administration was according to the Reitan instructions. All subjects were administered the Trailmaking Test first followed by

Table 14.12. TPT.10; Means and Standard Deviations for Time in Seconds to Execute the Task With the Preferred and Nonpreferred Hands Separately and Together, as Well as Means and Standard Deviations for Memory and Localization Scores, for Each Age Grouping and for the Total Sample

N	Age	Education	% Right Hand	FSIQ	Preferred	Non-Preferred	Combined	Memory	Localization
62	15-20	12.16 (1.75)	79.03	111.75 (10.16)	286.80 (101.90)	195.49 (84.93)	106.90 (43.71)	8.73 (1.07)	6.47 (2.44)
73	21-25	14.82 (1.88)	86.30	109.79 (9.97)	312.96 (131.61)	209.16 (86.44)	128.36 (74.42)	8.11 (1.29)	5.51 (2.10)
48	26-30	15.50 (2.65)	89.58	113.95 (10.61)	265.66 (92.45)	181.86 (67.06)	103.35 (42.34)	8.13 (1.55)	5.42 (2.23)
42	31-40	16.50 (3.11)	90.48	116.09 (9.51)	278.11 (101.94)	206.61 (69.08)	134.01 (53.13)	8.19 (1.35)	5.24 (1.97)
225	15-40	14.55 (2.78)	85.78	112.25 (10.25)	288.94 (111.22)	199.00 (79.26)	118.07 (57.75)	8.30 (1.33)	5.70 (2.24)

either the TPT or Booklet Category Test.

Mean times in minutes and standard deviations are reported for the preferred hand, nonpreferred hand, both hands, and total. In addition, mean number of blocks and standard deviations are presented for each time measure and for memory and localization. Using cutoffs of 15.7 minutes for total time, and five and four blocks for memory and localization, 77%, 36%, and 89%, respectively, of the sample were classified as impaired. Men outperformed women on memory, localization, and all time scores except dominant hand. No differences in TPT scores emerged between subjects with and without chronic disease although, of interest, participants taking medications scored better on memory and localization. Educational level did not appear to be related to TPT performance. A third of the sample (34.5%) failed to show superior nondominant hand performance on the second trial, and this subgroup was not overrepresented by men or women, older age (<70%), chronic illness, or medication usage, and did not show poorer scores on the TPT measures. Subjects administered the TPT prior to the Booklet Category Test obtained a higher mean number of blocks placed for the preferred hand, but no other test order effects were documented.

Study strengths

1. Large sample size in a restricted age range.
2. Presentation of the data by sex.

3. Information regarding education, geographic recruitment area, recruitment procedures, and ethnicity.
4. Information regarding test administration order effects.
5. Means and standard deviations are reported.

Considerations regarding use of the study

1. Approximately half of the subjects had at least one chronic illness, and over half were taking prescribed medications.
2. No information regarding IQ.
3. Low mean educational level.
4. Data were collected in Australia and may be unsuitable for clinical use in the United States (Table 14.13).

[TPT.12] Heaton, Grant, and Matthews, 1991

The authors provide normative data on the TPT from 486 (378 in the base sample and 108 in the validation sample) urban and rural subjects recruited in several states (California, Washington, Colorado, Texas, Oklahoma, Wisconsin, Illinois, Michigan, New York, Virginia, and Massachusetts) and Canada. Data were collected over a 15-year period through multicenter collaborative efforts; the authors trained the test administrators and supervised data collection. Exclusion criteria included history of learning disability, neurologic disease, illnesses affecting brain function, significant head trau-

Table 14.13. TPT.11; Mean Times in Minutes and Standard Deviations for the Preferred Hand, Nonpreferred Hand, Both Hands and Total Time°

N	Sex	Dominant		Nondominant		Both		Total		Memory	Localization
		Time	Blocks	Time	Blocks	Time	Blocks	Time	Blocks		
51	M	9.1	9.5	7.4	9.7	5.1	9.9	21.4	29.2	6.6	2.8
		(4.1)	(1.5)	(3.4)	(1.7)	(2.9)	(1.0)	(9.0)	(3.0)	(1.6)	(1.9)
59	F	10.3	9.0	10.1	9.1	6.6	9.8	26.9	28.0	5.9	2.0
		(4.1)	(2.2)	(4.2)	(2.0)	(3.8)	(0.9)	(10.9)	(3.8)	(1.6)	(1.8)

°In addition, mean number of blocks and standard deviations are presented for each time measure and for memory and localization.

ma, significant psychiatric disturbance (e.g., schizophrenia), and alcohol or the substance abuse. Mean age for the total sample was 42.0 ± 16.8, and mean educational level was 13.6 ± 3.5. Sixty-five percent of the sample were males. Mean WAIS FSIQ, VIQ, and PIQ were 113.8 ± 12.3, 113.9 ± 13.8, and 111.9 ± 11.6, respectively.

Subjects were generally paid for their participation, and they were judged to have provided their best efforts on the tasks. The TPT was administered according to Reitan and Wolfson's (1985) instructions, with the exception that TPT time trials were discontinued at 10 minutes unless the subject was progressing well or near to finishing the task or was judged to have the potential for becoming distressed if forced to discontinue before completion. Minutes per block (number of minutes divided by the number of blocks correctly placed) were the performance parameters employed for the preferred hand, nonpreferred hand, and both hands, and total time; number of blocks recalled and correctly located was used for memory and localization scores. A T-score system with demographic correction was developed on 378 subjects and cross-validated on 108 subjects. Extensive T-score tables corrected for age, education, and sex are provided, and the interested reader is referred directly to the handbook for these data.

Age accounted for 7% (dominant hand) to 29% (localization) of the variance in TPT scores; education was associated with 3% (dominant hand) to 14% (memory) of score variance; and sex only accounted for at most 1% of score variance. These demographic variables

in combination were associated with 7% (dominant hand) to 34% (total) of score variance. For the sample as a whole, minutes per block for the dominant hand, nondominant hand, both hands, and total were 0.7 ± 0.8, 0.6 ± 0.6, 0.4 ± 0.6, and 0.5 ± 0.3, respectively. Number of blocks recalled and correctly located were 7.6 ± 1.6 and 4.3 ± 2.5, respectively.

Study strengths
1. Large sample size.
2. *T* scores corrected for age, education, and sex.
3. Comprehensive exclusion criteria.
4. Information regarding IQ and geographic recruitment area.

Considerations regarding use of the study
1. Above average mean intellectual level (which is probably less of an issue given that these are WAIS rather than WAIS-R IQ data).

Other comments
1. The interested reader is referred to 1996 critique of Heaton et al. (1991) norms, and Heaton et al.'s 1996 response to this critique.

Control Groups in Clinical Studies

[TPT.13] Klove and Lochen (in Klove, 1974)

The authors obtained TPT data on 22 American controls from Wisconsin and 22 Norwegian controls as a part of a validation study on the ability of the Halstead-Reitan Battery to detect brain damage. The mean age, educational level, and IQ for the American subjects were 31.6, 11.1, and 109.3, respectively, and the mean age, educational level, and IQ for the Norwegian subjects were 32.1, 12.2, and 111.9, respectively.

The TPT data are presented in terms of mean for total time in minutes, and memory and localization scores for each group.

Study strengths
1. This publication is unique in providing TPT data on a Norwegian population.
2. Information regarding educational level, IQ, age, and geographic recruitment area reported.

Considerations regarding use of the study
1. The small sample size.
2. Undifferentiated age ranges.
3. No standard deviations reported.
4. No exclusion criteria are specified and no information regarding gender distribution of the sample is provided.
5. Individual times for each hand separately and combined are not reported.
6. No information on gender.
7. Relatively low educational level of the United States sample, although IQ is average (Table 14.14).

[TPT.14] Wiens and Matarazzo, 1977

The authors collected TPT data on 48 male applicants to a patrolman program in Portland, Oregon, as part of an investigation of the WAIS and MMPI correlates of the Halstead-Reitan Battery. All subjects passed a medical exam and were judged to be neurologically normal. Subjects were divided into two equal groups which were comparable in age (23.6 vs. 24.8), education (13.7 vs. 14.0), and WAIS FSIQ (117.5 vs. 118.3). Mean time in minutes and standard

deviations to complete the TPT with the preferred hand, nonpreferred hand, both hands, and total are provided, as well as means and standard deviations for memory and localization scores. A random subsample of 29 of the applicants was readministered the TPT 14 to 24 weeks following the original administration (Matarazzo et al., 1974) as a part of an examination of the Halstead Impairment Index. Means and standard deviations for TPT total time in minutes, and memory and localization, are reported for both the original testing and retest. One of the 29 subjects obtained a score outside Halstead's (1947) suggested cutoff for total time, while nearly a third (nine of 29) of the subjects scored below Reitan's cutoff on localization. Significant correlations were observed between the time scores and Performance IQ in both control groups (Wiens & Matarazzo, 1977), while significant correlations were documented between time scores and Full Scale IQ in only one control group; Verbal IQ was not associated with any of the TPT scores, and only the time scores were related to IQ measures.

Study strengths
1. Information on test/retest performance.
2. Adequate sample size for the small age range.
3. Adequate medical exclusion criteria.
4. Information provided regarding educational level, IQ, sex, occupation, and geographic recruitment area.
5. Means and standard deviations are reported.

Considerations regarding use of the study
1. High IQ level.
2. High educational level.
3. All-male sample (Table 14.15).

Table 14.14. TPT.13; Means for Total Time in Minutes, Memory, and Localization Scores for Each Group

	N	Age	Education	WAIS IQ	TPT Total	Memory	Localization
Americans	22	31.6	11.1	109.3	14.0	7.2	4.3
Norwegians	22	32.1	12.2	111.9	13.7	7.5	5.2

Table 14.15. TPT.14; Mean Time in Minutes and Standard Deviations to Complete the TPT With the Preferred Hand, Nonpreferred Hand, Both Hands, and Total, as Well as Means and Standard Deviations for Memory and Localization Scores for Two Equal Groups of Subjects°

				TPT					
N	Age	Education	WAIS FSIQ	Preferred	Nonpreferred	Both	Total	Memory	Localization
24	23.6	13.7	117.5	4.85	3.02	1.87	9.74	8.46	5.67
	(21–27)	(12–16)	(8.3)	(1.92)	(1.20)	(.89)	(3.16)	(.98)	(1.74)
24	24.8	14.0	118.3	4.38	2.97	1.83	9.18	8.67	6.13
	(21–28)	(12–16)	(6.8)	(1.24)	(1.03)	(.84)	(2.42)	(.76)	(2.61)

				TPT Test			Retest		
N	Age	Education	FSIQ	Total	Memory	Localization	Total	Memory	Localization
29	24	14	118	9.36	8.38	5.34	8.19	8.72	7.10
	(21–28)	(12–16)		(2.73)	(.82)	(2.41)	(2.70)	(.88)	(1.82)

°The data for a subset of 29 subjects include means and standard deviations for total time in minutes, memory, and localization scores for both the original testing and retest.

[TPT.15] Anthony, Heaton, and Lehman, 1980

The authors amassed TPT data on 100 normal volunteers from Colorado as a part of a cross-validation of two computerized interpretative programs for the Halstead-Reitan Battery. Subjects had no history of medical or psychiatric problems, head trauma, brain disease, or substance abuse. In addition, for 85% of the controls, normal EEGs and neurological exams were obtained; in the remaining 15% of the subjects it appears that this information was not available. Mean age was 38.88 ± 15.80 and mean years of education was 13.33 ± 2.56. Mean WAIS FSIQ, VIQ, and PIQ were 113.54 ± 10.83, 113.24 ± 11.59, and 112.26 ± 10.88, respectively.

The TPT data are presented in terms of mean time in minutes and standard deviation divided by the number of blocks placed, and mean and standard deviation for memory and localization scores. Subjects incorrectly identified as brain damaged (according to the Russell et al., 1970, system) were older, less educated, and less intelligent than subjects correctly classified as non-brain-damaged.

Study strengths
1. Large sample size.
2. Adequate exclusion criteria.

3. Information regarding education, IQ, age, and geographic recruitment area.
4. Means and standard deviations are reported.

Considerations regarding use of the study
1. The large undifferentiated age grouping.
2. The IQ range is high average.
3. No information regarding sex.
4. Individual times for each hand separately and together are not reported (Table 14.16).

[TPT.16] Bak and Greene, 1980

The authors gathered TPT data on 30 right-handed Texan subjects as a part of an investigation of the effect of age on performance on the Halstead-Reitan battery and the Wechsler Memory Scale. The participants were equally divided into two age groupings: 50–62 and 67–86. Subjects were fluent in English and denied history of CNS disorders, uncorrected sensory deficits, or illnesses or "incapacities" which might affect test results; subjects in poor health were excluded. The mean age of the two groups was 55.6 ± 4.44 and 74.9 ± 6.04, respectively. Subjects in the first group were born between the years 1916 and 1929, and subjects in the second group were born between 1892 and 1912. Nine individuals in the first group were female, and 10 subjects in the second group were female. Four WAIS subtests were administered (Information, Arithmetic, Block Design, Digit Symbol); the mean

Table 14.16. TPT.15; Mean Time in Minutes and Standard Deviation Divided by the Number of Blocks Placed, and Means and Standard Deviations for Memory and Localization Scores

N	Age	Education	WAIS			TPT		
			FSIO	VIQ	PIQ	Time	Memory	Localization
100	38.88	13.33	113.54	113.24	112.26	0.44	7.80	4.64
	(15.80)	(2.56)	(10.83)	(11.59)	(10.88)	(0.25)	(1.49)	(2.15)

scores on these measures suggested that IQ levels were within the high average range or higher. Mean educational levels for the two groups were 13.7 ± 1.91 and 14.9 ± 2.99, respectively.

Mean times in seconds and standard deviations for the right hand, left hand, both hands, and total are reported, as well as means and standard deviations for memory and localization. The groups differed significantly on all the time measures.

Study strengths
1. Data on a very elderly age group not found in other published reports.
2. Adequate exclusion criteria.
3. Information regarding education, IQ, sex, handedness, fluency in English, and geographic recruitment area.
4. Means and standard deviations are reported.

Considerations regarding use of the study
1. High IQ level.
2. High educational level.
3. The older age grouping spans nearly two decades and may be too broad for optimal clinical interpretive use.
4. Small sample sizes (Table 14.17).

[TPT.17] Russell, 1985

The author obtained data on the six-block children's version of the TPT (TPT-6) in a sample of 19 Caucasian "control" subjects as a part of his examination of the use of a shortened version of the TPT in adults. Participants had been admitted to a neurology ward of the Miami V.A. Medical Center for a suspected neurological condition but showed no evidence of brain damage upon neurological evaluation including brain CT scans. Mean age was 43.5 ± 13.6 and mean educational level was 14.8 ± 6.4. All but two subjects were male. Exclusion criteria included severe psychiatric disturbance (e.g., psychosis, severe depression), left-handedness, and inability to use one or both hands.

The TPT was administered according to the Rennick procedures (Russell et al., 1970); specifically, if a time trial was not completed after 10 minutes, the trial was discontinued and the score was prorated based on the number of blocks remaining to obtain a combined time score. The 19 control subjects were tested as a part of a group of 80 subjects administered both the 6-block and 10-block TPT. Forty subjects were given the 10-block version first, and the remaining sample was administered the six-block version first during the course of a com-

Table 14.17. TPT.16; Mean Time in Seconds and Standard Deviations for the Right Hand, Left Hand, Both Hands, and Total Time, as Well as Means and Standard Deviations for Memory and Localization Scores

N	Age	Education	TPT					
			Right	Left	Both	Total	Memory	Localization
15	50–62							
	55.6	13.7	365.20	306.80	169.80	841.80	5.27	2.07
	(4.44)	(1.91)	(151.49)	(161.51)	(71.03)	(326.01)	(1.49)	(1.53)
15	67–86							
	74.9	14.9	571.60	514.00	301.20	1,386.80	5.07	1.60
	(6.04)	(2.99)	(289.36)	(276.64)	(116.14)	(627.34)	(2.02)	(1.55)

prehensive neuropsychological evaluation. The interval between administration of the two versions ranged from 1 hour to 2 days.

Mean time in minutes and standard deviations are reported for the dominant hand, nondominant hand, both hands, and total, as well as mean and standard deviation for memory and localization for both the 6-block and 10-block versions. Correlations of the time scores between the two tests ranged from 0.62 (nondominant hand) to 0.82 (total time), suggesting that these scores "are measuring approximately the same attributes and the TPT 6 could be substituted for the TPT 10" (p. 73). The correlation for the memory scores was 0.71, but the correlation for localization was only 0.55. Despite the overall strong association between the two versions of the TPT, the TPT-10 was found to be much more difficult than the TPT-6; the time to complete the TPT-6 was approximately one-third that of the full TPT. The localization score was observed to have poor reliability due to its marked variability.

Study strengths

1. Data on the 6-block version in adults and its relationship to the 10-block test.

2. Information on educational level, geographic recruitment area, sex, ethnicity, handedness, and age.

3. Means and standard deviations are reported.

Considerations regarding use of the study

1. Small sample size.
2. Undifferentiated age range.
3. Insufficient exclusion criteria.
4. The mean score for the TPT-10 for both

hands appears to be in error since it is twice that of either hand alone.

5. High mean educational level.
6. No data on IQ.
7. Mostly male sample (Table 14.18).

[TPT.18] Heaton, Grant, and Matthews, 1986

The authors obtained TPT data on 553 normal controls in Colorado, California, and Wisconsin as a part of an investigation into the effects of age, education, and sex on Halstead-Reitan Battery performance. Nearly two-thirds of the sample were male (males = 356, females = 197). Exclusion criteria included history of neurologic illness, significant head trauma, and substance abuse. Subjects ranged in age from 15 to 81 (Mean = 39.3 ± 17.5), and mean number of years of education was 13.3 ± 3.4 with a range of 0 to 20 years. The sample was divided into three age categories (<40, 40–59, and ≥60) with sizes of 319, 134, 100, respectively, and classified into three education categories (<12 years, 12–15 years, and ≥16 years) with sizes of 132, 249, and 172, respectively.

Testing was conducted by trained technicians and all participants were judged to have expended their best effort on the task. TPT mean total time in minutes per block and mean memory/location scores are reported for the six subgroups, as well as percent classified as normal using Russell et al.'s (1970) criteria. Approximately 20% to 30% test score variance was accounted for by age, but only approximately 5% to 10% of test score variance was associated with education level. Significant group differences on all TPT scores were found across the three age groups; significant group differences

Table 14.18. TPT.17; Mean Time in Minutes and Standard Deviations for the Dominant Hand, Nondominant Hand, Both Hands, and Total Time, as Well as Mean and Standard Deviations for Memory and Localization Scores for the 10-Block and 6-Block Versions

				TPT					
	N	Age	Education	Dominant	Nondominant	Both	Total	Memory	Localization
10 blocks	19	43.5	14.8	6.88	5.67	13.33	15.68	7.42	4.10
		(13.6)	(6.4)	(3.36)	(3.25)	(2.03)	(6.94)	(1.64)	(2.57)
6 blocks				1.88	1.41	0.87	4.17	4.84	3.84
				(0.99)	(1.12)	(0.41)	(2.16)	(0.83)	(1.54)

across educational levels were only document-ed for the memory score, and a significant age by education interaction was documented for memory and location scores. Significant differ-ences in performance were found between males and females; men significantly outper-formed women on total time.

Study strengths

1. Large size of overall sample and individ-ual cells.

2. Information regarding education, sex, age, and geographic recruitment area.

3. Data grouped by age and also by educa-tion level.

4. Minimally adequate exclusion criteria.

Considerations regarding use of the study

1. No reporting of TPT score standard devi-ations.

2. Mean scores for individual WAIS subtest scaled scores reported, but not overall IQ scores.

3. Individual times for each hand separately and together are not reported (Table 14.19).

[TPT.19] Alekoumbides, Charter, Adkins, and Seacat, 1987

The authors report TPT data on 111 medical and psychiatric medical inpatients and outpa-tients without cerebral lesions or histories of al-coholism or cerebral contusion, from V.A. hos-pitals in Southern California, as a part of their development of standardized scores corrected for age and education for the Halstead-Reitan Battery. Among the 41 psychiatric patients, nine were diagnosed as psychotic and 32 were neurotic. In addition to psychiatry services, pa-tients were also drawn from medicine ($n = 57$), neurology ($n = 22$), spinal cord injury ($n = 9$), and surgery ($n = 6$) units. Mean age was 46.85 ± 17.17 (ranging from 19 to 82), and mean years of education were 11.43 ± 3.20 (ranging from 1 to 20). Frequency distributions for age and years of education are provided. Mean WAIS FSIQ, VIQ, and PIQ were within the av-erage range (105.89 ± 13.47, 107.03 ± 14.38, and 103.31 ± 13.02, respectively); means and standard deviations for individual age-correct-ed subtest scores are also reported. All subjects except one were males; the majority were Cau-casian (93%), with 7% African-American. The mean score on a measure of occupational at-tainment was 11.29.

No differences were found in test perfor-mance between the two psychiatric groups and the nonpsychiatric group and the data were collapsed. Mean time in minutes and standard deviation to correctly place all the blocks are presented for the preferred hand, nonpreferred hand, both hands, and total time, as well as memory and localization score. In addition, mean blocks correctly placed per minute and standard deviation are summa-rized for the preferred hand, nonpreferred hand, both hands, and total time. The latter scores were included because the first set of scores would not discriminate between sub-jects who successfully placed all the blocks ex-cept one in the allotted time vs. subjects who correctly placed no blocks. Both age and edu-cational level had significant associations with TPT scores in the expected direction, and re-gression equation information to allow correc-

Table 14.19. TPT.18; Mean Total Time in Minutes per Block, and Mean Memory and Localization Scores for the Six Subgroups, as Well as Percent Classified as Normal Using Russell et al.'s (1970) Criteria°

			WAIS	TPT			% Classified Normal		
N	Age	Education	Mean SS	Total Time	Memory	Localization	Total Time	Memory	Localization
319	<40		11.9	0.39	8.1	5.3	87.5	97.8	65.5
134	40–59		11.2	0.50	7.5	4.0	69.4	90.3	41.8
100	≥60		9.7	0.85	6.2	2.0	23.0	69.0	9.0
132		<12	9.5	0.64	6.9	3.6	53.7	78.8	35.6
249		12–15	11.2	0.47	7.7	4.4	75.9	93.2	49.0
172		≥16	12.9	0.43	8.0	5.0	78.5	96.5	61.1

°The mean WAIS scaled scores are also reported for each group.

tion of raw scores for age and education is included.

Study strengths
1. Large sample size.
2. Information regarding IQ, age, education, ethnicity, sex, occupational attainment, and geographic recruitment area.
3. Regression equation data for computation of age- and education-corrected scores.
4. Means and standard deviations are reported.

Considerations regarding use of the study
1. Data were collected on medical and psychiatric patients.
2. Undifferentiated age range (mitigated by the regression equation information).
3. Nearly all male sample (Table 14.20).

[TPT.20] Bornstein, Baker, and Douglass, 1987a

The authors collected TPT test-retest data on 23 volunteers (14 women, nine men) who ranged in age from 17 to 52 (Mean = 32.3 ± 10.3), as part of an examination of the short-term retest reliability of the Halstead-Reitan Battery. Exclusion criteria consisted of a positive history of neurological or psychiatric illness. Mean verbal IQ was 105.8 ± 10.8 (range = 88 to 128) and mean performance IQ was 105.0 ± 10.5 (range = 85 to 121).

Subjects were administered the Halstead-Reitan Battery in standard order both on initial testing and again 3 weeks later. Means, standard deviations, and ranges for time, memory, and localization scores for both testing sessions are provided, as well as raw score change and standard deviation, median raw score change, and mean percent of change. Significant improvements were noted in time, memory, and localization scores. Correlations between such demographic variables as age and education and mean percent of change and mean change were generally small, with education accounting for up to 17% of variance and age accounting for up to 8% of variance.

Study strengths
1. Information on short-term (3-week) retest data.
2. Information on IQ level, sex, and age.
3. Minimally adequate exclusion criteria.
4. Means and standard deviations are reported.

Considerations regarding use of the study
1. Undifferentiated age range.
2. No information regarding education.
3. TPT time score is not defined.
4. Individual times for each hand separately and together are not reported.
5. Small sample size (Table 14.21).

[TPT.21] El-Sheikh, El-Nagdy, Townes, and Kennedy, 1987

The authors reported TPT data on 32 undergraduate and graduate Egyptians at the Ameri-

Table 14.20. TPT19; Mean Time in Minutes and Standard Deviation to Correctly Place all the Blocks for the Preferred Hand, Nonpreferred Hand, Both Hands, and Total Time[°]

			WAIS		
N	Age	Education	FSIQ	VIQ	PIQ
111	46.85	11.43	105.89	107.03	103.1
	(17.17)	(3.20)	(13.47)	(14.38)	(13.02)

Time				Blocks per Minute					
Preferred	Nonpreferred	Both	Total	Preferred	Nonpreferred	Both	Total	Memory	Localization
7.80	6.18	4.31	18.29	1.58	2.10	3.42	2.05	6.28	2.67
(3.73)	(3.51)	(3.43)	(9.87)	(0.90)	(1.20)	(2.08)	(1.06)	(2.01)	(2.29)

[°]Mean number of blocks correctly placed per minute and standard deviation are summarized for the preferred hand, nonpreferred hands, both hands, and total time. Memory and localization scores as well as demographic information are also provided.

Table 14.21. TPT.20; Means and Standard Deviations for Total Time, Memory and Localization Scores for Both Testing Sessions, as Well as Raw Score Change and Standard Deviation, Median Raw Score Change, and Mean Percent of Change

				Test			Retest		
N	Age	VIQ	PIQ	Time	Memory	Localization	Time	Memory	Localization
23	32.3 (10.3)	105.8 (10.8)	105.0 (10.5)	10.7 (4.2)	8.4 (0.9)	5.1 (2.3)	7.4 (2.6)	8.9 (1.0)	6.3 (2.9)

Raw Score Change			Median Raw Score Change			Mean % of Change		
Time	Memory	Localization	Time	Memory	Localization	Time	Memory	Localization
3.25 (3.3)	0.65 (0.61)	0.88 (1.9)	2.2	1.0	1.0	27	6	34

can University at Cairo as a part of their cross-cultural investigation of the Luria-Nebraska and Halstead-Reitan battery. The average age was 20.6 (range = 17–24). No subject had a history of known brain damage. Participants were described as "Arabic and English speaking." TPT instructions were translated in Egyptian Colloquial Arabic by the first author and checked by two independent judges fluent in both Arabic and English. In the case of disagreement between these two judges, a third judge was consulted.

The TPT was administered in English to 23 subjects and in Arabic to nine subjects and readministered 2 weeks later. Mean time in minutes and standard deviations are reported for the preferred hand, nonpreferred hand, both hands, and total, as well as means and standard deviations for memory and localization. No differences in performance were found between subjects administered the test in English or Arabic. Significant practice effects were documented for time for both hands, total time and localization.

Study strengths
1. Data obtained on an Arabic sample.
2. Information on test–retest scores.
3. Information regarding educational level, age, and geographic recruitment area.
4. Means and standard deviations are reported.

Considerations regarding use of the study
1. Small sample size.
2. Minimal exclusion criteria.

3. No information regarding intellectual level.

4. Undifferentiated age range although it can be assumed it is fairly restricted (Table 14.22).

[TPT.22] Clark and Klonoff, 1988

The authors obtained data on the six-block children's version of the TPT (TPT-6) in a sample of 79 male, right-handed, coronary-by-pass-surgery subjects in Canada as a part of their evaluation of the reliability and construct validity of the shortened TPT in adults. Exclu-

Table 14.22. TPT.21; Mean Times in Minutes and Standard Deviations for the Dominant Hand, Nondominant Hand, Both Hands, and Total, as Well as Means and Standard Deviations for Memory and Localization Scores for Both Test and Retest

		Test	Retest
N	32		
Age	20.6 (1.4)		
Dominant hand		4.95 (1.96)	3.32 (1.43)
Nondominant hand		3.68 (1.28)	2.83 (1.43)
Both hands		2.35 (.84)	1.74 (.71)
Total		11.01 (3.38)	7.71 (3.03)
Memory		8.34 (1.41)	8.59 (1.93)
Localization		5.53 (2.59)	6.88 (2.46)

sion criteria included postsurgical complications and stroke or other neurological conditions. Apparently all of the sample were prescribed coronary medications (β blockers = 75%; calcium channel blockers = 65%; long-acting nitrates = 59%; nitroglycerin = 47%; antiarrhythmics = 7%; digitalis = 7%). In addition, six subjects were prescribed antianxiety medication, two were receiving sleeping medication, and one was on an antidepressant. Also, several were receiving treatment for chronic medical illnesses such as diabetes (two), ulcers (three), gout (two), allergies (three), and arthritis (two). Mean age was 55.5 ± 8.0 (range = 35–68), and mean WAIS-R FSIQ was 105.9 ± 12.2 (range = 77–137). The majority of the sample had completed at least nine years of education (84%), and nearly one-third had completed some post–high school work (29.1%).

The TPT-6 was administered according to the instructions for the 10-block TPT to each subject 3 weeks before surgery, and 3, 12, and 24 months postsurgery. Mean time in minutes and standard deviations for time to complete the task with each hand, both hands, and total are reported, as well as mean and standard deviation for the localization and memory for each of the four testing sessions. No significant correlations were noted between measures of presurgical cardiac status and TPT scores, and only one significant difference in test performance was noted across the four largest cardiac medication groups, but this may have been a chance result given the multiple comparisons. The authors argue that "these findings suggest that the sample is an appropriate normative group in that the stress of a disease state and upcoming surgical intervention was present but the disease per se or specific medications were not directly related to test performance" (p. 177). The authors note that the 6-block TPT had good test–retest reliability, with little practice effect across the four testing sessions. Construct validity appeared to be consistent with that of the 10-block TPT.

Study strengths
1. Data for the six-block version.
2. Test–retest data (although it is technical-

ly not a true test–retest study since the subjects underwent an intervening surgical procedure).
3. Information regarding education, sex, age, IQ, geographic recruitment area, and handedness.
4. Large sample size.
5. Means and standard deviations are reported.

Considerations regarding use of the study
1. All patients were medically ill and receiving various medications.
2. Undifferentiated age range.
3. Low overall educational level, although IQ is average.
4. Data collected in Canada raising concerns regarding usefulness for clinical interpretive purpose in the United States.
5. All male sample (Table 14.23).

[TPT.23] Thompson and Heaton, 1991

The authors report TPT data on 489 subjects apparently recruited from California, Colorado, Ohio, and/or Michigan as a part of their examination of the relationship between patterns of TPT performance and other neuropsychological test scores. Exclusion criteria included history of head trauma, neurologic illness, substance abuse, "serious" psychiatric illness, and peripheral injury which could interfere with test performance. Mean age and years of education were 39.43 ± 17.76 and 13.19 ± 3.46, respectively. Mean WAIS FSIQ was 113.09 ± 12.07.

The TPT was administered by trained technicians according to standard procedures. Mean times in minutes and standard deviations for dominant hand, nondominant hand, both hands, and total are provided as well as number of blocks correctly recalled and located. A reversal in the expected pattern of improvement from dominant to nondominant hand performance occurred in 30% of subjects and was associated with relatively poorer scores on some WAIS Performance subtests.

Study strengths
1. Large sample size.
2. Information regarding education, IQ, age, and geographic recruitment area.

Table 14.23. TPT.22; Mean Time in Minutes and Standard Deviations for Time to Complete the Task With the Right Hand, Left Hand, Both Hands, and Total, as Well as Mean and Standard Deviation for the Memory and Localization for Each of the Four Testing Probes for the Six-Block TPT Version

| | Age | WAIS-R FSIQ | TPT | | | | | |
			Right	Left	Both	Total	Memory	Localization
Presurgery	55.5	105.9	2.37	1.74	1.05	5.16	4.46	3.33
	(8.01)	(12.2)	(1.16)	(0.86)	(0.59)	(2.29)	(1.11)	(1.59)
Postsurgery								
3 months			2.07	1.83	0.97	4.87	4.64	3.47
			(0.86)	(1.10)	(0.49)	(2.16)	(1.09)	(1.67)
12 Months			2.06	1.63	1.05	4.73	4.78	3.69
			(0.82)	(0.81)	(0.60)	(1.87)	(1.05)	(1.48)
24 months			2.19	1.65	0.92	4.77	4.72	3.44
			(1.01)	(0.91)	(0.42)	(1.87)	(1.10)	(1.65)

3. Adequate exclusion criteria.

4. Means and standard deviations are reported.

Considerations regarding use of the study

1. Undifferentiated age range.

2. No information regarding sex distribution.

3. High mean educational and IQ levels (Table 14.24).

CONCLUSIONS

The review of the validity studies and normative data for the TPT reveals considerable controversy regarding the utility of this test. Although some authors found the TPT to be sensitive to different aspects of brain dysfunction, many investigators point to notable drawbacks limiting its practical utility. One of the major liabilities of this test is that it is long, difficult, and requires the examiner to blindfold the examinee. This often creates consid-

erable psychological discomfort for the examinee (see Lezak, 1995, pp. 490–493). Use of the 6-block version of this test can alleviate some of the problems associated with the full 10-block version. However, data should be collected on the validity/reliability of the short version and on its comparability to the full version if the short version is to be used in clinical practice.

The clinical usefulness of the TPT would be improved by adjusting cutoffs relative to subject's age, intellectual level, and, possibly, education and sex, although the effect of the latter two demographic variables on TPT performance needs to be further explored. Taking demographic factors into account in assigning subjects to impaired vs. nonimpaired groups would improve the specificity of the TPT. This would also reduce excessively high rates of misclassification of "normal" subjects in the impaired range reported in the studies reviewed.

Another aspect of the test which would benefit from further attention of researchers is

Table 14.24. TPT.23; Mean Times in Minutes and Standard Deviations for Dominant Hand, Nondominant Hand, Both Hands, and Total Time, as Well as Memory and Localization Scores

| N | Age | Education | WAIS IQ | TPT | | | | | |
				Dominant	Nondominant	Both	Total	Memory	Localization
489	39.43	13.9	113.09	6.78	5.72	3.51	14.85	7.59	4.43
	(17.76)	(3.46)	(12.07)	(7.56)	(6.13)	(5.72)	(10.20)	(1.58)	(2.45)

standardization of the procedure for test administration.

The above suggestions address major criticisms voiced by investigators regarding the validity of the TPT. With further improvements in administration and refinement in interpretation guidelines, perhaps the utility of this widely used test would be considerably improved.

V

VERBAL AND VISUAL LEARNING AND MEMORY

15

Wechsler Memory Scale[1]

BRIEF HISTORY OF THE TEST BATTERY

The Wechsler Memory Scale (WMS) was one of the first standardized memory batteries and has remained one of the most popular since its appearance in 1945. Revisions of the WMS test battery were published in 1987 and 1997. (Please see Appendix 1 for ordering information).

WMS (1945)

Wechsler developed the original test battery with the intention of providing "a rapid, simple and practical memory examination" (p. 87). The test takes about 30 minutes to administer and consists of seven subtests: (1) *Personal and Current Information*, which includes six relatively simple general and personal information questions; (2) *Orientation*, which asks five questions relating to place and time; (3) *Mental Control*, which requires the patient to count backward from 20, recite the alphabet, and count by threes; bonus points are awarded for fast, perfect performance; (4) *Logical Memory*, which tests immediate auditory memory for two separate orally presented stories; (5) *Digits Forward and Digits Backwards*, which assesses attention span and immediate auditory memory; (6) *Visual Reproduction*, which tests imme-

diate visual memory for geometric designs after a 10-second exposure; and (7) *Associate Learning*, which tests recall for an orally presented list of five semantically related (easy) and five unrelated word pairs (hard) over three trials.

Although Wechsler (1945) originally introduced two forms of the WMS, only form I has been adequately normed for clinical use. We still lack sufficient data to draw inferences about the integrity of a person's memory based on assessment with form II of the WMS, although it has frequently been used in test–retest situations. Researchers and clinicians, therefore, have relied on form I of the WMS to provide evidence for the integrity of memory function. See Lezak (1995, pp. 500–502) and Spreen and Strauss (1998, pp. 373–387) for further information regarding characteristics of the WMS battery and neuropsychological findings.

WMS-R (1987)

The Wechsler Memory Scale-Revised (WMS-R) was introduced in 1987 and is described by the test publisher as a "diagnostic and screening device for use as part of a general neuropsychological examination, or any other clinical examination requiring the assessment of memory functions" (Wechsler, 1987, p. 1). Several changes were made in this first major revision of the WMS, including modifications of test items and administration procedures. New subtests were added to assess spatial and figural memory, and

[1] The authors gratefully acknowledge the contributions of Paul Satz and David Schretlen to an early version of this chapter as it originally appeared in D'Elia, Satz & Schretlen (1989).

delayed recall testing on most subtests is incorporated as standard procedure. Scoring accuracy was greatly improved by the provision of detailed scoring procedures.

Overall, the significant improvements in scoring criteria and administration procedures for the WMS-R permit a more valid assessment of memory than was possible with the original WMS.

A brief overview of the WMS-R follows. The full battery includes information and orientation questions, eight short-term memory tasks, and four delayed recall trials, all of which take about 45 minutes to 1 hour to administer. Four of the six information and all five of the orientation questions from the original WMS were retained, and three new questions were added, so there are a total of 14 scorable information and orientation questions (as opposed to 11 in the original WMS). The presentation of the Mental Control subtest was left unchanged, except that bonus points are no longer assigned for fast, perfect performance.

The Digit Span subtest uses a different sequence of numbers from the original WMS and begins with series that are shorter by one digit. Paragraph 1 of the WMS-R Logical Memory subtest is similar to the one used in the original WMS with only slight modification. It seems that Anna found new employment, but unfortunately still in the old neighborhood. Although she appears to have a bit more spendable income, she is still having difficulty making ends meet. Regarding paragraph 2, the American liner New York was scrapped and in its place a new story about a trucking company accident which undoubtedly left the driver with "egg on his face." Immediate and 30-minute delay recall are assessed. A detailed scoring method awards full credit for either a verbatim *or* "gist" response. The WMS-R Verbal Paired Associates subtest uses four of the six easy and all four of the hard pairs found on the Associate Learning subtest of the original WMS. The revised edition provides up to six trials to correctly learn all the pairs, and equal credit is awarded to all pairs, regardless of difficulty. Delayed recall for the pairs is assessed after 30 minutes.

The Visual Reproduction subtest is also familiar in that two of the three original WMS stimulus cards were retained. Two additional cards were added: one containing one design, the other containing two designs. Although this subtest was intended to assess nonverbal learning and memory, all stimulus cards are, unfortunately, easy to verbally encode. Immediate and 30-minute delay recall for the designs are assessed. A detailed set of scoring criteria for the designs was developed.

Three additional subtests were added to the WMS-R which purport to assess aspects of nonverbal (visual) memory. The Visual Paired Associates subtest was developed as an analog to the Verbal Paired Associates (word pairs) subtest. This test presents six colors, one at a time, in association with a different design. Immediately following presentation of the six pairs, the design is presented alone and the subject is to remember the name of the color paired with the design. Although this subtest was developed with the intention to "minimize the role of verbal mediation in memorizing and responding to the figure–color pairs," it appears that four of the six designs can be readily verbally encoded. A 30-minute delay recall of the figure–color pairs is also assessed.

The Figural Memory subtest was developed as a measure of nonverbal (visual) recognition memory. The subject is shown a set of shaded geometric designs which *are* difficult to verbally encode. After the designs are removed, multiple-choice recognition memory for the design is assessed.

The Visual Memory Span subtest is a variant of the Corsi Cube Test, which is itself a variant of the Knox Cube Imitation Test. (See Lezak, 1995, pp. 361–363, for discussion of Knox Cube and Corsi Block-Tapping tests.) For this WMS-R subtest, eight like-colored squares are printed on a card in random order. As in Corsi's task, every time the examiner taps the squares in a prearranged sequence, the subject attempts to copy the tapping pattern. Part two requires the subject to tap out the pattern in the reverse order.

The original WMS Memory Quotient (MQ) was replaced with five composite scores intended to differentiate separate memory mechanisms. However, it should be noted that the scores bottom out at 50, so the test may generate an overestimation of memory functioning in individuals with severe memory impairments.

The WMS-R is purported to provide norms for individuals aged 16 years 0 months to 74 years 11 months; however, close inspection of the technical manual reveals that the norms for the age groups 18–19, 25–34, and 45–54 were interpolated on the basis of the scores of the adjacent sampled age groups.

Although the WMS-R is a better battery of memory tests than the original WMS, several reviews of the test suggested there was still room for improvement (D'Elia et al., 1989; Chelune et al., 1989; Elwood, 1991). Please refer to Lezak (1995, pp. 502–505) and Spreen and Srauss (1998, pp. 391–415) for information regarding neuropsychological findings as well as further presentation of the merits and limitations of the WMS-R.

WMS-III (1997)

The WMS-III is an individually administered battery of 11 subtests of learning, memory, and working memory. Six of the subtests are included in the core battery, and five subtests are considered optional/supplemental. In comparison with the WMS-R, administration time has been reduced. Administering the WMS-III core battery (i.e., six subtests) takes approximately 30–35 minutes, and administering the five supplementary scales adds another 30 minutes to the process. All the memory subtests include a delayed recognition procedure to enable the differentiation of retrieval vs. encoding deficits. The WMS-III was co-normed with the WAIS-III, and their joint factor index scores permit ability/memory comparisons.

The WMS-III includes six subtests from the WMS-R, although most have been altered and improved (Information and Orientation, Digit Span, Mental Control, Verbal Paired Associates, Logical Memory, and Visual Reproduction). The scoring sensitivities of these subtests have been generally improved by extending the floor and raising the ceiling. The WMS-R Figural Fluency and Visual-Paired Associate subtests have been deleted from the WMS-III battery. Four new subtests have been added to the test battery (Faces, Family Pictures, Word Lists and Letter-Number Sequencing).

A brief description of the WMS-III subtests follows: With the exception of minor changes to

the wording of one question, the Information and Orientation subtest is essentially unchanged from the WMS-R version. Regarding the Logical Memory subtest, in story A, poor old Anna is still living in the same neighborhood and experiencing the same problems. One very minor change to the description of her plight was made. Regarding story B, the macho truck driver from the WMS-R was evidently fired, and now a new story is offered about a man living in San Francisco who prefers watching old movies. The new story B was reportedly developed so that it would "be less likely to evoke an emotional reaction from some examinees" (p. 13).

Regarding the immediate recall condition, similar to the WMS-R, the examiner separately requests recall for story A and story B following each presentation. However, unlike the WMS-R, the WMS-III examiner presents story B a second time, to increase the likelihood of learning story B details. Immediate recall for story B is then reassessed. Following an approximately 30-minute delay, recall for stories A and B is again captured.

Scoring procedures for verbatim or near-verbatim recall of the stories have been tightened; numerous examples are offered in the manual to improve interrater reliability. A supplemental scoring procedure has also been developed to allow examiners to characterize the subjects' "gist" or thematic recall of the stories. Following free recall for both stories after an approximately 30 minute delay, recognition memory is tested utilizing 30 questions probing for details about stories A and B.

The WMS-III manual does not present any standardized administration guidelines regarding the speed (slow, medium, fast) of reading the stories to the subject; nor does it comment on the intonation, pauses, or inflection of the presentation. It is known that the speed of presentation of similar prose passages can affect delayed recall performance (Shum et al., 1997). In order to ensure a standardized administration and improve the reliability and validity of the subtest (especially when the test is being administered by trainees, interns, etc.), a cassette-taped version of the two stories using a medium speed (Shum et al., 1997) should be considered for future versions of this subtest.

The Faces subtest is new to the WMS-III but will be familiar to anyone who has used the Warrington Faces Test (Warrington, 1984) or the Denman Neuropsychology Memory Scale (Denman, 1984). The WMS-III Faces subtest uses a recognition paradigm to assess visual immediate and visual delayed memory by presenting a series of 24 faces to the subject and then showing them a second series of 48 faces and requesting that they identify only the 24 faces that they had been previously shown. Approximately 30 minutes later, the subject is again shown the series of 48 faces and again requested to identify the 24 faces they had initially seen.

All eight Verbal Paired Associates word pairs from the WMS-R have been replaced with novel, unrelated word pairs. The ceiling has been raised by an expanded word-pair list. The WMS-R provided for eight learning trials; however, only four learning trials of the word-pair list are administered for the WMS-III. Following an approximately 30-minute delay, cued recall is elicited, with the examiner offering the first word of each pair and the subject expected to provide the second or "associated" word. There is also a subsequent recognition task, where the examiner reads a list of 24 word pairs, and the subject must identify the pair as either "new" or from the previous condition.

The Family Pictures subtest is new to the WMS-III, is purported to be the visual analog to the Logical Memory subtest, and requires recall of the characters, their scene activity, and spatial location. The Family Pictures subtest is a multimodality test of memory in that the family scenes are visually presented but can also be verbally encoded. The subject is initially shown a "family portrait" card of six family members along with the family dog and told that these will be the characters on four subsequent scene cards. The subject is then shown the four cards for 10 seconds each and requested to try and recall as much about each of the scenes as possible. After all four cards have been exposed, recall for the characters in the scene, their location, and their action is elicited for each card. Approximately 30 minutes later, the recall paradigm is repeated for all four cards.

The Word Lists subtest is new to the scale and is considered optional; however, it will be familiar to anyone who has administered the Rey Auditory Verbal Learning Test (Rey, 1964) or California Verbal Learning Test (Delis et al., 1987). The WMS-III version presents a list of 12 semantically unrelated words to be learned across four learning trials. Following the learning trials, the subject is presented with a one-trial distractor list to learn, followed by recall for the first, original list. The subject is told that recall for the first list will be later assessed. Approximately 30 minutes later, recall for the first list is obtained, followed by an auditory recognition protocol.

The Visual Reproduction subtest, a former core WMS-R subtest, is optional for the WMS-III and consists of five design cards, some of which are easy to verbally encode. Cards A , C, and D remain from the WMS-R; however, card B has been dropped. Two additional design cards are offered—one of which is a modification of a card resurrected from the original WMS (1945). Similar to the WMS-R, immediate and ~30-minute delay recall for the designs is assessed. However, unlike the WMS-R, following the delay condition there is a 48-item recognition task, a direct copy condition and a seven-item discrimination condition, allowing for evaluation of motor vs. memory performance. The scoring criteria have been improved to allow for partial credit, rather than the all-or-nothing WMS-R approach.

The Letter-Number Sequencing subtest is new to the WMS-III and is a measure of auditory working memory. The subject is read seven, ever-increasing, strings of letters and numbers, the first starting with just a single number–letter pair, and the final string containing eight elements in four pairs (e.g., 7-N-1-Q-4-V,-3-O). Following each string presentation, the subject must remember the numbers and letters and then repeat them, saying the numbers first in ascending order and then the letters in alphabetical order.

The WMS-III Spatial Span subtest stimuli have been modified from the WMS-R two-dimensional, eight-like colored square format, to a three-dimensional 10-block board format patterned after the WAIS-R NI Spatial Span Board (Kaplan et al., 1991a). The administration is otherwise identical to the WMS-R—namely, the subject is asked to replicate an increasingly long series of visually presented spatial locations that are tapped out on the stimulus block tops. Every time the examiner taps the blocks in a prearranged sequence, the subject attempts to copy the tapping pattern. Part two of the test requires the subject to tap out the pattern in the reverse order.

The Mental Control subtest is considered an optional test and consists of eight items. The ceiling has been raised by expanded content. Counting backwards by 3's has been deleted, and six new tasks have been created. As was true for the WMS (1945) but not for the WMS-R (1987), bonus points are awarded for fast, perfect performance. As a result, a possible 40 points can be generated from the eight items.

The Digit Span subtest is optional on the WMS-III and is identical to the WAIS-III version. It is similar to the WMS-R version with the exceptions that the Digit Span Forward test now begins with a two-digit sequence and ends with a nine-digit sequence. For Digit Span Backwards, an eight-digit sequence has been added. The administration and scoring procedures are otherwise identical to the WMS-R. This subtest is identical to that found on the WAIS-III.

Only six of the WMS-III subtests are considered primary subtests (Logical Memory, Verbal Paired Associates, Faces, Family Pictures, Letter–Number Sequencing, and Spatial Span), and all these must be administered in order to calculate the WMS-III index scores. The primary subtests can be administered in 30 to 35 minutes.

The Information and Orientation, Word Lists, Visual Reproduction, Digit Span, and Mental Control subtests are considered optional subtests and do not contribute to the WMS-III index scores but are utilized to obtain supplementary information.

The structure of the WMS-III is substantially different from the WMS-R in that the number of summary indexes has been increased from five to eight and they reflect the significant revisions to the content of the test. The WMS-III provides for the calculation of eight Primary index scores and four Auditory Process Composite scores. The Primary indexes are considered by the publishers to be core to evaluating memory functioning, whereas the Auditory Process Composites are considered sup-

plementary scales to be utilized in helping to better isolate and characterize various processes in memory functioning, such as single trial learning vs. learning over trials, retention, and retrieval.

The method of calculating the WMS-III index scores is also different from the WMS-R (see pp. 190–197, *WMS-III Technical Manual,* 1997). There are three primary indexes for auditorily processed material (Auditory Immediate, Auditory Delayed, and Auditory Recognition Delayed), two primary indexes for visually processed materials (Visual Immediate, Visual Delayed), and three primary indexes assessing multimodality memory functioning (Immediate Memory, Working Memory, and General Memory).

The WMS-III and WAIS-III were co-normed, with the WMS-III randomly administered to approximately one half of the WAIS-III standardization participants within each standardization stratification variable category. The standardization sample for the WAIS-III included 2,450 adults selected to be representative of the U.S. population of adults aged 16–89 years in the year 1995. The collected sample was stratified for age, sex, race/ethnicity, education level, and geographic region. The standardization test sites were divided into four regions of the country: Northeast, North Central, South, and West. The WMS-III standardization sample includes 1,250 individuals ranging in age from 16 to 89 years, divided into 13 age-group categories as presented in Table 15.1.

Table 15.1. WMS.Standard; Sample Sizes for 13 Age Groupings for the WMS-III Standardization Sample

Age Category	Sample Size
16–17	100
18–19	100
20–24	100
25–29	100
30–34	100
35–44	100
45–54	100
55–64	100
65–69	100
70–74	100
75–79	100
80–84	75
85–89	75

Although previous research with the WMS and WMS-R showed that better performance was positively correlated with higher education, currently, age/education normative information for the WMS-III is not separately available. However, because the WAIS-III and WMS-III were co-normed, one can readily compare performance on the WMS-III with IQ. Both tests have summary indexes with means of 100 and standard deviation scores of 15 points.

The WMS-III represents a significant improvement over previous incarnations of Wechsler's Memory battery and should be considered a welcome addition to the neuropsychologist's armamentarium.

RELATIONSHIP BETWEEN WMS PERFORMANCE AND DEMOGRAPHIC FACTORS

It has long been accepted that memory functions decline with age (Botwinick, 1981). Advancing age appears to have a differentially negative effect on WMS performance, with short- and long-term term memory for new information (i.e., as generally reflected in the performance on Visual Reproduction, Logical Memory and Associate Learning subtests) impacted more strongly than memory for old information (i.e., Personal & Current Information, Orientation, Mental Control subtests). On delayed recall tasks, normal elderly tend to retain more than 80% of the material originally learned (Spreen & Strauss, 1991).

The WMS and WMS-R Visual Reproduction (VR) subtest appears to be the most sensitive to deterioration with age (Ivnik et al., 1992b; Lezak, 1995), whereas immediate recall performance on the Logical Memory subtest remains relatively stable through middle age, and then starts to decline. However, Logical Memory delay recall performance begins to gradually decline in the 30s through 50s, after which the decline accelerates (Wechsler, 1987). Lezak (1995) cautions that for older age groups in the WMS-R standardization, education and age are strongly negatively correlated, thereby making it difficult to disentangle their individual impact on performance. The WMS-R manual, however, notes that "the user should keep the effects

of age in mind when interpreting Index scores (p. 77)," since these scores reflect performance relative to an age-peer group. Wechsler (1987) notes that an index score of 100 obtained by an older adult in their 70s, although average, would not reflect the same level of *absolute* performance when compared to a young adult in his or her 20s also obtaining the same index score.

The question of gender differences in performance has been more controversial. On the VR subtest, while some authors have reported no gender effects (Trahan et al., 1988), Ivison (1977) found that women performed slightly worse than men. The WMS-R manual reports that males and females do not significantly differ on the WMS-R indexes. Moderate correlations have been generally reported between education and memory functioning (Lezak, 1995; Wechsler, 1987). Ivnik et al. (1992b), in examining VR performance, found it was a significant variable in older adults, with better performance noted for those who were better educated. Years of education were found to be significantly correlated with all WMS-R indexes (Wechsler, 1987). Richardson and Marottoli (1996) note that adjustment for lower levels of education is especially important when testing the elderly, since the "educational attainment of both White and non White Americans aged 75 years and older is less than 12 years (median for Whites = 11.6 years, median for non Whites < 8 years, median for all ethnic = 10.9 years). As Stern et al. (1992) have emphasized, "utilization of standard non-education corrected normative data will frequently result in normal subjects being misclassified as impaired or demented, especially if they are older and have low education (e.g., <8 years)."

The effect of IQ on subtest performance remains controversial. However, an examination of correlation tables provided in the WMS-R manual suggests modest correlations with IQ for many of the WMS-R subtests.

The WMS-III manual does not specifically present information on the effects of sex and education/IQ on individual aspects of subtest performance; however, examination of the normative data tables does show the expected decline in performance starting in the 30s and accelerating in the 50s through 70s.

METHOD FOR EVALUATING THE NORMATIVE REPORTS

In order to adequately evaluate the WMS, WMS-R, and WMS-III normative reports, eight key criterion variables were deemed crucial. The first five of these relate to *subject* variables, and the remaining three dimensions relate to *procedural* variables.

Minimal requirements for meeting the criterion variables were as follows:

Subject Variables

Age-Group Interval

Since Wechsler's original intention was to tie memory to IQ, and because of the well-documented correlation between memory and age, WAIS-R age-interval groupings were adopted as the standard against which to compare the WMS and WMS-R studies, whereas the age group intervals of the WAIS-III were utilized for the WMS-III.

Sample Size

As Wechsler (1987) noted, 50 cases have generally been recommened (Hayes, 1963; Guilford, 1965) as providing a reliable estimate of the population mean. Following Wechsler's (1987) lead and for the purpose of review, a minimum of 50 subjects per age-group interval was deemed adequate.

Sample Composition Description

Pertinent information should minimally include data regarding medical and psychiatric exclusion criteria and geographic area.

Reporting of IQ and/or Education Levels

Since performance on the WMS, WMS-R and WMS-III is known to be positively correlated with IQ and education, the means and standard deviations for years of education and/or estimated IQ should be reported.

Reporting of Gender

Given equivocal evidence of an effect of gender on performance, at the least, information on the gender distribution of the sample should be reported.

Procedural Variables

Inclusion of a Delayed Recall Condition

In order to assess storage and rates of forgeting over time, the addition of a delayed recall condition to assess long-term memory is essential.

Description of Scoring Procedures

A clear statement of the method used for scoring the WMS, WMS-R, and WMS-III is critical. Several methods are currently available for scoring the original WMS and WMS-R (Crosson et al., 1984b; Power et al., 1979; Schear, 1986; Schwartz & Ivnik, 1980; Wechsler, 1945). It is important to keep in mind that application of any one of these scoring procedures to the same protocol will result in a different score reflecting the patient's performance. *Therefore, the scoring method used in the normative report must be identical to that used by the clinician in order to insure appropriate comparison.*

Data Reporting

Mean and standard deviation scores should be provided at minimum.

With these requirements for reporting in mind, the normative studies for the WMS, WMS-R, and WMS-III were examined.

SUMMARY OF THE STATUS OF THE NORMS FOR THE WMS, WMS-R, AND WMS-III

Of the 27 reviewed reports for the original WMS, form I, 15 present data for groups residing in the United States (Abikoff et al., 1987; Bak & Greene, 1980; Bigler et al., 1981; Haaland et al., 1983; Heaton et al., 1991; Hulicka, 1966; Ivnik et al., 1991; Mitrushina & Satz, 1991; Russell, 1975; Russell & Starkey, 1993; Ryan et al., 1987; Schaie & Strother, 1968a; Trahan et al., 1988; Van Gorp et al., 1989; Wechsler, 1945). Nine studies report data for individuals living elsewhere, including three studies for Canadian individuals (Klonoff & Kennedy, 1965, 1966; Cauthen, 1977), four for Australian groups (Ivinskis et al., 1971; Ivison, 1977, 1986; desRosiers & Ivison, 1986), and one study each for British (Kear-Colwell & Heller, 1978) and Turkish populations (Gilleard & Gilleard, 1989).

Performance on the Wechsler Memory Test batteries is known to be positively correlated with IQ (Lezak, 1995); however, reports of WMS and WMS-R comparison data which control for IQ are surprisingly unavailable. Ivnik et al. (1991) provide IQ and education norms for the WMS for a very broadly defined age group (i.e., 65–97). In addition to the age category being too broad, the sample size within each of the age/education categories was very small (i.e., <30 subjects per cell). Cauthen (1977) reports WMS and Mittenberg et al. (1992) reports WMS-R scores for subjects grouped by IQ estimates within each age-group interval; however, these results were also based on small sample sizes. Almost every study compensates, to some degree, for this limitation by reporting mean IQ and/or educational level for subject groups. Still, an empirical basis for judgments about the range of normal variance in memory that is attributable to variation in IQ cannot be found in the literature at this time for the original WMS or WMS-R or WMS-III.

Almost without exception, WMS studies published subsequent to Russell's (1975) article include a delayed recall condition on one or more subtests, usually Logical Memory and Visual Reproduction. However, some investigators (Bak & Greene, 1980; Haaland et al., 1983; Trahan et al., 1988; Ivnik, et al., 1991) follow Russell's procedure of interposing 30 minutes between the immediate and delayed recall conditions, while others have used delays of 45 minutes (Van Gorp et al., 1990; Mitrushina & Satz, 1991a,b), 1 hour (Cauthen, 1977), and even 24 hours (Abikoff et al., 1987). For subjects under 50 years of age, only Abikoff et al. (1987) provide WMS normative data for delayed recall of the Logical Memory subtest. Trahan et al. (1988), Ryan et al. (1987), and Ivnik et al. (1991) provide normative data for the delayed recall of the Visual Reproduction subtest of the original WMS. There are no studies that provide reliable WMS delayed recall normative data for the Associate Learning subtest for U.S. populations. Delayed recall data for any subtest of the original WMS are scant for subjects under 20 years of age.

All seven of the WMS-R normative reports reviewed present data from U.S. populations, with one presenting data for low education, rural-residing individuals (Marcopulous et al., 1997).

There are currently *no* published data available regarding recognition testing on delay for any of the original WMS or WMS-R subtests. Without assessing delay recognition for the material not freely recalled, one is unsure whether the patient primarily has an *encoding* or a *retrieval* problem. Fortunately, the WMS-III corrects this problem by providing a recognition component following the delayed recall condition on the memory subtests. However, the WMS and WMS-R tests should be considered as providing a limited assessment of memory functioning until similar procedures are developed and data become available.

The WMS-III is adequately normed from ages 16 to 89 years.

Table 15.2 summarizes information provided in the studies described in this chapter.

SUMMARIES OF THE STUDIES

This section presents critiques of the various normative and clinical studies for the WMS, WMS-R, and WMS-III. The studies are reviewed in chronological order.

Wechsler Memory Scale

[WMS.1] Wechsler, 1945

This is the standardization of the original WMS. This report provides data for 20–29 ($N = 50$)- and 40–49 ($N = 46$)-year-olds. Wechsler-Bellevue *IQ scores* are provided for each age group interval. Wechsler did not provide information regarding the population from which his normative sample was drawn, with the exception that they were "not hospital patients." No delayed recall condition was included in Wechsler's original report because the concept of secondary memory had not been formulated at the time.

Study strengths
  1. Reported age-group intervals are adequate.
  2. Sample size is adequate.
  3. IQ scores are reported.

4. Data reporting included mean and standard deviation scores.

5. Scoring procedures are adequately described.

Considerations regarding use of the study
1. Data were collected almost a half-century ago, raising questions of cohort effects.
2. No delayed recall condition.
3. Sample composition is not adequately described in terms of exclusion criteria.
4. No information on years of education is provided.
5. No information on gender.

Other comments
1. There is an inconsistency in Wechsler's data reporting. The methods section notes that subjects were aged 25 to 50 years. However, in the tabular presentation of the results, data were shown for two groups: 20–29 (n = 50) and 40–49 (n = 46) years of age.
2. Wechsler's estimate of IQ was based on the Wechsler-Bellevue scale, which is not equivalent to WAIS, WAIS-R, or WAIS-III values (Table 15.3).

[WMS.2] Klonoff and Kennedy, 1965

This article is entitled "Memory and Perceptual Functioning in Octogenarian and Nonagenarians in the Community" and was intended to provide normative data for the WMS and the Benton Visual Retention Test. The composition of the sample was described as "Canadian veterans able to manage well on their own in the community" (p. 328) (Vancouver, B.C.). Indeed, this is a healthy (self-report = 76.2% very good/good; 23.8% fair), and active (self report = 73.83% very/moderately; 26.17% minimally) sample. The sample consisted of retired community residents and un/semiskilled laborers. The scoring procedures followed those described by Wechsler (1945). Mean education of the sample was 7.04 years.

Although this study was conducted in Canada, only 19.19% of the sample were born in Canada; 72.68% were born in the British Isles and 8.13% in other countries of Europe. This is basically a "blue-collar" sample (skilled, semiskilled = 35.47%; unskilled = 47.10%; professional, semiprofessional, service = 17.43%).

Because only mean values are reported (no standard deviation values available), the data from this study should be used with caution.

Study strengths
1. Age-group intervals are adequate.
2. Scoring procedures are adequately described.
3. Information about education was obtained for 155 of the 172 subjects.
4. The description of the sample composition is adequate with information regarding SES and geographic area provided.

Considerations regarding use of the study
1. Sample size is small.
2. No IQ data are provided.
3. No delayed recall testing was administered.
4. Data reporting is insufficient, in that only mean performance scores (no standard deviations) are presented.
5. Data collected in Canada, raising questions regarding clinical utility for use in the United States.
6. No medical or psychiatric exclusion criteria.
7. No information on gender.
8. This is a generally low educated sample.

Other comments
1. These investigators were the first to extend Wechsler's original norms, by providing data for seniors aged 80–92 years (Table 15.4).

[WMS.3] Klonoff and Kennedy, 1966

This study compared memory and perceptual functioning in two matched groups of military veteran octogenerians and nonagenerians—one residing in the community (e.g., subjects from WMS.2), the other hospitalized and under custodial care. The age-group category for both the community (80–92; Mean = 83.6 [2.48] years) and custodial-care group (80–93; Mean = 84.1 [2.9] years) is broad. No data on education or IQ was provided; however, since the community sample was drawn from the previous study (see WMS.2), it is probably safe to assume a mean educational level of about 7 years for this group. Educational level of the custodial care group is unknown.

Table 15.2. WMS.L; WMS, WMS-R, WMS-III Normative Data Locator Table

Study	Age Groups	Sample Size	Sample Composition	IQ and/or Education	Length of Delay	Scoring Method	Subtests Administered	Special Notes	Country/Locale
WMS.1 Wechsler, 1945 page 274	20–29 40–49	50 46	"Not hospital patients" both men and women	Mean IQ 102.9 (5.5) 102.0 (6.6) Wechsler-Bellevue IQ's	No delay condition	All or none	Full WMS		USA (New York)
WMS.2 Klonoff & Kennedy 1965 page 275	80 81 82 83 84–85 86+	35 34 23 27 26 27	Male Canadian vets able to manage well on their own in the community. Random sample of vets living in Vancouver. 75% in good/very good health; 23% fair health	Group mean education = 7.04 years	No delay condition	All or none	Full WMS	Scores do not provide information on standard deviation, so difficult to use data for inferential purposes	Canada (Vancouver)
WMS.3 Klonoff & Kennedy, 1966 page 275	Community sample 80–92 Hospital sample 80–93	115 115	Randomly selected from 1965 data base (all males) Randomly selected from a testable group of custodial care residents at a veterans hospital (all male)	No information No information	No delay condition No delay condition	All or none All or none	Full WMS Full WMS	93% blue collar, 72% good/very good health; 28% fair health 88% blue collar, 43% fair health, 57% poor/very poor health	Canada (Vancouver)
WMS.4 Hulicka, 1966 page 288	15–17 30–39 60–69 70–79 80–89	43 53 70 46 25	High school students or recent dropouts. Hospitalized vets. Composite of hospitalized vets, residents of senior homes, and members of senior clubs	Education = 11.6 (0.9) years 10.7 (2.3) 8.9 (3.1) 8.6 (2.6) 8.6 (2.8)	No delay condition No delay condition	No information	Full WMS except that Orientation subtest was not administered	Perfect scores for orientation subtest were substituted in calculating WMS total raw score	USA
WMS.5 Schaie & Strother, 1968a page 289	70–88	50	25 males, 25 females optimally functioning retired university professors and	All had minimum of B.A. degree (e.g., ≥16 years)	No delay condition	No information	Full WMS	No standard deviation scores reported, so difficult to use data for inferential purposes	USA

Study	Age range	N	Sample	IQ / Education	Delay condition	Scoring method	WMS version	Notes	Country
WMS.6 Ivinskis et al., 1971 page 289	10–14	30	professional workers who responded to appeals in newspapers / Male and female students from local primary and high schools	WISC IQ = 108.5 (12.2)	No delay condition	No information	Full WMS		Australia
	16–18	44	Male and female students from local high schools	WAIS IQ = 107.7 (7.7)					
WMS.7 Russell, 1975 page 290	Controls: No range reported. Age = 36.5 (14.2) years	30	Controls referred from neurology. psychiatry and extebded care services with no history of brain damage. 93% male	Education 12.5 (2.9) years		Russell method	Logical memory & visual Reproduction subtests only		USA (Miami)
	Brain-damaged sample No range reported. Age = 42.0 (14.3) years	75	Referred from neurology wards, psychiatric outpatient and extended care clinics with verified brain damage (heterogeneous etiology)	Education 11.6 (2.9) years	30-minute delay				
WMS.8 Cauthen, 1977 page 291	20–29	15	Healthy male & female volunteers. No further info on S's provided	WAIS IQ 100–135		No informaiton	Logical memory subtest only		Canada (Calgary)
	30–39	14		100–135					
	40–49	13		100–135					
	50–59	9		107–135	1-hour delay		Full WMS		
	60–69	20	Healthy male & female volunteers, the majority of whom were living in institutional settings	80–140					
	70–79	18		80–140					
	80–89	22		80–140					
	90–94	4		no information					
WMS.9 Ivison, 1977 page 292	20–69	500	Male and female in-patients suffering from no known memory, neurological or psychiatric impairment recruited from general medical/surgical wards	No information	No delay condition	According to Ivison	Full WMS	Alterations made to test content to avoid American idioms or references	Australia (Sydney)

continued

Table 15.2. (*Continued*)

Study	Age Groups	Sample Size	Sample Composition	IQ and/or Education	Length of Delay	Scoring Method	Subtests Administered	Special Notes	Country/ Locale
WMS10. Kear-Colwell & Heller, 1978 page 293	17–34	56	Stratified quota sample of health service employees in a hospital in England	No information	No delay condition	No information	Full WMS		England
	35–64	60							
WMS.11 Bak & Greene, 1980 page 294	50–62	15	Male and female active, healthy adults recruited from large metropolitan areas	Education 13.7 (1.9) years	30 minute delay	Russell (1975) method	Logical memory visual repro-duction, & associate learning subtests only	Scoring procedure for the Associate Learning subtest not described, but is available from authors	USA (Texas)
	67–86	15		14.9 (3.0) years					
WMS.12 Bigler et al., 1981a page 295	16–20	10	Selected group of male and female patients from a neurology clinic with complaints of head-ache but subsequently found to have no serious neurological disorder. Oldest group stringently selected to assure maximally healthy sample	WAIS IQ = 113.2 (11.6) Education = 11.1 (0.9) years			Full WMS	Cutoff scores between last two age groups were inconsistently reported in the text tables	USA (Texas)
	21–35	15		WAIS IQ = 112.2 (14.6) Educaiton = 13.9 (2.1) years	No delay condition	No informaiton			
	36–50	12		WAIS IQ = 110.3 (10.1) Education = 14.4 (3.3) years					
	51–75	14		WAIS IQ = 118.6 (7.9) Educaiton = 14.4 (4.1) years					
WMS.13 Haaland et al., 1983 page 295	65–69	49	A group of healthy, highly educated, motivated, non-institutionalized primarily Caucasian aged adults—both males and females	No information	30-minute delay	Wechsler (1945)	Logical memory & visual repro-duction subtests only	Informed Ss that delay recall would be assessed. Half-points were given for incomplete LM responses only if retained original wording	USA (New Mexico)
	70–74	74							
	75–79	40							
	80+	13							

Study	Type	Age	N	Sample	Education/Demographics	Delay	Subtest	Comments	Location
WMS. 14 Crosson et al., 1984 page 296	Meta-analytic study							Meta-analytically derived clinical comparison data.	
WMS.15 Margolis & Scialfa, 1984 page 297	Meta-analytic study							Meta-analytically derived "norms"	
WMS.16 Wallace, 1984 page 297	Meta-analytic study							Meta-analytically derived "norms"	
WMS.17 Ivison, 1986 page 297		20–29 / 30–39 / 40–49 / 50–59 / 60–69	100 / 100 / 100 / 100 / 100	See Ivison (1977)	No information	No delay condition	See Ivison (1977) Logical memory subtest only	See Ivison (1977) Reanalysis of 1977 data	Australia (Sydney)
WMS.18 desRosiers & Ivison, 1986 page 297		20–29 / 30–39 / 40–49 / 50–59 / 60–69	M 50 F 50 / M 50 F 50 / M 50 F 50 / M 50 F 50 / M 50 F 50	Medical and surgical inpatients with no known neurological or psychiatric impairment	No information	No delay conditions According to Ivison (1977)	Paired associates subtest only	This article presents reanalyzed data from Ivison's 1977 paper. It provides comparison data for the recall of high and low associate pairs	Australia (Sydney)
WMS. 19 Ryan et al., 1987 page 298		21–30 / 31–40 / 41–50 / 51–59	55 / 45 / 44 / 38	182 Caucasian native English-speaking blue-collar workers with exposure to heavy metals and toxic substances with no reported psychiatric or neurological problems	Education 12.3 (1.4) / 11.9 (2.2) / 11.3 (1.8) / 11.0 (1.8)	30-minute delay	Wechsler (1945) Visual reproduction subtest scoring procedure was modified allowing bonus points for accuracy of spatial relationship		USA (eastern Pennsylvania)

continued

Table 15.2. (*Continued*)

Study	Age Groups	Sample Size	Sample Composition	IQ and/or Education	Length of Delay	Scoring Method	Subtests Administered	Special Notes	Country/Locale
WMS.20 Abikoff, et al., 1987 page 299	18–29 30–39 40–49 50–59 60–69 70–80+	74 67 41 54 56 47	Male and female paid volunteers recruited from local businesses community organizations, or employee pool of the medical center in New York	Data are presented for five separate educational levels (e.g., 8 years) thru graduate school)	30-minute 24-hour delay scores are available	Wechsler (1945) & Schwartz & Ivnik (1980)	Logical memory subtest only	Data are presented for Forms I and II of the WMS for logical memory subtest "Gist" scoring procedure for Form II not described	USA (New York)
WMS.21 Trahan, et al., 1988 page 300	18–29 30–41 42–53 54–65 66–77 78–89	96 40 36 19 29 11	Neurologically normal, healthy adults—both male and female	Education = 13.7 (1.9) years 14.7 (2.4) years 14.3 (2.9) years 13.8 (1.8) years 16.5 (3.1) years 13.9 (2.8) years	30-minute delay	Wechsler (1945)	Visual Reproduction subtest only		USA (Texas)
WMS.22 Gilleard & Gilleard, 1989 page 301	20–39 40–59	120 80	Turkish subjects from a variety of urban and rural areas	Each age group partitioned into two educational groups (1) nil or elementary, (2) secondary or above	No delay condition	No information	Full WMS	The study purpose was to compare Turkish and Anglo-American normative data on the WMS, using Turkish translation of form 1, and employing minor procedureal modifications	Turkey
WMS.23 van Gorp, et al., 1987 page 302	58–65 66–70 71–75	28 45 57	Group of very intelligent, healthy males and females residing in a retirement community	VIQ = 117.2 (11.3) PIQ = 109.2 (11.6) VIQ = 114.8 (17.0) PIQ = 111.5 (16.8) VIQ = 122.9 (11.4) PIQ =	45-minute delay	No information	Logical memory & visual reproduction subtests only	Group mean education 14.1 (2.9) years	USA (California)

Study	Age	N	Sample description	IQ / Education	Delay	Method	Subtest	Comments	Country
	76–85	26		115.1 (11.9) VIQ = 110.5 (11.2) PIQ = 101.0 (8.8) All above are Satz-Mogel WAIS-R estimates					USA (Rochester, Minnesota)
WMS.24 Ivnik et al., 1991 page 303	65–97	99	"Neither unusually healthy nor unhealthy" older Caucasian adult patients recruited from a community-based internal medicine private practice in Rochester, Minnesota. All volunteer subjects were screened medically and psychiatrically for absence of cognitive difficulty (Folstein MMSE >23)	WAIS-R FIQ = 100.4 (11.1) VIQ = 97.5 (12.3) PIQ = 99.3 (11.6) mean education = 12.4 (3.3) years	30-minute delay. Russell (1975) protocol	Schwartz & Ivnik (1980) "gist" method	Full WMS with delay for logical memory and visual reproduction subtests only	This study provides IQ and educational norms for a broadly defined age group (i.e., 65–97). Norms reported by WAIS-R FIQ ranges are <90; 90–100; 101–110; >110. Education ranges are <12; 12–15; and >15 years. Sample size within these various IQ and education groups are generally quite small (i.e., <30 subjects). Therefore, use caution in interpretation	USA (Rochester, Minnesota)
WMS.25 Heaton et al., 1991 page 304	20–34 35–39 40–44 45–49 50–59 60–64 65–69 70–74 75–80 X̄ = 46.4 years	378 (no information on sample size within each of the age groups)	Volunteers: urban and rural. Data collected over 15y through multi-center collaboration. Strict exclusion criteria, 65% M. Data are presented in T-score equivalents for M and F separately across 10 age groupings by 6 educational groupings	Education for the whole sample; 13.6 (3.5) years. Range 6–18+ years	4-hour delay	Wechsler & Stone, 1945, production	Visual Reproduction subtest	Data are provided on the Figure Memory Test, which utilizes the figures from the WMS Visual reproduction subtest. Tables provide T-scores corrected for age, education, and sex	USA & Canada (California, Texas, Washington, Oklahoma, Wisconsin, Illinois, Michigan, New York, Virginia, Massachusetts, Canada—provinces unknown)

continued

Table 15.2. (*Continued*)

Study	Age Groups	Sample Size	Sample Composition	IQ and/or Education	Length of Delay	Scoring Method	Subtests Administered	Special Notes	Country/Locale
WMS.26 Mitrushina & Satz, 1991 page 307	57–65	19	Group of healthy, intelligent (49) males and (73) females residing in a planned retirement community	14.4 (2.0) years WAIS-R FSIQ 115.0 (12.1)		Schwartz & Ivnik (1980) "gist" method	WMS logical memory & visual reproduction subtests only	Provides test–retest norms for two annual follow-ups.	USA (California, Camarrilo)
	66–70	40		13.7 (1.8) years WAIS-R FSIQ 119.4 (15.2)	45-minute delay				
	71–75	47		14.5 (3.1) years WAIS-R FSIQ 119.8 (11.3)					
	75–85	16		14.0 (3.8) years WAIS-R FSIQ 114.4 (12.3)					
WMS.27 Russell & Starkey, 1993 page 307	20–29 30–39 40–49 50–59 60–69 70–79 80–89	$n = 200$ for total sample	Neurology patients at the V.A. determined to be "neurologically normal" after a neurological exam.	Data reported at 4 educational/IQ levels	30-minute delay	WMS Russell version or WMS-R version		The authors provide data for the HRNES battery	USA (Cincinatti, Ohio, and Miami Florida)
WMS-R.1 Wechsler, 1987 page 309	16–17	53	Sample designed to represent the normal population of the U.S. Stratified sample based on age, sex, race, and geographic region	Mean WAIS-R FSIQ was 110(15), however, the full WAIS-R was administered only to the 35–44 and 55–69 groups. A 4-test short form was given to the other 4 age groups on whom data were collected	30-minute delay	Wechsler (1987)	Full WMS-R	"Normative data for 18–19, 25–34 and 45–54 age groups were statistically interpolated (i.e., no data were actually collected)	USA (standardization)
	18–19	0							
	20–24	50							
	25–34	0							
	35–44	54							
	45–54	0							
	55–64	54							
	65–69	55							
	70–74	50							

Study	Age	N	Sample description	IQ	Delay	Source	Test	Comments	Country
WMS-R.2 Cullum et al., 1990 page 310	50–70 75–95	47 32	Group of healthy, well-educated community-dwelling older adult volunteers recruited via flyers, newspaper, and subsequently screened via telephone "for neuropsychological risk factors, history of neurological disorder learning disability, major psychiatric disorder, major medical illness or substance abuse." Also excluded if taking any medications which might negatively affect performance on memory tests. Low-dose antihypertensives were allowed		30-minute delay	Wechsler (1987)	Full WMS-R	Provides WMS-R "preliminary norms" for "normal elderly subjects." Forgetting rates for verbal and nonverbal material is also provided	USA (San Diego)
WMS-R.3 Mittenberg et al., 1992 page 310	25–34	50	Sample designed to match 1980 U.S. census data stratified on age, gender ethnicity and education. Differs from WMS-R standardization in that all subjects reside in Florida. Recruited from "local businesses, weekend/evening adult education and vocational/technical classes"	Prorated WAIS-R FSIQ based on Vocabulary and Block Design subtests only. Mean = 101.3 (14.6) Range = 72–131. Median = 100	30-minute delay	Wechsler (1987)	Full WMS-R		USA (Florida)

continued

Table 15.2. (*Continued*)

Study	Age Groups	Sample Size	Sample Composition	IQ and/or Education	Length of Delay	Scoring Method	Subtests Administered	Special Notes	Country/Locale
WMS-R.4 Lichtenberg & Christensen, 1992 page 312	70–74 75–79 80–99	25 23 18	Consecutive admission sample of cognitively intact geriatric medical patients from an urban hospital. About 1/3 had hip fractures, 1/3 had knee replacement due to arthritis, 1/3 showed "deconditioning from lengthy illness." Sample comprised of 43 women, 23 men; 35 Caucasian, 31 black	No information, however, Mattis Dementia Rating Scale cutoff was 129 to insure intact cognition	30-minute delay	Wechsler (1987)	WMS-R logical memory subtest only	Provides clinical comparison data (not normative data) for geriatric medical patients seeking treatment in an urban medical setting	USA (Detroit, Michigan)
WMS-R.5 Ivnik et al., 1992, page 313	Total sample 56–74 75–94 Data tables use midpoint interval method: 56–66 59–69 62–72 65–75 68–78 71–81 74–84 77–87 80–90 83–94	274 167 154 161 169 168 178 160 151 123 84 53	Sample represents a combination of 1). Patients who had a medical exam at the Mayo Clinic and deemed 'normal' because they lacked active neurologic or psychiatric conditions that would compromise cognitive functioning. Chronic medical illness was not an exclusion criterion. All were able to function independently; 2). 'Normal controls' from a research project at Mayo's Alzheimer's	For total sample n = 441 *WAIS-R IQ* VIQ = 105.5 (10.0) PIQ = 107.3 (11.4) FSIQ = 106.6 (10.5) Years of Education ≤7 0.7% 8–11 13.6% 12 39% 13–15 22% 16–17 15%	30-minute	WMS-R converted to Mayo summary scores	Full WMS-R however only allowed 3 learning trials during both the Visual and Verbal Paired Associates 1 subtests. No additional trials were administered if criterion not reached by third trial	Data are reported using the midpoint interval technique (Pauker, 1988) in order to "maximize available information." This research provides a statistically derived estimate of probable WMS-R values for individuals >74 years. NOTE: Mayo and WMS-R summary scores are not interchangeable.	USA (Rochestor and Olmstead County, Minnesota)

Reference	N	Sample	Age	Education	Delay	Source	Subtests	Notes	Location
		Disease Patient Registry. Criterion for normality determination was as above	≥18	9.8% Sample primarily well educated Caucasian older adults from a primarily agricultural region					
WMS-R.6 Richardson & Marottoli, 1996 page 315	101	All autonomously living elderly Ss, current drivers; 48 F, 53 M. Ss are free from neurologic and psychiatric illness	81.5 (3.3) 76–80 81–91	Education for sample 11.0 (3.7) years	30-minute delay	Wechsler (1987)	Logical memory and visual reproduction subtests	Data are presented in age by education cells: <12, ≥12 years	USA (New Haven, Connecticut
WMS-R.7 Marcopullos et al., 1997 page 316	131	Ss were healthy adults over 55 years of age, living in a rural setting	Mean age = 76.48 (7.87) years. 55–64 65–74 75–84 ≥85	Education mean = 6.65 (2.14) years. Range = 0–10 years	30-minute delay	Presumably Wechsler (1987)	Logical memory and visual reproduction subtests	The sudy aimed at development of normative data for rural community-dwelling older adults with no more than 10 years of formal education. Data are reported by age, and age by education. Percent retention was calculated	USA (rural central Virginia
WMS-R abnorms.1 Fox, 1994 page 317	100	37M; 63F	18–63		30-minute delay	Wechsler (1987)	Logical memory	Workers' compensation claimants	USA
WMS-III.1 Wechsler, 1997 page 318	1,250	Nationally collected standardization sample	16–79, partitioned into 11 age groupings		Approximately 30-minute delay	Wechsler (1997)	Full WMS-III	Raw scores are reported which can be converted to scaled scores	USA national standardization

Table 15.3. WMS.1

Age	Infomation	Mental Control	Logical Memory (LM)	LM-A	LM-B	Digits Forward	Digits Back	Visual Reproduction	Paired Associates	Easy	Hard	Memory Score
20–29 (n = 50)	5.96 (0.02)	7.50 (1.97)	9.28 (3.10)	9.80 (3.74)	8.76 (3.37)	7.04 (1.22)	5.26 (1.13)	11.00 (2.73)	15.72 (2.81)	8.56 (0.45)	7.16 (2.63)	68.1 (6.47)
Age	Infomation	Mental Control	Logical Memory (LM)	LM-A	LM-B	Digits Forward	Digits Back	Visual Reproduction	Paired Associates	Easy	Hard	Memory Score
40–49 (n = 46)	5.70 (0.40)	6.61 (1.90)	8.09 (2.52)	8.65 (3.46)	7.54 (2.66)	5.98 (1.12)	4.30 (1.11)	8.35 (3.17)	13.91 (3.12)	8.26 (0.24)	5.70 (2.73)	58.78 (7.12)

Table 15.4. WMS.2

Age	Information	Orientation	Mental Control	Logical Memory (LM)	LM-1	LM-2	Digits Forward	Digits Back	Digits Total	Visual Reproduction	Paired Associates	Memory Quotient (MQ)
80 $n = 35$	5.00	4.57	6.31	5.94	3.03	2.91	6.03	3.89	9.91	4.57	10.34	110.51
81 $n = 34$	5.62	4.88	6.21	6.82	3.53	3.29	6.26	4.24	10.5	3.97	10.24	113.53
82 $n = 23$	5.09	4.87	6.57	7.04	3.61	3.43	6.17	4.04	10.22	4.00	10.7	113.3
83 $n = 27$	5.41	4.59	6.26	5.07	2.44	2.63	6.48	4.04	10.52	3.07	9.04	105.96
84–85 $n = 26$	5.15	4.81	5.00	5.42	3.04	2.38	5.85	4.08	9.92	3.58	10.81	107.62
86+ $n = 27$	4.89	4.56	5.81	5.37	2.48	2.89	5.89	3.74	9.63	3.37	9.56	108.22

The community group is composed of "Canadian male veterans randomly selected from their earlier study (see WMS.2). The hospitalized group consists of male subjects, selected from a testable group group of custodial-care residents at a veterans hospital in Vancouver, British Columbia." Information regarding occupational status (93% blue collar for community group, 88% blue collar for hospital group) and overall health ratings (community = 72% good/very good, 28% fair; hospital group = 43% fair, 57% poor/very poor) were presented.

Study strengths
1. Sample size was adequate.
2. Sample composition description was adequate.
3. Scoring procedures were described (Wechsler, 1945).
4. Data reporting included mean and standard deviation scores.
5. Some information regarding gender is provided.

Considerations regarding use of the study
1. No data on education or IQ were provided.
2. No delayed recall testing was administered.
3. No exclusion criteria of the normative group are reported.
4. Age group interval for both the community and custodial care group is too broad.

Other comments
1. This study provides comparison data for a group of elderly custodial care residents (Table 15.5).

[WMS.4] Hulicka, 1966

This article is entitled, "Age Differences in Wechsler Memory Scale Scores." Data from this study are difficult to apply because, as Hulicka acknowledges, the sample was not representative of a clearly identifiable population. For example, the 15–17-year-old group included high school students or recent dropouts. The 60–90-year-olds comprised a composite of hospitalized veterans, residents of homes for the aged, and members of Golden Age clubs.

Information on years of education and mean raw WAIS Vocabulary subtest scores is provided for each age group:

15–17 group, education = 11.6 years, Vocabulary = 40.2 (12.2)

30–39 hospitalised veterans group, education = 10.7 years, Vocabulary = 41.5 (16.7)

60–69 group, education = 8.9 years, Vocabulary = 42.2 (16.8)

70–79 group, education = 8.6 years, Vocabulary = 39.5 (15.8)

80–89 group, education = 8.6 years, Vocabulary = 40.5 (14.6)

Study strengths
1. Age-group intervals are adequate.
2. Information on years of education and mean raw WAIS Vocabulary subtest scores are provided for each age group.
3. Data reporting included mean and standard deviation scores.

Table 15.5. WMS.3

Normative Sample

Age	Information	Orientation	Mental Control	Logical Memory	Digit Span	Visual Reproduction	Paired Associates	MQ
80–92	5.23	4.76	5.92	5.72	10.20	3.76	10.15	109.91
N = 115	(1.21)	(0.57)	(2.07)	(2.91)	(1.97)	(2.70)	(3.80)	(19.21)

Clinical Comparison Sample

Age	Information	Orientation	Mental Control	Logical Memory	Digit Span	Visual Reproduction	Paired Associates	MQ
80–93	3.43	3.63	4.69	3.56	9.05	2.78	6.74	91.31
N=115	(2.20)	(1.54)	(2.17)	(2.86)	(2.42)	(2.37)	(4.54)	(20.93)

Table 15.6. WMS.4

Age	Information	Mental Control	Logical Memory	Digit Span	Visual Reproduction	Paired Associates
15–17	5.91	7.09	10.37	11.37	10.60	15.71
N = 43	(0.48)	(1.96)	(3.50)	(1.80)	(2.84)	(2.96)
30–39	5.56	6.75	7.99	11.02	10.09	15.48
N = 53	(0.72)	(1.92)	(2.95)	(1.93)	(3.01)	(3.48)
60–69	5.47	6.24	7.34	9.91	6.03	11.94
N = 70	(1.16)	(2.29)	(2.90)	(1.58)	(3.72)	(4.53)
70–79	5.24	5.63	7.35	9.91	4.95	10.98
N = 46	(1.03)	(2.46)	(3.83)	(2.51)	(3.42)	(4.78)
80–89	5.60	6.92	6.80	10.00	4.00	9.98
N = 25	(0.24)	(2.02)	(3.19)	(2.35)	(2.38)	(3.28)

Considerations regarding use of the study

1. Sample size generally did not meet review criteria (N ≥ 50); however, sample size within two of the five age group intervals met criteria, and two others almost met criteria.

2. No exclusion criteria are reported.

3. Scoring procedures were not described.

4. No delayed recall procedure was administered.

5. No information on gender.

6. Sample composition not representative of any identifiable population.

7. Low educational level.

Other comments

1. Lezak (1987) notes, "Hulicka's (older) subjects would have attended school around the turn of the century when relatively few Americans completed high school and many had less than eight years of schooling." This fact probably helps explain why Hulicka's normative data are about one standard deviation lower than scores reported more recently by other researchers across the same age-group intervals.

2. Hulicka did not administer the Orientation subtest to her sample because it "irritated" patients. Therefore, in calculating the WMS raw score, perfect Orientation scores were substituted, which likely inflated overall WMS raw performance scores for her group (Table 15.6).

[WMS.5] Schaie and Strother, 1968a

The goal of this article, "Cognitive and Personality Variables in College Graduates of Advanced Age," was to provide normative data on an optimally functioning older adult group. Subjects were aged 70–88 (n = 50; 25 men, 25 women) and consisted of a group of retired university professors and of retired academic or professional workers responding to a newspaper advertisement. Requirements included at least a B.A. degree, previous employment at a professional level, not residing in an institution for the aged or infirm, and in "good enough physical shape to visit the project office without any help or assistance." (p. 284).

Study strengths

1. Sample size was adequate.

2. Some information regarding education (i.e., at least 16 years).

3. Information regarding gender.

4. Sample composition was adequately detailed.

Considerations regarding use of the study

1. The age-group interval was broad.

2. No information on IQ was provided (although IQ level can be assumed to be high given the occupations).

3. No delay recall testing was administered.

4. Scoring procedures were not described.

5. Data reporting included only presentation of mean scores without standard deviations.

6. Minimal exclusion criteria are reported (Table 15.7).

[WMS.6] Ivinskis, Allen and Shaw, 1971

This article is entitled, "An Extension of Wechsler Memory Scale Norms to Lower Age

Table 15.7. WMS.5

Age	Information	Orientation	Mental Control	Logical Memory	Digits Forward	Digits Backward	Visual Reproduction	Paired Associates
70–88 n = 50	5.72	4.86	7.46	8.52	6.86	5.04	7.90	13.64

Groups." Subjects were male and female primary and high school students living in Australia (near University of Newcastle). The data were reported in two age categories: 10–14 years (*N* = 30) and 16–18 years (*N* = 44).

The report extends "WMS norms down to the 10 year old level." A comparison of WMS subtest scores with the WISC and WAIS subtest scores is also made.

Study strengths

1. Age-group intervals are small and well delineated.

2. IQ data are presented.

3. Data reporting included mean and standard deviation scores.

4. Information on gender and geographic area is provided.

5. Sample composition description is minimally adequate.

Considerations regarding use of the study

1. Individual cell sizes are less than 50.

2. Mean years of education are not reported although all subjects were in school.

3. No delayed recall testing was administered.

4. Scoring procedures were not described.

5. No exclusion criteria were reported.

6. Data were collected in Australia raising

questions regarding appropriateness for clinical interpretive use in the United States.

Other comments

1. This is the first published study to provide WMS adolescent norms (Table 15.8).

[WMS.7] Russell, 1975

This is the preliminary report of Russell's scoring method for the WMS. Subjects were patients tested with the full Halstead Reitan Battery at the Cincinnati Veterans Administration Hospital between October 1969 and August 1971 and at the Miami Veterans Administration Hospital from August 1971 to August 1973. The group "consisted of patients with suspected neurological disease who had a negative neurological examination, including a normal EEG and brain scan, and medical patients without neurological disease who volunteered as subjects" (p. 802). Education level of the sample was as follows: Neurologically normal = 12.5 (2.9) years; "organic" = 11.6 (2.9) years. The majority of subjects were male (28/30 neurological normal; 71/76 "organics"). Delayed recall (e.g., 30 minute) for the Logical Memory and Visual Reproduction subtests is assessed.

Table 15.8. WMS.6

Age/IQ	Information	Orientation	Mental Control	Logical Memory	Digits Forward	Digits Backward	Visual Reproduction	Paired Associates Total Score	Easy	Hard
10–14 n = 30 WISC IQ = 108.5 (12.2)	4.4 (1.4)	4.8 (0.6)	5.4 (1.9)	7.3 (3.1)	6.6 (1.1)	4.0 (1.1)	10.2 (2.5)	16.9 (2.2)	8.5 (0.8)	8.4 (1.9)
16–18 n = 44 WAIS IQ = 107.7 (7.7)	5.4 (0.8)	4.9 (0.4)	7.1 (2.0)	7.7 (2.1)	6.7 (1.2)	5.0 (1.2)	10.3 (1.4)	15.9 (2.1)	8.4 (0.5)	7.5 (2.2)

Study strengths

1. The description of sample composition is adequate. Data on education, gender, and geographic area are provided.
2. Delayed recall is assessed.
3. Scoring procedures are well described.
4. Data reporting included mean and standard deviation scores.

Considerations regarding use of the study

1. Only information regarding the sample mean age and standard deviation is reported. No age-group interval data are provided.
2. Sample size (*N* = 30) for the neurologically normal clinical comparison group did not meet review criteria.
3. No IQ data are provided.
4. Insufficient exclusion criteria.

Other comments

1. Russell reported a new administration and scoring procedure for the Logical Memory and Visual Reproduction subtests of the WMS. His revision included a 30-minute delay recall condition for these two subtests. Russell was the first investigator to include a delay recall condition. It should be noted that Russell's scores for the Logical Memory subtest were based on the *total* information recalled from both paragraphs, rather than the *average* amount recalled, as Wechsler suggested.
2. Since data are provided for a group of pa-tients seeking evaluation for medical/neurological complaints, this study presents *clinical comparison data* rather than *normative data* (Table 15.9).

[WMS.8] Cauthen, 1977

Cauthen's (1977) study had three objectives: to extend the WMS norms to adults in the 60–94-year age range, to obtain delayed recall scores on the Logical Memory subtest across the greater part of the adult life span (20–94), and to report these scores across age-group intervals that were further subdivided into IQ ranges. The data were collected in Calgary, Canada, and English was the first language for all subjects. Full-scale IQ estimates are provided using the Satz-Mogel (1962) short form of the WAIS. Delay recall (e.g., 1 hour) is assessed for the Logical Memory subtest only.

The majority of the sample age ≥60 lived in institutional settings, and therefore these data should be considered clinical comparison, rather than normative data. No information on sample characteristics of the younger groups was provided. Sample size is generally small (between four and 22 subjects), and subdividing the different age intervals by three different IQ (80–106, 107–118, 119–140) levels further compounded the problem of small sample size.

Table 15.9. WMS.7

Neurologically Intact Subjects

Age	Logical Memory Immediate	Logical Memory 30-Minute Delay	Logical Memory % Retained	Visual Repro Immediate	Visual Repro 30-Minute Delay	Visual Repro % Retained
36.5	23.1	20.8	89.5	10.4	9.1	87.6
(14.2)	(6.1)	(6.4)	(8.8)	(2.7)	(2.9)	(13.2)
n = 30						

Clinical Comparison ("Organic")

Age	Logical Memory Immediate	Logical Memory 30-Minute Delay	Logical Memory % Retained	Visual Repro Immediate	Visual Repro 30-Minute Delay	Visual Repro % Retained
42.0	14.9	10.5	56.0	5.6	3.7	51.4
(14.3)	(8.0)	(8.2)	(34.2)	(3.7)	(3.7)	(37.3)
n = 76						

Table 15.10. WMS.8a

Age	WAIS IQ Range		Logical Memory A	Logical Memory B	1-Hour Delay LM-A	1-Hour Delay LM-B
20–29	100–106	n = 4	13.8 (6.0)	8.8 (2.4)	13.0 (5.0)	7.8 (2.8)
	107–118	n = 8	11.0 (3.4)	6.6 (3.4)	8.4 (3.7)	6.0 (3.7)
	119–135	n = 3	16.7 (2.1)	11.3 (4.0)	16.7 (2.1)	10.0 (3.6)
30–39	100–106	n = 3	13.0 (3.6)	6.0 (1.0)	10.3 (2.5)	5.3 (0.6)
	107–118	n = 5	12.2 (4.7)	7.0 (3.6)	9.8 (2.2)	6.4 (3.0)
	119–135	n = 6	15.0 (4.2)	11.8 (4.8)	13.0 (4.0)	11.2 (4.5)
40–49	100–106	n = 1	9.0 (—)	6.0 (—)	7.0 (—)	3.0 (—)
	107–118	n = 7	13.7 (3.4)	6.8 (3.8)	10.6 (4.6)	7.0 (3.4)
	119–135	n = 5	12.6 (3.6)	11.6 (2.7)	10.6 (2.3)	10.8 (2.9)
50–59	107–118	n = 5	13.0 (2.3)	7.4 (2.9)	10.2 (0.4)	5.2 (2.5)
	119–135	n = 4	10.8 (2.1)	7.8 (3.0)	8.5 (4.0)	4.2 (3.3)

Study strengths

1. Information regarding IQ is reported.
2. Delay recall is assessed.
3. Data reporting included mean and standard deviation scores.

Considerations regarding use of the study

1. Age group intervals were not fully described.
2. Sample sizes within each age group category were small.
3. The sample exclusion criteria were not sufficient to meet review criteria.
4. No information on education or gender is provided.
5. Scoring procedures were not described.
6. Data collected in Canada, raising questions regarding appropriateness for clinical interpretive use in the United States (Tables 15.10–15.12).

[WMS.9] Ivison, 1977

The goal of this article was to present normative data for the WMS based on an Australian population. Data are provided for a sample of inpatients, "suffering from no known memory, . . . neurological or psychiatric impairment, (p. 304) recruited from general medical and surgical wards of a large teaching hospital in Sydney, Australia. Therefore, this study actually presents clinical comparison data on hospitalized Australian-educated patients, rather than normative data. Ivison notes that there were 100 subjects in each of the five age group intervals (20–29, 30–39, 40–49, 50–59, 60–69) with equal numbers of males and females in each age group. However, the normative data are presented for the *whole* group of 500 and not broken down by these age-group intervals. Because the age-group interval is so

Table 15.11. WMS.8b

Age	WAIS IQ Range		Logical Memory Average	Logical Memory A	Logical Memory B	1-Hour Delay LM-A	1-Hour Delay LM-B
60–69	80–106	n = 8	7.3 (3.3)	8.8 (4.6)	5.9 (2.8)	5.8 (4.1)	2.6 (3.7)
	107–118	n = 6	7.4 (2.6)	10.0 (4.7)	4.8 (2.6)	7.0 (4.5)	2.7 (2.6)
	119–140	n = 6	10.1 (1.3)	10.8 (1.5)	9.3 (2.0)	8.7 (2.2)	5.8 (3.9)
70–79	80–106	n = 4	4.9 (1.9)	5.5 (2.4)	4.2 (1.5)	2.0 (2.3)	0.75 (1.5)
	107–118	n = 5	6.4 (3.1)	6.6 (5.2)	6.2 (1.3)	3.0 (4.2)	3.0 (2.5)
	119–140	n = 9	9.6 (2.1)	11.0 (3.4)	8.2 (2.2)	9.3 (3.4)	5.7 (2.8)
80–89	80–106	n = 9	5.0 (3.6)	7.1 (5.0)	3.0 (2.8)	2.0 (3.0)	0.6 (1.3)
	107–118	n = 7	7.8 (1.5)	9.3 (2.8)	6.4 (2.6)	4.0 (3.6)	1.9 (2.4)
	119–140	n = 6	8.4 (3.3)	9.5 (4.6)	7.3 (2.6)	4.7 (5.6)	4.0 (3.3)
90–94		n = 4	6.8 (1.6)	9.8 (1.0)	4.0 (2.2)	1.8 (3.5)	0.2 (.5)

Table 15.12. WMS.8c

Age	WAIS IQ	Information	Orientation	Mental Control	Digits Forward	Digits Backward	Visual Repro	Paired Associates Total	Easy	Hard
60–69	80–106	5.2	4.4	5.0	4.9	4.1	5.2	10.9	7.1	3.8
	n = 8	(0.7)	(0.7)	(1.7)	(0.8)	(0.6)	(3.0)	(4.3)	(1.2)	(3.4)
	107–118	5.7	4.8	6.5	6.0	5.2	11.2	12.3	8.5	3.8
	n = 6	(0.5)	(0.4)	(1.9)	(1.1)	(1.0)	(2.0)	(2.1)	(0.8)	(1.6)
	119–140	5.5	5.0	7.8	5.8	4.0	9.5	15.2	8.6	6.7
	n = 6	(0.5)	(0.0)	(1.6)	(1.0)	(0.6)	(2.6)	(2.0)	(0.4)	(1.9)
70–79	80–106	5.2	4.5	5.2	5.2	2.2	2.2	10.5	7.2	3.2
	n = 4	(1.0)	(0.6)	(3.8)	(0.5)	(1.5)	(2.6)	(5.1)	(2.9)	(2.4)
	107–118	5.2	4.6	5.2	6.2	3.2	5.4	12.2	8.0	4.2
	n = 5	(1.3)	(0.5)	(0.4)	(1.5)	(0.8)	(3.6)	(2.0)	(0.9)	(1.3)
	119–140	5.3	4.8	6.6	5.6	4.6	7.0	13.1	8.3	4.8
	n = 9	(0.7)	(0.4)	(1.9)	(0.5)	(1.1)	(1.0)	(3.2)	(0.6)	(3.0)
80–89	80–106	4.4	4.0	4.9	5.4	2.9	4.7	9.6	7.8	1.8
	n = 9	(1.5)	(0.7)	(1.8)	(1.0)	(0.3)	(2.4)	(2.2)	(1.0)	(1.6)
	107–118	5.4	4.6	7.6	5.6	5.1	4.3	12.6	8.3	4.3
	n = 7	(0.5)	(0.5)	(1.3)	(1.1)	(0.7)	(2.3)	(2.2)	(0.8)	(1.6)
	119–140	5.3	5.0	7.7	6.3	5.2	5.3	12.5	8.2	4.3
	n = 6	(0.8)	(0.0)	(0.8)	(1.2)	(1.5)	(2.2)	(3.7)	(1.4)	(2.7)
90–94	n = 4	5.5	4.5	5.8	7.2	5.0	4.8	11.5	7.8	3.8
		(0.6)	(0.6)	(2.2)	(1.0)	(0.8)	(1.5)	(2.6)	(0.6)	(2.9)

broad (e.g., 20–69), the data are of questionable utility.

Study strengths
1. The sample composition description is adequate.
2. Sample size is adequate.
3. Scoring procedures are well described (see *Other Comments*).
4. Data reporting included mean and standard deviation scores.
5. Information regarding gender and geographic area is provided.

Considerations regarding use of the study
1. The age-group interval was too broad.
2. No information on IQ and/or education is provided.
3. A delayed recall condition was not administered.

4. Data were collected in Australia, raising questions regarding clinical interpretive use in the United States.
5. Subjects were medically ill.

Other comments
1. In administering the WMS, some alterations in the test content were made to avoid the use of American idioms or references. For instance, the first paragraph of the Logical Memory subtest substituted "East Sydney" for "South Boston" and in the Information Subtest, "Who is the Prime Minister of Australia?" was substituted for the question, "Who is the President of the United States?" Ivison described several other such changes in his article. Scoring criteria were also changed for the Mental Control and Visual Reproduction subtests, and these changes were also well documented (Table 15.13).

Table 15.13. WMS.9

Age	Information	Orientation	Mental Control	Logical Memory	Digit Span	Visual Reproduction	Paired Associates
20–69	4.41	4.63	6.63	7.77	10.42	8.46	12.89
n = 500	(1.22)	(0.56)	(2.05)	(3.70)	(1.96)	(3.25)	(3.93)

[WMS.10] Kear-Colwell and Heller, 1978

This article is entitled, "A Normative Study of the Wechsler Memory Scale." The sample consisted of health service employees at St. Luke's Hospital in Cleveland, England, "collected on a stratified quota sample basis, i.e., the incidence by social class, age group and sex was broadly representative of that in the population at large. . . . As far as possible, equal numbers of older and younger subjects were tested in each social class" (p. 438). Two age categories are presented: 17–34 (mean age = 24.8 [5.4] years] and 35–64 years (mean age = 48.2 [8.2] years).

The authors report a positive relationship between social class and memory skill. In comparing their data with previously published norms they suggest that there has been an "upward drift" in cognitive performance associated with aging over the prior three decades.

Study strengths

1. Sample size is adequate.
2. Sample composition description is adequate.
3. Data reporting includes mean and standard deviation scores.

Considerations regarding use of the study

1. Age-group intervals are broad.
2. No information on IQ, education, or gender is provided.
3. No delayed recall condition was administered.
4. Scoring procedures are not described.
5. Data were collected in England raising questions regarding clinical interpretive use in the United States.
6. No exclusion criteria are reported (Table 15.14).

[WMS.11] Bak and Greene, 1980

The purpose of this study was to develop preliminary reference data for the WMS for older adults and compare performance of two older groups of healthy, normally functioning adults on portions of the Halstead-Reitan Battery. The sample consists of healthy, active, older male and female adults recruited from two large metropolitan areas in Texas. All were fluent in English. Subjects with less than nine or greater than 18 (e.g., M.A.) years of education were excluded from the study. None had history of CNS disorder or illness, incapacity, or uncorrected sensory deficits. A 30-minute delayed recall condition for the Logical Memory, Associate Learning, and Visual Reproduction subtests is assessed. Russell's (1975) scoring procedures were followed for recall of the Logical Memory and Visual Reproduction subtests (see Lezak, 1995).

Study strengths

1. The description of the sample composition is adequate and the exclusion criteria are adequate.
2. Information on education, fluency in English, and geographic area is provided.
3. Delayed recall is assessed.
4. Scoring procedures are described.
5. Data reporting include mean and standard deviation scores.

Considerations regarding use of the study

1. Age-group intervals are broad.
2. Sample size is small.
3. No IQ data are provided.
4. No information on gender.
5. High educational level.

Other comments

1. Scoring procedures were not detailed for the delay recall of the Associate Learning Test.
2. Mean and standard deviation scores for performance on the Information, Arithmetic, Block Design, and Digit Symbol subtests from the WAIS are reported for both age groups.
3. Although not specified, it appears that all

Table 15.14. WMS.10

Age	Information	Orientation	Mental Control	Logical Memory	Digit Span	Visual Reproductive	Paired Associates	Digit Forward	Digit Backward	MQ
17–34	5.48	4.98	7.11	13.57	12.23	10.39	18.26	6.96	5.13	114.32
n = 56	(0.67)	(0.20)	(1.52)	(2.97)	(1.53)	(1.47)	(1.16)	(1.13)	(1.36)	(15.46)
35–64	5.53	4.97	6.85	10.39	11.08	7.98	15.28	6.53	4.70	115.17
n = 60	(.85)	(0.03)	(1.70)	(3.12)	(2.52)	(2.79)	(3.82)	(1.08)	(1.28)	(19.60)

Table 15.15. WMS.11

Age	Education Years	Logical Memory Immediate	Visual Reproductive Immediate	Paired Associates Immediate	30-Minute Logical Memory Delay	30-Minute Visual Reproductive Delay	30-Minute Paired Associates Delay
50–62	13.7	9.63	9.60	16.33	16.13	8.93	5.80
n = 15	(1.91)	(2.00)	(2.72)	(3.19)	(3.89)	(3.35)	(0.94)
67–86	14.9	10.30	6.20	16.53	16.33	5.33	6.07
n = 15	(2.99)	(3.06)	(3.07)	(2.75)	(7.08)	(2.72)	(0.80)

immediate recall data are scored according to Wechsler's (1945) method (Table 15.15).

[WMS.12] Bigler, Steinman and Newton, 1981a

This article is entitled, "Clinical Assessment of Cognitive Deficit in Neurologic Disorder: Effects of Age and Degenerative Disease." The sample was comprised of selected cases (male and female) from the Austin (Texas) Neurological Clinic. "All patients had no known neurologic history and their referral for neurological examination was for routine purposes only. All had minor neurological symptoms (e.g., simple headache) but were found to have no serious neurological disorder." (p. 5). All had normal EEG and CAT scans. The older group was selected to assure a maximally healthy sample. Information regarding full-scale WAIS IQ and years of education is provided for the sample:

Age 16–20 years, VIQ 114.8 (9.1), PIQ 111.7 (12.9), FSIQ 113.2 (11.6), education 11.1 (.9) years

Age 21–35 years, VIQ 113.9 (16.5), PIQ 108.2 (12.6), FSIQ 112.2 (14.6), education = 13.9 (2.1) years

Age 36–50 years, VIQ 108.7 (10.7), PIQ 111.3 (11.6), FSIQ 110.3 (10.1), education = 14.4 (3.3) years

Age 51–75 years, VIQ 122.8 (10.1), PIQ 112.1 (7.1), FSIQ 118.6 (7.9), education = 14.4 (4.1) years

Because this study uses patients as subjects, clinical comparison data are actually being presented rather than normative data.

Study strengths
1. Adequate exclusion criteria. Sample composition is adequate.
2. Information regarding IQ, education, and geographic area is provided.
3. Data reporting includes mean and standard deviation scores.

Considerations regarding use of the study
1. Age-group intervals are generally broad.
2. Sample size is small.
3. No delayed recall condition was presented.
4. Scoring procedures were not described.
5. No information regarding gender.
6. High IQ and educational level.

Other comments
1. The upper range of the age-group category is inconsistently reported between the text and a table as either 49 or 50 years (Table 15.16).

[WMS.13] Haaland, Linn, Hunt and Goodwin, 1983

This article is entitled, "A Normative Study of Russell's Variant of the WMS in a Healthy Elderly Population." The sample consists of a group of healthy, highly educated, motivated, noninstitutionalized, primarily Caucasian, older adults (male and female) living in Albuquerque, New Mexico. Fifty-eight percent of the sample had a college or advanced degree. Years of education for each age group were provided (65–69 group mean education = 14.8 [2.6] years; 70–74 group = 14.6 [2.7] years; 75–79 group = 13.7 [2.7] years; 80+ group = 13.9 [2.1] years). With the exception of the 80+ group, sample size is probably large enough to

Table 15.16. WMS.12

Age	Information	Orientation	Mental Control	Logical Memory	Digit Total	Digit Forward	Digit Backward	Visual Reproduction	Paired Associates	MQ
16–20	5.1	4.9	7.6	12.4	12.8	7.0	5.8	11.3	18.3	112.9
n = 10	(0.8)	(0.4)	(1.5)	(2.7)	(2.2)	(0.9)	(1.3)	(2.7)	(1.4)	(10.4)
21–35	5.4	4.9	6.9	10.6	11.6	6.6	5.1	11.6	16.9	108.4
n = 15	(0.8)	(0.3)	(1.6)	(3.2)	(2.6)	(1.5)	(1.4)	(2.1)	(3.4)	(16.3)
36–50	5.4	5.0	7.3	10.0	10.8	6.2	4.4	9.3	16.0	111.8
n = 12	(0.9)	(0.0)	(1.0)	(2.8)	(1.9)	(1.3)	(0.9)	(3.1)	(3.3)	(15.2)
51–75	5.5	4.8	7.3	10.3	11.3	6.6	4.7	10.8	14.2	121.4
n = 14	(0.8)	(0.5)	(2.0)	(3.1)	(1.2)	(0.9)	(0.8)	(4.0)	(4.5)	(16.3)

support provisional inferences. Thirty-minute delay recall for Logical Memory and Visual Reproduction subtests was assessed. Scoring procedures were according to Russell's (1975) protocol.

Study strengths

1. The age group intervals generally met review criteria, however, the 80+ group did not.

2. Sample composition description is adequate.

3. Information on education and geographic area is provided.

4. Delay recall is assessed.

5. Scoring procedures are described.

6. Data reporting included mean and standard deviation scores.

Considerations regarding use of the study

1. Sample size generally did not meet review criteria, however, two of the four age groupings exceeded Ns of 50.

2. No IQ or gender data are provided.

3. Alteration in test administration procedure (see below).

4. High educational level.

Other comments

1. The investigation deviated significantly from Russell's procedure by informing subjects that their delayed recall would be assessed.

2. In scoring the LM subtest, half-points were awarded for incomplete responses if they retained the original wording. Wechsler's (1945) scoring criteria were followed for the VR subtests. "Extra points for accuracy were given rarely" (p. 879).

3. Percentage Retained is a ratio of total number of details recalled on delay to the total number of details recalled immediately (Table 15.17).

[WMS.14] Crosson, Hughes, Roth and Monkowski, 1984a

This report pools data from several studies where the subjects were "neurotics, victims of

Table 15.17. WMS.13

Age	Logical Memory Immediate	30-Minute Logical Memory Delay	% Retained Logical Memory Delay	30-Minute Visual Reproduction Immediate	30-Minute Visual Reproduction Delay	% Retained Visual Reproduction
65–69	7.4	4.8	63.1	6.0	5.4	89.3
n = 49	(2.5)	(2.4)	(21.3)	(2.1)	(2.5)	(27.6)
70–74	6.7	4.2	60.2	5.1	4.3	83.4
n = 74	(2.6)	(2.4)	(23.0)	(2.0)	(2.3)	(37.2)
75–79	5.9	3.6	56.3	4.9	4.2	86.8
n = 40	(2.5)	(2.5)	(23.9)	(2.0)	(1.9)	(31.5)
80+	6.1	4.0	65.7	3.3	2.8	92.6
n = 13	(1.7)	(1.4)	(13.2)	(2.3)	(1.9)	(42.8)

personality disorders, medical patients, community volunteers and patients referred for neuropsychological assessment whose diagnostic tests were negative" (p. 639). A *T*-score table for immediate recall performance for the Logical Memory and Visual Reproduction subtests is presented. The authors note that the *T* scores "must be used with caution."

This report provides meta-analytically derived clinical comparison data, rather than normative data. Further, because of the considerable heterogeneity regarding the subject and procedural variables employed across the studies entered into the analysis, the *T*-score values from this report probably should be used with caution.

[WMS.15] Margolis and Scialfa, 1984

This report provides meta-analytic derived normative data. However, because of the considerable heterogeneity regarding the subject and procedural variables employed across the studies entered into the meta-analysis, the data from this report probably should be used with caution.

[WMS.16] Wallace, 1984

This report provides meta-analytic derived normative data. However, because of the considerable heterogeneity regarding the subject and procedural variables employed across the studies entered into the meta-analysis, the data from this report probably should be used with caution.

[WMS.17] Ivison, 1986

This article is entitled, "Anna Thompson and the American Liner New York: Some Normative Data." This study presents data for the Logical Memory subtest only. Ivison reanalyzed data from his 1977 report with attention to performance differences between paragraph A and B and noted that performance on paragraph was better on A. He concludes that the Logical Memory subtest might serve as a screening device for pathological levels of proactive inhibition, "provided that other factors such as fluctuating motivation can be discounted." In order to help the clinician "determine how abnormal an obtained difference is," Ivison presented the average discrepancy score between the two paragraphs broken down by age and sex.

The data are obtained from a sample of inpatients from general medical and surgical wards, "with no known neurological or psychiatric impairment" (Ivison, 1977, p. 304), so this study actually presents data on Australian-educated hospitalized patients, rather than normative data.

Study strengths
1. Sample composition was well described (see WMS.9, p. 292).
2. Age-group intervals generally met review criteria.
3. Sample size is adequate.
4. Information on gender and geographic area was provided.
5. Scoring procedures are well described (see WMS.9, p. 292).
6. Data reporting includes mean and standard deviation scores.

Considerations regarding use of the study
1. No education or *IQ* data were provided.
2. No delay recall condition was administered.
3. Data were collected in Australia raising questions regarding clinical use in the United States.
4. Subjects were ill (Table 15.18).

[WMS.18] desRosiers and Ivison, 1986

DesRosiers reanalyzed Ivison's data from his 1977 report to provide comparison data regarding the "difference scores" in the recall of High Associate and Low Associate word pairs from the WMS Paired Associate Learning subtest. DesRosiers and Ivison also present the average discrepancy score between High and Low Associates broken down by age. The data are from a sample of inpatients from general medical and surgical wards, "with no known neurological or psychiatric impairment" (Ivison, 1977, p. 304). Data were collected at a large teaching hospital in Sydney, Australia. Therefore, this study actually presents data on Australian-educated hospitalized patients, rather than normative data.

Study strengths
1. Age-group intervals generally met review criteria.
2. Sample size is adequate.
3. Sample composition was well described (see WMS.9, p. 292).

Table 15.18. WMS.17

Age			Logical Memory A	Logical Memory B	Difference Score (A Minus B)
20–29	Male	n = 50	11.62 (4.39)	8.60 (4.85)	3.02 (4.22)
	Female	n = 50	12.16 (4.92)	7.40 (3.50)	4.76 (3.98)
30–39	Male	n = 50	9.94 (4.46)	7.66 (3.93)	2.28 (4.06)
	Female	n = 50	10.38 (4.26)	6.10 (3.46)	4.28 (3.34)
40–49	Male	n = 50	9.16 (4.61)	6.12 (3.86)	3.04 (3.26)
	Female	n = 50	9.26 (4.53)	6.18 (3.42)	3.08 (3.58)
50–59	Male	n = 50	8.72 (4.73)	5.26 (3.99)	3.46 (3.88)
	Female	n = 50	8.02 (4.13)	4.96 (2.93)	3.06 (3.84)
60–69	Male	n = 50	6.58 (4.27)	5.06 (3.10)	1.52 (3.20)
	Female	n = 50	7.80 (4.68)	4.32 (3.48)	3.48 (2.83)

4. Information on gender and geographic area is provided.

5. Scoring procedures are well described (see WMS.9, p. 292).

6. Data reporting includes mean and standard deviation scores.

Considerations regarding use of the study

1. No education or IQ data were provided.

2. No delay recall condition was administered.

3. Data were collected in Australia, raising questions regarding clinical use in the United States.

4. Subjects were ill (Table 15.19).

[WMS.19] Ryan, Morrow, Bromet, and Parkinson, 1987

This study presents data from the Pittsburgh Occupational Exposures Test Battery (POET) and offers clinical comparison data for the performance of 182 blue-collar workers with exposure to heavy metals and toxic substances. The POET was designed to be sensitive to the subtle cognitive changes that are associated with exposure to toxic chemicals or heavy metals in the workplace. This report presents clinical comparison data for the following neuropsychological tests, which are part of the POET battery: the WMS Visual Reproduction subtest (form I), the Trail-Making Test, and the Grooved Pegboard Test.

The sample consists of 182 Caucasian, native English-speaking, male, blue-collar workers randomly recruited from a plant in eastern Pennsylvania that manufactures truck and auto chassis. All recruits had been working at the plant for at least 1 year, and of this group, 67% had no previous exposure to heavy metals, mixtures of organic solvents, or toxic inhalents before working for this company. Exclusion

Table 15.19. WMS.18

Age			High Associates M(SD)	Low Associates M(SD)	Difference Score M(SD)
20–29	Male	n = 50	16.65 (1.70)	7.45 (3.29)	9.20 (2.83)
	Female	n = 50			
30–39	Male	n = 50	16.19 (2.35)	5.59 (3.25)	10.60 (2.83)
	Female	n = 50			
40–49	Male	n = 50	15.28 (2.75)	4.61 (3.28)	10.67 (2.98)
	Female	n = 50			
50–59	Male	n = 50	15.52 (2.35)	4.13 (3.03)	11.39 (2.75)
	Female	n = 50			
60–69	Male	n = 50	15.05 (2.62)	3.32 (2.89)	11.73 (2.75)
	Female	n = 50			

criteria included the presence of medical or psychiatric disorders, a history of neurologic or psychiatric disorder, or renal or hepatic disease. Most participants consumed alcohol on a regular basis, although the authors note that "there was no meaningful association between performance on various tests and subjects' report of number of drinks consumed daily" (p. 671). Mean number of drinks per day, according to age group, was as follows: 21–30 years, 1.9 (2.4) drinks; 31–40 years, 2.0 (2.9) drinks; 41–50 years, 1.4 (1.8) drinks; 51–59 years, 1.5 (1.9) drinks. All subjects were asked to refrain from drug or alcohol use 12 hours prior to testing. Their self-report was confirmed by alcohol and drug screens, all of which were negative.

With the exception of the 21–30 category, where the $n = 55$, the sample sizes are below 50. The sample size for the other age groupings are as follows: 31–40, $n = 45$; 41–50, $n = 44$; 51–59, $n = 38$. Education information for the age-group samples was reported as follows: age 21–30, 12.3 (1.4) years education; age 31–40, 11.9 (2.2) years education; age 41–50, 11.3 (1.8) years education; age 51–59, 11.0(1.8) years education.

Study strengths
1. Sample composition is well described.
2. Age-group intervals are adequate.
3. Data regarding education, gender, ethnicity, occupation, and geographic area are reported.
4. Delayed recall is assessed for the Visual Reproduction subtest.
5. Scoring and administration criteria are well described. (See *Other Comments #1*.)
6. Data reporting included the presentation of means and standard deviation scores.

Considerations regarding use of the study
1. Sample sizes generally fall below 50.
2. Toxic exposures plus alcohol use.

Other comments
1. Administration of immediate recall of the WMS (form I) design cards was according to Wechsler (1945). Without warning, delayed recall was assessed 30 minutes later. The scoring procedure was modified, allowing bonus points for accuracy and spatial relationship. The Immediate and Delay recall conditions each have a maximum of 17 points (Table 15.20).

[WMS.20] Abikoff, Alvir, Hong, Sukoff, Orazio, Solomon and Saravay, 1987

This article is entitled, "Logical Memory Subtest of the WMS: Age and Education Norms and Alternate-Form Reliability of Two Scoring Systems." Data are presented for the Logical Memory subtest, Forms 1 and 2. The sample consists of male and female paid volunteer recruits from local (Hyde Park, New York), businesses and community organizations or from the staff of the community medical center. Over 95% were Caucasian. Education level is presented for each age group: (Gist Recall, form 1: 18–29 = 14.3 [1.3] years; 30–39 = 14.7 [2.2] years; 40–49 = 14.9 [2.0] years; 50–59 = 14.3 [2.2] years; 60–69 = 13.4 [2.5] years; 70–83 = 12.4 [2.5] years.

For Verbatim Recall, form 1: 18–29 = 14.3 [1.5] years; 30–39 = 14.6 [2.3] years; 40–49 = 14.9 [1.7] years; 50–59 = 14.5 [2.1] years; 60–69 = 13.4 [2.5] years; 70–81 = 12.1 [2.3] years.

For form 2: 18–29 = 14.5 [1.2] years; 30–39 = 14.9 [2.1] years; 40–49 = 15.1 [2.2] years; 50–59 = 14.2 [2.5] years; 60–69 = 13.3 [2.5] years; 70–81 = 13.0 [2.5] years.)

For forms 1 and 2, Wechsler's (1945) verbatim scoring system was used. Form 1 was also scored using the "gist" (i.e,: Schwartz & Ivnik, 1980) scoring method. Delayed recall was assessed twice—the first averaging 20 to 30 minutes after the initial presentation (approximate

Table 15.20. WMS.19; Mean Neuropsychological Test Scores (±Standard Deviation) Statified by Age

Age Range	21–30	31–40	41–50	51–59
Mean age	26.1 ± 2.3	36.8 ± 2.7	45.7 ± 2.9	54.8 ± 2.8
Years of education	12.3 ± 1.4	11.9 ± 2.2	11.3 ± 1.8	11.0 ± 1.8
Number of subjects	55	45	44	38
Immediate visual reproductions	13.0 ± 2.3	11.9 ± 2.5	11.0 ± 3.2	9.4 ± 3.2
Delayed visual reproductions	13.2 ± 2.8	12.1 ± 3.1	10.4 ± 3.8	9.7 ± 2.8

mean delay for form 1 = 25.20 (3.16) minutes; form 2 delay = 25.36 (3.01 minutes) and the second 24 hours later, via telephone. The later assessment was intended to provide a more "meaningful index of long-term memory."

Study strengths
1. Sample size is generally adequate.
2. Sample composition description is adequate.
3. Data regarding education and geographic area are reported.
4. Delayed recall is assessed.
5. The scoring procedure is described.
6. Data reporting included mean and standard deviation scores.

Considerations regarding use of the study
1. No IQ data are provided.
2. Exclusion criteria are not detailed.
3. No information on gender.
4. High educational level.
5. The youngest and oldest age group intervals are too broad. However, the age group intervals 30–39, 40–49, 50–59 and 60–69 are adequate.

Other comments
1. These investigators also present tables (not shown here) for mean verbatim and gist recall responses for five educational levels. However, the data are reported for the whole sample aged 18–83; making the norms unusable for inferential purposes. Further complicating

use of the data is that when the data were grouped by educational level, the resulting sample sizes were generally very small (Tables 15.21 and 15.22).

[WMS.21] Trahan, Quintana, Willingham and Goethe, 1988

This study provides normative data for a delayed recall procedure using the Visual Reproduction subtest from form 1 of the WMS. Subjects were a group of healthy, nonhospitalized, neurologically normal, male and female adults with no evidence of major psychiatric illness or mental deficiency. Information regarding education is reported

Age 18–29 = 13.73 (1.89) years

Age 30–49 = 14.79 (2.42) years

Age 50–69 = 14.12 (2.67) years

Age 70–91 = 15.69 (3.31) years

Study strengths
1. With the exception of the 70–91 group, sample size is adequate.
2. Sample composition description is adequate.
3. Adequate exclusion criteria.
4. Information on education was reported.
5. Delay recall condition (30 minute) without prior warning was assessed.
6. Scoring procedures were according to Wechsler (1945).

Table 15.21. WMS.20a; Gist Recall Scores

Age	Logical Memory Immediate	25-Minute Logical Memory Delay	24-Hour Logical Memory Delay
18–29 n = 74	22.99 (6.33)	19.84 (6.67)	19.31 (5.52) n = 73
30–39 n = 67	24.57 (6.97)	22.16 (7.57)	21.92 (7.53) n = 64
40–49 n = 41	23.44 (5.01)	21.07 (5.91)	20.10 (6.11)
50–59 n = 54	23.63 (6.14)	20.13 (6.48)	18.79 (7.36) n = 53
60–69 n = 56	20.48 (6.42)	17.34 (6.71)	15.75 (6.35) n = 53
70–80+ n = 47	19.11 (6.74)	15.33 (7.57) n = 46	14.31 (7.61) n = 45

Table 15.22. WMS.20b; Verbatim Recall Scores

Age	Logical Memory Immediate	25-Minute Logical Memory Delay	24-Hour Logical Memory Delay
18–29			
Form1	11.18 (5.34) $n = 39$	8.46 (4.50) $n = 39$	7.87 (3.61) $n = 38$
Form2	12.51 (4.58) $n = 39$	9.62 (4.05) $n = 39$	9.44 (3.86) $n = 39$
30–39			
Form1	13.79 (5.82) $n = 33$	9.85 (4.87) $n = 33$	8.88 (4.64) $n = 32$
Form2	14.31 (4.94) $n = 36$	11.78 (4.72) $n = 36$	12.00 (5.09) $n = 34$
40–49			
Form1	12.79 (3.31) $n = 24$	8.58 (3.92) $n = 24$	8.79 (3.51) $n = 24$
Form2	13.23 (3.68) $n = 22$	10.36 (3.72) $n = 22$	10.27 (3.34) $n = 22$
50–59			
Form1	11.73 (4.73) $n = 30$	8.07 (4.45) $n = 30$	7.13 (4.70) $n = 30$
Form2	12.90 (4.22) $n = 29$	10.00 (4.23) $n = 29$	8.86 (3.87) $n = 29$
60–69			
Form1	9.88 (4.84) $n = 32$	6.72 (4.67) $n = 32$	5.03 (3.30) $n = 32$
Form2	12.00 (4.13) $n = 29$	8.83 (4.02) $n = 29$	7.38 (3.84) $n = 29$
70–80+			
Form1	9.11 (4.52) $n = 28$	5.32 (3.61) $n = 28$	4.86 (3.19) $n = 28$
Form2	11.83 (4.92) $n = 24$	8.13 (4.21) $n = 23$	6.73 (3.41) $n = 22$

7. Data reporting included mean and standard deviation scores.

Considerations regarding use of the study

1. The age group intervals are broad; however, they may be used for cautious interpretation.

2. No IQ data are provided.

3. No reporting of gender distribution.

Other comments

1. The data from the 70–91 group are of questionable utility because of large age interval and small sample size (Table 15.23).

[WMS.22] Gilleard and Gilleard, 1989

The purpose of this study was to compare Turkish and Anglo-American normative data on the Wechsler Memory Scale. Performance of the Turkish sample was compared to Wechsler's (1945), Hulicka's (1966), and Kear-Colwell and Heller's (1978) normative data. This study uses the Turkish translation of the WMS form 1. There were some "minor modifications to the Information subtest" that were not described,

and story B of the Logical Memory subtest was replaced with story A from Form 2.

The study sample consists of 200 Turkish subjects, aged 20 to 59, recruited from a variety of urban and rural areas in the provinces of Ankara and Izmir. The age and sample size for the decade age spans are as follows: 20–29 ($n = 60$); 30–39 ($n = 60$); 40–49 ($n = 42$); 50–59 ($n = 38$). Of the 120 individuals aged 20–39, 72 have no formal education or elementary education, and 47 have a secondary or greater education. (See *Other Comments* regarding dis-

Table 15.23. WMS.21

Age	Visual Reproduction Immediate	30-Minute Visual Reproduction Delay
18–29	10.48	9.84
$n = 97$	(1.93)	(2.21)
30–49	10.10	9.26
$n = 81$	(2.55)	(2.74)
50–69	8.73	7.35
$n = 51$	(2.59)	(2.46)
70–91	6.46	5.62
$n = 26$	(2.79)	(2.79)

crepancy.) Of the 80 individuals aged 40–59, 59 have no formal education or elementary education, and 21 have a secondary or greater education.

Study strengths

1. Sample size is generally adequate, with the exception of the group of 40–59-year-olds with secondary or greater education.
2. Sample composition description is adequate.
3. Education levels are highlighted in presenting the normative data by age ranges.
4. Data reporting included mean and standard deviation scores.

Considerations regarding use of the study

1. Age-group intervals are broad.
2. No delayed recall procedure was administered.
3. Scoring procedures were not described.
4. Exclusion criteria were not fully described.
5. No information on IQ or gender.
6. Alterations in test administration format.

Other comments

1. Although it was reported that data were collected on 120 20–39-year-olds, data are only reported for 119 subjects (e.g., nil or secondary education, $n = 72$; secondary education or above, $n = 47$) (Table 15.24).

[WMS.23] Van Gorp, Satz and Mitrushina, 1990

This study reports cross-sectional data on 156 normal adults, aged 57–85 years, in the initial phase of a longitudinal study addressing neuropsychological processes associated with normal and abnormal aging. The sample consists of normal, healthy, active, well-educated male and female volunteers recruited from an independent-living retirement community in Camarillo, California. This is a sample of healthy, very intelligent (e.g., High Average to Superior IQ) older adults. WAIS-R VIQ, PIQ, and FSIQ estimates were derived using the Satz-Mogel (1962) short-form procedure. Full-scale IQ estimates were as follows (personal communication):

Age	WAIS-R FSIQ	VIQ	PIQ
57–65	115.8 (12.6)	117.2 (11.3)	109.2 (11.6)
66–70	119.3 (14.5)	114.8 (17.0)	111.5 (16.8)
71–75	118.7 (10.8)	122.9 (11.4)	115.1 (11.9)
76–85	112.0 (11.7)	110.5 (11.2)	101.0 (8.8)

Education for each age group—not reported in the paper—is as follows (personal communication):

Age	Education
57–65	14.2 (2.0)
66–70	14.0 (2.0)
71–75	14.6 (3.4)
76–85	13.3 (3.6)

Table 15.24. WMS.22; Performance on the Wechsler Memory Scale by Age and Education Status

	Age						
	20 to 39 $N = 120$				40 to 59 $N = 80$		
	Nil or Elementary $N = 72$		Secondary or Above $N = 47$		Nil or Elementary $N = 59$		Secondary or Above $N = 21$
Information	4.96 (1.22)		5.83 (0.38)		4.68 (1.58)		6.00 (0.00)
Orientation	4.62 (0.62)		5.00 (0.00)		4.25 (0.96)		4.89 (0.31)
Mental control	3.17 (2.45)		5.87 (2.38)		2.61 (2.41)		6.03 (1.95)
Logical memory	4.74 (2.21)		9.88 (4.01)		4.27 (2.85)		10.00 (3.14)
Digit span	7.35 (1.46)		10.21 (2.36)		6.86 (1.48)		10.21 (1.69)
Visual reproduction	6.25 (3.20)		10.49 (3.06)		4.14 (3.50)		10.10 (2.64)
Paired associates	11.22 (3.16)		15.49 (3.05)		9.42 (4.15)		14.00 (0.00)
Raw score total	42.29 (9.60)		62.70 (10.90)		36.20 (13.72)		60.92 (7.61)

The investigators used a 45-minute delay interval for assessing recall of the Logical Memory and Visual Reproduction subtests.

Study strengths
1. With the exception of the oldest group, the study met the age group interval criteria.
2. The sample composition is well described.
3. Information regarding IQ, education, and geographic area is reported.
3. Delay recall is assessed.
4. Data reporting includes mean and standard deviation scores.

Considerations regarding use of the study
1. Sample size generally did not meet review criteria. However, it is still sufficiently large to allow cautious interpretation.
2. Scoring procedures were not described in the article; however, the authors used the Power et al. (1979) procedures (personal communication).
3. Unclear exclusion criteria.
4. No information regarding gender.

Other comments
1. Subjects were administered the WMS subtests as part of a larger neuropsychological battery used in a longitudinal study of normal and abnormal aging (Table 15.25).

[WMS.24] Ivnik, Smith, Tangalos, Petersen, Kokmen and Kurland, 1991

The study sample consists of older Caucasian adult patients "neither unusually healthy nor unhealthy," aged 65 to 97 years, recruited from a community-based internal medicine practice in Rochester, Minnesota, who had been randomly selected to serve as controls matched on age and gender with dementia patients in the Mayo Clinics' Alzheimer Disease Patient Registry. Potential controls were screened for *active* CNS or psychiatric conditions or complaints of cognitive difficulty (Folstein MMSE>23). Exclusion also occurred if during history-taking or system review any condition was discovered that would compromise cognition. Psychoactive medications were allowed, as well as chronic medical illness and history of head injury or substance abuse, as long as the condition was stable, controlled, and judged by the examining internist to be cognitively benign.

The age-group interval (65–97 years) is broad—covering a 32-year span. The mean age of the sample (80.9 [7.4] years) suggests the majority of subjects were over age 75.

IQ and Education levels are reported for the whole sample.

$$\text{WAIS-R FSIQ} = 100.4 \ (11.1)$$

$$\text{VIQ} = 97.5 \ (12.3)$$

$$\text{PIQ} = 99.3 \ (11.6)$$

Mean years of education = 12.4 (3.3) years. Norms are separately presented by FSIQ and education groupings. In summary, the data presented here are for a sample of middle-class, educated, urban-dwelling Caucasian elderly individuals.

Study strengths
1. Sample size is adequate ($n = 99$). See *Other Comments* #1.
2. Sample composition description is adequate and exclusion criteria are detailed.

Table 15.25. WMS.23

Age	Logical Memory Immediate	Visual Reproduction Immediate	45-Minute Logical Memory Delay	45-Minute Visual Reproduction Delay
57–65 n = 28	9.75 (2.39)	9.6 (2.76)	7.8 (2.16)	6.6 (2.46)
66–70 n = 45	8.47 (2.65)	8.67 (3.81)	5.73 (2.24)	6.33 (3.83)
71–75 n = 57	9.27 (3.15)	7.79 (2.99)	6.31 (3.16)	4.37 (3.93)
76–85 n = 26	8.05 (2.19)	4.09 (2.26)	5.32 (2.48)	1.64 (1.69)

3. IQ and education levels are reported.

4. Delayed recall condition (30 minutes) is available for the Logical Memory and Visual Reproduction subtests only.

5. Scoring procedures are according to Schwartz and Ivnik (1980).

6. Data reporting include mean and standard deviation scores.

7. Data on geographic area and ethnicity is reported.

Considerations regarding use of the study
1. The age-group interval is broad.
2. No information regarding gender.

Other comments
1. Normative sample size within the reported IQ and education groupings is generally small (i.e., <30 subjects).

2. The normals for this study represent a subset of the total control subject pool from Mayo's Alzheimer Disease Patient Registry (ADPR). Specifically, the subjects were patients from a community-based internal medicine practice who had been randomly selected to serve as controls matched on age and gender with dementia patients in the ADPR. As the authors note, this control sample, therefore, is not representative with respect to the age and gender distribution of older adults in the community of Rochester, Minnesota. Since this sample consists of patients who were being seen for non-memory-related problems (i.e., yearly physical checkup, etc), the data are appropriate for normative purposes.

4. Delay recall of Paired Associates not provided.

5. Correlation with age was only found on the Mental Control subtest and the Total Raw Score. IQ was found to correlate with WMS performance, and to a lesser extent with education. The authors therefore recommend use of IQ tabled norms, rather than education norms, when possible (Tables 15.26 and 15.27).

[WMS.25] Heaton, Grant and Matthews, 1991

The authors provide normative data on the Figure Memory Test, which utilizes the figures from the 1945 version of the WMS Visual Reproduction subtest. The normative data are derived from a larger sample of urban and rural subjects recruited in several states (California, Washington, Colorado, Texas, Oklahoma, Wisconsin, Illinois, Michigan, New York, Virginia, and Massachusetts) and Canada who were involved in research with the authors and completed a battery of tests. Most subjects were paid for their participation in the research. Data were collected over a 15-year period through multicenter collaborative efforts. The authors trained the test administrators and supervised data collection. Exclusion criteria included history of learning disability, neurologic disease, illness affecting brain function, significant head trauma, significant psychiatric disturbance (e.g., schizophrenia), and alcohol or other substance abuse. The sample size of the larger norming study contained 378 individuals. Mean age for the total subsample ($n = 155$) completing the Figural Memory Test was was 46.4(20.3) years, and mean educational level was 14.4(3.0) years. Sixty-five percent of the sample were males.

Data are separately reported for males and females across 10 age *and* six educational ranges. The age categories are 20–34, 35–39, 40–44, 45–49, 50–54, 55–59, 60–64, 65–69, 70–74, and 75–80 years old. The education categories are 6–8, 9–11, 12, 13–15, 16–17, and 18+ years of education. Data are presented by age and education. As a result, the manual contains 120 age/education tables: 60 tables for males and 60 tables for females.

The administration procedure for the Figural Memory Test (FMT) differs significantly from the WMS protocol. Specifically, in the FMT, the stimulus cards can be presented up to five times, or "until the subject reaches a criterion of 15 points on a single trial." Immediate recall for all three cards is assessed following exposure of *all* three cards, and not after presentation of each card as is required in the WMS protocol. Subjects are also warned that they will be required to recall the figures again at a later time. Indeed, recall is again assessed 4 hours later. Scoring is according to the Wechsler and Stone (1945) protocol.

Study strengths
1. The age-group intervals are adequate.
2. The sample composition is well described and the exclusion criteria are adequate.

Table 15.26. WMS.24a; Normative Sample by WAIS-R Full Scale IQ

Age Range 65–97 Years	IQ	Education	WAIS-R FSIQ	Information	Orientation	Mental Control	Logical Memory	Digit Span	Visual Reproduction	Paired Associates	30-Minute Delay LM	30-Minute Delay VR
84.5 (7.0) n = 27	<90	9.7 (3.1)	84.6 (3.5)	4.5 (1.3)	4.7 (0.5)	4.9 (2.2)	5.6 (2.3)	9.0 (1.5)	3.4 (2.1)	10.8 (2.8)	3.8 (2.5)	2.8 (2.3)
79.7 (7.5) n = 22	90–100	12.3 (3.0)	95.9 (3.0)	5.2 (0.7)	4.8 (0.4)	6.0 (1.5)	7.9 (2.6)	10.2 (1.5)	6.1 (2.6)	13.1 (3.2)	6.3 (2.6)	5.0 (3.2)
78.6 (7.2) n = 34	101–110	13.6 (2.2)	105.6 (3.1)	5.5 (0.6)	4.9 (0.3)	6.8 (1.6)	9.1 (2.7)	11.0 (1.8)	7.1 (3.0)	13.3 (3.4)	7.0 (2.8)	6.1 (3.3)
80.8 (4.9) n = 15	>110	14.6 (3.1)	116.7 (4.4)	5.7 (0.7)	6.0 (0.0)	7.9 (1.4)	10.5 (2.9)	10.9 (2.0)	9.3 (2.6)	14.4 (3.4)	8.1 (3.1)	8.1 (3.5)

Table 15.27. WMS.24b; Normative Sample by Years of Education

Age Range 65-97 Years	Education	WAIS-R FSIQ	Information	Orientation	Mental Control	Logical Memory	Digit Span	Visual Reproduction	Paired Associates	30-Minute Delay LM	30-Minute Delay VR
83.3 (8.0) n = 29	<12	89.9 (9.2)	4.6 (1.3)	4.8 (0.5)	5.6 (2.3)	6.8 (3.3)	9.6 (1.9)	4.4 (2.4)	11.7 (3.3)	5.1 (3.4)	3.5 (3.6)
79.0 (6.8) n = 48	12–15	101.5 (9.4)	5.3 (0.7)	4.9 (0.4)	6.3 (1.8)	8.5 (3.1)	10.6 (1.7)	6.4 (3.3)	13.9 (3.2)	6.4 (3.1)	5.5 (3.2)
82.1 (6.7) n = 22	>15	107.2 (10.8)	5.5 (0.7)	5.0 (0.2)	7.0 (1.8)	8.6 (2.3)	10.6 (1.9)	8.0 (3.2)	13.4 (3.9)	6.8 (2.5)	6.9 (3.8)

3. Information regarding education, gender, and demographic area is provided.

4. Delayed recall (4 hours) for the Visual Reproduction subtest was assessed.

5. Scoring procedures were described.

Considerations regarding use of the study

1. Sample size could not have meet criteria, since the total $N = 115$ and this data are reported across 120 age/education tables.

2. Data reporting does not include mean and standard deviation scores; however, T scores corrected for age, education, and sex can be determined with reference to the tables in the manual.

Interested readers are referred to the manual for data presentation.

[WMS.26] Mitrushina and Satz, 1991a

The sample is composed of active, primarily upper middle class, healthy, elderly Caucasian volunteers recruited from an independent retirement community in Camarillo, California, screened for history of neurological or psychiatric disorders. IQ and education levels for each age group are as follows:

Age	FSIQ (Time 1)	Education (Years)
57–65	115.0 (12.1)	14.4 (2.0)
66–70	119.4 (15.2)	13.7 (1.8)
71–75	119.9 (11.3)	14.5 (3.1)
76–85	114.4 (12.3)	14.0 (3.6)

WAIS-R FSIQ estimates are based on Satz-Mogel administration (see Lezak, 1995, pp. 700–701 for description). VIQ and PIQ estimates are also provided in the paper. The data for this study represent a subset ($n = 122$) of the larger ($n = 156$) sample of older adults participating in a longitudinal study on aging who completed three consecutive yearly neuropsychological evaluations lasting 2 hours. (See WMS.18.)

Test–retest changes on the Logical Memory subtest showed improvement between the first and third probes for the 57–65 and 66–70 groups, relative stability for the 71–75 group, and a general pattern of decline for the 76–85 group. Consistent test–retest improvement, however, was noted across all four age groups on the Visual Reproduction subtest.

Study strengths

1. With exception of the oldest group, the study met age group interval criteria.

2. Adequate exclusion criteria, and the sample composition is well described.

3. Information regarding IQ, education, and geographic area is provided.

4. Delayed recall (45 minute) for the Logical Memory and Visual Reproduction subtests was assessed.

5. Data reporting includes mean and standard deviation scores.

Considerations regarding use of the study

1. Sample size generally did not meet review criteria; however, the 66–70 ($n = 40$) and 71–75 ($n = 47$) age groupings came close. Caution should be employed when using the data reported for the other two age groupings.

2. Scoring procedures were not described in the paper; however, the authors used the Power et al. (1979) protocol (personal communication).

3. High IQ and educational level of the sample.

Other comments

1. This paper reports the only test–retest WMS norms available for older adults.

2. The investigators used a 45-minute delay interval for assessing recall of the Logical Memory and Visual Reproduction subtests. The Paired Associates subtest was not part of their study protocol (Tables 15.28 and 15.29).

[WMS.27] Russell and Starkey, 1993

The HRNES battery consists of 22 tests; however, any subset of tests can be administered, scored, and "interpreted" according to this system. Tests included in the battery are as follows: Lateral Dominance Examination (parts 1 & 2, including Grip Strength), Trail-Making Test A & B, Wechsler Memory Scale, Russell version or Wechsler Memory Scale-Revised, Finger Tapping Test, Tactual Performance Test (Seguin-Goddard Form Board), Halstead Category Test or the Short Category Test (booklet format), Speech Perception Test, Rhythm Test, Perceptual Disorders Examination, Aphasia Screening Test, Miami Selective Learning Test, H-Words Test, HRNES Analogies Test, Peabody Picture

Table 15.28. WMS.26a; Logical Memory Subtest Performance

Age	Immediate Recall 1st Administration	45-Minute Delay 1st Administration	Immediate Year 2	Delay Year 2	Immediate Year 3	Delay Year 3
57–65	9.7	6.5	9.3	6.9	10.5	8.3
n = 19	(2.5)	(3.0)	(3.1)	(2.7)	(3.2)	(2.9)
66–70	10.1	6.8	9.9	7.2	10.5	7.9
n = 40	(2.6)	(2.7)	(3.0)	(3.1)	(3.0)	(3.3)
71–75	9.2	6.0	8.9	6.0	9.2	6.6
N = 47	(3.2)	(3.2)	(3.1)	(3.6)	(3.4)	(3.8)
76–85	9.4	6.6	8.4	4.8	8.8	5.8
N = 16	(2.2)	(2.5)	(1.8)	(2.4)	(1.8)	(2.8)

Vocabulary Test-Revised, Boston Naming Test, Grooved Pegboard Test, Gestalt Identification Test, Design Fluency Test, Corsi Board, Wide Range Achievement Test-Revised, Wechsler Adult Intelligence Scale-Revised. The HRNES scales all have a mean of 100 and standard deviation of 15. The authors note, however, that the HRNES was designed for the assessment of individuals who may be impaired; therefore, scores only extend upward to 112, whereas the floor goes down to 55.

The HRNES evaluates a patient's performance relative to the HRNES clinical comparison group of 576 brain-damaged individuals, as well as the HRNES normative group of 200 "normals" recruited from V.A. Hospitals in Cincinnati and Miami. However, close inspection of the manual reveals that the "normal" sample is actually composed of patients who were initially suspected of having brain damage, but a neurological examination at the V.A. failed to reveal any significant findings. These individuals were therefore determined to be "neurologically normal." This sample is disproportionately male (86%) and is primarily white (94%; 6% African-American).

The HRNES brain-damaged comparison group comprises various neurological and psychiatric disorders. Exclusion criteria included schizophrenia, severe depression requiring hospitalization, and systemic vascular disease, or any doubt about the presence or absence of a brain lesion. This brain-damaged sample is also primarily male (95%) and white (95%), 4% African-American, 1% "other."

HRNES test data are grouped according to the following age categories: 20–29, 30–39, 40–49, 50–59, 60–69, 70–79, 80–89. Education/IQ data are reported for four levels: "less than highschool [sic] corresponding to a WAIS-R FSIQ of <98; highschool graduation through 3 years of college, corresponding to a FSIQ of

Table 15.29. WMS.26b; Visual Reproduction Subtest Performance

Age	Immediate Recall 1st Administration	45-Minute Delay 1st Administration	Immediate Year 2	Delay Year 2	Immediate Year 3	Delay Year 3
57–65	8.8	5.8	10.3	7.4	11.2	8.5
n = 19	(2.6)	(3.4)	(2.6)	(4.4)	(2.5)	(3.4)
66–70	8.8	6.3	10.3	8.1	10.5	8.3
n = 40	(3.4)	(3.5)	(2.6)	(3.6)	(2.8)	(3.0)
71–75	8.1	4.9	9.3	5.8	9.0	6.3
n = 47	(3.0)	(3.8)	(2.9)	(3.8)	(3.1)	(3.7)
76–85	6.1	4.1	7.3	4.8	7.1	5.4
n = 16	(3.6)	(4.0)	(3.7)	(3.8)	(3.1)	(3.3)

98–107; 16 years of education, corresponding to a FSIQ >118." Sample size for each of the age group categories is not specified. The sample size in any event would most probably be quite small for the "neurologically normal" comparison group when spread across the seven age-group categories. The small sample-size problem is further compounded when data are reported by age *and* education/IQ. The HRNES system provides a computer-assisted scoring program. Please see Lezak (1995, pp. 714–715) for further description of the HRNES.

Study strengths
1. The age-group intervals are adequate.
2. Sample composition is adequately described (see *Other Comments #1*).
3. Information on education, IQ, gender, ethnicity, and geographic area is provided.
4. Delayed recall procedures are provided for the Logical Memory and Visual Reproduction subtests.
5. Scoring procedures are described.

Considerations regarding use of the study
1. Sample sizes are not specified.
2. Data reporting includes means and standard deviation scores for the whole group of 20–89-year-olds on all the test measures; however, they are not separately presented by age decade groups.
3. Insufficient exclusion criteria.

Other comments
1. Although the sample composition of the "normal comparison" and "brain-damaged" groups is described, because both groups are not distinct in their composition, it is uncertain how either group could be reasonably utilized for comparison purposes. The data from HRNES, therefore, should be used with caution.

Due to the large amount of normative data, it is not reproduced here. The reader is referred to the HRNES manual.

Wechsler Memory Scale-Revised

[WMS-R.1] Wechsler, 1987

This is the standardization of the WMS-R. The standardization sample was "designed to represent the normal population of the United States." Each case needed for the standardization sample was prespecified according to age, sex, race, and geographic regions. Education level of the standardization sample included those with "0–11 years, 12 years (high school graduation or its equivalent), and 13 years or more." The mean full-scale *IQ* estimate of the sample at each age group was reported to be 100, with a standard deviation of 15. (See *Other Comments #1*.) Although the manual reports that the WMS-R provides "norms stratified at nine age levels" (p. 2), close inspection reveals that normative data were only collected for six of the nine age groups–the other "normative data" has been estimated statistically by interpolation. Specifically, no data were collected for three of the nine reported age groups (18–19, 25–34, and 45–54 years). The WMS-R is a proprietary test and the interested reader is referred to the manual for normative data presentation.

Study strengths
1. Age-group intervals mirror WAIS-R intervals.
2. Sample size generally met criteria.
3. Information regarding gender, ethnicity, and geographic region is provided.
4. Delayed recall procedures are followed for four of the nine subtests.
5. Scoring procedures are well described in the manual.
6. Data reporting include mean and standard deviation scores.
7. Sample composition description is adequate.

Considerations regarding use of the study
1. Normative data not available by education and/or IQ level, although information regarding IQ and educational characteristics of the sample was described.
2. Exclusion criteria were not fully detailed.

Other comments
1. IQ scores were generally estimated. The complete WAIS-R was only administered to the 35–44 and 55–69-year-olds. A four-subtest short form (Vocabulary, Arithmetic, Picture

Completion, Block Design) was administered to the other four age groups on which normative data were collected.

[WMS-R.2] Cullum, Butters, Troster and Salmon, 1990

The sample is described as a group of healthy, "above average" educated, community-dwelling older adult volunteers recruited via flyers and newspaper advertisements and screened over the telephone for neuropsychological, neurological, psychiatric, and medical disorders. The author's stated intention was to provide "preliminary" WMS-R norms for healthy elderly individuals over age 74, since the WMS-R standardization cutoff at age 74 years. Education level is presented for each age group.

50–70 years, mean = 14.4(2.7) years

75–95 years, mean = 14.6(3.0) years

Delayed recall for Logical Memory, Verbal Paired Associates, Visual Reproduction, and Visual Paired Associates was assessed at 30 minutes.

Study strengths
1. Adequate exclusion criteria. Sample composition description is adequate.
2. Information regarding education is provided.
3. Delayed recall is assessed.
4. Scoring and method of administration were according to Wechsler (1987).
5. Data reporting included mean and standard deviation scores.

Considerations regarding use of the study
1. The age-group intervals are broad; however, they are probably sufficiently narrow to allow cautious interpretation.
2. Sample size did not meet review criteria; however, it is sufficiently large to allow cautious interpretation.
3. High educational level.
4. No information regarding gender.

Other comments
1. Forgeting rates (i.e., "savings scores") are also provided. Savings scores (SS) were calculated for Logical Memory, Visual Reproduc-

tion, Verbal Paired Associates, and Visual Paired Associates using the formula:

$$SS = \text{delayed recall/immediate recall} \times 100$$

2. The subject's *last* learning trial was used as the measure of immediate recall.
3. All subjects were administered the Dementia Rating Scale (DRS) (Mattis, 1976) to assess overall cognitive status.

DRS	Total Score
50–40	141.1 (3.7)
75–95	139.8 (4.3)

4. The authors caution against the application of the standard WMS-R index scores for individuals over age 74 because use "would likely result in an underestimation of older subject's true abilities." Therefore, the WMS-R Index scores "must be used only as approximate estimates of memory function" in individuals over age 74 (Tables 15.30 and 15.31).

[WMS-R.3] Mittenberg, Burton, Darrow and Thompson, 1992

This study provides empirically derived normative data for an age group (25–34) neglected in the WMS-R standardization. The WMS-R manual reports estimated "norms" statistically interpolated from adjacent age groups in the standardization sample.

Subjects were volunteers recruited in Florida from "local businesses, evening/weekend adult education and vocational/technical classes" and were screened to exclude neurologic, psychiatric, and alcohol problems. The sample was designed to match 1980 U.S. Census data stratified on age, gender, ethnicity and education. Education level of the sample was described as 0–11 years ($n = 12$); 12 years ($n = 20$); 13+ years ($n = 18$). WAIS-R estimated FSIQ Mean = 101.3 (14.58), range 72–131, Median = 100. The WAIS-R FSIQ estimate was based upon administration of the Vocabulary and Block Design subtests only.

Study strengths
1. Age-group interval is adequate.
2. Sample size met minimal criteria.
3. Exclusion criteria are well described and sample composition description is adequate.

Table 15.30. WMS-R.2a; Data For Younger and Older Age
Groups

	Age 50–70 (N = 47)		Age 75–95 (N = 32)	
	M	SD	M	SD
WMS-R Subtest				
Digit Span	14.9	3.7	15.3	3.7
Visual Span	14.7	2.4	14.1	2.5
Logical Memory I	29.2	7.7	25.0	7.5
Logical Memory II	25.6	7.9	20.9	8.4
Verbal Paired Associates I	19.7	2.9	18.3	2.8
Verbal Paired Associates II	7.6	0.7	6.9	1.2
Visual Reproduction I	34.3	3.9	29.1	7.3
Visual Reproduction II	29.1	6.1	20.1	9.1
Visual Paired Associates I	14.1	3.7	12.7	3.5
Visual Paired Associates II	5.6	0.9	4.8	1.4
Figural Memory	6.5	1.7	6.5	1.5
WMS-R Raw Summary Scores				
Attention/Concentration	64.7	9.3	64.5	11.2
Verbal Memory	78.0	16.3	68.5	16.8
Visual Memory	55.0	7.1	48.3	9.7
General Memory	133.0	20.7	116.6	22.0
Delayed Memory	81.1	12.8	64.5	17.4

4. Education level and IQ estimate of the sample are described.

5. Delayed recall procedures were according to Wechsler (1987).

6. Scoring procedures were according to Wechsler (1987).

7. Data reporting include mean and standard deviation scores.

8. Information provided regarding geographic area and recruitment procedures.

Considerations regarding use of the study

1. Normative data are not reported by education or IQ level because sample size is small relative to this purpose.

2. No information regarding gender.

Other comments

1. The authors note that the interpolated WMS-R norms presented in the manual underestimate performance on the "Attention/

Table 15.31. WMS-R.2b; Savings Scores for Younger
and Older Age Group

Savings Score	Age 50–70 (N = 47)		Age 75–95 (N = 32)	
	M%	SD	M%	SD
Logical Memory	87	13	83	18
Verbal Paired Associates	96	8	88	13
Visual Reproduction	85	15	68	25
Visual Paired Associates	97	20	84	23

Table 15.32. WMS-R.3a; Raw-Score Means and Standard Deviations for the Wechsler Memory Scale-Revised

Subtest	M	SD	Range
Information/Orientation	13.88	0.33	13–14
Mental Control	4.98	1.13	2–6
Figural Memory	7.20	1.49	4–10
Logical Memory 1	26.04	6.81	11–40
Visual Paired Associates 1	15.12	3.39	5–18
Verbal Paired Associates 1	20.80	3.16	12–24
Visual Reproduction 1	34.52	5.39	16–41
Digit Span	14.96	3.71	7–22
Visual Memory Span	17.66	3.62	10–25
Logical Memory 2	22.38	7.38	9–37
Visual Paired Associates 2	5.60	0.95	2–6
Verbal Paired Associates 2	7.62	0.86	4–8
Visual Reproduction 2	32.88	6.59	13–41

Concentration Index at the lower end of the score distribution and overestimate scores on the Visual Memory and Delayed Recall Indexes at the upper end of the distribution" (Tables 15.32 and 15.33).

[WMS-R.4] Lichtenberg and Christensen, 1992

This study entitled, "Extended Normative Data for the Logical Memory Subtests of the WMS-R: Responses From a Sample of Cognitively Intact Elderly Medical Patients," provides clinical comparison data for a group of cognitively intact geriatric medical patients, aged 70 to 99 years old seeking treatment in a hospital in Detroit, Michigan, one-third of whom were being seen for hip fractures from falling, one-third for knee replacements due to arthritis, and one-third for stabilization and recovery from a lengthy illness. The sample was comprised of 25 men, 43 women (35 Caucasian and 31 African-Americans), screened for the absence of neurological dysfunction. Information on years of education is provided for each age group interval:

70–74 group, education = 12.0 (3.7) years

75–79 group, education = 10.5 (2.8) years

80–99 group, education = 11.2 (3.1) years

Although the title of this report suggests that normative data are being supplied, the authors actually provide WMS-R Logical Memory subtest clinical comparison data for a sample of cognitively intact geriatric medical inpatients. Indeed, the author's caution that "the data presented here will be best used when applied to geriatric medical patients seeking treatment in an urban medical setting" (p. 746).

Study strengths
1. Age-group intervals are generally adequate; however, the 80–99 age category is broad.
2. Information regarding years of education is provided for each age-group interval.
3. Delayed recall for the Logical Memory subtest is assessed according to Wechsler 1987.
4. Scoring procedures were acccording to Wechsler (1987).

Table 15.33. WMS-R.3b; Wechsler Memory Scale–Revised Weighted Raw Score Composites

Subtest	Subtest	
Verbal Memory	72.58	15.30
Visual Memory	56.46	8.91
General Memory	129.04	20.25
Delayed Recall	80.74	15.16
Attention/Connection	69.58	13.40

5. Data reporting included mean and standard deviation scores.

6. Information regarding gender, ethnicity, and geographic area is provided. Sample composition description is adequate.

Considerations regarding use of the study

1. Sample size within each age group interval did not meet review criteria.

Other comments

1. Medical history ruled out suspected cerebral damage, and the the Mattis Dementia Rating Scale (cutoff score = 129) was administered to insure intact cognitive functioning.

70–74 group, Mattis = 134.7 (3.6),

75–79 group, Mattis = 134.9 (4.2),

80–99 group, Mattis = 133.3 (3.9)

(Table 15.34).

[WMS-R.5] Ivnik, Malec, Smith, Tangalos, Petersen, Kokmen and Kurland, 1992b

This study presents age-corrected (aka: age-specific) norms for the WMS-R derived from a sample of 441 cognitively normal individuals age 56 to 94 who are participants in Mayo's Older American Normative Studies (MOANS). Total sample $n = 441$; 56–74 years, $n = 274$; 75–94 years, $n = 167$. Information regarding the IQ of the sample was provided; however, *valid* WAIS-R verbal, performance, and full-scale IQs could only be calculated for 274 individuals that were age 56–74, since the standardization data could be obtained from the WAIS-R manual. For this group, the actual WAIS-R IQ summary data are as follows: VIQ = 106.1 (10.0), PIQ = 108.0 (11.7), and FSIQ = 107.3 (10.6). The MAYO cal-

culated values for the entire sample of 441 are as follows: VIQ = 105.5 (10.0), PIQ = 107.3 (11.4), and FSIQ = 106.6 (10.5).

The MOANS recruits participants from two ongoing research projects at the Mayo Clinic in Rochester, Minnesota. One of the goals of Research Project 1 is to obtain age-specific norms on traditional and experimental cognitive tests. Potential normal volunteers were captured by sampling all recent medical examinations performed at Mayo's Division of Community Internal Medicine. A participant was deemed "normal" if able to function independently and lacked any active neurologic or psychiatric conditions that might compromise cognitive status. All subjects had a thorough medical screening; however, chronic medical illness was not an exclusion criterion. For instance, persons with diabetes, cardiac problems, and hypertension were included in the "normal" sample. Individuals deemed normal by chart review were added to a possible participants list. Participants culled from research project 1 were willing to undergo a 4-hour outpatient clinic visit, during which a battery of neuropsychological tests were administered.

Research Project 2 is a component of the Mayo Clinic's ongoing Alzheimer's Disease Patient Registry. This project follows up all newly diagnosed persons with dementia who present for examination at Mayo's Department of Community Internal Medicine (CIM). Every patient is demographically matched to a normal control. The normal control is obtained by recruiting individuals who present for a general medical examination to any CIM internist. To be considered "normal," the individual must have a Mini-Mental State Exam (Folstein et al., 1975) score above 24, and the internist must satisfy "him or herself that the patient is indeed

Table 15.34. WMS-R.4; Means and Standard Deviations for Logical Memory I and II from the Wechsler Memory Scale-Revised

Group	Years	N	M_I	SD_I	M_{II}	SD_{II}
				Logical Memory Scores		
Overall		66	17.8	5.8	13.7	6.6
Group 1	70–74	25	19.4	5.4	15.7	6.7
Group 2	75–79	23	16.5	6.3	12.9	6.3
Group 3	80+	18	17.3	5.4	12.1	6.6

cognitively normal" (Ivnik et al., 1990). These individuals also received a neurological examination. Data from a potential recruit was reviewed by a team which included a geriatrician, neurologists, and neuropsychologists. These individuals had also been administered a battery of neuropsychological tests, but the results from this evaluation were not used in determining the normality of the potential subject. The criteria for normality were otherwise the same as for project 1.

Potential participants were randomly solicited from projects 1 and 2, and approximately 34% agreed to participate. A further exclusion criterion included inability to complete any neuropsychological test that was administered, regardless of reason.

The obtained MOANS normative sample consists of primarily well-educated (high school or greater) Caucasian adults living in Rochester, Minnesota, and the immediately surrounding "primarily agricultural" communities of Olmstead County.

Study strengths

1. Age-group intervals are generally adequate, with the exception of the table listing data for an 88-year-old midpoint. (The age-group interval for this midpoint value table is actually 83–94 years.)

2. Sample size is adequate.

3. Sample composition description is well detailed in the current and prior reports (Ivnik et al., 1990, 1991, 1992a; Malec et al., 1992).

4. Reporting of IQ and education levels was detailed.

5. Delayed recall conditions were administered according to the WMS-R manual.

6. The scoring procedure is well described according to standardized procedures detailed in the test manual.

7. Adequate exclusion criteria with the exception of chronic medical illness.

Considerations regarding use of the study

1. Data reporting does not include presentation of mean and standard deviation scores. Rather, tables are provided which convert WMS-R raw scores to percentile ranks and age-specific scaled scores for midpoint ages occurring at 3-year intervals from midpoint ages 61

through 88. The age range around each midpoint age is plus or minus 5 years.

Other comments

1. The sample consists of primarily well-educated, urban-residing, Caucasian adults, which should be considered when using these data.

2. One of the purposes of this study was to extend the norms on the WMS-R above age 74. In order to accomplish the extension, data were collected on normal volunteers aged 56–74. Data collected from this younger sample was then compared to the actual 56–74-year WMS-R norms available in the test manual to determine how the two groups differed. Knowing how the younger sample differed allowed Ivnik and colleagues to "correct" the norms collected from their 74–94-year-old sample so that they would correspond with what probably would have been the WMS-R norms for 74–94-year-olds had they actually been collected during the WMS-R standardization. In other words, this research provides a statistically derived estimate of probable WMS-R values for individuals older than age 74. The differences noted in performance values between the WMS-R standardization sample and the MOANS sample most probably reflect the different sampling procedures employed in the two studies as well as the differences in sampling national vs. regional populations.

MAYO procedures convert all WMS-R subtest raw scores to age-corrected, normalized scaled scores "before any other algebraic or tabular conversions" are undertaken.

Regarding the "normalizing" procedure, each raw score in the MAYO sample was first converted to a percentile rank "based upon the actual cumulative percent distribution." Each percentile rank was then converted to a scaled score ($M = 10$, $SD = 3$). Within each age group, "the percentile range encompassed by each scaled score was set so that the resultant distribution of scaled scores was as normal as possible," resulting in age-corrected scaled scores. In determining age-corrected MOANS WMS-R summary indices, linear transformations of the sums of MOANS scaled scores were computed to convert the distribution to the accepted WMS-R standard (i.e., $M = 100$, $SD =$

15). The resulting summary scores are referred to as MAYO Verbal Memory Index, MAYO Visual Memory Index, MAYO General Memory Index, MAYO Attention/Concentration Index, MAYO Delayed Recall Index, MAYO Percent Retention Index. The MAYO Percent Retention Index is a new index and is computationally derived.

3. A major assumption of Ivnik and colleagues is that the "persons above age 74 who agreed to serve as normal volunteers are demographically similar to those age 56 through 74, since they were drawn from the same population via identical sampling procedures. We further assume that the differences which exist between our younger sample and the [WMS-R] national sample would be similar for the persons above age 74 if we were able to compare these older persons to a national normative sample of like age (p. 5)."

4. The administration and scoring procedures for the MAYO system are identical to the WMS-R with the exception of the Verbal and Visual Paired Associates I subtests. Specifically, for the Verbal and Visual Paired Associates I subtests, if the criterion was not reached by the third learning trial, additional trials were not administered as required by the WMS-R manual. As a result, the MAYO Delayed Recall Index is not directly comparable to the WMS-R Delayed Recall Index.

5. Since Ivnik and colleagues are applying the same norming procedure to each test in their extensive neuropsychological battery, this should enhance the comparability of test scores across tests.

6. MAYO indices differ from WMS-R indices, even for the 56–74-year olds. Therefore, if you are evaluating someone who was previously tested when they were 74 or younger, and you are now examining them at an age above 74, you will need to convert the prior exam scores to MOANS equivalents in order to compare old vs. current performance.

7. MAYO and Wechsler summary scores are *not* interchangeable. Ivnik et al. (1993) notes that the difference can be as large as plus or minus 17 points.

Due to the innovative nature and the voluminous amount of the normative data, they are not reproduced here. The reader is referred to the original article.

[WMS-R.6] Richardson and Marottoli, 1996

This study provides education-corrected normative data for the performance of adults, aged 75 to 91 years, on commonly administered neuropsychological tests. The sample consists of a subset of 101 adults (53 males, 48 females) recruited from a larger longitudinal study (Project Safety, n = 1,103), aged 76–91 years who were active drivers, free from neurologic and psychiatric disease, and living independently in an urban community in the northeastern United States (e.g., New Haven, CT).

Education levels were reported as follows:

Age	76–80 years	81–91 years
Education	10.44 (3.86)	11.59 (3.45)
Sample size	50	51

Range for entire sample: 4th grade through college

Sample size for the age education categories are as follows:

Age	76–80		81–91	
Education	<12 years	≥12 years	<12 years	≥12 years
Sample size	26	24	18	33

Study strengths
1. Age-group intervals are adequate.
2. Adequate exclusion criteria. The sample description was adequate.
3. Education for the sample was reported.
4. Delayed recall was assessed for the Logical Memory and Visual Reproduction subtests.
5. Description of the administration and scoring procedures was according to the WMS-R test manual.
6. Data reporting included mean and standard deviation scores.
7. Information regarding gender and geographic area is reported.

Considerations regarding use of the study
1. Sample size is adequate for data reported by age category; however, it becomes quite small when data are presented by age and education.

Other comments
1. Use of the Logical Memory subtest performance data for the less well educated 81–91-

Table 15.35. WMS-R.6; Means and Standard Deviations of Test Scores for Age and Education Subgroups ($N = 101$)

	Age 76–80		Age 81–91	
	Education <12 (n = 26)	Education ≥12 (n = 24)	Education <12 (n = 18)	Education ≥12 (n = 33)
WMS-R				
LMI	14.17 (6.48)	19.24 (5.62)	14.29 (4.70)	19.57 (7.13)
LMII	8.88 (5.24)	12.70 (5.49)	9.12 (4.41)	12.69 (8.44)
VRI	20.29 (6.91)	28.24 (4.77)	20.31 (7.96)	23.70 (6.80)
VRII	8.63 (6.57)	16.15 (7.33)	11.56 (10.16)	11.97 (8.57)

year-olds should be used with caution due to small sample size and the finding that the norms deviated significantly from normality when compared to other available normative data.

2. The authors note that since their sample was not medically screened, and individuals were not ruled out if they had more common medical diseases (such as hypertension and diabetes) the "data should be viewed as reflecting the 'normative' population of urban drivers older than age 75 rather than the performance of 'normal' individuals" (Table 15.35).

[WMS-R.7] Marcopulos, McLain and Giuliano, 1997

The goal of this study was to develop normative data for rural community-dwelling adults aged 55 and older with no more than 10 years of formal education. Participants were administered a battery of nine neuropsychological tests.

The data were obtained from a biracial sample ($n = 133$; white = 64, African-American = 69) of nondemented, healthy adults, aged 55 and older (mean age = 76.48; SD = 7.87; range unknown), who attended school for 10 years or less (mean education = 6.65 years; SD = 2.14; range 0–10 years) and who were educated and primarily lived in a rural community setting (central Virginia). Subjects were excluded if they reported the presence of chronic or severe psychiatric disorder, history of extensive psychotropic drug use, long-term substance abuse, neurological disease, electroconvulsive therapy (ECT), head injury, or loss of consciousness. Subjects were paid $10 and received a certificate of appreciation for completing a 2-hour test battery which was administered in one test

session. Data were reported by age and again by age/education. The age group categories were as follows: 55–64, 65–74, 75–84, and 85+. The upper range of the oldest age category is not known. Education data were reported by age category as follows: 0–4 years, 5–6 years, 7–8 years, and 9–10 years. The sample contains primarily females.

Study strengths

1. Age-group intervals are generally adequate.

2. Adequate exclusion criteria. Sample composition description is adequate.

3. Education data were reported and grouped by age category.

4. Delayed recall for the Logical Memory and Visual Reproduction subtests is assessed.

5. Data reporting included presentation of mean and standard deviation scores.

6. Information on gender, ethnicity, and geographic area is provided.

Considerations regarding use of the study

1. Sample size is generally too small to allow valid use of the normative data.

2. Description of the scoring procedures was not specifically mentioned, but presumably followed the protocol in the WMS-R manual.

3. The sample is primarily female; therefore caution is suggested when applying the data to performance of males.

Other comments

1. The percent retention as a measure of the rate of forgetting (i.e., savings score) was calculated by using the following formula:

Savings score % = [delayed recall/immediate recall] × 100

The authors found the savings score to be relatively impervious to the effects of age and suggested that it may be "the most sensitive and specific indicator of abnormal memory functioning."

2. The authors highlight the fact that most of the normative data in the literature are based on urban high-school-educated, white, urban-residing adults. They caution that "the use of extant norms with lower educated, rural-dwelling, older adults can overestimate degree of cognitive impairment." Since 26% of the elderly live in nonurban areas and rural dwelling individuals tend to be disadvantaged in regard to education, the authors urge the development of more normative data for this group (Tables 15.36–15.39).

[WMS-R Abnorms. 1] Fox, 1994

The sample consists of 100 workers' compensation claimants (37 men, 63 women), aged 18–63, with alleged orthopedic or emotional injuries and without "potential neuropsychological sequelae (e.g., head injury, toxic exposure)." Education level is reported for the sample (13.5 [2.2] years; range 6–20 years). The WMS-R Logical Memory I was administered followed by approximately 30 minutes of nonmemory testing. Recall for the two paragraphs (Logical Memory II) was then elicited. This study examined a sample of neuropsychologically normal worker's compensation claimants performance on the Logical Memory subtest of the WMS-R. The sample had a mean MMPI Depression Scale T score of 78.8 (16.3). This sample performed significantly worse than the norms provided in the WMS-R manual. The author of this study makes the point that clinical comparison norms need to be developed for individuals involved in litigation. This study suggests that standard norms may inappropriately generate an impaired finding, especially if there are depressive complaints present.

Table 15.36. WMS-R.7a; Means and Standard Deviations for WMS-R Logical Memory I by Age and Education Level[*]

| Age | Education Level | | | | | |
| | 0–4 Years | | | 5–6 Years | | |
	N	M	(SD)	N	M	(SD)
55–64	1	4.0	(—)	2	19.0	(11.3)
65–74	5	11.2	(5.9)	8	14.0	(7.9)
75–84	12	11.8	(6.4)	15	13.4	(7.4)
85+	5	7.4	(2.4)	1	0.0	(—)
Total by Education	23	10.4	(5.7)	26	13.5	(8.0)
	7–8 Years			9–10 Years		
Age	N	M	(SD)	N	M	(SD)
55–64	2	16.5	(3.5)	2	14.0	(1.4)
65–74	20	16.9	(5.8)	10	16.7	(5.3)
75–84	28	14.1	(6.6)	8	19.4	(9.3)
85+	10	7.9	(6.4)	2	12.5	(12.0)
Total by Education	60	14.1	(6.8)	22	17.0	(7.3)
	Total by Age					
Age	N	M	(SD)			
55–64	7	14.7	(7.1)			
65–74	43	15.7	(6.2)			
75–84	63	14.2	(7.3)			
85+	18	7.8	(6.1)			

[*]Note: Total sample ($N = 131$); Mean = 13.8, SD = 7.2, Range = 0–32.

Table 15.37. WMS-R.7b; Means and Standard Deviations for WMS-R
Logical Memory II by Age and Education Level°

| Age | Education Level | | | | | |
| | 0–4 Years | | | 5–6 Years | | |
	N	M	(SD)	N	M	(SD)
55–64	1	2.0	(—)	2	14.0	(4.2)
65–74	5	4.4	(3.0)	8	8.9	(7.5)
75–84	12	7.4	(5.0)	15	8.5	(6.1)
85+	4	1.8	(2.1)	1	0.0	(—)
Total by Education	22	5.5	(4.6)	26	8.7	(6.5)

| Age | 7–8 Years | | | 9–10 Years | | |
	N	M	(SD)	N	M	(SD)
55–64	2	11.0	(1.4)	2	11.0	(0.0)
65–74	20	11.4	(6.7)	10	12.7	(5.4)
75–84	28	9.4	(7.1)	8	14.1	(9.2)
85+	10	3.8	(3.7)	2	10.5	(13.4)
Total by Education	60	9.2	(6.8)	22	12.9	(7.1)

| Age | Total by Age | | |
	N	M	(SD)
55–64	7	10.6	(4.4)
65–74	43	10.4	(6.6)
75–84	63	9.4	(6.9)
85+	17	3.9	(5.2)

°Note: Total sample ($N = 130$): Mean = 9.1, SD = 6.5, Range = 0–28.

Study strengths

1. Sample composition description is adequate.
2. Sample size is adequate.
3. Information reported on gender.
4. Data regarding education is provided.
5. Delayed recall procedure is well described.
6. The scoring procedures was according to the WMS-R manual.
7. Data recording include the reporting of mean and standard deviation scores.

Considerations regarding use of the study

1. Age-group interval is too broad (age 18–63 years).
2. Sample of patients with medical and/or psychiatric illness.

Other comments

1. Given the litigation setting, it is likely that the patients were not motivated to provide their best effort (Table 15.40).

Wechsler Memory Scale-III

[WMS-III.1] Wechsler, 1997

This is the standardization of the WMS-III. The normative information was generated from an age, sex, race/ethnicity, education level, and geographic region, nationally collected stratified sample representative of the 1995 U.S. population. The data are a subset ($n = 1,250$) of a larger stratified sample collected while norming the WAIS-III ($n = 2,450$). Subjects were located "primarily through the use of marketing research firms in 28 U.S. cities in the Northeast, North Central, South, and West regions." Subjects were recruited by random telephone calls, newspaper ads, and via flyers posted at senior centers and with various community organizations. Additionally, several independent examiners recruited and tested additional subjects. Standardization sampling sites (marketing researchers and independent researchers) were located in 47 of the 50 states (Hawaii, Utah, and North Carolina were evidently not included).

Table 15.38. WMS-R.7c; Means and Standard Deviations for WMS-R Visual Reproduction I by Age and Education Level.

| | Education Level | | | | | |
| | 0–4 Years | | | 5–6 Years | | |
Age	N	M	(SD)	N	M	(SD)
55–64	1	12.0	(—)		25.0	(1.4)
65–74	5	8.0	(5.4)	8	15.3	(7.5)
75–84	13	12.8	(5.9)	15	12.7	(5.7)
85+	5	10.2	(4.2)	2	3.5	(2.1)
Total by Education	24	11.2	(5.5)	27	13.7	(7.2)
	7–8 Years			9–10 Years		
Age	N	M	(SD)	N	M	(SD)
55–64	2	25.5	(4.9)	2	31.5	(4.9)
65–74	20	18.6	(7.7)	10	21.6	(9.2)
75–84	28	18.4	(8.8)	8	14.9	(8.1)
85+	10	9.2	(6.1)	2	15.0	(5.7)
Total by Education	60	17.2	(8.7)	22	19.5	(9.3)
	Total by Age					
Age	N	M	(SD)			
55–64	7	25.1	(7.1)			
65–74	43	17.4	(8.5)			
75–84	64	15.5	(7.9)			
85+	19	9.5	(5.7)			

°Note: Total sample ($N = 133$): Mean = 15.8, SD = 8.4, Range = 0–35.

All participants were paid for taking the tests. Participants were excluded if they were color-blind, had uncorrected hearing loss or visual impairment, were in current treatment for drug or alcohol dependence or consumed more than three alcoholic beverages on more than two nights a week, were taking any psychiatric medications, were seeing any professional for thinking or memory problems, had a disability that would affect motor performance, reported a history of unconsciousness for 5 minutes or more, or had a history of any medical or psychiatric condition that could potentially alter cognitive functioning (see *WAIS-III & WMS-III Technical Manual*, p. 22 for full details). Performance scores are reported for 11 age groupings in the range 16 to 79 years. Each of these age group categories contain data on 100 participants. The two oldest age groupings in the range 80 to 89 years each have a sample size of 75.

This is a proprietary test, and the normative data are available in the test manual. Scaled scores can be converted to percentiles by examining Table E.1 on page 200 of the *WMS-III Administration and Scoring Manual.*

Study strengths
1. Age-group intervals are adequate.
2. Sample size met criteria.
3. Information on education, gender, ethnicity, geographic area, and recruitment procedures is provided.
4. Delayed recall and recognition procedures are standard on all appropriate subtests.
5. Scoring procedures are well described in the manual.
6. Adequate exclusion criteria. Sample composition description is adequate.

Considerations regarding use of the study
1. Data reporting did not include mean and standard deviation scores; however, raw scores and their corresponding scaled score equivalents can be obtained from the tables.

Table 15.39. WMS-R.7d; Means and Standard Deviations for WMS-R Visual Reproduction II by Age and Education Level[°]

| | Education Level | | | | | |
| | 0–4 Years | | | 5–6 Years | | |
Age	N	M	(SD)	N	M	(SD)
55–64	1	2.0	(—)	2	22.5	(4.9)
65–74	5	4.6	(5.9)	8	6.1	(4.8)
75–84	13	5.5	(5.3)	15	6.2	(5.9)
85+	4	5.8	(4.3)	2	0.0	(0.0)
Total by Education	23	5.2	(5.0)	27	6.9	(7.0)
	7–8 Years			9–10 Years		
Age	N	M	(SD)	N	M	(SD)
55–64	2	18.0	(7.1)	2	12.5	(17.7)
65–74	20	11.3	(7.9)	10	11.7	(7.5)
75–84	28	9.9	(10.9)	8	6.9	(4.3)
85+	10	2.4	(4.4)	2	2.5	(3.5)
Total by Education	60	9.4	(9.5)	22	9.2	(7.5)
	Total by Age					
Age	N	M	(SD)			
55–64	7	15.4	(10.8)			
65–74	43	9.7	(7.4)			
75–84	64	7.7	(8.4)			
85+	18	2.9	(4.2)			

[°]Note: Total sample (N = 132): Mean = 8.1, SD = 8.2, Range = 0–34.

Other comments

1. Although education is well known to be positively correlated with performance on memory tests (Lezak, 1995), WMS-III normative data are not available by age *and* education. Data are also not available by age *and* IQ; however, some comparisons can be made with the WAIS-III since the two tests were co-normed.

2. The WMS-III battery, similar to the WMS and WMS-R, is designed so that individual subtests can be administered, scored, and interpreted as needed.

3. For the ages 16–64 years, an equal number of males and females participated; however, for the ages 65–89 years, the proportions reflected the 1995 Census data.

CONCLUSIONS

There have been three published versions of the WMS: the original WMS (1945), the WMS-R (1987), and WMS-III (1997). The strength and considerations regarding use of the extant comparison data for the various versions of the test battery are summarized below:

WMS (1945)

Idiosyncratic administration and scoring procedures generally limit the usefulness of many of the WMS normative studies. Additionally, many of the normative studies are over 20 years old, raising concerns regarding possible cohort effects. If the old WMS must be used, the test

Table 15.40. WMS-R Abnorms.1

| | M | SD | % Recalled | |
			M	SD
LMI	19.5	6.1	30.2	22.6
LMII	17.1	6.1	36.9	23.3
% Recall	88.3	17.1		

user is advised to select the "best" normative study before the evaluation takes place, so the test may be administered and scored according to how the selected norms were originally collected. For example, for the evaluation of memory function with the WMS in an adult who is 65 or older, the comparison data reported by Haaland et al. (1983), Van Gorp et al. (1990), Mitrushina & Satz (1991) probably represent the most appropriate norms available (including 30- or 45-minute delayed recall), especially if the individual is American, lives independently, comes from an upper socioeconomic status (SES) background, and is of at least average intelligence.

With respect to assessments of Americans, caution is recommended in the use of norms provided by studies conducted in other English-speaking countries, regardless of their merit, because of cultural differences. It is strongly advised that the normative data reported by any study be used only after a careful review of the subject and procedural variables employed, since the population to which the reported findings apply may be either restricted or ambiguous. Some investigators have reported only mean performance scores and provide no information on dispersion of performance scores (e.g., standard deviation). As a result, data from the reports of Klonoff & Kennedy (1965), Schaie & Strother (1968), and Ivison (1977) are difficult to apply for inferential purposes. There is considerable heterogeneity regarding the subject and procedural variables employed across the 28 normative studies for the original Wechsler Memory Scale. Therefore, reliance on "norms" derived from attempts to summarize or otherwise combine and/or reanalyze data from the various normative reports (Margolis & Scialfa, 1984; Wallace, 1984) and tables summarizing data from various normative reports (Piersma, 1986; Crosson et al., 1984a) requires appropriate caution.

WMS-R (1987)

Because the WMS-R has remained popular since its introduction over a decade ago, WMS-R subtests have been included in numerous research protocols, which insures that we will continue to see data published utilizing this test for years to come. As such, it is likely that the WMS-R will continue to be relied upon by clinicians and researchers during the phase-in period of acceptance of the WMS-III.

For Americans of average intelligence in the age ranges 16–17, 20–24, 35–44, 55–64, 65–69, and 70–74, the norms provided with the Wechsler Memory Scale Revision (WMS-R) should receive the strongest attention and generally be relied upon. The data presented for age groups 18–19, 25–34, and 45–54 most probably should only be utilized with appropriate caution since the values were estimated by statistical interpolation. Although "test standardization of necessity involves interpolation between points on a continuous variable like age" (Bowden & Bell, 1992, p. 34), granting permission to a commercial test developer/distributor to interpolate data across *decade* increments seems unjustified. We feel strongly that reliance upon such estimated normative data for interpretative purposes raises professional concerns. Highlighting our concern, Mittenberg et al. (1992) provided empirically derived provisional norms for the 25–34 age group. Differences between Mittenberg's norms and the WMS-R published index scores appeared to be clinically significant.

The normative data developed by Ivnik et al., (1992b) are also recommended as long as the demographics of Ivnik's participants match closely the demographic characteristics of the subject you are studying.

Despite the fact that educational level was significantly related to test performance in the standardization sample, WMS-R normative data stratified by age and education, as well as data for various ethnic and cultural groups, is lacking. Although four of the nine subtests of the WMS-R require delayed recall of the material presented, a recognition testing format was not provided, making it impossible to determine whether a poor recall score is due to an encoding problem or to a retrieval problem, or both. The interested reader is referred to work by Fastenau (1996), who has developed multiple-choice recognition stimuli for the WMS-R Logical Memory and Visual Reproduction subtests.

Over 10 years have passed since the introduction of the WMS-R, and considerable research has accumulated regarding its utility with various clinical populations. Although the WMS-R is a better instrument than the old WMS, the WMS-III should be considered the preferred version of the test for the assessment of memory functions. Research using the original WMS has generally ended, and new research using the WMS-R will soon cease. Therefore clinicians and researchers are encouraged to use the WMS-III. However, it still may be necessary to occasionally use sections of the original WMS or WMS-R when evaluating a patient previously assessed on an old form of the test.

WMS-III (1997)

The WMS-III standardization norms provided in the manual appear to be adequate for the ages 16 to 89, especially if applied to individuals born and educated in the United States. Since education has been consistently found to enhance performance on WMS test performance, future normative studies involving the WMS-III should report data by *age/education* categories. Although the WMS-III only recently appeared on the market, it will likely, and deservingly, become one of the most popular test batteries utilized to assess memory functioning.

16

Rey Auditory-Verbal Learning Test

BRIEF HISTORY OF THE TEST

The Rey Auditory-Verbal Learning Test (AVLT) has been extensively used to evaluate memory functioning in normal samples and in a variety of clinical samples representing different medical and psychiatric conditions. The test was introduced by the Swiss psychologist Andre Rey (1941) as a measure useful in assessing inconsistency in relative performance on the recall task vs. the recognition task. The test was described in English by Taylor (1959). The English translation of the AVLT does not correspond exactly with the original French version: Three French words were substituted in the translation ("bell" for "belt," "moon" for "sun," and "nose" for "mustache"). Later, Rey (1964) modified the procedure to include five free recall trials and a recognition task. Contemporary versions of this test (described in Lezak, 1976, 1983, 1995) include an interference trial (first introduced by Taylor, 1959) and postinterference recall; the most recent additions have been the delayed recall and delayed recognition trials (Lezak, 1983, 1995; Spreen & Strauss, 1991, 1998).

Variability in Administration of the AVLT

Due to its usefulness in detection and identification of faulty memory mechanisms, the AVLT gained remarkable popularity among clinicians. Interpretations of clinical data, however, are obscured by remarkable variability in administration of the test. There is very little uniformity in various procedural aspects:

1. The administration procedure varies widely. The standard administration includes five successive presentations of the original list of 15 words followed by free recall on each trial; an interference trial involving presentation and free recall of another list of 15 words; a postinterference free recall of the words from the original list; and a recognition trial (Lezak, 1995). A number of studies also utilized a delayed recall and delayed recognition trial (Lezak, 1995).

In contrast to this standard, some studies utilize a different number of recall trials, which varies from three (White, 1984) to six (Madison et al., 1986). The interference trial is omitted in several studies (Miceli et al., 1981; Bolla-Wilson & Bleecker, 1986; Bleecker et al., 1988). Uzzell and Oler (1986) omitted the postinterference recall trial and presented recognition immediately following recall of the interference list. Squire and Shimamura (1986) and Shimamura et al. (1987) modified their procedure to present a recognition trial after each of the five acquisition trials, without using free-recall trials. Shimamura et al. (1987) presented the words in a different order on each acquisition trial.

2. The format of the recognition trial varies widely: Rey (1964) and Lezak (1995) described a story format in which all 15 words from the original list are imbedded. The original story described by Rey contained twice as many distractor nouns as the one being utilized in current studies. According to Rey (1964), the story was to be read to the subject, who was instructed to stop the examiner when a word was recognized. The story described by Lezak was to be read by the subject with the instructions to circle recognized words. In addition to the story format, Lezak described other versions of the recognition trial, consisting of lists of 50 words which include words from list A, the interference list, and 20 words phonemically and/or semantically similar to the words from both lists presented to the subjects. Presentation of the lists can be either auditory or visual. It should be noted that other versions of the recognition list have been proposed. For example, Ivnik et al. (1987, 1990, 1992c) used a 30-word list for recognition.

The order of administration of the recognition trial also varies between studies. The recognition trial is administered after the postinterference recall trial, after the delayed recall trial (with varying delay intervals), or after both—postinterference and delayed recall trials, which influences performance on the last recognition trial.

3. The interval for the delay varies from 15 minutes (Miceli et al., 1981) to 60 minutes (Ivnik, et al., 1987). Geffen et al. (1990, 1994), and Selnes et al. (1991) used a 20-minute delay, whereas Ivnik et al. (1990, 1992) and Savage and Gouvier (1992) used a 30-minute delay. These differences in delay intervals should be taken into consideration, even though Lezak (1995) reports a minimal decline in recall over a 30 minute interval.

In addition, the delay interval is filled with various activities in different studies, which may influence performance on the delayed recall and recognition trials.

4. The rate of presentation differs across studies. According to Rey (1964) and Taylor (1959), each word should be separated by a 1-second interval. Rey also suggested recording the number of words remembered in each 15-second block to provide an indication of the rhythm of recall. According to Lezak (1995), the rate of the presentation should be one word per second. Some authors utilized a slower rate of presentation, e.g., one word every 2 seconds (White, 1984).

5. Time allowed for recall differs between studies. According to Rey's (1964) instructions, the first presentation of the list should be followed by recall within 60 seconds, and on subsequent acquisition trials, 90 seconds should be allowed for recall. The majority of investigators, however, allow unlimited time for recall. This aspect of administration is not usually described by the authors.

The degree of encouragement on the part of the examiner to elicit maximal effort from the subject also varies between the studies.

6. The extent of feedback on subject's performance on each trial might influence the results. According to Rey (1964) and Taylor (1959), the feedback had to be given to the subject each time the word was repeated within one trial. Rey also instructed test administrators to provide the subject with the feedback on the number of words recalled on each trial and to inform the subject on the fifth recall trial that this is the last trial. The current standard administration does not follow these guidelines. According to Lezak, the examiner should not volunteer information about repetition of the same words within one trial unless this information is solicited by the subject, because this might cause distraction.

Additional information on the history and procedural aspects of the AVLT is provided in several sources (Fabry, in press; Lezak, 1995; Peaker & Stewart, 1989; Spreen & Strauss, 1991; Wiens et al., 1988).

Functioning of Different Memory Mechanisms, as Assessed by the AVLT

The advantage of the AVLT is that it does not only provide a measure of rote verbal memory; it allows partitioning of memory processes into their components and identifying faulty memory mechanisms which lead to memory loss.

The AVLT was reported to load on a verbal learning and memory factor in a factor-analytic study conducted by Ryan et al. (1984). Vakil and Blachstein (1993) factor-analyzed the Rey AVLT performance of 146 normal subjects. The basic factors extracted were acquisition and retention. The latter factor was further subdivided into storage and retrieval. This information suggests that verbal memory functioning can be subdivided into separate mechanisms, which is consistent with empirical data accumulated in the field of experimental psychology. Integrity of these mechanisms is reflected in different indices derived from AVLT performance.

Recall on trial I represents immediate memory span for words. It is expected to be roughly similar to recall on the interference trial, because both of them present equivalent word lists for the first time. Superiority in recall on trial I over the interference trial may indicate the effects of proactive interference on the latter. The opposite pattern might suggest difficulties in changing response set (Lezak, 1995). In most cases immediate memory span for words is expected to be consistent with the immediate memory span for digits. Discrepancy between recall on trial I and digit span in favor of digit span can be attributed to information overload (Geffen et al., 1990).

Change in performance over five acquisition trials indicates a learning curve, and its slope provides a measure of verbal learning. Verbal learning over five acquisition trials is also commonly identified as the difference between recall on trial V vs. trial I. Some authors define learning as the difference between the highest recall on any trial vs. recall on trial I (Query & Megran, 1984).

Analysis of the recall pattern might shed light on the use of memory strategies and organization of the material. Mungas (1983) introduced a measure of consistency of sequential organization, reflecting the degree to which pairs of words that are recalled consecutively on one trial are recalled consecutively on the next trial.

Serial position effects have been reported to provide information on the functioning of certain memory mechanisms. Primacy and recency effects in the recall pattern provide another index of vulnerability to proactive and retroactive interference. These indices are useful in distinguishing amnesias affecting encoding mechanisms (in which case the predominance of the recency effect would be evident) and those conditions which compromise the efficiency of recall but spare basic encoding processes (demonstrating intact primacy and recency effects). For example, Tierney et al. (1994) reported greater recency than primacy effects in Alzheimer's patients, whereas Parkinson's dementia patients

as well as control subjects demonstrated intact primacy and recency effects. Similarly, Bigler et al. (1989) reported only recency effects in a sample of Alzheimer's patients. In contrast, Crockett et al. (1992) did not find differences in the magnitude of the primacy–recency effect in patients with anterior and posterior brain damage and in psychiatric inpatients. The serial position effect also reflects the predictive role of recall efficiency from the middle segment of the list. Ryan et al. (1992) reported a significantly lower recall of words from the middle segment in AIDS subjects in comparison to controls in a federal corrections sample.

Comparison of performance on acquisition and other trials provides another avenue for exploring memory mechanisms. Comparison of recall on trial V vs. the postinterference trial provides a measure of retention for newly learned information and its loss due to retroactive interference. The rate of forgetting over time can be explored through comparison between recall on the postinterference trial and the delayed recall trial. A comparison of performance on recall vs. recognition conditions provides additional insight into assessing faulty encoding, storage, or retrieval mechanisms. A comparison of the number of words recognized from list A and the interference list suggests differences in storage of overlearned vs. oncelearned material.

Analysis of errors also provides useful information on integrity of different memory mechanisms. Rey (1964) instructed that in addition to the number of correct responses, the number of false responses, repetitions, and repetitions where the subject questioned recalling the word previously should be recorded. Spreen and Strauss (1991) and Lezak (1995) suggest a notation system to identify the quality of errors on recall and recognition trials.

Quality of intrusion errors can be analyzed. Intrusions of words from list A on recall of interference list or from interference list on postinterference recall provides evidence of proactive interference and weakness in source or context memory (Geffen et al., 1990). Extralist intrusions reveal a tendency for semantic or phonetic confusion or confabulatory responses. Intrusions, as well as the tendency to repeat words from the list more than once, reflects impairment in self-monitoring functions (Lezak, 1995).

Ivnik et al. (1990, 1992c) and Geffen et al. (1990, 1994) developed additional measures of performance which allow exploration of the effect of different memory mechanisms on memory functioning. Similarly, Vakil and Blachstein (1994) developed a measure assessing incidental learning of temporal order which provides an additional index of retention.

Contribution of the Rey AVLT to accuracy of diagnostic determination in head injuries, dementias, amnesias, and frontal lobe syndrome has been well documented in the literature (Armstrong et al., 1996; Bigler et al., 1989; Blachstein et al., 1993; Glennerster et al., 1996; Guilmette & Rasile, 1995; Heubrock, 1995; Janowsky et al., 1989; Lezak, 1995; Lucas & Sonnenberg, 1996; Mitrushina et al., 1994, Mitrushina et al., 1995b).

In addition to its usefulness in the identification of faulty memory mechanisms, several AVLT indices can be used as measures of motivational level and cooperation in the testing procedures (Bernard, 1990, 1991; Bernard et al., 1993; Binder et al., 1993; Greiffenstein et al., 1994).

Practice Effect and Alternate Forms of the AVLT

The effect of repeated administration of the AVLT was investigated by several authors. Lezak (1982) reported a small but statistically significant practice effect observed at 6- and 12-month retest in a group of normal subjects. Mitrushina and Satz (1991a) reported improvement in recall on trial I (attributed to the practice effect) over repeated annual probes, which was consistent for all age groups in a sample of healthy elderly.

Crawford et al. (1989) hypothesized that two factors can lead to practice effects on memory tests: (1) retention of specific test material, and (2) metamemoric factor—i.e., effect of exposure to a similar task may facilitate development of optimal strategy. Comparison of the test–retest performance for those subjects who were presented with the same vs. different forms of the AVLT on the retest (27±3 days after original testing) indicated that the practice effect was evident only in the group exposed to the same list. Therefore, the practice effect is largely due to the retention of specific test material rather than to the metamemoric factor and can be overcome by using an alternate form on the retest. Shapiro and Harrison (1990) suggested that when the test–retest sessions are spaced very close to each other (5 days apart), there remains a general practice effect due to repeated administrations in healthy college students but not among the older patient population.

These results indicate a need for alternate forms of the AVLT which can be used in longitudinal evaluation of changes over time in patients' verbal memory. A number of investigators have developed alternate forms and reported their psychometric properties (Crawford et al., 1989; Geffen et al., 1994; Ryan et al., 1986; Shapiro & Harrison, 1990). Lezak (1995) provides several alternate forms. Ryan and Geisser (1986) reported high comparability between form A and form C provided by Lezak.

Criteria for generation of alternate word lists vary between different studies; however, the most salient requirements include a match between the original and alternate lists with regard to the following characteristics: probability of the occurrence of the word in English usage, which is assessed using Thorndike-Lorge tables (1944); word length (one- or two-syllable nouns); serial position; the imagery value of the words based on Paivio et al.'s (1968) tables; and control for semantic or phonetic associations between words. A good match of the word lists on the first criterion is especially important, since according to Fuller et al. (1997), low-frequency words result in lower recall and higher recognition than high-frequency words.

Different studies yielded a wide array of alternate form reliability coefficients, but generally coefficients fell within acceptable range (above 0.60).

Other Verbal and Nonverbal List Learning Tests

A number of more recent tests assessing verbal and nonverbal memory follow the same paradigm as the Rey AVLT.

The California Verbal Learning Test (CVLT; Delis et al., 1987) utilizes a structure similar to that of the Rey AVLT. The stimuli are presented in a shopping list format with words drawn from four categories. In addition to presentation of 16 nouns according to the standard procedure described above, the CVLT includes short-delay and long-delay cued recall (which aids recall by providing category cues), and a 44-word list for the recognition trial. The test is based on constructs developed in the context of cognitive psychology. Numerous measures aimed at assessment of cognitive strategies underlying subjects' performance are derived from test scores. In contrast to the Rey AVLT, the CVLT measures more than rote verbal memory; it also assesses subjects' ability to conceptualize information into categories, which facilitates learning. Normative data for seven age groups between ages of 17 and 80 are provided in the test manual (Delis et al., 1987).

A number of studies provide additional normative information on the CVLT and evaluate its clinical utility. Wiens et al. (1994) expand the normative database for normal subjects, whereas Otto et al. (1994) present data on CVLT performance for a large sample of depressed individuals. Keenan et al. (1996) and Kramer et al. (1988) discuss the effect of demographic variables on CVLT performance. Cullum et al. (1995), Stallings et al. (1995), and Vanderploeg et al. (1994) address memory mechanisms assessed by this test and its utility in clinical practice.

Based on a comprehensive review of the literature on the CVLT, Elwood (1995) reported limited utility of this test due to flaws in its design and standardization. The author concluded, however, that the CVLT can make a useful contribution to the clinical assessment if its limitations are recognized.

A shopping list format is also used in other list-learning tests because it presents an "ecologically valid" measure of learning and memory, especially in evaluation of older individuals. For example, Anschutz et al. (1985) report use of shopping list in assessment of mnemonic strategies utilized by elderly.

Lezak (1995) describes a new test recently developed by UCLA investigators for the World Health Organization (WHO/UCLA-AVLT; Maj et al., 1993), which is designed to minimize the cultural bias inherent in the Rey AVLT, while preserving its original format. The new test consists of two lists containing words from five categories: body parts, animals, tools, household objects, and vehicles. Similar to the Rey AVLT, the test requires the subject to learn 15 words across five learning trials. For each of the five categories, there are three exemplars. The WHO/UCLA-AVLT utilizes exemplars selected from the 250-item lexicon of universally familiar concepts as compiled by Snodgrass & Vanderwart (1980). A copy of the WHO/UCLA-AVLT and administration instructions can be found in Appendix 3. Due to "universal familiarity" of the words used in this test, its intercultural variability is low (Lezak, 1995), which warranted its use by the WHO in the study on cognitive sequelae of HIV-1 infection across different countries. Normative data stratified by age and education are available for a Spanish translation of the WHO/UCLA-AVLT test (Ponton et al., 1996).

Assessment of some patients with memory disorders using a list of 15 to-be-remembered words might be an overwhelming task. Lezak recommends administration of a shortened version of the Rey AVLT (10 words) in these cases. Similarly, the Consortium to Establish a Registry for Alzheimer's Disease (CERAD) battery includes a word-list learning task which taps immediate recall after one acquisition trial, recall after interference, and recognition of a 10-word list (Morris et al., 1989).

Toglia and Battig (1978) developed the Affective Auditory Verbal Learning Test, which consists of positively and negatively valenced word lists in addition to affectively neutral Rey AVLT. Snyder and Harrison (1997) suggested that the affective valency of the word list yielded different magnitudes of primacy vs recency effect, which may be useful in the evaluation of individuals suffering from affective disorders. Effect of positively and negatively valenced words on physiological measures of arousal was described by Snyder et al. (1998).

Majdan et al. (1996) developed a nonverbal analog of the Rey AVLT, the Aggie Figures Learning Test (AFLT). The three forms of the AFLT described by the authors were constructed according to the Rey AVLT format using abstract figures which do not lend themselves to verbal encoding. The authors emphasize that the AFLT is superior to the Rey Visual Design Learning Test (see Lezak, 1995), which has only one version and is designed to assess learning over five acquisition trials and recognition only. The Rey's analog does not contain an interference list, which precludes evaluation of retention rates. In addition, Rey's stimuli represent simple geometrical designs which can be easily encoded verbally.

In addition to these nonverbal analogs, Lezak (1995) described the Pictorial Verbal Learning Test (PVLT) which follows the five-trial learning format characteristic for the Rey AVLT.

For more information on list-learning tests, such as the CAVLT-2 for children, the Hopkins Verbal Learning Test, the Buschke Selective Reminding test, etc., refer to Lezak (1995).

RELATIONSHIP BETWEEN REY AVLT PERFORMANCE AND DEMOGRAPHIC FACTORS

The effect of demographic variables on AVLT performance has been extensively explored in the literature. Studies consistently demonstrate the effect of age on recall, and some studies report the effect of age on recognition (Bleecker et al., 1988; Geffen et al., 1990; Graf & Uttl, 1995; Mitrushina et al., 1991; Mitrushina & Satz, 1991; Savage & Gouvier, 1992; Selnes et al., 1991; Query and Berger, 1980; Query & Megran, 1983; Wiens et al., 1988). Some investigators suggest that age only impacts specific AVLT scores. For example, total number of words recalled on the five learning trials may be lower in older subjects, and they may show more information overload (forward digit span > trial 1), confusion regarding information source (e.g., misclassify list B words as list A words), and less efficient retrieval. However, rate of learning (learning curve), loss of information over a distractor or an extended delay, recognition ability, and false-positive errors may be resistant to aging (Bleecker et al., 1988; Bolla-Wilson & Bleecker, 1986; Cohen et al.,

personal communication; Geffen et al., 1990; Mitrushina et al., 1991; Wiens et al., 1988). Salthouse et al. (1996) suggested the presence of direct age-related influences on memory independent of speed of performance, based on the existence of the direct path from age to memory in their structural equation model.

The effect of education is somewhat more controversial. Cohen et al. (personal communication), Delaney et al. (1992), Query and Berger (1980), and Query and Megran (1983) observed a relationship between education and AVLT scores, while Mitrushina et al. (1991), Bolla-Wilson and Bleecker, 1986), and Wiens et al. (1988) could not detect a significant association. Bolla-Wilson and Bleecker (1986) argue, based on their multiple regression analyses, that education does not account for AVLT test score variance over that associated with IQ. The other studies reporting a relationship between education and AVLT performance either did not include an examination of the effects of IQ on scores or simply reported correlations between education and AVLT scores without controlling for the significant association between education and IQ.

Interestingly, the effect of IQ is not consistently seen across all studies. Bolla-Wilson and Bleecker (1986) and Query and Megran (1983) reported an association between IQ and AVLT measures, although there has been some discrepancy in the literature regarding which specific scores are affected. Wiens et al. (1988) reported an effect of FSIQ and age on recall, but not recognition, which suggests utility of recognition in assessment of pathological conditions, free of confounds from demographic and IQ factors. Similarly, Bleecker et al. (1988) did not find an effect of age, sex or vocabulary storage on recognition performance.

Sex differences on the AVLT have recently been reported. Women outperformed men on learning, interference, and delayed recall trials (Bleecker et al., 1988; Bolla-Wilson & Bleecker, 1986; Cohen et al., personal communication; Geffen et al., 1990; Vakil & Blachstein, 1997). Other studies, however, did not demonstrate an effect of gender on any of the AVLT measures (Savage & Gouvier, 1992; Wiens et al., 1988).

To account for the effect of demographic

variables on test performance, Tuokko and Woodward (1996) developed a demographic correction system (using Heaton, Grant and Matthews, 1991, procedure), which incorporates various neuropsychological measures, including Rey AVLT. It was developed and validated on samples of community-dwelling and institutionalized Canadian elderly over the age of 65 years. In the context of this system, raw scores are converted to T scores corrected for age and education, which can be plotted on a profile sheet containing suggested optimal cutoff points for impairment. The set-up of the profile sheet allows grouping of data in accordance with the DSM-III-R criteria for dementia. The authors suggest that application of demographic correction system considerably improves accuracy of diagnostic interpretations of test scores.

METHOD FOR EVALUATING THE NORMATIVE REPORTS

The studies reporting normative data on the Rey AVLT vary in description of procedural and subject variables and in the grouping of obtained data into categories.

In order to adequately evaluate the AVLT normative reports, seven key criterion variables were deemed critical. The first five of these relate to *subject* variables, and the remaining two dimensions refer to *procedural* issues.

Minimal requirements for meeting the criterion variables were as follows:

Subject Variables

Age Group Intervals

This criterion reflects the grouping of data into limited age intervals. Age proved to be highly related to performance on this test (see above), which warrants careful attention to appropriate age grouping of the data.

Sample Size

The data based on small sample sizes are highly influenced by individual differences and do not provide an accurate estimate of the population parameters. However, it is difficult to specify an adequate number of subjects which would be universal for all studies, since it depends on the purpose of the study and the characteristics of the population subjects are drawn from. These factors were taken into consideration when assessing adequacy of the sample size for the studies reviewed in this chapter. In general, at least 50 subjects for normative grouping is preferable.

Sample Composition Description

Information regarding medical and psychiatric exclusion criteria is important; it is unclear if information regarding geographic recruitment region, socioeconomic status or occupation, ethnicity, handedness, and recruitment procedures is relevant, so until this is determined, it is best that this information be provided.

IQ and Educational Levels

Whereas there is some controversy in the literature as to the effect of the intellectual and educational levels on Rey AVLT performance, it is important that individual scores be viewed in the context of persons with similar intellectual and educational background.

Sex Distribution

Given the possible relationship between gender and AVLT performance, gender distribution of the sample needs to be taken into consideration, and data should preferably be presented for males and females separately.

Procedural Variables

Description of Administration Procedures

As pointed out above, administration procedures differ widely among studies. Detailed description of administration procedures allows selection of the most appropriate norms or corrections in interpretation of the data to account for differences in administration procedure.

Data Reporting

In order to facilitate interpretation of the data, the group mean and the standard deviation for all AVLT trials should be presented at minimum.

Table 16.1. RAVLT.L; Locator Table for the RAVLT

Study[*]	Age[**]	N	Sample Composition	IQ,[**] Education	Trials Reported	Country/ Location
RAVLT.1 Rey, 1941, 1964 page 333	—	132	French speaking, Swiss Ss classified into 5 occupational groups	—	I–V	Sweden
RAVLT.2 Query & Megran, 1983 page 333	19–81 15–24 25–29 30–34 35–39 40–44 45–49 50–54 55–59 60–64 65–69 70+	677 54 88 109 54 50 52 83 81 57 26 23	The study provides norms for male ambulatory inpatients treated for a variety of physical complaints at a VA Medical Center	Education 11.44 WAIS IQ 93.83	I & V, postinter- ference, recall, recognition	North Dakota
RAVLT.3 Rosenberg, et al., 1984 page 334	48.62 (16.60) 47.51 (13.59)	47 45	VAMC psychiatric and neurological inpatients classified as memory- impaired and non- memory-impaired	Education 10.81 (3.01) 11.87 (2.58)	1–5, postinter- ference, recall, recognition	Illinois
RAVLT.4 Cohen, et al., personal communication page 335	60–64 65–69 70–74 ≥75	81	Normative data are provided for elderly volunteers per age group, for males and females separately	Education 13.8	Trials I–V, interference, postinter- ference recall, immediate recognition, 30-minutes delayed recall, delayed recognition	Peoria, Illinois
RAVLT.5 Ryan et al., 1986 page 336	45.86 (14.05)	85	VAMC inpatients served as subjects in a study assessing alternate form relibility for AVLT	Educ. 11.85	I–V, Postinter- ference, recall, recognition for alternate forms	Kansas
RAVLT.6 Bleecker et al., 1988 page 337	40–49 50–59 60–69 70–79 80–89	196	The study presents norms for healthy subjects broken down by age group and gender	Means range from 13 to 18 years for different groups	I–V recognition	Maryland
RAVLT.7 Wiens et al., 1988 page 338	19–51 29.1 (6.0)	222	The study presents norma- tive data for healthy job applicants, representing an occupational cross- section of the community; 193 M, 29 F. The data were stratified by FSIQ, age, and education	≥12 for all groups	I–V, postinter- ference recall, recognition	Oregon
RAVLT.8 Crawford		60	The study compared test–		Trials I–V, inter-	UK

continued

Table 16.1. (*Continued*)

Study[°]	Age[°°]	N	Sample Composition	IQ,[°°] Education	Trials Reported	Country/ Location
et al., 1989 page 339			retest performance over 27 days with the same form of RAVLT and with a parallel version developed by the authors. Subjects were healthy adults.		ference, post-interference recall, recognition	
RAVLT.9 Nielsen et al., 1989 page 343	20–54 Groups: 20–29 30–39 40–54	101 35 27 39	53 M, 48 F; the majority of Ss had undergone minor surgery and were tested several weeks postsurgery	VIQ 98.6 (12.2)	I–V, total for trials I–V, delayed recall	Denmark
RAVLT.10 Roth et al., 1989 page 344	27.5 (SE=1.0)	61	45 M, 16 F; control Ss in a study on neuropsy-chological deficits in acute spinal cord injury	Education 12.8 (SE=0.2)	I–V, interference, postinter-ference, recognition, (means and SEs are reported)	Detroit, Ann Arbor, Michigan
RAVLT.11 Geffen et al., 1990 page 345	16–86 16–19 20–29 30–39 40–49 50–59 60–69 70–86	153 25 20 23 23 20 22 20	Norms are provided for adults ranging in age 16 to 86. Variety of perfor-mance indices are derived to explore different memory mechanisms	Education 11.2	All standard recall, delayed recall and recognition trials, serial position and functional indices	Australia
RAVLT.12 Ivnik et al., 1990 page 346	55–97 55–59 60–64 65–69 70–74 75–79 80–84 85–97	394 45 53 64 67 69 49 47	The study provides age-specific norms for elderly	Education range ≥7 years to ≥18 years	Trials I–V, inter-fer, postinter-ference recall, 30-minute delayed recall, and 4 summary scores	Omstead County, Minnesota
RAVLT.13 Miller et al., 1990 page 349	Age range 21–72 37.20 (7.52) 35.66 (6.47) 36.90 (7.04)	769 727 84	The study compared performance of the 3 groups of homosexual/ bisexual men: 1. Seronegative 2. Asymptomatic seropositive 3. Symptomatic seropositive	16.36 (2.34) 15.70 (2.44) 16.06 (2.50)	Trial V, total for trials I–V	MACS Centers at Baltimore, Chicago, L.A., & Pittsburgh
RAVLT.14 Shapiro & Harrison, 1990 page 350	66 19	17 25	Four alternate forms of RAVLT were compared. Two of these forms were generated according to the criteria developed by the authors. Two subject samples were used: VAMC patients and undergraduate students		Trials I–V, inter-ference, post-interference recall	Virginia

continued

Table 16.1. (*Continued*)

Study°	Age°°	N	Sample Composition	IQ,°° Education	Trials Reported	Country/ Location
RAVLT.15 Mitrushina & Satz, 1991a page 351	57–65 66–70 71–75 76–85	19 40 47 16	Performance of highly functioning elderly sample is compared over three longitudinal annual probes	Education 14.4 13.7 14.5 14.0	Trial I, Trial V, postinterference recall	California
RAVLT.16 Mitrushinaet al., 1991 page 355	57–65 66–70 71–75 76–85	28 45 57 26	Norms are provided for highly functioning elderly sample broken down into four age groups	Education 14.2 14.0 14.6 13.3	Trials I–V, postinterference recall, recognition, false positives, computed rates of acquisition and forgetting, primacy/ recency effect	California
RAVLT.17 Selnes et al., 1991 page 356	25–34 35–44 45–54	733	The study reports normative data collected on a large sample of seronegative homosexual/bisexual men. The data are stratified by age, education, and age/education	<college College >college	Trial V, total for Trials I–V, Postinterference recall, delayed recall, Delayed recognition	MACSCenters at Baltimore, Chicago, L.A., & Pittsburgh
RAVLT.18 Delaney et al., 1992 page 357	45.8 22–67	42	Control SS w/out histories of neurologic or psychiatric problems	Education 12.8 6–16	I, III, IV delayed recall, delayed recognition	Conneticut, California, Florida, Virginia, Massachusetts, New York, Minnesota
RAVLT.19 Ivnik et al., 1992c page 358	Age range 56–97 divided into groups based on midpoint interval technique	530	The study provides age-specific norms for elderly. Scoring procedures were developed which convert raw scores and computed scores into scaled scores	Education range ≥7 years to ≤ 18 years	Raw scores for various recall and recognition trials are reported in the earlier article. Conversion tables from raw scores to scaled scores are presented in this article	Minnesota
RAVLT.20 Savage & Gouvier, 1992 page 361	16–19 20–29 30–39 40–49 50–59 60–69 70–76	134	The study provides norms for RAVLT recall, memory and recognition trials broken down by age group and gender	≥12 years	Trials I–V, interference, Postinterfer ence recall, recognition, 30-minute delayed recall, delayed recognition	Louisiana
RAVLT.21 Crossen & Wiens, 1994 page 366	29.9 (6.2)	60	Performance on RAVLT and CVLT was compared for a group of healthy adults	Education 14.7 FSIQ 106.3	Trials I–V, interference, Postinterference recall, recognition	

continued

Table 16.1. (*Continued*)

Study[a]	Age[b]	N	Sample Composition	IQ,[b] Education	Trials Reported	Country/Location
RAVLT.22 Geffen et al., 1994 page 367	31.3 (12.7)	51	The study explored equivalence between the orginal form of RAVLT and a new form on a sample of healthy volunteers	Education 12.2	Trials I–V, interference, Postinterference recall, 20-minute delayed recall, recognition	Brisbane, Australia

[a]The study number corresponds to the number provided in the text of the chapter.

[b]Age column and IQ/education column contain information regarding range, and/or mean and standard deviation for the whole sample and/or separate groups, whichever information is provided by the authors.

SUMMARY OF THE STATUS OF THE NORMS

Table 16.1 summarizes information provided in the studies described in this chapter.[1] The majority of the studies present data in number of words produced by subjects on different RAVLT trials. When reported units deviate from this format, the system used will be described in the context of that particular table.

SUMMARIES OF THE STUDIES

Normative Studies

[RAVLT.1] Rey, 1941, 1964

The author provided normative data for the five learning trials on a sample of 132 French-speaking Swiss subjects. The AVLT performance of five groups is reported: manual laborers ($n = 25$), professionals ($n = 30$), students ($n = 47$), elderly laborers ($n = 15$), and elderly professionals ($n = 15$). Age ranges are specified only for the last two groups: The elderly laborers ranged in age from 70 to 90, and the elderly professional ranged from 70 to 88. No other descriptive data are provided, such as mean educational or intellectual level and exclusion criteria. Mean scores and standard deviations across the five learning trials are reported. No other data are available.

Study strengths
1. Large overall sample size.

[1] Normative data for children and adolescents are provided by Spreen and Strauss (1998).

Considerations regarding use of the study
1. Data were collected more than 50 years ago on French-speaking subjects.
2. No data are available for the interference trials or delayed recall.
3. No description of exclusion criteria, IQ levels, years of education, or composition of the sample by sex.
4. Subjects were French-speaking, and as discussed earlier, the French test stimuli differ from the currently used English words (i.e., "moustache," "sun," and "belt" were included in the French stimuli).

Other comments
1. Chiulli et al. (1985) reported that use of Rey's norms led to a misclassification of 22% of their control group as impaired (using criteria of 1 standard deviation below the appropriate age and education mean). They recommend caution in using Rey's norms, and this concurs with our own clinical experience (Table 16.2).

[RAVLT.2] Query and Megran, 1983

The study provides norms for 677 male ambulatory inpatients between ages 19 and 81 treated at North Dakota VAMC for a variety of physical complaints. The mean education was 11.44; the mean IQ was 93.83. Psychotic, severely brain damaged patients and those suffering from major depressive disorder were not included in the study. The sample was divided into age groups.

The standard administration procedure was used; recognition was measured with a story in which the subject was instructed to circle words from the learned list. Learning was measured

Table 16.2. RAVLT.1

Subject Groups		Trial				
		I	II	III	IV	V
Manual Laborers	Mean	7.0	10.5	12.9	13.4	13.9
(n = 25)	SD	2.1	1.9	1.6	2.0	1.2
Professionals	Mean	8.6	11.8	13.4	13.8	14.0
(n = 30)	SD	1.5	2.0	1.4	1.1	1.0
Students	Mean	8.9	12.7	12.8	13.5	14.5
(n = 47)	SD	1.9	1.8	1.5	1.3	0.7
Elderly laborers	Mean	3.7	6.6	8.4	8.7	9.5
(70–90 years)	SD	1.4	1.4	2.4	2.3	2.2
(n = 15)						
Elderly professionals	Mean	4.0	7.2	8.5	10.0	10.9
(70–88 years)	SD	2.9	2.9	2.5	3.3	2.9
(n = 15)						

by the difference in number of words recalled on the highest trial from the lowest trial.

Study strengths
1. The data were broken down by age group.
2. Administration procedure was well outlined.
3. Sample size was large and most individual cells exceed Ns of 50.
4. Means and standard deviations are reported.
5. Information on gender, education, IQ, and geographic area was presented.

Considerations regarding use of the study
1. Data for acquisition trials 2–4 and postinterference trial were not provided.
2. Demographic characteristcs for each group were not reported, even though some of them were used in the analyses.
3. The exclusion criteria indicate that "severely brain damaged" individuals were not included in the sample. This implies that mildly to moderately brain-damaged patients were included.
4. The data were collected on medical patients in an acute care hospital.
5. Mean IQs nearly fell within the low average range of intellectual ability, and mean educational level was below average. Thus, the data may be relevant only for individuals with IQs in the 80s and 90s.
6. Data are available only for males.

Other comments
1. The data suggest effect of education and IQ on maintenance of learning ability for younger men. A more complicated relationship was found for older men. The authors concluded that there is a progressive short-term memory loss with advancing age, which results in decline in recall, then in recognition, followed by decline in learning ability. Recognition is highly affected by IQ in older men (Table 16.3).

[RAVLT.3] Rosenberg, Ryan and Prifitera, 1984

Ninety-two male psychiatric and neurological inpatients from V.A. Medical Center in Chicago were divided into memory-impaired and non-memory-impaired groups. Those subjects whose memory quotient (MQ) based on WMS was ≥12 points lower than the WAIS FSIQ and/or those whose MQ was <85 were classified as memory impaired. The groups did not differ significantly with respect to age or education. Subjects were referred to the psychology service for routine psychological and/or neuropsychological evaluation and were selected without regard to diagnostic classification. Mean age, education, and FSIQ for the entire sample were 48.05 (14.03), 11.37 (2.82), and 93.11 (13.43), respectively.

The test was administered according to Lezak's description. The paragraph was used for the recognition task.

Table 16.3. RAVLT.2°

Age	N	Trial I M	Trial I SD	Trial V M	Trial V SD	Interference M	Interference SD	Recognition M	Recognition SD	V–I Difference
15–24	54	6.15	1.46	11.50	0.63	9.80	1.66	12.81	2.26	5.35
25–29	88	5.98	1.43	11.27	1.87	9.91	2.36	12.16	2.51	5.29
30–34	109	5.68	1.17	10.71	4.19	9.08	2.94	13.03	1.57	5.03
35–39	54	5.49	1.77	11.80	1.94	9.55	2.05	13.45	1.12	6.31
40–44	50	5.51	1.44	11.14	1.59	9.37	2.60	12.86	2.25	5.63
45–49	52	5.10	1.27	10.43	1.92	8.18	2.91	12.23	1.70	5.33
50–54	83	5.01	1.62	9.38	2.66	7.12	3.40	11.48	2.67	4.37
55–59	81	4.53	2.50	8.80	5.04	5.96	4.28	10.75	6.41	4.27
60–64	57	4.09	1.61	7.54	2.57	5.81	2.64	9.96	2.62	3.45
65–69	26	4.12	1.26	7.29	6.12	5.21	2.58	9.50	3.33	3.17
70+	23	3.14	1.50	5.86	2.04	3.45	2.92	8.91	3.64	2.72

°The table provides data for males only.

Study strengths

1. Information on age, education, IQ, gender, recruitment procedures, and geographic area is provided.
2. Sample sizes were sufficient.
3. Test administration procedures and the type of the recognition task were identified.
4. Means and standard deviations are reported.

Considerations regarding use of the study

1. Data were not partitioned into age groups.
2. The "normal control" sample is not representative of the overall population. It consists of neurological and psychiatric patients.
3. All male patient sample.
4. Somewhat low IQ level (Table 16.4).

[RAVLT.4] Cohen, Andres and Smolen, Personal communication

Subjects (Ss) were elderly volunteers (53 women and 28 men) from Peoria, Illinois and the surrounding communities, ranging in age from 60 to 89 years. Mean education was 13.8 years; 30.6% of the sample were suffering from hypertensive illness and 18.8% reported a history of head trauma. These subjects were included in the study since the results of the preliminary regression analyses indicated a lack of association between test performance and these conditions. However, gender was found to be related to performance. Therefore, norms are presented for males and females separately.

Administration procedure included acquisition trials with immediate recognition, and 30-minute delayed recall followed by delayed recognition trial.

Study strengths

1. The data are partitioned into age groups.
2. The data are presented for males and females separately.
3. A comprehensive set of scores is presented.
4. Information regarding education, gender, and geographic area is provided.

Table 16.4. RAVLT.3

	N	Years Age	Years Education	RAVLT Trial I	II	III	IV	V	Recall After Interference	Recognition
N°	45	47.51 (13.59)	11.87 (2.58)	4.96 (1.78)	6.81 (2.31)	8.66 (2.33)	9.40 (2.53)	9.71 (3.04)	7.81 (3.71)	11.53 (3.06)
I	47	48.62 (16.60)	10.81 (3.01)	3.91 (1.93)	5.00 (2.06)	5.71 (2.27)	6.13 (2.77)	6.89 (2.91)	4.07 (2.79)	8.18 (4.05)

°N—Normal; I—Impaired.

5. Test administration procedures are generally specified.

6. Means and standard deviations are reported.

Considerations regarding use of the study

1. Sample sizes are small.

2. High mean educational level.

3. The exact recognition procedure was not specified.

4. No reported exclusion criteria. Subjects with histories of head trauma and chronic illnesses (e.g., hypertension) were included.

5. No information on IQ.

6. An immediate recognition trial was used, which facilitates performance on delayed recall and delayed recognition.

Other comments

1. The authors concluded that gender, age, and education were related to performance, with women performing better than men (Tables 16.5 and 16.6).

[RAVLT.5] Ryan, Geisser, Randall, and Georgemiller, 1986

The study provides alternate form reliability and equivalency in a group of diagnostically heterogeneous inpatients from the V.A. Medical Center in Kansas (82 males and 3 females) referred for psychological and/or neuropsycho-logical assessment. The sample represented a wide range of psychiatric and neurological diagnoses, including undiagnosed patients and vocational counseling clients. This sample, therefore, is not representative of any identifiable diagnostic group.

For the original administration of the test, the authors followed the standard procedure described in Lezak (1983). The recognition trial consisted of a list of 50 words which included words from list A and list B (interference list) and 20 words phonemically and/or semantically similar to those in lists A and B.

For the alternate form, the authors used list C provided by Lezak (1983) and Taylor (1959). Interference and recognition stimuli were constructed by the authors following Lezak's model.

The original and alternate forms were presented in a counterbalanced order with the mean test–retest interval of 140 minutes.

Study strengths

1. Administration procedure is well identified.

2. Information on age, education, IQ, gender, ethnicity, recruitment procedures, and geographic area is provided.

3. Sample size is large.

4. Information on alternate form.

5. Means and standard deviations are reported.

Table 16.5. RAVLT.4a: Females

	Age Group			
	60–64 (n = 23)	65–69 (n = 13)	70–74 (n = 12)	≥75 (n = 9)
Subtest	M(SD)	M(SD)	M(SD)	M(SD)
Trial I	5.70 (1.48)	5.46 (1.39)	5.67 (1.23)	4.94 (1.63)
Trial II	8.13 (1.69)	8.88 (2.08)	8.42 (1.38)	8.17 (1.80)
Trial III	10.00 (1.84)	10.31 (1.81)	10.04 (1.48)	9.33 (1.92)
Trial IV	11.58 (2.35)	11.00 (1.97)	10.67 (1.66)	10.72 (2.28)
Trial V	11.83 (2.39)	11.54 (2.61)	10.71 (1.82)	11.33 (2.12)
List B	6.13 (2.20)	5.81 (1.93)	5.17 (1.48)	5.50 (1.17)
List B errors	0.00 (0.00)	0.23 (0.44)	0.33 (0.65)	0.44 (0.73)
Trial VI postinterference recall (PostIR)	10.15 (2.94)	9.23 (3.21)	8.21 (2.23)	7.78 (3.87)
Intrusions from list B	0.09 (0.29)	0.08 (0.28)	0.25 (0.45)	0.33 (0.71)
Trial V − I	6.04 (1.60)	6.08 (2.17)	5.04 (1.32)	6.39 (2.00)
Trial VI − V	1.67 (1.87)	2.31 (1.75)	2.50 (1.17)	3.56 (2.60)
Total errors	0.70 (1.40)	1.38 (1.80)	2.08 (2.61)	2.00 (2.24)
Immediate Recognition	12.65 (2.10)	12.46 (2.40)	12.25 (2.05)	12.22 (3.67)
Delayed (30-minute) recall	9.98 (2.66)	9.38 (2.95)	9.00 (3.08)	8.61 (3.00)
Delayed (30-minute) recognition	12.61 (1.70)	12.69 (1.75)	11.58 (2.50)	11.33 (3.88)

Table 16.6. RAVLT.4b: Males

	Age Group			
Subtest	60–64 (n = 8) M (SD)	65–69 (n = 7) M (SD)	70–74 (n = 9) M (SD)	≥75 (n = 4) M (SD)
Trial I	5.24 (1.50)	6.00 (1.00)	4.22 (1.32)	3.75 (2.50)
Trial II	6.88 (1.46)	8.36 (1.49)	6.44 (1.13)	6.50 (0.58)
Trial III	8.25 (2.38)	9.79 (1.78)	7.22 (1.80)	8.25 (1.71)
Trial IV	9.38 (1.92)	10.71 (2.36)	8.22 (1.64)	9.75 (2.22)
Trial V	10.50 (1.69)	12.14 (1.86)	8.72 (0.90)	9.25 (1.89)
List B	5.38 (1.22)	5.57 (1.40)	4.06 (1.55)	4.25 (1.71)
List B errors	0.25 (0.46)	0.43 (0.54)	0.11 (0.33)	0.25 (0.50)
Trial VI (PostIR)	6.75 (2.71)	8.57 (3.50)	5.94 (1.98)	8.50 (1.73)
Intrusions from list B	0.00 (0.00)	0.14 (0.38)	0.11 (0.33)	0.25 (0.50)
Trial V − I	5.25 (2.19)	6.14 (1.95)	4.61 (1.87)	5.50 (1.73)
Trial VI − V	3.75 (2.12)	3.57 (1.99)	2.78 (1.50)	0.75 (0.50)
Total errors	4.38 (6.68)	1.29 (0.95)	1.67 (3.08)	1.25 (1.89)
Immediate recognition	9.71 (1.89)	11.43 (2.22)	11.89 (1.27)	11.75 (2.50)
Delayed (30-minute) recall	7.71 (1.80)	7.71 (2.98)	4.89 (1.54)	8.25 (2.63)
Delayed (30-minute) recognition	10.43 (1.72)	11.14 (3.08)	11.89 (2.03)	11.50 (2.08)

Considerations regarding use of the study

1. The sample was clinically heterogeneous, consisted of inpatients, and cannot be considered "normal"; no exclusion criteria.

2. Undifferentiated age group.

3. Predominantly male sample.

4. Low IQ level of the sample.

Other comments

1. Alternate form reliability coefficients ranged from 0.60 to 0.77. The differences between means were less than one point on each of the five acquisition trials, postinterference trial, and recognition trials. The forms were judged to be equivalent measures (Table 16.7).

[RAVLT.6] Bleecker, Bolla-Wilson, Agnew, and Meyers, 1988

The authors report AVLT data on a large sample (n = 196) of Maryland subjects aged 40 to 89 drawn from the Johns Hopkins Teaching Nursing Home Study of Normal Aging as a part of an investigation of the contribution of age, sex, vocabulary range, and depression to AVLT performance. The sample used for this article

Table 16.7. RAVLT.5

	N	Gender	Race	WAIS-R FSIQ	Age	Education
	85	82 M 3 F	61 W 24 Non-W	89.74 (11.11)	45.86 (14.05)	11.85 (2.51)

		Trial							Total
Form		I	II	III	IV	V	Postinterference	Recognition°	I–V
Original	M	4.69	6.34	7.29	8.35	8.87	6.18	9.82	35.55
	SD	1.70	2.08	2.55	3.03	3.20	3.75	3.64	11.08
Alternate	M	4.46	6.05	6.93	7.39	7.99	5.44	10.39	32.81
	SD	1.78	2.39	2.59	2.87	2.81	3.27	2.91	11.18
	r	0.63	0.62	0.60	0.62	0.71	0.66	0.65	0.77

°For this variable n = 84.

includes subjects described in Bolla-Wilson and Bleecker (1986).

Subjects with histories of head trauma with loss of consciousness, stroke, seizures, uncontrolled hypertension, congestive heart failure, abnormal thyroid function, electroconvulsive therapy, sleep disorders, coma, psychiatric disorders, or alcohol or drug abuse were excluded. All participants had Mini-Mental State Examination scores above 23. WAIS-R Vocabulary raw scores were used to estimate verbal intelligence. The presence of depressive symptomatology was assessed with the Beck Depression Scale. Means and standard scores are presented for males ($n = 87$) and females ($n = 109$) separately by five age decades: 40–49, 50–59, 60–69, 70–79, and 80–89.

Test administration generally followed the instructions recommended by Lezak (1983) and involved presentation of the words at the rate of one per second for five acquisition trials, each followed by a free-recall period. After the fifth trial, subjects were presented with a recognition trial containing 50 words including the 15 test words and phonemically and semantically similar distractor words. No interference or delayed recall trials were employed.

Means and standard deviations for the five acquisition trials and recognition trial are reported for each decade for males and females separately. In addition, means and standard deviations for number of words learned (trial 5 minus trial 1) are reported separately for men and women aged 40 to 65 and 66 to 89. Although males and females were comparable in verbal intelligence, women outperformed men on the acquisition trials, especially in the older subjects. Older participants scored more poorly than younger subjects, except on the recognition trials. Perseverations, confabulations, and intrusions were not associated with age or sex.

Study strengths

1. Large sample size, but the individual cells do not approach Ns of 50.

2. Presentation of the data by age decades and by sex.

3. Stringent medical and psychiatric exclusion criteria.

4. Use of a screening instrument for depressive symptomatology.

5. Information regarding educational level, estimated verbal intelligence, and geographic recruitment area.

6. Specification of an administration format.

7. Means and standard deviations are reported.

Considerations regarding use of the study

1. Very high educational and IQ (at least high average) levels, which was particularly true for the older age groups.

2. Test administration did not include an interference or delayed recall trial. In addition, the recognition trial followed trial V and thus the normative data derived from this recognition trial may not be representative of recognition performance associated with the traditional administration format involving an interference trial prior to the recognition trial.

Other comments

1. A stepwise regression analysis showed that age and sex accounted for a significant portion of the variance on each acquisition trial. Vocabulary accounted for a significant portion of the variance only on trials IV and V. The performance on recognition trial was not affected by age, sex or vocabulary. Overall performance was higher for women in comparison to men, with increase in this tendency with age (Table 16.8).

[RAVLT.7] Wiens, McMinn and Crossen, 1988

The study reports normative data for 222 job applicants, currently employed in a variety of occupations (white collar and blue collar), who had previously passed basic-academic-skills tests and physical examinations and were free from physical illness or limitations. The applicants represented an occupational cross-section of the community. Subjects were free from alcohol and other substance abuse. Subjects ranged in age between 19 and 51 years, with a mean age of 29.1 (SD = 6.0). Sample composition was 87% male, 13% female; 94.6% Caucasian, 5.4% racial minority.

Standard administration was used with 1-second interval between each word during word presentation. On the recognition trial, subjects were to circle words from the learned list in a paragraph.

Table 16.8. RAVLT.6

N	Age	Sex	Education	Vocabulary	Beck	AVLT I	II	III	IV	V	Recognition
15	40–49	M	15 (3.1)	55 (8.3)	3 (2.5)	7.2 (1.6)	9.5 (2.3)	10.7 (3.0)	11.6 (2.6)	12.3 (2.6)	14.1 (1.3)
16	40–49	F	15 (3.0)	55 (10.2)	5 (4.5)	7.7 (1.6)	10.9 (2.1)	12.3 (2.0)	12.6 (1.8)	13.6 (1.7)	14.5 (0.9)
20	50–59	M	13 (3.2)	51 (10.2)	5 (5.4)	6.5 (1.6)	9.8 (2.0)	11.5 (2.0)	11.8 (2.0)	12.8 (2.2)	14.4 (0.9)
22	50–59	F	14 (2.9)	54 (10.2)	5 (3.6)	7.4 (1.3)	10.0 (1.5)	12.0 (1.5)	12.8 (1.6)	13.6 (1.7)	14.5 (0.8)
23	60–69	M	13 (2.8)	52 (7.0)	5 (5.4)	5.6 (1.8)	8.0 (1.9)	9.9 (1.9)	10.3 (2.5)	11.3 (1.8)	13.9 (1.7)
29	60–69	F	14 (2.6)	55 (9.0)	6 (4.7)	6.6 (1.8)	9.6 (2.0)	11.1 (2.1)	12.2 (2.2)	12.6 (2.3)	14.4 (1.0)
18	70–79	M	15 (2.8)	56 (7.7)	3 (3.0)	6.3 (1.6)	8.2 (2.2)	9.6 (2.2)	10.0 (2.3)	10.8 (2.2)	14.2 (0.6)
29	70–79	F	15 (3.4)	59 (9.8)	5 (5.1)	6.3 (1.7)	9.4 (2.2)	10.4 (2.2)	11.8 (2.3)	12.5 (2.1)	14.5 (0.8)
11	80–89	M	18 (1.9)	61 (6.4)	5 (3.4)	5.0 (1.2)	7.1 (1.4)	8.0 (2.1)	8.7 (1.9)	9.2 (2.1)	13.0 (4.1)
13	80–89	F	15 (2.0)	58 (7.0)	7 (3.5)	5.6 (1.6)	8.2 (1.5)	9.7 (2.3)	11.0 (1.8)	11.1 (1.4)	13.9 (1.4)

The data were stratified by WAIS-R FSIQ, age, and education.

Study strengths

1. The data were stratified by age, education, and IQ levels.
2. Administration procedures were well outlined.
3. Exclusion criteria appear to be adequate.
4. Sample sizes vary between the groups, but for majority of the groups they are adequate.
5. Information regarding recruitment procedures, gender, and ethnicity and geographic area is provided.
6. Means and standard deviations are reported.

Considerations regarding use of the study

1. Age groups are restricted to younger range.
2. Some sample sizes are very small.

Other comments

1. The authors noted better recall at higher IQ levels and inverse trend between age and all

acquisition and delayed recall trials. A proactive interference effect was observed for all groups; recall for the second word list was inferior to initial recall of the first word list. Performance on recognition trial was unrelated to age and IQ, which suggests its importance in studying pathological memory loss (Tables 16.9–16.11).

[RAVLT.8] Crawford, Stewart and Moore, 1989

The study compared test–retest performance with the same form of Rey AVLT and using a parallel version of the AVLT. The parallel version was developed by the authors based on the criteria identified in the article.

Sixty subjects, free of neurological, psychiatric, and sensory disability, were recruited from nonmedical health service personnel and the fire service. Subjects were divided into pairs matched for sex, age (±3 years) and years of education (±1 year) to form two groups. There were no significant differences between groups in mean estimated IQ based on National Adult Reading Test (NART) scores (106 and 108, respectively).

One group was administered the original

Table 16.9. RAVLT.7a; Rey Auditory-Verbal Learning Test Scores by WAIS-R Full Scale IQ

WAIS-R FSIQ	N	Trial					Postinterference Recall	Recognition	Distractor Trial List(B)	Words Learned (Trial V − I)	Percentage Recall	Errors	Repetitions	Total (Trials I ... V)
		I	II	III	IV	V								
80–89	5	8.0	10.4	10.8	11.0	11.0	10.6	14.0	6.6	3.0	99.5	2.2	2.6	51.2
		(2.5)	(1.7)	(2.2)	(2.1)	(3.0)	(2.4)	(0.7)	(2.6)	(1.7)	(22.0)	(1.8)	(3.2)	(10.9)
90–99	29	7.1	9.7	11.4	12.2	13.0	11.2	14.0	6.0	5.9	86.7	3.2	5.6	53.4
		(1.6)	(1.8)	(2.1)	(1.8)	(2.0)	(2.2)	(1.1)	(1.6)	(2.2)	(14.5)	(3.9)	(5.7)	(7.4)
100–109	81	7.2	9.9	11.8	12.4	12.9	11.6	14.2	6.5	5.7	90.1	2.2	5.2	54.2
		(1.8)	(2.5)	(2.0)	(1.9)	(1.8)	(2.3)	(0.9)	(1.5)	(1.9)	(12.0)	(2.9)	(5.8)	(8.2)
110–119	55	7.5	10.4	11.9	13.1	13.2	12.1	14.0	6.8	5.7	91.8	2.1	7.0	56.1
		(1.7)	(2.2)	(1.9)	(1.4)	(1.6)	(2.3)	(1.2)	(1.5)	(2.1)	(12.1)	(2.4)	(6.9)	(7.0)
120–129	38	7.7	10.7	12.7	13.3	13.7	12.6	14.4	7.2	6.0	92.5	2.0	5.4	58.1
		(1.8)	(2.2)	(1.7)	(1.5)	(1.7)	(1.9)	(0.8)	(1.9)	(1.8)	(9.9)	(2.3)	(6.3)	(7.2)
130–139	3	10.0	12.3	13.7	15.0	14.7	14.3	15.0	7.7	4.7	97.9	2.0	0.7	65.7
		(2.6)	(2.5)	(1.5)	(0)	(0.6)	(1.2)	(0)	(1.5)	(2.5)	(10.4)	(1.7)	(1.2)	(6.7)

Table 16.10. RAVLT:7b; Rey Auditory-Verbal Learning Test Scores by Age

Age	N	Trial					Postinterference Recall	Recognition	Distractor Trial List B	Words Learned (Trial V − I)	Percentage Recall	Errors	Repetitions	Total (Trials I … V)
		I	II	III	IV	V								
20–29	126	7.4	10.4	12.2	13.0	13.4	12.1	14.2	6.8	6.0	90.4	2.2	5.8	56.3
		(1.7)	(2.2)	(1.9)	(1.7)	(1.7)	(2.2)	(1.0)	(1.6)	(2.0)	(12.4)	(3.0)	(6.1)	(7.4)
30–39	71	7.4	9.9	11.7	12.4	12.7	11.7	14.2	6.5	5.3	92.0	2.3	5.0	54.2
		(1.9)	(2.5)	(2.0)	(1.8)	(1.8)	(2.2)	(1.1)	(1.7)	(1.9)	(12.7)	(2.5)	(5.5)	(8.3)
40–49	12	7.3	9.8	11.4	12.3	12.5	11.2	13.8	6.6	5.5	88.9	2.7	7.3	53.3
		(2.2)	(2.7)	(2.6)	(1.8)	(2.5)	(3.1)	(0.9)	(1.8)	(2.6)	(10.8)	(2.3)	(10.1)	(10.3)

Table 16.11. RAVLT:7c; Rey Auditory-Verbal Learning Test Scores by Education

Years of Education	N	Trial					Postinterference Recall	Recognition	Distractor Trial List B	Words Learned (Trial V − I)	Percentage Recall	Errors	Repetitions	Total Words (Trials I . . . V)
		I	II	III	IV	V								
12	34	7.0	9.9	11.7	11.9	12.4	11.4	13.9	6.6	5.3	93.1	1.9	6.6	52.9
		(1.6)	(3.5)	(2.0)	(3.5)	(2.3)	(2.4)	(1.2)	(1.8)	(2.0)	(13.5)	(1.9)	(6.7)	(7.9)
13	25	7.5	10.1	11.9	12.7	13.2	12.1	13.9	6.0	5.7	91.4	1.4	7.1	55.3
		(1.2)	(2.4)	(2.4)	(1.7)	(1.6)	(2.1)	(1.2)	(1.6)	(1.6)	(10.4)	(1.7)	(7.3)	(7.7)
14	50	7.2	9.9	11.8	13.0	13.2	12.3	14.4	6.7	6.0	93.3	2.5	6.5	55.2
		(1.9)	(2.3)	(2.1)	(1.9)	(2.0)	(2.2)	(0.8)	(1.8)	(2.2)	(11.0)	(3.2)	(6.9)	(8.4)
15	19	7.4	10.3	12.4	12.6	13.2	11.4	14.3	6.6	5.7	86.0	2.3	2.6	55.8
		(2.2)	(2.9)	(2.0)	(2.1)	(1.9)	(2.7)	(.7)	(.9)	(2.1)	(50.7)	(3.5)	(2.7)	(9.5)
16	80	7.6	10.5	12.1	13.0	13.3	12.0	14.2	6.8	5.7	90.0	2.6	5.0	56.5
		(1.9)	(2.2)	(1.8)	(1.4)	(1.5)	(2.1)	(.9)	(1.7)	(2.0)	(11.8)	(3.0)	(5.6)	(7.2)
≥17	5	7.8	10.4	12.4	13.8	13.4	11.2	13.4	5.8	5.6	83.0	1.2	4.2	57.8
		(2.6)	(3.0)	(1.1)	(1.3)	(1.7)	(3.1)	(1.8)	(1.1)	(3.0)	(16.6)	(1.6)	(1.6)	(7.7)

Table 16.12. RAVLT.8a; Mean Scores (SDs) for Matched Groups Receiving the Original AVLT and the Parallel Version

	Trials					List B	Trial 6	Recognition
	1	2	3	4	5			
Original	8.30	11.00	11.80	12.73	13.20	6.90	11.90	25.37
	(1.80)	(2.11)	(2.36)	(2.02)	(1.61)	(2.22)	(2.55)	(2.68)
Parallel	7.37	10.50	11.70	12.63	13.00	6.43	11.43	25.13
	(1.67)	(2.52)	(2.25)	(1.50)	(1.48)	(1.89)	(2.00)	(2.96)

AVLT, the other the parallel version. Subjects were retested following a delay of 27 days (±3 days) with half of each group receiving the same version, the other half the alternative version.

The standard administration procedure was used. On the recognition condition, subjects were asked to inform the examiner of the stimulus words that had been contained in the previously presented word lists. A recognition score was obtained by subtracting the number of false-positive identifications from the number of words correctly identified.

Study strengths

1. Information on an alternate form and practice effects.
2. Administration procedure was described.
3. Adequate exclusion criteria.
4. Information on IQ and geographic recruitment area.
5. Means and standard deviations are reported.

Considerations regarding use of the study

1. Demographic characteristics of the sample are not described.
2. Relatively small sample sizes.
3. Data are not presented by age groupings.
4. Data were collected in the UK and it is unclear to what extent this is appropriate for clinical use in the United States.

Other comments

1. The authors concluded that the parallel version can be used as an equivalent form of the AVLT. Significant practice effect was seen for subjects who were administered the same versions (Tables 16.12 and 16.13).

[RAVLT.9] Nielsen, Knudsen, and Daugbjerg, 1989

The authors gathered AVLT normative data on 101 Danish subjects aged 20 to 54. The majority of the participants (87) had undergone minor surgery (primarily arm and leg) and were

Table 16.13. RAVLT.8b; Mean Scores (SDs) for Groups Receiving Either the Same or Different AVLT Version at 27-Day Retest

	Trial					List B	Postinterference Recall	Recognition
	1	2	3	4	5			
Test	7.87	11.10	11.93	13.03	13.33	6.70	11.93	25.30
	(1.76)	(2.19)	(2.00)	(1.59)	(1.56)	(2.40)	(1.95)	(2.47)
Same Version Retest	10.53	12.87	13.67	13.90	14.13	7.70	13.43	26.67
	(2.39)	(1.81)	(1.40)	(1.35)	(1.14)	(2.29)	(1.68)	(2.47)
Test	7.53	10.40	11.57	12.33	12.87	6.63	11.40	25.20
	(1.76)	(2.43)	(2.56)	(1.88)	(1.80)	(1.70)	(2.58)	(3.15)
Different Version Retest	7.50	10.27	11.87	12.70	12.90	6.23	11.93	24.57
	(2.13)	(2.16)	(2.00)	(1.82)	(2.11)	(1.91)	(2.77)	(3.67)

tested several weeks postsurgery "when they were free of post-surgical inconveniences": Fourteen recruits were hospital laundry workers. Exclusion criteria included history of head trauma, alcohol abuse, prolonged exposure to organic solvents or other toxic agents; presence of somatic or psychiatric disease "which might adversely affect neuropsychological functioning"; or use of medications "which could affect intellectual capacity." Fifty-three subjects were male and 48 were female, and 91% were right-handed. The sample was classified into three age groupings: 20–29 (n = 35), 30–39 (n = 27), and 40–54 (n = 39); only two subjects were older than age 50. Mean prorated verbal IQ (based on a translation of the WAIS-R) was 98.61 ± 12.21 (range = 78 to 140); means and standard deviations for seven subtests are reported for the three age groupings. Information on occupational status indicated that skilled workers were somewhat overrepresented in the sample compared to the general population, while self-employed individuals were under-represented.

Test administration appeared to be based on the Lezak (1983) instructions. Specifically, "a list of 15 discrete nouns was read aloud at a rate of one per second for five consecutive learning trials, each followed by a free recall test. Delayed recall was tested 15 min after completion of the fifth learning trial" (p. 39). It is not reported if the words were translated.

Means, standard deviations, and ranges are reported for the five acquisition trials, total score across the five trials, and delayed recall.

Study strengths
1. Data presented by age groupings
2. Information presented regarding sex, IQ, geographic recruitment area, age, handedness, and occupation
3. Adequate exclusion criteria.
4. Means and standard deviations are reported.
5. Administration procedure is specified.

Considerations regarding use of the study
1. No information regarding educational level.
2. Some information regarding occupational status is reported but not all of the categories are defined.
3. It is unknown if the stimulus words were translated.
4. No interference trial was administered; thus the delayed recall information may not be comparable to that obtained if any interference trial had been administered prior to the delayed trial.
5. Individual cell sizes are rather small.
6. Data were collected on a Danish sample. This might limit their clinical use in the United States (Table 16.14).

[RAVLT.10] Roth, Davidoff, Thomas, Doljanac, Dijkers, Berent, Morris, and Yarkony, 1989

The authors obtained AVLT data on 61 paid control subjects as a part of their examination of neuropsychological deficits in acute spinal cord injured patients. Mean age was 27.5 (standard

Table 16.14. RAVLT.9; Means, Standard Deviations, and Ranges for RAVLT Indices for Three Age Groups

N	Age	Trial					Total	15-Minute Delayed Recall
		I	II	III	IV	V		
35	20–29	6.31	9.77	11.31	12.31	12.74	52.46	11.91
		(1.53)	(2.00)	(1.97)	(1.79)	(1.46)	(7.21)	(1.76)
		4–10	6–14	7–14	8–15	9–15	37–68	9–15
27	30–39	5.85	9.04	10.26	11.59	12.22	48.96	11.22
		(1.15)	(1.55)	(1.60)	(1.71)	(1.76)	(6.19)	(2.56)
		4–8	6–12	6–14	7–15	8–15	33–64	5–15
39	40–54	5.67	8.18	10.08	10.77	11.41	46.10	9.92
		(1.31)	(1.89)	(2.29)	(2.02)	(2.14)	(7.99)	(2.73)
		4–9	4–12	5–15	6–15	7–15	27–63	4–15

error = 1.0) and mean years of education was 12.8 (standard error = 0.2). Forty-five subjects were male, 16 female; 39 subjects were recruited in Detroit and 22 in Ann Arbor. Exclusion criteria included history of closed head injury and recent high-frequency alcohol or substance abuse.

The AVLT appeared to have been administered according to the Lezak (1983) instructions. Means and standard errors are reported for the five acquisition trials, list B, the postinterference trial, and recognition.

Study strengths
  1. Information regarding age, sex, education, and geographic recruitment area.
  2. Minimally adequate exclusion criteria.
  3. Adequate sample size.
  4. Means and standard errors are reported.
  5. Test instructions are not specified but appear to be standard.

Considerations regarding use of the study
  1. Undifferentiated age range, although the small standard error would suggest that the age spread was not large.
  2. Recognition procedure was not specified (Table 16.15).

[RAVLT.11] Geffen, Moar, O'Hanlon, Clark and Geffen, 1990

The article provides norms for 153 adults residing in Australia, in age groups spanning seven decades (from 16 to 86 years, M = 44.5 years, SD = 20.2). Age groups included approximately equal number of males and females and were matched for intelligence, education, and occupation. All participants were physically healthy and free of neurological symptoms by self-report. Subjects' occupations (current or preretirement) ranged from unskilled workers to professionals. The average years of education completed was 11.2 years (±2.2), with a range from 7 to 22 years. Estimates of FSIQ were derived from error scores on the National Adult Reading Test (NART, Nelson, 1982). Average estimated IQ was 111.5 (±7.3) with a range from 94 to 127. All subjects spoke English as a first language.

Standard administration procedures were used for recall trials. Twenty-minute delayed recall followed by a recognition condition was used. The delay was filled with the Digit Span, WMS Logical Memory subtest, and NART. The recognition condition consisted of a list of 50 words which included words from lists A and B as well as 20 phonemically or semantically similar distractor words. The subjects were to identify as many of the previously learned words as possible, as well as the specific list of origin (list A or B). Scoring sheets were scored using a specially designed computer program.

The following variables were included in the analyses:
  1. Recall trials: recall of list A on trials I–V; total recall over five trials; total number of repeated words; extralist intrusions; recall of list B; postinterference recall (retention); and 20-minute delayed recall.
  2. Recognition trial: number of words recognized from lists A and B; a nonparametric signal detection measure of recognition performance $p(A) = 0.5[1 + \text{hit rate (HR)} − \text{false positive (FP)}]$, which corrects the recognition score by taking into account misassignments from list A to list B and vice versa; and total number of FP misidentifications.
  3. Serial position effect was measured for list A averaged over the five acquisition trials. Serial positions of the words were collapsed into

Table 16.15. RAVLT.10

| N | Age | Education | Trial | | | | | | Postinterference Recall | Recognition |
			I	II	III	IV	V	B		
61	27.5	12.8	7.4	10.4	11.9	12.8	13.7	6.7	12.4	14.0
	(1.0)°	(0.2)	(0.2)	(0.3)	(0.3)	(0.2)	(0.2)	(0.3)	(0.3)	(0.2)

°Standard errors.

five groupings (words 1–3, 4–6, 7–9, 10–12, 13–15).

4. Functional indices, such as proactive and retroactive interference effects, forgetting, retrieval efficiency, and item information overload were computed as ratios of pairs of trials. All of the above indices were presented for males and females separately.

Study strengths

1. Demographic characteristics of the sample are well described in terms of age, occupation, education, IQ, fluency in English, and geographic area.

2. The normative data were presented by age group and separately for males and females.

3. The administration procedure was well described. Additional indices were developed to explore different memory mechanisms.

4. Large overall sample size.

5. Adequate exclusion criteria.

6. Means and standard deviations are reported.

Considerations regarding use of the study

1. The 20-minute delay interval was filled with verbal memory tasks, which might serve as a source of interference.

2. The sample had high estimated IQ values, which might limit generalizability of the data.

3. The estimated IQs of the youngest age group were up to 10 points lower than the other age groups; however, this may have been an artifact of the NART since the teenagers probably had not yet been exposed to all the vocabulary items on the NART and as a result the NART, may have underestimated their IQs.

4. Sample sizes per group are small.

5. Data obtained in Australia which may limit usefulness for clinical interpretative purposes in the United States.

Other comments

1. Based on subjects' performance on different trials, the authors make inferences regarding memory mechanisms involved.

2. The authors noted significant association between age, gender, and Rey AVLT performance, with females consistently outperforming males. Performance of younger subjects was superior to that of older subjects (Tables 16.16–16.19).

[RAVLT.12] Ivnik, Malec, Tangalos, Peterson, Kokmen and Kurland, 1990

The study provides age-specific norms for the Rey AVLT, derived from a sample of 394 cognitively intact volunteers ages 55 years and older living in Omsted County, Minnesota. Subjects received general medical examinations performed by their primary care physicians prior to the enrollment in the study. Subjects were excluded from the study if they had active psychiatric or central nervous system condition; complaints of cognitive difficulty during history taking and systems review; findings on physical examination suggesting disorders with potential to affect cognition; certain types and dosages of psychoactive medication use; or prior histories of disorders causing residual cognitive deficit; chronic medical illnesses were excluded only when they were reported by the physician to compromise cognition. These normative data are believed to be a reasonably unbiased representation of the elderly living in this geographic region.

The standard administration procedure was used including 30-minute delayed recall and recognition trials. Standard scoring procedure was used. The scores were also provided for the number of errors on recognition trial. In addition, four summary measures (two "learning" and two "memory" scores) were computed:

1. Total Learning (*TL*) score represents a total of five acquisition trials.
2. Learning Over Trials [$LOT = TL - (5 \times$ trial I)] is an estimate of an individual's improvement over trials.
3. Short-Term Percent Retention (*STPR*) represents trial VI recall as a proportion of trial V recall.
4. Long-Term Percent Retention (*LTPR*) reflects the Delayed Recall as a proportion of trial V recall.

The data for the raw scores are broken down into seven age groups. The data for the summary scores are organized using overlapping intervals at specified age midpoints. The authors

Table 16.16. RAVLT.11a; Means and Standard Deviations (in Parentheses) for Acquisition Trials, Recall and Recognition:° *Males:*

	Age Group						
Trials	16–19 (13)	20–29 (10)	30–39 (10)	40–49 (11)	50–59 (11)	60–69 (10)	≥70 (10)
I	6.9 (1.8)	8.4 (1.2)	6.0 (1.8)	6.4 (1.8)	6.5 (2.0)	4.9 (1.1)	3.6 (0.8)
II	9.7 (1.7)	10.8 (1.9)	8.0 (2.4)	9.0 (2.3)	8.6 (2.0)	6.4 (1.2)	5.7 (1.7)
III	11.5 (1.2)	11.3 (1.6)	9.7 (2.7)	9.8 (2.0)	10.1 (1.6)	8.0 (2.6)	6.8 (1.6)
IV	12.8 (1.5)	12.2 (1.8)	10.9 (2.8)	11.5 (1.9)	10.7 (1.9)	8.5 (2.7)	8.3 (2.7)
V	12.5 (1.3)	12.2 (2.2)	11.4 (2.6)	10.9 (2.0)	11.8 (2.6)	8.9 (2.0)	8.2 (2.5)
Total	53.4 (5.4)	54.9 (7.0)	46.0 (10.9)	47.5 (8.3)	47.6 (8.5)	36.7 (8.4)	32.6 (8.3)
Total repeats	5.9 (5.6)	8.0 (4.6)	3.0 (3.6)	4.1 (2.9)	7.3 (7.5)	5.0 (3.6)	5.1 (8.6)
Extra list intrusions	0.39 (0.65)	0.90 (1.29)	1.20 (3.12)	0.55 (0.82)	0.73 (1.19)	0.30 (0.68)	0.90 (1.67)
List B	6.9 (1.9)	6.5 (1.8)	5.3 (1.6)	6.1 (2.1)	5.0 (2.3)	4.9 (1.6)	3.5 (1.3)
Postinterference recall	11.2 (1.6)	11.1 (1.7)	9.7 (2.3)	9.7 (2.5)	9.6 (2.9)	7.2 (2.8)	6.4 (1.7)
20-minute delayed recall	11.3 (1.7)	10.6 (2.4)	10.4 (2.3)	10.5 (2.7)	10.0 (2.6)	7.1 (3.8)	5.6 (2.6)
Recognition							
List A	14.4 (0.9)	14.2 (0.8)	13.5 (1.5)	14.2 (1.0)	13.9 (0.9)	12.4 (2.8)	11.5 (2.6)
List B	8.4 (2.8)	8.2 (2.7)	4.4 (2.0)	6.9 (2.6)	4.7 (2.9)	4.9 (2.7)	3.0 (2.5)
p(A) List A	0.95 (0.04)	0.90 (0.05)	0.92 (0.04)	0.92 (0.06)	0.90 (0.06)	0.82 (0.13)	0.81 (0.10)
p(A) List B	0.77 (0.09)	0.76 (0.09)	0.64 (0.01)	0.71 (0.09)	0.65 (0.10)	0.65 (0.09)	0.59 (0.08)
Misassignments							
A to B	0.77 (1.01)	1.00 (1.89)	0.70 (1.25)	1.18 (1.33)	1.18 (1.54)	2.20 (1.32)	0.80 (1.03)
B to A	0.08 (0.28)	0.40 (0.84)	0.60 (0.70)	0.18 (0.60)	0.27 (0.65)	1.40 (1.78)	1.00 (1.25)
Total false positives	1.39 (1.76)	3.20 (1.99)	1.50 (1.35)	2.64 (2.66)	2.91 (2.55)	4.30 (3.95)	3.10 (2.96)

°Data for the additional indices developed by the authors are included.

Table 16.17. RAVLT.11b; Means and Standard Deviations (in Parentheses) for Acquisition Trials, Recall and Recognition:° *Females:*

				Age Group			
Trials	16–19 (12)	20–29 (10)	30–39 (13)	40–49 (11)	50–59 (9)	60–69 (12)	≥70 (10)
I	7.8 (1.9)	7.7 (1.0)	8.0 (2.0)	6.8 (1.5)	6.4 (1.5)	6.0 (2.2)	5.6 (1.4)
II	10.5 (2.0)	10.5 (2.0)	10.8 (2.1)	9.4 (1.5)	8.2 (2.4)	9.0 (2.0)	6.9 (2.1)
III	12.3 (1.2)	12.2 (2.3)	11.5 (1.7)	11.4 (1.7)	10.2 (2.1)	10.8 (2.0)	8.9 (1.9)
IV	12.5 (1.7)	12.0 (1.6)	12.9 (1.3)	11.7 (2.1)	11.1 (1.9)	11.3 (1.4)	10.1 (1.9)
V	13.3 (1.5)	12.9 (1.5)	12.7 (1.3)	12.8 (1.4)	11.6 (2.1)	11.9 (1.6)	10.1 (1.2)
Total	56.5 (6.0)	55.3 (6.6)	55.9 (6.3)	52.1 (7.1)	47.6 (7.7)	49.0 (7.1)	41.6 (6.6)
Total repeats	5.5 (6.5)	10.6 (14.3)	5.0 (5.8)	8.0 (4.8)	4.9 (3.7)	4.8 (2.8)	3.5 (4.8)
Extra list intrusions	0.92 (1.38)	1.20 (1.40)	1.23 (1.74)	0.83 (1.19)	0.78 (1.30)	0.67 (1.07)	0.50 (0.97)
List B	7.7 (1.3)	7.9 (2.0)	6.5 (1.5)	5.2 (1.3)	4.6 (1.9)	5.3 (1.1)	4.2 (1.9)
Postinterference recall	11.9 (2.5)	11.6 (2.5)	12.1 (1.9)	11.1 (2.4)	9.9 (2.8)	9.8 (1.6)	7.8 (1.8)
20-minute delayed recall	11.4 (2.5)	11.0 (2.0)	12.2 (2.5)	11.1 (2.3)	10.2 (2.7)	10.3 (2.3)	8.3 (2.1)
Recognition							
List A	13.8 (2.0)	14.4 (0.8)	14.2 (1.7)	14.4 (0.8)	13.7 (1.1)	13.8 (1.1)	13.6 (2.0)
List B	7.8 (3.1)	8.0 (2.9)	8.9 (4.1)	7.4 (2.8)	5.7 (2.4)	7.5 (3.6)	7.5 (3.7)
p(A) List A	0.92 (0.08)	0.91 (0.09)	0.89 (0.08)	0.88 (0.07)	0.88 (0.08)	0.90 (0.06)	0.84 (0.11)
p(A) List B	0.74 (0.10)	0.75 (0.10)	0.78 (0.13)	0.73 (0.09)	0.68 (0.07)	0.74 (0.11)	0.73 (0.10)
Misassignments							
A to B	0.33 (0.49)	0.40 (0.97)	0.31 (0.63)	1.17 (1.64)	1.56 (1.94)	1.42 (1.44)	0.90 (1.37)
B to A	0.25 (0.45)	0.30 (0.48)	0.00 (0.00)	0.17 (0.58)	0.33 (0.71)	0.58 (0.67)	1.10 (0.88)
Total false positives	2.33 (2.96)	3.60 (3.92)	4.23 (3.37)	4.58 (2.68)	3.67 (3.71)	2.92 (3.12)	5.60 (5.72)

°Data for the additional indices developed by the authors are included.

Table 16.18. RAVLT.11c; Mean (SD) Number of Words Recalled in Five Grouped Serial Positions of Words in List A Averaged Over the Five Acquisition Trials

Males

Serial Position	16–19	20–29	30–39	40–49	50–59	60–69	≥70
1 (1–3)	12.7 (2.2)	12.3 (2.1)	10.3 (2.9)	12.9 (1.9)	11.2 (3.5)	9.0 (2.7)	9.3 (2.3)
2 (4–6)	10.3 (1.9)	11.1 (1.8)	8.6 (3.1)	9.0 (2.7)	10.5 (2.2)	6.2 (3.7)	5.2 (2.6)
3 (7–9)	7.8 (2.7)	7.7 (3.0)	6.7 (3.4)	6.0 (3.0)	7.2 (3.2)	3.5 (2.4)	2.4 (2.5)
4 (10–12)	10.6 (1.9)	12.0 (2.4)	10.0 (2.1)	8.8 (2.6)	8.7 (3.0)	8.6 (3.2)	7.6 (3.8)
5 (13–15)	12.0 (1.9)	11.8 (2.1)	10.4 (3.3)	10.8 (2.3)	10.1 (2.1)	9.4 (1.4)	8.1 (2.8)

provide justification for this approach, asserting its advantage over more conventional group assignment.

Study strengths

1. Demographic characteristics of the sample are well described in terms of geographic area, age, handedness, gender, education, IQ, and marital status.
2. The data are partitioned by age group based on midpoint interval technique.
3. The scoring system was well described.
4. The sample sizes for each group are large.
5. Stringent exclusion criteria were utilized.
6. Means and standard deviations are reported.

Considerations regarding use of the study

1. The procedure for the recognition trial was not specified.
2. The measures proposed by the authors are quite complicated and might be difficult to compute in clinical practice (Tables 16.20–16.26).

[RAVLT.13] Miller, Selnes, McArthur, Satz, Becker, Cohen, Sheridan, Machado, VanGorp, and Visscher, 1990

The article described the results obtained for homosexual/bisexual males recruited in the MACS study, an epidemiologic project designed to assess the natural history of HIV-1 infection. The article explores the effect of HIV

Table 16.19. RAVLT.11d; Mean (SD) Number of Words Recalled in Five Grouped Serial Positions of Words in List A Averaged Over the Five Acquisition Trials

Females

Serial Position	16–19	20–29	30–39	40–49	50–59	60–69	≥70
1 (1–3)	12.5 (1.9)	12.4 (2.3)	13.2 (1.6)	12.6 (2.7)	11.7 (3.5)	11.9 (1.7)	10.3 (2.6)
2 (4–6)	11.6 (1.7)	11.0 (1.8)	11.2 (2.1)	9.8 (2.4)	8.9 (2.3)	10.1 (1.8)	8.1 (2.3)
3 (7–9)	10.2 (2.3)	8.4 (3.8)	8.7 (2.8)	8.2 (2.6)	7.3 (3.4)	8.0 (2.9)	4.9 (2.0)
4 (10–12)	11.3 (1.5)	11.5 (1.8)	11.2 (2.7)	10.9 (2.5)	9.0 (2.9)	9.1 (1.6)	8.4 (2.8)
5 (13–15)	11.0 (2.9)	12.0 (2.7)	11.6 (2.4)	10.6 (2.1)	10.7 (1.9)	9.9 (3.1)	9.9 (3.3)

Table 16.20. RAVLT.12a; Frequency and Percentage of Total Sample for Different Demographic Strata°

	Count	% of Total	Full Scale IQ
Age			
55–59	45	11.4	110.9 (12.4)
60–64	53	13.5	107.7 (10.2)
65–69	64	16.2	104.8 (9.8)
70–74	67	17.0	106.2 (10.1)
75–79	69	17.5	
80–84	49	12.4	
85–87	47	11.9	
Handedness			
Right-handed	369	93.7	
Left-handed	14	3.6	
Mixed/both	11	2.8	
Sex			
Men	145	36.8	
Women	249	63.2	
Marital Status			
Single	51	12.9	
Married	235	59.6	
Divorced	7	1.8	
Widowed	100	25.4	
No response	1	0.3	
Education(years)			
<8	9	2.3	
8–11	60	15.2	
12–15	226	57.4	
16–17	60	15.2	
>17	39	9.9	

°WAIS-R FSIQs for age groups below age 75 are also provided.

serostatus and symptom status on cognitive and motor functioning. Administration procedures outlined in Lezak (1983, 1995) were employed.

Study strengths
1. Sample sizes are large.
2. Demographic characteristics of each sample are described in terms of gender, race, age, education, and geographic location.
3. Means and standard deviations reported.
4. Administration procedures are specified.

Considerations regarding use of the study
1. The study recruited subjects ranging in age from 21 to 72. Norms are presented for all ages combined. They would be most accurate for young and middle adults.
2. The data are presented only for trial V and total for trials I–V.
3. High educational level of the samples.
4. All-male sample.
5. Exclusion criteria are not specified.

Other comments
1. In addition to other demographic variables, the paper reports race composition (white, black, Hispanic, other), CES Depression Scale scores, and CD4 cells/mm^3 count (Table 16.27).

[RAVLT.14] Shapiro and Harrison, 1990

The authors developed criteria for word selection to generate new lists to be used as alternate forms of AVLT. Four AVLT forms were compared on two samples of subjects:

1. Seventeen elderly subjects were recruited from the patient population at the VAMC at Salem, Virginia, with mean age of 66 years. They were rehabilitating primarily from stroke or limb surgery but also had associated medical illness. Seven of these subjects carried a clinical diagnosis of dementia. The exclusion criteria were as follows: acute illness, change in their psychotropic medication during the study, and being present on the ward for less than 2 weeks.

2. Twenty-five subjects were undergraduate students with mean age of 19 years.

Four alternate forms of the AVLT (forms AB, CD, EF, and GH) were used (one trial for the acquisition and interference lists, respectively). List pair AB represented the standard form used for Rey AVLT; form CD was the alternate list pair provided by Lezak. The remaining two list pairs were generated based on their match to the above lists according to the criteria developed by the authors. The order of administration of the forms was counterbalanced across dates and subjects. Only one form was used per session. The interval between sessions varied from 2 to 13 days (Mean = 5 days, SD = 3.6). Standard administration procedure was used for each form.

Study strengths
1. Established reliability indices for alternate forms.

Table 16.21. RAVLT.12b

Age Group	N	Trials					List B	Trial 6	30-Minute Delayed Recall	Recognition	Errors
		1	2	3	4	5					
55–59	45										
M		6.8	9.5	11.4	12.4	13.1	5.3	11.2	10.4	14.0	0.6
SD		1.6	2.2	2.0	1.9	1.9	1.7	2.5	3.1	1.3	0.9
R		4–10	6–14	6–15	7–15	7–15	2–9	5–15	0–15	10–15	0–3
60–64	53										
M		6.4	9.0	10.6	11.7	11.9	4.9	10.0	9.9	13.9	0.8
SD		1.9	2.3	2.3	2.7	2.0	1.5	3.1	3.1	1.5	1.2
R		3–13	3–14	6–14	7–15	7–15	3–9	4–15	3–15	8–15	0–5
65–69	64										
M		5.7	8.6	9.7	10.6	11.2	4.7	9.1	8.3	13.3	0.9
SD		1.6	2.1	2.3	2.4	2.4	1.5	3.2	3.5	2.0	0.9
R		1–10	5–13	4–15	6–15	6–15	1–9	0–15	0–15	8–15	0–3
70–74	67										
M		5.5	7.8	9.1	10.2	10.5	4.1	8.3	7.4	12.7	1.0
SD		1.5	1.8	2.1	2.3	2.6	1.5	2.9	3.1	2.1	1.2
R		2–9	3–12	4–13	3–14	5–15	1–8	1–14	0–13	6–15	0–5
75–79	65										
M		5.0	7.0	8.2	9.2	10.1	4.2	7.8	6.9	12.5	1.5
SD		1.5	1.9	2.2	2.2	2.2	2.0	2.7	2.9	2.4	1.6
R		1–8	3–12	3–15	4–15	5–15	1–10	2–15	0–14	6–15	0–7
80–84	49										
M		4.4	6.5	7.7	8.6	9.0	3.5	6.7	5.5	12.3	1.2
SD		1.2	1.5	2.1	2.5	2.5	1.6	2.5	3.3	2.4	1.4
R		2–7	3–10	3–12	1–14	4–15	0–8	1–14	0–12	2–15	0–7
≥85	47										
M		4.0	6.0	7.4	7.9	9.1	3.1	6.2	5.4	12.3	1.5
SD		1.5	1.8	2.2	2.4	2.3	1.4	2.6	2.7	2.3	1.6
R		0–7	2–10	2–12	3–15	3–14	0–7	2–14	0–13	6–15	0–7

2. Means and standard deviations are reported.

3. Test administration procedures are specified.

Considerations regarding use of the study

1. Sample sizes are small.

2. Demographic characteristics of the subjects are scarcely described (no information on gender, educational level of the older group, IQ or age ranges).

3. No exclusion criteria are reported for the younger group.

4. Subjects in the older group had either neurological or medical illness.

Other comments

The authors concluded that all four forms yielded comparable mean recall scores. Alternate

form reliability coefficients for each comparison varied from 0.67 to 0.90.

The results suggested that the use of alternate forms may eliminate direct practice effects; however, there remains a general practice effect due to repeated administrations when the tests are spaced as much as 5 days apart. This effect persisted for a number of days in healthy college students but not among the older patient population (Tables 16.28–16.30).

[RAVLT.15] Mitrushina and Satz, 1991a

The study explored the magnitude of practice effects in repeated administration of neuropsychological measures in a sample of 122 healthy elderly subjects (49 males and 73 females) between the ages of 57 and 85 recruited in Southern California. This study represents a longitu-

Table 16.22. RAVLT.12c; Means, Standard Deviations, and Ranges (R) for AVLT Summary Scores

Age	N	Total Learning	Learning Over Trials	Short-Term Percent Retention	Long-Term Percent Retention
55–59	45				
M		53.2	19.3	85.0	79.1
SD		8.2	5.8	12.9	18.7
R		33–67	3–34	45–100	0–108
60–64	53				
M		49.7	17.8	82.8	81.7
SD		9.1	7.0	18.3	18.0
R		32–68	2–30	44–118	30–118
65–69	64				
M		45.8	17.2	80.5	72.3
SD		9.5	6.1	21.2	23.6
R		22–66	(−3)–28	0–133	0–125
70–74	67				
M		43.1	15.6	78.7	68.4
SD		9.1	6.9	18.4	23.6
R		19–61	(−1)–33	12–120	0–111
75–79	69				
M		39.6	14.5	76.5	67.1
SD		8.7	6.6	18.9	21.6
R		21–63	2–31	25–133	0–110
80–84	49				
M		36.2	14.3	74.0	60.1
SD		7.4	7.3	21.7	33.4
R		21–51	1–30	25–133	0–150
≥85	47				
M		34.4	14.4	69.1	58.7
SD		8.6	6.6	22.7	23.4
R		1–56	0–31	25–133	0–100

Table 16.23. RAVLT.12d; Percentile Ranks for AVLT Total Learning (TL) Scores by Midpoint Age Groupings

	Midpoint Age Groupings									
Percentile Ranges	61 56–66	64 59–69	67 62–72	70 65–75	73 68–78	76 71–81	79 74–84	82 77–87	85 80–90	90 83–97
N	114	126	140	148	159	143	130	107	84	64
90–100	>62	>58	>57	>55	>54	>52	>48	>47	>45	>46
80–89	59–62	57–58	55–57	53–55	49–54	48–52	45–48	44–47	43–45	43–46
70–79	56–58	54–56	51–54	49–52	47–48	45–47	43–44	42–43	40–42	39–42
60–69	54–55	50–53	48–50	46–48	45–46	43–44	41–42	40–41	38–39	37–38
50–59	51–53	48–49	46–47	44–45	42–44	41–42	39–40	37–39	35–37	35–36
40–49	49–50	45–47	43–45	41–43	39–41	39–40	36–38	35–36	33–34	33–34
30–39	46–48	43–44	41–42	39–40	36–38	36–38	34–35	33–34	31–32	31–32
20–29	43–45	39–42	37–40	36–38	34–35	33–35	32–33	30–32	29–30	29–30
10–19	37–42	35–38	33–36	32–35	30–33	29–32	28–31	26–29	25–28	25–28
0–9	<37	<35	<33	<32	<30	<29	<28	<26	<25	<25

Table 16.24. RAVLT.12e; Percentile Ranks for AVLT Learning Over Trials (LOT) Scores by Midpoint Age Groupings

	Midpoint Age Groupings									
Percentile Ranges	61 56–66	64 59–69	67 62–72	70 65–75	73 68–78	76 71–81	79 74–84	82 77–87	85 80–90	90 83–97
90–100	>25	>25	>25	>24	>23	>24	>23	>24	>24	>22
80–89	23–25	23–25	23–25	21–24	21–23	21–24	21–23	22–24	22–24	19–22
70–79	22	21–22	21–22	20	19–20	19–20	19–20	18–21	18–21	18
60–69	20–21	19–20	19–20	18–19	17–18	17–18	17–18	16–17	16–17	15–17
50–59	19	18	17–18	16–17	15–16	15–16	13–16	13–15	14–15	14
40–49	17–18	16–17	15–16	14–15	14	13–14	11–12	11–12	12–13	12–13
30–39	16	14–15	14	13	11–13	11–12	10	10	11	11
20–29	14–15	12–13	11–13	10–12	10	9–10	9	9	9–10	9–10
10–19	10–13	9–11	9–10	8–9	8–9	7–8	6–8	6–8	6–8	5–8
0–9	<10	<9	<9	<8	<8	<7	<6	<6	<6	<5

Table 16.25. RAVLT.12f; Percentile Ranks for AVLT Short-term Percent Retention (STPR) Scores by Midpoint Age Groupings

	Midpoint Age Groupings									
Percentile Ranges	61 56–66	64 59–69	67 62–72	70 65–75	73 68–78	76 71–81	79 74–84	82 77–87	85 80–90	90 83–97
90–100	>99	>93	>93	>93	>93	>93	>93	>93	>91	>90
80–89	—	—	—	93	93	92–93	90–93	93	91	89–90
70–79	93–99	92–93	93	90–92	88–92	88–91	84–89	87–92	86–90	83–88
60–69	90–92	88–92	87–92	85–89	83–87	83–87	82–83	82–86	80–85	80–82
50–59	86–89	83–87	83–86	80–84	78–82	79–82	74–81	75–81	71–79	71–79
40–49	83–85	79–82	78–82	75–79	74–77	74–78	71–73	69–74	66–70	65–70
30–39	78–82	72–78	73–77	71–74	71–73	70–73	69–70	63–68	61–65	57–64
20–29	70–77	67–71	67–72	65–70	64–70	63–69	61–68	56–62	51–60	47–56
10–19	60–69	56–66	57–66	58–64	58–63	58–62	50–60	43–55	42–50	40–46
0–9	<60	<56	<57	<58	<58	<58	<50	<43	<42	<40

Table 16.26. RAVLT.12g; Percentile Ranks for AVLT Long-term Percent Retention (LTPR) Scores by Midpoint Age Groupings

	Midpoint Age Groupings									
Percentile Ranges	61 56–66	64 59–69	67 62–72	70 65–75	73 68–78	76 71–81	79 74–84	82 77–87	85 80–90	90 83–97
90–100	>93	>93	>93	>93	>92	>91	>92	>92	>92	>91
80–89	—	93	91–93	90–93	87–92	87–91	85–92	86–92	84–92	80–90
70–79	91–93	90–92	85–90	83–89	81–86	81–86	78–84	75–85	75–83	71–79
60–69	86–90	83–89	80–84	78–82	75–80	75–80	72–77	71–74	71–74	65–70
50–59	80–85	78–82	75–79	72–77	71–74	70–74	68–71	66–70	64–70	60–64
40–49	76–79	74–77	70–74	65–71	65–70	64–69	62–67	61–65	56–63	55–59
30–39	72–75	65–73	61–69	61–64	59–64	60–63	58–61	50–60	48–55	50–54
20–29	63–71	59–64	59–60	51–60	51–58	53–59	45–57	41–49	32–47	36–49
10–19	56–62	50–58	45–55	42–50	40–50	40–52	25–44	20–40	13–31	20–35
0–9	<56	<50	<45	<42	<40	<40	<25	<20	<13	<20

Table 16.27. RAVLT.13

	Race[°]				CES Depression Scale	CD4	Age	Education	RAVLT Trial V	Trials Total Trial I–V
	W	B	H	O						
Seronegative	92	2	4	2	9.08 (9.03)	970.42 (332.46)	37.20 (7.52)	16.36 (2.34)	12.83 (1.85)	52.75 (8.05)
Asymptomatic Seropositive	91	2	6	2	9.44 (9.27)	561.90 (277.98)	35.66 (6.47)	15.70 (2.44)	12.64 (1.88)	52.18 (8.30)
Symptomatic Seropositive	90	2	5	3	15.21 (11.19)	277.22 (269.45)	36.90 (7.04)	16.06 (2.50)	12.40 (2.20)	50.51 (9.52)

[°]W, white; B, black; H, Hispanic; O, others—percentages.

dinal follow-up of the sample described in Mitrushina et al. (1991). Subjects with a history of neurological or psychiatric illness (per self-report) were excluded from the study. Mini-Mental State Exam score for all subjects was above 24. All subjects were native English speakers and were active in the community. Mean age of the sample was 70.4 years (SD = 5.0), mean education 14.1 years (SD = 2.7), and a mean WAIS-R FSIQ 118.2 (SD = 13.0). The sample was partitioned into four age groups, which did not differ significantly in level of education or gender.

Standard administration procedures were followed. The longitudinal data over three annual probes for trial 1, trial 5, and postinterference recall trial are presented.

Study strengths

1. The data were divided into age groups.
2. Sample composition was well described in terms of age, gender, education, IQ, English fluency, and geographic area.
3. Administration procedure was described.
4. Adequate exclusion criteria.
5. Means and standard deviations are reported.

Considerations regarding use of the study

1. The sample represents highly functioning, well-educated elderly individuals, which might limit generalizability of the results.
2. Sample sizes for the youngest and the oldest groups are relatively small.
3. No data for trials II to IV.

Table 16.28. RAVLT.14a; The Original AVLT (List AB), the Alternate List (List CD) and Two New Lists (List EF and List GH)

List AB[°]		List CD[°°]		List EF		List GH	
Drum	Desk	Book	Bowl	Street	Baby	Tower	Sky
Curtain	Ranger	Flower	Dawn	Grass	Ocean	Wheat	Dollar
Bell	Bird	Train	Judge	Door	Palace	Queen	Valley
Coffee	Shoe	Rug	Grant	Arm	Lip	Sugar	Butter
School	Stove	Meadow	Insect	Star	Bar	Home	Hall
Parent	Mountain	Harp	Plane	Wife	Dress	Boy	Diamond
Moon	Glasses	Salt	County	Window	Steam	Doctor	Winter
Garden	Towel	Finger	Pool	City	Coin	Camp	Mother
Hat	Cloud	Apple	Seed	Pupil	Rock	Flag	Christmas
Farmer	Boat	Chimney	Sheep	Cabin	Army	Letter	Meat
Nose	Lamb	Button	Meal	Lake	Building	Corn	Forest
Turkey	Gum	Key	Coat	Pipe	Friend	Nail	Gold
Color	Pencil	Dog	Bottle	Skin	Storm	Cattle	Plant
House	Church	Glass	Peach	Fire	Village	Shore	Money
River	Fish	Rattle	Chair	Clock	Cell	Body	Hotel

[°]Rey (1964).

[°°]Lezak (1995).

Table 16.29. RAVLT.14b; Means and Standard Deviations for the Original and Three Alternate Forms of the AVLT for University Undergraduates

Trial	List AB	List CD	List EF	List GH
I	7.00 ± 1.63	7.40 ± 1.63	6.84 ± 1.93	7.28 ± 2.39
II	10.20 ± 2.24	10.08 ± 1.87	9.76 ± 1.90	10.00 ± 2.25
III	11.76 ± 2.45	11.40 ± 1.71	11.12 ± 2.26	11.80 ± 2.08
IV	12.40 ± 2.20	12.40 ± 1.68	12.16 ± 1.82	12.52 ± 1.78
V	13.04 ± 2.09	12.80 ± 1.55	12.92 ± 2.14	13.40 ± 1.35
List B	7.20 ± 1.89	6.76 ± 1.59	7.04 ± 1.62	7.52 ± 1.50
Postinterference	12.00 ± 2.61	11.64 ± 2.12	11.68 ± 2.64	12.24 ± 2.31

Other comments

1. The authors concluded that recall on trial I improved over repeated probes for all age groups which might be attributed to practice effect, whereas cross-sectional comparisons revealed decrease in scores on this trial with age.

2. Effect of longitudinal testing on verbal learning and forgetting (trials V and postinterference recall trial) was negated by the effect of immediate rehearsal of to-be-remembered information over five trials (Tables 16.31 and 16.32).

[RAVLT.16] Mitrushina, Satz, Chervinsky and D'Elia, 1991

The study explored effect of age on different memory mechanisms in a sample of 156 healthy elderly subjects (62 males and 94 females) between ages of 57 and 85. The sample was partitioned into four age groups, which do not differ significantly in level of education or FSIQ. Subjects with a history of neurological or psychiatric illness (per self-report) were excluded from the study. Mini-Mental State Exam score for all subjects was above 24. All subjects were native English speakers and were active in the community.

The standard administration procedure was used. The recognition trial, consisting of a paragraph, followed a 10-minute interval after the last recall trial, during which nonverbal tests were administered.

The authors reported recall on five acquisition trials, postinterference recall (trial 6), recognition, number of false-positive misidentifications, forgeting rates (loss of information from trial 5 to trial 6), and acquisition rates (trial 5 minus trial 1 score).

In addition, serial position effect was explored by dividing the list into three segments: beginning (words 1–5), middle (6–10), and end (11–15).

Study strengths

1. The data were divided into age groups.

2. Sample composition was described in terms of gender, native language, age, IQ, education, and geographic area.

3. Administration procedure was described.

4. Adequate exclusion criteria.

5. Data on a comprehensive set of the RAVLT scores are provided.

6. Means and standard deviations are reported.

Table 16.30. RAVLT.14c; Means and Standard Deviations for the Original and Three Alternate Forms of the AVLT for the VAMC Population

Trial	List AB	List CD	List EF	List GH
I	4.06 ± 1.43	3.29 ± 1.96	3.52 ± 1.55	3.41 ± 1.37
II	5.52 ± 1.66	4.94 ± 2.08	4.76 ± 2.61	4.71 ± 1.57
III	6.12 ± 2.00	5.59 ± 2.09	5.76 ± 2.31	5.76 ± 2.44
IV	6.41 ± 2.12	5.71 ± 2.26	6.47 ± 2.65	5.65 ± 2.18
V	6.47 ± 2.72	6.47 ± 2.83	6.88 ± 3.16	6.47 ± 3.24
List B	3.35 ± 1.66	3.41 ± 1.66	3.18 ± 1.55	3.41 ± 1.97
Postinterference	4.06 ± 3.65	3.29 ± 2.87	3.71 ± 3.67	4.17 ± 2.96

Table 16.31. RAVLT.15a; Demographic Characteristics for Four Age Groups

	57 to 65	66 to 70	71 to 75	76 to 85
Mean age	62.2 (2.5)	68.2 (1.2)	72.9 (1.4)	78.3 (2.5)
Mean education	14.4 (2.0)	13.7 (1.8)	14.5 (3.1)	14.0 (3.6)
Male/female %	10/90	15/85	30/70	22/78
N	19	40	47	16

Considerations regarding use of the study

1. The sample represents highly functioning, well-educated elderly individuals which might limit generalizability of the results.

2. Sample sizes for the youngest and the oldest groups are relatively small.

Other comments

1. The authors concluded that significant effect of age is evident in recall on five acquisition trials, whereas rates of acquisition, forgetting, and recognition are not affected by age. In addition, primacy/recency effect was equally strong for all groups (Tables 16.33–16.35).

[RAVLT.17] Selnes, Jacobson, Machado, Becker, Wesch, Miller, Visscher and McArthur, 1991

The study used subjects from the MACS study, described above (see Miller, 1990). The article presents results of seronegative homosexual and bisexual males for the purpose of establishing normative data for neuropsychological test performance based on a large sample.

The standard procedure was used for administration. In addition, recall after 20-minute delay was tested, followed by delayed recognition trial. (Recognition was not tested after administration of a postinterference trial.)

Study strengths

1. Data are stratified by age, education, and age × education.

2. The demographic composition of the sample is well described in terms of age, gender, ethnicity, education, and geographic area.

3. The administration procedure is well outlined.

4. Sample sizes are large.

5. Means, SDs, as well as scores for percentiles 5 and 10 are presented.

Considerations regarding use of the study

1. The generalizability of the results is limited due to high educational level of the majority of the sample.

2. Data on trials I–IV are not reported.

3. All male sample.

4. No exclusion criteria were reported.

Other comments

1. The authors concluded that age and education are important determinants of performance on Rey AVLT (Table 16.36).

Table 16.32. RAVLT.15b; Comparison of Three Longitudinal Probes

	57–65 (N = 16)			66–70 (N = 40)			71–75 (N = 47)			76–85 (N = 16)		
	T1	T2	T3°	T1	T2	T3	T1	T2	T3	T1	T2	T3
Trial I	6.7	6.4	7.9	6.0	6.2	7.3	5.1	5.4	6.4	5.1	5.8	6.0
	(1.6)	(1.3)	(2.3)	(1.6)	(1.8)	(1.8)	(2.0)	(1.7)	(1.8)	(1.5)	(1.2)	(1.9)
Trial V	12.4	12.3	11.9	11.8	11.7	12.1	10.4	10.1	10.4	10.3	10.6	9.8
	(2.6)	(2.5)	(2.8)	(2.5)	(2.5)	(2.3)	(2.7)	(3.3)	(3.2)	(2.4)	(3.2)	(4.0)
Postinterference recall	10.7	10.8	10.5	9.5	9.9	10.4	8.7	8.4	8.9	8.4	8.5	7.9
	(3.2)	(3.2)	(3.4)	(3.0)	(3.2)	(2.8)	(3.5)	(3.6)	(3.6)	(3.5)	(3.8)	(4.7)

°Three annual probes.

Table 16.33. RAVLT.16a; Demographic Characteristics of the Sample

| | All | Age Groups | | | |
		57–65	66–70	71–75	76–85
Age	70.7	62.8	68.2	72.9	78.7
(SD)	(5.4)	(2.3)	(1.3)	(1.4)	(2.7)
Education	14.1	14.2	14.0	14.6	13.3
(SD)	(2.9)	(2.0)	(2.0)	(3.4)	(3.6)
WAIS-R FSIQ	117.2	115.8	119.3	118.7	112.0
(SD)	(12.6)	(12.6)	(14.5)	(10.8)	(11.7)
N	156	28	45	57	26

Table 16.34. RAVLT.16b; Average Recall for Four Age Groups on the RAVLT

| Age Group | Trials | | | | | Recall Postinterference | Recognition | FP | T5 − T6 | T5 − T1 |
	1	2	3	4	5					
57–65	6.4	8.8	10.4	11.4	12.1	10.3	13.2	0.8	1.9	5.7
SD	1.5	2.4	2.5	2.3	2.4	3.0	1.3	1.4	1.7	2.0
66–70	5.9	8.5	9.8	11.3	11.5	9.1	13.0	1.0	2.4	5.6
SD	1.6	2.3	2.3	2.3	3.0	3.3	1.1	1.6	2.5	2.9
71–75	5.1	7.5	8.7	9.7	10.3	8.4	12.7	1.1	1.9	5.2
SD	1.8	2.2	2.4	2.7	2.9	3.5	1.9	1.7	2.2	2.5
76–85	5.1	6.8	8.3	9.5	9.7	7.7	12.6	0.8	2.0	4.7
SD	1.6	2.1	2.3	2.8	2.8	3.4	1.9	1.2	2.6	2.7

In another table resulting from the same study, the investigators presented data broken down by age and education. This table has not been published (personal communication) (Table 16.37).

[RAVLT.18] Delaney, Prevey, Cramer, and Mattson, 1992

The authors collected data on 42 control subjects as a part of an investigation on partial com-

Table 16.35. RAVLT.16c; Primacy/Recency Effects for the Entire Sample*

| | Trial | | | | |
	1	2	3	4	5
Beginning	1.9	3.0	3.4	3.9	3.9
Middle	1.1	1.7	2.3	2.7	3.1
End	2.6	3.0	3.3	3.6	3.6

*Provides mean number of words recalled within each segment of the list across five acquisition trials.

plex and generalized seizures and memory, and anticonvulsant efficacy. The subjects were recruited in Connecticut, California, Florida, Virginia, Massachusetts, New York, and Minnesota. Exclusion criteria included history of neurologic or psychiatric disorder or "current drug history that could affect performance." Mean age was 45.8 (range = 22 to 67) and mean years of education was 12.8 (range = 6 to 16).

The administration format detailed in Lezak (1983, 1995) was employed with the exception that subjects were forewarned that a 20-minute delayed recall would occur. During the 20-minute delay period, additional testing involving motor, attentional, and verbal fluency tasks was conducted. An alternate list (C; Lezak, 1983, 1995) was administered 1 month later.

Means and standard deviations for trials I, III, V; interference; 20-minute delayed recall; and recognition are reported for both test forms. The two forms correlated highly (acqui-

Table 16.36. RAVLT.17a

	By Age		
		Age Group	
Variable	25–34	35–44	45–54
N	309	290	97
Education	16.1 (2.2)	16.4 (2.3)	16.7 (2.6)
Race	96.4%C°	96.6%C	95.9%C
Total score	54.4 (7.8)	51.4 (8.1)	49.5 (7.9)
Trial V	13.0 (1.8)	12.6 (1.8)	12.3 (1.8)
Recall after Interference	11.3 (2.4)	10.7 (2.6)	10.6 (2.8)
Delayed recall	11.1 (2.5)	10.4 (2.9)	10.2 (3.2)
Delayed recognition	14.4 (0.9)	14.1 (1.2)	14.0 (1.2)

	By Education		
		Education	
Variable	<College	College	>College
N	229	202	302
Mean age	36.1 (7.4)	35.6 (7.2)	38.4 (7.8)
Race	94.8%C	96.0%C	96.7%C
Total score	50.7 (7.5)	53.2 (8.1)	53.3 (8.3)
Trial V	12.6 (1.7)	12.8 (1.9)	12.9 (1.8)
Recall after Interference	10.5 (2.5)	10.9 (2.5)	11.2 (2.6)
Delayed recall	10.1 (2.7)	10.8 (2.9)	10.9 (2.8)
Delayed recognition	14.1 (1.2)	14.4 (0.9)	14.2 (1.1)

°C, Caucasian.

sition trials: $r = 0.61$ to 0.86; delayed recall trials: $r = 0.51$ to 0.72), providing support for their comparability. Significant correlations were documented between test scores and age ($r = -0.22$ to -0.55) and education ($r = 0.14$ to 0.54).

Study strengths
1. Information on alternate forms.
2. Adequate exclusion criteria.
3. Information regarding age, education, and geographic recruitment area.
4. Most test administration procedures are specified.
5. Means and standard deviations are reported.

Considerations regarding use of the study
1. The exact recognition procedure was not specified.
2. Subjects were forewarned regarding delayed recall.

3. Undifferentiated age range.
4. No information regarding IQ or sex.
5. Somewhat small sample.
6. No data for trials II and IV (Table 16.38).

[RAVLT.19] Ivnik, Malec, Smith, Tangalos, Petersen, Kokmen, and Kurland, 1992c

The study provides age-specific norms for the Rey AVLT obtained in Mayo's Older Americans Normative Studies (MOANS). Information provided in this article updates previous normative data reported by Ivnik et al. (1990). The present study extends the normative base from 394 to 530 subjects, refines scoring procedures, and develops a uniform methodology for producing normative information on many different tests. There were no changes in the administration procedure in comparison to the earlier publications.

The sample consisted of cognitively normal volunteers aged 56 to 97. Age categorization utilized the midpoint interval technique.

Table 16.37. RAVLT.17b

<*College*

	Age Group		
Variable	25–34	35–44	45–54
N	107	93	42
Total score	51.9 (7.5)	50.0 (7.6)	49.0 (7.4)
Trial V	12.8 (1.7)	12.4 (1.8)	12.2 (1.8)
Recall after	10.9 (2.4)	10.2 (2.8)	9.8 (2.6)
Interference			
Delayed recall	10.6 (2.6)	9.8 (2.8)	9.5 (2.9)
Delayed recognition	14.3 (1.0)	14.0 (1.5)	13.6 (1.6)

College

	Age Group		
Variable	25–34	35–44	45–54
N	104	77	35
Total score	54.6 (8.0)	51.3 (8.0)	53.3 (8.5)
Trial V	12.9 (2.0)	12.5 (2.0)	13.0 (1.7)
Recall after	11.4 (2.1)	10.7 (2.8)	10.3 (3.0)
Interference			
Delayed recall	11.1 (2.4)	10.8 (3.1)	9.8 (3.5)
Delayed recognition	14.5 (0.8)	14.1 (1.4)	14.5 (0.8)

>*College*

	Age Group		
Variable	25–34	35–44	45–54
N	111	150	64
Total score	56.4 (7.1)	52.2 (8.7)	51.5 (7.9)
Trial V	13.3 (1.6)	12.8 (1.9)	12.8 (1.8)
Recall after	11.6 (2.4)	10.9 (2.6)	11.1 (2.7)
Interference			
Delayed recall	11.5 (2.3)	10.4 (2.9)	11.0 (2.9)
Delayed recognition	14.4 (0.9)	14.1 (1.3)	14.1 (1.1)

Mean MAYO VIQ, PIQ, and FSIQ (which differ somewhat from standard WAIS-R IQs) for the whole sample were 104.8 (10.4), 106.6 (11.5), and 105.8 (10.8), respectively. The sample is almost exclusively Caucasian and living in an economically stable region.

The standard administration procedure was used for recall trials. In addition, 30-minute delayed recall followed by a recognition trial was administered. The recognition trial presented 30 words italicized in Lezak's 1976 paragraph as a two-column list, which the subject reads. The subjects indicates recognition of a learned word by crossing it off the list.

The AVLT component scores were converted to age-corrected and normalized scaled scores with a mean of 10 and a SD of 3, which are derived from the cumulative frequency distributions of each raw score within each midpoint age group. The scaled scores are grouped and summed within groups to allow derivation of three summary indices: MAVLEI, MAVDRI, and MAVPRI.

The following measures derived from Rey AVLT performance were summarized in the tables provided by the authors:

1. The MAYO Auditory-Verbal Learning Efficiency Index (MAVLEI) consists of the following measures:

    a. Recall on trial I.

    b. Learning Over Trials (LOT) calculated as Total Learning (the sum of words remembered across trials I through V) corrected for immediate word span (trial I): LOT = TL − (5 × trial I score). This index represents ability to improve upon Trial I performance during each of the subsequent four learning trials.

2. Recall of list B represents an index of proactive interference on later word span.

3. The MAYO Auditory-Verbal Delayed Recall Index (MAVDRI) includes the following measures:

    a. Recall on trial VI, representing memory status after a brief delay.

    b. Recall after 30-minute delay represents memory functioning after an extended delay.

Table 16.38. RAVLT.18

Form	N	Age	Education	Trial			Interference	20-Minute Delayed Recall	Recognition
				I	III	V			
A	42	45.8	12.8	6.0	10.1	11.6	9.9	9.9	13.6
		(22–67)	(6–16)	(2.1)	(2.4)	(2.5)	(3.2)	(3.1)	(1.8)
C				6.1	10.0	11.8	9.9	9.2	14.0
				(2.2)	(2.4)	(2.8)	(3.3)	(3.5)	(1.2)

4. Recognition efficiency.

5. The MAYO Auditory-Verbal Percent Retention Index (MAVPRI) reflects the common clinical practice of evaluating information recalled after a delay as a function of the amount of data originally learned, and includes the following measures:

   a. Short-Term Percent Retention (STPR) expresses trial VI recall as a proportion of trial V recall: STPR = 100 × (Trial VI recall/trial V recall).

   b. Long-Term Percent Retention (LTPR) expresses delayed recall score as a proportion of trial V recall: LTPR = 100 × (delayed recall score/trial V recall).

Conversion of raw and computed scores into scaled scores allows greater comparability of these indices to each other and to performance on other tests.

Study strengths

1. Demographic characteristics of the sample are well described in terms of geographic area, age, gender, education, IQ, handedness, and ethnicity.

2. The data were broken down by age group based on midpoint interval technique.

3. The administration procedure was well described.

4. The innovative scoring system was well described. The authors developed new indices of performance to explore different memory mechanisms.

5. The sample sizes for each group are large.

Considerations regarding use of the study

1. The measures proposed by the authors are quite complicated and might be difficult to compute in clinical practice.

2. Subjects with prior history of neurological, psychiatric, or chronic medical illnesses were included.

Other comments

The theoretical assumptions underlying this normative project have been presented in Ivnik et al. (1992a,b).

The authors cautioned that validity of the MAYO AVLT indices depends heavily on the match of demographic features of the individual to the normative sample presented in this article (Table 16.39).

In the following tables (Tables 16.40–16.50) MOANS Scaled Scores are corrected for age influences.

The following abbreviations are used:

MOANS = Mayo's Older Americans Normative Studies

LOT = Learning Over Trials

Recog. = Recognition

STPR = Short-Term Percent Retention

Table 16.39. RAVLT.19a; Demographic Data

	Count	Percent of Total
Age		
56–59	41	7.7
60–64	72	13.6
65–69	83	15.7
70–74	82	15.5
75–79	105	19.8
80–84	76	14.3
85–89	49	9.2
≥90	22	4.1
Handedness		
Right-handed	501	94.5
Left-handed	16	3.0
Mixed/both	13	2.5
Sex		
Males	200	37.7
Females	330	62.3
Marital Status		
Single	69	13.0
Married	318	60.0
Divorced	12	2.3
Widowed	131	24.7
Race		
Caucasian	528	99.6
Black	1	0.2
Hispanic	1	0.2
Education		
≤7 years	8	1.5
8–11 years	84	15.8
12 years	192	36.2
13–15 years	117	22.1
16–17 years	82	15.5
≥18 years	47	8.9

Table 16.40. RAVLT.19b; Midpoint Age = 61 (Age Range = 56–66, n = 143)

MOANS Scaled Score	Learning Efficiency Index Measures			Delayed Recall Index Measures			Percent Retention Index Measures		
	Trial 1	LOT	List B	Trial 6	30-Minute Recall	Recognition	STPR	LTPR	PR
2	0–2	0	0	0–2	0	0–5	0–30	0–10	<1
3	—	1	1	3	—	6–7	31–42	11–13	1
4	—	2–3	2	—	—	—	43–44	14–15	2
5	3	4–6	—	4	1–3	8–9	45–50	16–37	3–5
6	—	7–8	—	5	4	10	51–58	38–53	6–10
7	4	9–11	3	6	5–6	11	59–69	54–58	11–18
8	—	12–13	—	7	7	12–13	70–75	59–64	19–28
9	5	14–16	—	8–9	8	—	76–80	65–75	29–40
10	6	17–19	4	10	9	14	81–87	76–83	41–59
11	—	20–21	5	11	10–11	—	88–91	84–88	60–71
12	7	22–23	—	12	12	15	92–93	89–93	72–81
13	8	24–26	6	13	13	—	94–95	94+	82–89
14	—	27	7	14	14	—	96+	—	90–94
15	9	28–29	8	15	15	—	—	—	95–97
16	—	—	9	—	—	—	—	—	98
17	10–12	30–32	—	—	—	—	—	—	99
18	13–15	33+	10–15	—	—	—	—	—	>99

LTPR = Long-Term Percent Retention

PR = Percentile ranges

[RAVLT.20] Savage and Gouvier, 1992

The study explored effect of age and gender on Rey AVLT performance. Subjects were 134 undergraduate students, senior citizens from community programs, and others (66 males and 68 females), forming seven age groups ranging from the late teens through the seventh decade. Only those subjects who completed 12th grade were included in the study (with the exception

Table 16.41. RAVLT.19c; Midpoint Age = 64 (Age Range = 59–69, n = 168)

MOANS Scaled Score	Learning Efficiency Index Measures			Delayed Recall Index Measures			Percent Retention Index Measures		
	Trial 1	LOT	List B	Trial 6	30-Minute Recall	Recognition	STPR	LTPR	PR
2	0–1	0	0	0–1	0	0–5	0–20	0–10	<1
3	2	1	—	2	—	6	21–25	11–13	1
4	—	2–3	1	3	—	7	26–33	14–15	2
5	3	4–5	2	4	1–2	8	34–40	16–30	3–5
6	—	6–7	—	5	3	9–10	41–57	31–45	6–10
7	—	8–9	3	6	4	11	58–63	46–54	11–18
8	4	10–12	—	7	5–6	12	64–72	55–62	19–28
9	5	13–15	—	8	7	13	73–76	63–71	29–40
10	—	16–18	4	9	8–9	14	77–86	72–82	41–59
11	6	19–20	5	10	10	—	87–91	83–88	60–71
12	—	21–23	—	11–12	11	15	92–93	89–92	72–81
13	7	24–25	6	—	12	—	94–95	93–95	82–89
14	8	26	—	13	13	—	96+	96+	90–94
15	9	27	7	14	14	—	—	—	95–97
16	—	28–29	8	15	—	—	—	—	98
17	10–12	30–32	9	—	15	—	—	—	99
18	13–15	33+	10–15	—	—	—	—	—	>99

Table 16.42. RAVLT.19d; Midpoint Age = 67 (Age Range = 62-72, n = 182)

MOANS Scaled Score	Learning Efficiency Index Measures			Delayed Recall Index Measures			Percent Retention Index Measures		
	Trial 1	LOT	List B	Trial 6	30-Minute Recall	Recognition	STPR	LTPR	PR
2	0–1	0	0	0	—	0–5	0–20	—	<1
3	—	1	—	1	0	6	21–25	0–5	1
4	2	2–3	1	2	—	7	26–33	6–12	2
5	—	4–5	—	3	1	8	34–40	13–21	3–5
6	3	6–7	2	4	2–3	9	41–57	22–42	6–10
7	—	8–9	—	5	4	10	58–63	43–53	11–18
8	4	10–11	3	6	5	11	64–71	54–60	19–28
9	—	12–13	—	7	6–7	12	72–76	61–70	29–40
10	5	14–18	4	8–9	8	13	77–86	71–80	41–59
11	6	19–20	—	10	9	14	87–91	81–94	60–71
12	—	21–22	5	11	10	15	92–93	85–90	72–81
13	7	23–25	—	12	11–12	—	94–95	91–94	82–89
14	—	26	6	13	13	—	96+	95+	90–94
15	8	27	7	—	—	—	—	—	95–97
16	—	28–29	8	14	14	—	—	—	98
17	9–10	30–32	9	15	15	—	—	—	99
18	11–15	33+	10–15	—	—	—	—	—	>99

of the 16–19-year-old group). All subjects completed an extensive medical history questionnaire. Subjects with a history of head injury, alcoholism, mental illness, cardiovascular disease, or other conditions associated with impaired memory functioning were excluded.

Standard administration procedure was used, including recall after 30-minute delay during which subjects filled out personal and medical questionnaires. The number of correctly recalled words from list A, as well as the number of commission errors or words incor-

Table 16.43. RAVLT.19e; Midpoint Age = 70 (Age Range = 65–75, n = 194)

MOANS Scaled Score	Learning Efficiency Index Measures			Delayed Recall Index Measures			Percent Retention Index Measures		
	Trial 1	LOT	List B	Trial 6	30-Minute Recall	Recognition	STPR	LTPR	PR
2	0–1	0	0	0	—	0–5	0–20	—	<1
3	—	1	—	1	0	6	21–25	0–5	1
4	2	—	—	—	—	7	26–33	6–12	2
5	—	2–4	1	2–3	1	8	34–40	13–21	3–5
6	3	5–6	—	4	2–3	9	41–54	22–38	6–10
7	—	7–8	2	5	4	10	55–62	39–49	11–18
8	4	9–10	—	6	5	11	63–69	50–59	19–28
9	—	11–13	3	7	6	12	70–73	60–65	29–40
10	5	14–16	4	8	7	13	74–83	66–76	41–59
11	—	17–19	—	9	8	14	84–88	77–83	60–71
12	6	20–21	5	10	9	–	89–93	84–89	72–81
13	—	22–23	—	11	10–11	15	94–95	90–92	82–89
14	7	24–26	6	12	12	—	96+	93–94	90–94
15	—	27	7	13	13	—	—	95+	95–97
16	8	28–29	8	14	—	—	—	—	98
17	9	30–32	9	—	14	—	—	—	99
18	10–15	33+	10–15	15	15	—	—	—	>99

Table 16.44. RAVLT.19f; Midpoint Age = 73 (Age Range = 68–78, n = 214)

MOANS Scaled Score	Learning Efficiency Index Measures			Delayed Recall Index Measures			Percent Retention Index Measures		
	Trial 1	LOT	List B	Trial 6	30-Minute Recall	Recognition	STPR	LTPR	PR
2	0	0	0	0	—	0–5	0–20	—	<1
3	1	1	—	1	—	—	21–25	—	1
4	—	—	—	—	0	—	26–33	0–10	2
5	2	2–4	1	2	1	6–7	34–40	11–19	3–5
6	—	5–6	—	3–4	2	8–9	41–54	20–36	6–10
7	3	7–8	2	5	3	10	55–61	37–49	11–18
8	—	9–10	—	—	4	11	62–66	50–56	19–28
9	4	11–12	3	6	5	12	67–71	57–63	29–40
10	5	13–16	—	7	6–7	13	72–80	64–74	41–59
11	—	17–18	4	8	8	—	81–86	75–80	60–71
12	—	19–20	5	9	9	14	87–92	81–86	72–81
13	6	21–23	—	10	10	15	93–95	87–90	82–89
14	7	24–26	6	11–12	11	—	96+	91–94	90–94
15	—	27	7	13	12	—	—	95+	95–97
16	8	28–29	8	14	13	—	—	—	98
17	—	30–32	9	—	14	—	—	—	99
18	9–15	33+	10–15	15	15	—	—	—	>99

rectly identified as being on the list, was recorded. Immediate and delayed recognition trials were used, which consisted of underlining the learned words in the same paragraph for both recognition trials.

Study strengths

1. Administration procedures were well described.
2. The data were partitioned by age and gender.

Table 16.45. RAVLT.19g; Midpoint Age = 76 (Age Range = 71–81, n = 203)

MOANS Scaled Score	Learning Efficiency Index Measures			Delayed Recall Index Measures			Percent Retention Index Measures		
	Trial 1	LOT	List B	Trial 6	30-Minute Recall	Recognition	STPR	LTPR	PR
2	0	0	—	0	—	0–5	0–20	—	<1
3	1	1	0	1	—	—	21–25	—	1
4	—	—	—	—	0	—	26–33	0–5	2
5	2	2–4	1	2	1	6–7	34–40	6–20	3–5
6	—	5–6	—	3–4	2	8–9	41–54	21–36	6–10
7	3	7–8	2	—	3	10	55–61	37–49	11–18
8	—	9	—	5	4	11	62–63	50–56	19–28
9	4	10–11	3	6	5	12	64–71	57–62	29–40
10	—	12–15	—	7	6	13	72–80	63–74	41–59
11	5	16–18	4	8	7–8	—	81–86	75–80	60–71
12	—	19–20	—	9	9	14	87–90	81–86	72–81
13	6	21–23	5	10	—	15	91–95	87–90	82–89
14	7	24–26	6	11–12	10–11	—	96+	91–94	90–94
15	—	27	7	13	—	—	—	95+	95–97
16	8	28–29	8	14	12	—	—	—	98
17	—	30–32	9	—	13	—	—	—	99
18	9–15	33+	10–15	15	14–15	—	—	—	>99

Table 16.46. RAVLT.19h; Midpoint Age = 79 (Age Range = 74–84, n = 196)

MOANS Scaled Score	Learning Efficiency Index Measures			Delayed Recall Index Measures			Percent Retention Index Measures		
	Trial 1	LOT	List B	Trial 6	30-Minute Recall	Recognition	STPR	LTPR	PR
2	0	0	—	0	—	0–4	0–20	—	<1
3	1	1	—	1	—	5	21–25	—	1
4	—	—	—	—	—	—	26–33	—	2
5	2	2–3	0	2	0	6–7	34–38	0–7	3–5
6	—	4–5	1	3	1	8	39–46	8–27	6–10
7	3	6–7	2	4	2–3	9–10	47–58	28–44	11–18
8	—	8	—	5	4	11	59–63	45–56	19–28
9	—	9–10	—	—	5	—	64–70	57–61	29–40
10	4	11–14	3	6–7	6	12–13	71–78	62–71	41–59
11	5	15–17	4	8	7	–	79–84	72–79	60–71
12	—	18–19	—	—	8	14	85–89	80–86	72–81
13	6	20–22	5	9	9	15	90–93	87–90	82–89
14	—	23–25	6	10	10	—	94+	91–94	90–94
15	7	26–27	7	11–13	11	—	—	95+	95–97
16	8	28–29	8	14	12	—	—	—	98
17	—	30–32	9	—	13	—	—	—	99
18	9–15	33+	10–15	15	14–15	—	—	—	>99

3. Adequate exclusion criteria.

4. Information regarding education, recruitment sources, and geographic area was provided.

5. Means and standard deviations are reported.

Considerations regarding use of the study

1. Immediate recognition trial was used, which facilitates performance on delayed recall and recognition.

2. No information on mean educational level.

Table 16.47. RAVLT.19i; Midpoint Age = 82 (Age Range = 77–87, n = 168)

MOANS Scaled Score	Learning Efficiency Index Measures			Delayed Recall Index Measures			Percent Retention Index Measures		
	Trial 1	LOT	List B	Trial 6	30-Minute Recall	Recognition	STPR	LTPR	PR
2	—	—	—	0	—	0–2	0–10	—	<1
3	0	0	—	1	—	3–4	11–20	—	1
4	1	1	—	—	—	5	21–30	—	2
5	—	2–3	0	2	—	—	31–36	—	3–5
6	2	4–5	1	—	0–1	6–8	37–40	0–24	6–10
7	—	6–7	—	3–4	2	9–10	41–50	25–36	11–18
8	3	8	2	—	3	11	51–61	37–49	19–28
9	—	9–10	—	5	4	—	62–69	50–60	29–40
10	4	11–14	3	6	5	12–13	70–78	61–69	41–59
11	—	15–17	—	7	6	—	79–84	70–75	60–71
12	5	18–19	4	8	7–8	14	85–89	76–84	72–81
13	—	20–22	5	9	—	—	90–93	85–90	82–89
14	6	23–25	6	10	9–10	15	94+	91–94	90–94
15	7	26–27	7	11–13	11	—	—	95+	95–97
16	8	28–29	8	14	12	—	—	—	98
17	—	30–32	9	—	13	—	—	—	99
18	9–15	33+	10–15	15	14–15	—	—	—	>99

Table 16.48. RAVLT.19j; Midpoint Age = 85 (Age Range = 80–90, n = 131)

| MOANS Scaled Score | Learning Efficiency Index Measures | | | Delayed Recall Index Measures | | | Percent Retention Index Measures | | |
	Trial 1	LOT	List B	Trial 6	30-Minute Recall	Recognition	STPR	LTPR	PR
2	—	—	—	—	—	0–2	0–10	—	<1
3	0	—	—	0	—	3–4	11–20	—	1
4	1	0–1	—	1	—	5	21–25	—	2
5	—	2–3	—	2	—	—	26–33	—	3–5
6	2	4–5	0–1	—	0	6–8	34–40	0–24	6–10
7	—	6–7	—	3	1–2	9	41–44	25–32	11–18
8	—	8	2	4	3	10	45–58	33–49	19–28
9	3	9–10	—	5	4	11	59–66	50–59	29–40
10	4	11–14	3	6	5	12	67–78	60–69	41–59
11	—	15–17	—	7	6	13	79–84	70–75	60–71
12	5	18–19	4	8	7–8	—	85–89	76–84	72–81
13	—	20–22	—	9	—	14	90–93	85–90	82–89
14	6	23–25	5	10	9–10	15	94+	91–94	90–94
15	7	26–27	6	11–13	11	—	—	95+	95–97
16	—	28–29	7	14	12	—	—	—	98
17	8	30–31	8	—	13	—	—	—	99
18	9–15	32+	9–15	15	14–15	—	—	—	>99

3. Sample sizes for each group are small.

4. Normative data for older groups (60–69 and 70–76) are not reported for the delayed recall trials.

Other comments

The authors concluded that there was no effect of gender for any of the trials. Effect of age was evident for all trials with the exception of

Table 16.49. RAVLT.19k; Midpoint Age = 88 (Age Range = 83 and Above, n = 98)

| MOANS Scaled Score | Learning Efficiency Index Measures | | | Delayed Recall Index Measures | | | Percent Retention Index Measures | | |
	Trial 1	LOT	List B	Trial 6	30-Minute Recall	Recognition	STPR	LTPR	PR
2	—	—	—	—	—	0–2	—	—	<1
3	0	—	—	0	—	3–4	0–10	—	1
4	—	0	—	1	—	5	11–25	—	2
5	1	1–3	—	2	—	—	26–30	—	3–5
6	2	4–5	0	—	0	6–8	31–38	0–19	6–10
7	—	6–7	1	3	1–2	9	39–44	20–32	11–18
8	—	8	2	4	3	10	45–55	33–45	19–28
9	3	9–10	—	—	4	11	56–64	46–54	29–40
10	4	11–14	3	5–6	5	12	65–77	55–65	41–59
11	—	15–16	—	7	6	13	78–81	66–70	60–71
12	5	17–18	—	8	7	—	82–87	71–80	72–81
13	—	19–20	4	9	8	14	88–92	81–86	82–89
14	6	21–22	5	10	9–10	15	93+	87–92	90–94
15	7	23–25	—	11–13	11	—	—	93+	95–97
16	—	26	6	14	12	—	—	—	98
17	8	27	7	—	13	—	—	—	99
18	9–15	28+	8–15	15	14–15	—	—	—	>99

Table 16.50. RAVLT.19l; Table for Converting AVLT MOANS Scaled Score Sums to MAYO Indices

MAYO Index Score	AVLT MOANS Scaled Score Sums			MAYO Index Score
	Learning Efficiency Sum	Delayed Recall Sum	Percent Retention Sum	
<65	≤13	≤8	≤9	≤65
65		9		65
66				66
67	14		10	67
68		10		68
69				69
70			11	70
71		11		71
72	15			72
73		12	12	73
74				74
75				75
76	16	13	13	76
77				77
78				78
79		14		79
80			14	80
81	17			81
82		15		82
83			15	83
84				84
85		16		85
86	18		16	86
87				87
88		17		88
89			17	89
90	19			90
91		18		91
92				92
93			18	93
94		19		94
95	20			95
96			19	96
97		20		97
98				98
99	21		20	99
100		21		100
101				101
102			21	102
103		22		103
104	22			104
105				105
106		23	22	106
107				107
108	23			108
109		24	23	109
110				110
111				111
112		25	24	112
113	24			113

continued

Table 16.50. *(Continued)*

MAYO Index Score	AVLT MOANS Scaled Score Sums			MAYO Index Score
	Learning Efficiency Sum	Delayed Recall Sum	Percent Retention Sum	
114				114
115		26	25	115
116				116
117	25			117
118		27		118
119			26	119
120				120
121		28		121
122	26		27	122
123		29		123
124				124
125			28	125
126		30		126
127	27			127
128			29	128
129		31		129
130				130
131	28			131
132		32	30	132
133				133
134				134
135		33	31	135
>135	≥29	≥34	≥32	135

trials I and II and list B (Tables 16.51 and 16.52).

[RAVLT.21] Crossen and Wiens, 1994

The study compares performance on Rey AVLT and California Verbal Learning Test (CVLT). Subjects were 60 individuals (52 men and eight women) who had applied for jobs in the civil service involving public safety and passed medical screening examinations. Their mean age was 29.9 years (SD = 6.2), mean education was 14.7 years (SD = 1.6), and mean WAIS-R FSIQ was 106.3 with a range of scores from 88 to 133.

All subjects were administered both forms in a counterbalanced order, with an interval of about 2 to 4 hours between administrations. The Rey AVLT was administered according to standard procedure. On the recognition trial the subjects were to read a paragraph and circle the learned words. The CVLT was administered according to the instructions in the manual (Delis et al., 1987).

Table 16.51. RAVLT.20a; Trials I Through V

Gender/Age	N	Trials				
		I	II	III	IV	V
Males 16–19	10	6.2 (0.78)	7.7 (1.8)	9.9 (1.5)	11.1 (2.3)	12.3 (1.6)
Females	10	6.5 (1.7)	7.7 (2.3)	10.6 (2.4)	11.7 (1.2)	12.9 (0.2)
Males 20–29	10	6.4 (2.0)	8.4 (2.4)	9.6 (2.3)	10.1 (3.1)	10.5 (1.9)
Females	9	5.7 (0.97)	7.3 (1.3)	8.0 (2.7)	9.6 (2.3)	10.3 (2.0)
Males 30–39	9	5.5 (1.1)	7.6 (1.0)	9.0 (2.3)	9.5 (2.7)	9.8 (2.1)
Females	10	6.2 (3.2)	8.6 (3.8)	10.8 (2.3)	10.7 (2.2)	11.8 (1.9)
Males 40–49	9	6.0 (1.2)	7.3 (2.0)	9.1 (1.8)	9.8 (1.2)	10.4 (2.1)
Females	10	5.7 (1.5)	7.3 (2.2)	9.1 (2.7)	9.4 (3.2)	10.4 (3.1)
Males 50–59	9	5.7 (0.83)	8.1 (1.0)	9.1 (1.8)	9.4 (2.5)	9.3 (2.2)
Females	10	5.6 1.6)	7.9 (1.5)	8.8 (2.2)	11.3 (2.4)	11.6 (2.2)
Males 60–69	9	5.0 (1.0)	6.0 (1.1)	7.4 (2.5)	8.2 (2.3)	8.4 (2.3)
Females	10	5.6 (1.2)	7.4 (1.5)	7.0 (2.7)	9.0 (2.5)	9.3 (1.9)
Males 70–76	10	5.3 (1.4)	6.3 (1.2)	7.5 (1.6)	7.9 (2.4)	8.1 (2.4)
Females	9	5.6 (1.1)	6.5 (1.7)	6.5 (1.8)	6.7 (1.6)	7.4 (1.6)

Study strengths

1. Information regarding age, gender, IQ, and educational level.
2. Administration procedure was outlined.
3. Sample size is sufficient.
4. Adequate exclusion criteria.
5. Means and standard deviations are reported.

Considerations regarding use of the study

1. Undifferentiated age range.
2. High educational level.
3. Mostly male sample.

Other comments

1. The authors concluded that CVLT yielded higher scores than Rey AVLT. There were significant differences in performance on all parameters of the AVLT and corresponding variables of the CVLT, which amounted to one-half to one full word difference on every trial. The results suggested no order effect and minimal practice effect for different list-learning tests administered in the same test battery (Table 16.53).

[RAVLT.22] Geffen, Butterworth and Geffen, 1994

The study explored the equivalence between the original form of the Rey AVLT (form 1) and a new form (form 4), as well as test–retest reliability of both forms. Subjects were 51 volunteers (25 males and 26 females) living in Australia with no self-reported history of head

Table 16.52. RAVLT.20b; Trials B Through Delayed Recognition

Gender	Age	List B	Postinterference Recall	Immediate Recognition	Delayed Recall	Commission Errors	Delayed Recognition
M	16–19	5.9 (0.74)	10.6 (2.5)	14.1 (1.2)	9.9 (2.5)	0.60 (0.96)	13.9 (1.2)
F		5.4 (1.2)	12.1 (2.6)	14.4 (0.51)	11.4 (2.6)	0.60 (0.96)	14.3 (0.67)
M	20–29	4.7 (1.6)	10.1 (3.0)	14.2 (1.6)	10.0 (3.4)	0.30 (0.67)	14.0 (1.6)
F		5.3 (2.1)	8.7 (2.3)	14.0 (1.1)	8.6 (2.1)	0.55 (0.88)	13.8 (1.6)
M	30–39	4.6 (2.1)	8.3 (2.7)	13.1 (2.0)	9.0 (3.3)	0.11 (0.33)	12.6 (2.4)
F		5.0 (2.2)	10.7 (2.9)	14.0 (0.94)	11.7 (2.8)	0.40 (0.52)	13.6 (2.8)
M	40–49	5.0 (1.0)	8.1 (1.9)	13.1 (1.9)	7.6 (2.0)	0.11 (0.33)	13.5 (2.1)
F		4.7 (1.4)	8.2 (3.4)	13.3 (2.2)	7.6 (3.5)	0.90 (1.4)	12.9 (2.8)
M	50–59	4.3 (2.0)	8.3 (2.4)	12.8 (1.7)	7.5 (2.7)	0.88 (1.4)	12.5 (2.1)
F		4.5 (1.6)	9.2 (1.9)	12.0 (2.8)	9.4 (2.3)	0.60 (1.1)	13.3 (2.4)

Table 16.53. RAVLT.21; Comparion of AVLT and CVLT Scores

	AVLT		CVLT	
	M	SD	M	SD
Trial I	7.0	1.6	7.5	1.6
Trail II	9.7	2.0	10.5	1.9
Trial III	11.1	2.0	11.7	2.1
Trial IV	11.7	2.1	12.5	2.0
Trial V	12.2	1.8	13.0	1.8
Total Words	51.7	7.5	55.1	7.7
List B	7.0	2.0	7.9	1.9
Postinterference Recall	10.6	3.1	11.7	2.3
Recognition	13.4	1.2	14.7	1.4

injury or neurological abnormality. The mean age was 31.3 (SD = 12.7), education varied from 6 to 20 years with a mean of 12.2 years (SD = 2.4), and estimated IQ (based on NART) ranged from 100 to 128 with a mean of 115.6 (SD = 6.26).

Table 16.54. RAVLT.22a; Recall and Recognition Scores on the Rey AVLT for Each Form (1 and 4)

	Form 1	Form 4
Trial 1	6.82	6.82
	(1.47)	(1.58)
Trial 2	9.35	8.90
	(1.98)	(1.98)
Trial 3	10.92	10.76
	(1.97)	(1.99)
Trial 4	11.55	11.53
	(2.12)	(2.05)
Trial 5	12.47	12.00
	(1.91)	(1.99)
Total (1 to 5)	51.12	50.02
	(7.42)	(7.68)
List B	6.02	5.68
	(1.73)	(1.68)
Postinterference	10.88	10.65
	(2.91)	(2.71)
Delayed recall	10.82	10.33
	(2.99)	(2.83)
Recognition A total	13.71	13.65
	(1.60)	(1.48)
Recognition A p[A]	0.90	0.90
	(0.08)	(0.07)
Recognition B total	6.94	7.59
	(2.92)	(2.77)
Recognition B p[A]	0.71	0.73
	(0.10)	(0.09)

A new form of AVLT (form 4) was generated by the authors based on criteria developed by them. All subjects were tested on both form 1 and form 4 in a counterbalanced order with an interval of 6 to 14 days between the sessions.

The standard administration procedure was used with the exception of using a 20-minute delay interval filled with verbal cognitive and verbal memory tests. A list of 50 words was used for delayed recognition trial. Subjects were asked to identify words from lists A and B and to specify their list of origin.

The authors reported recall on five acquisition trials, the total number of words recalled over five trials, the interference trial, postinterference recall, delayed recall trial, number of words recognized from lists A and B, and a nonparametric measure of recognition performance, $p[A] = .5(1 + HR\text{-}FP)$, which corrects the recognition score (hit rate, HR) by taking into account false positives (FP).

Study strengths

1. Demographic characteristics of the sample were described in terms of geographic area, gender, age, education, and IQ.

2. Administration and scoring system were described.

3. Sample size was adequate.

4. A comparison of two alternate forms is provided.

5. Means and standard deviations are reported.

Considerations regarding use of the study

1. The 20-minute delay interval was filled with verbal cognitive and verbal memory tests

Table 16.55. RAVLT.22b; Frequency (Approximate Occurrence per Million) and Length (Number of Letters) of Words, Comparing Rey AVLT Form 1 With Form 4, List A

	Form 1			Form 4	
List A	Frequency	Length	List A	Frequency	Length
Drum	11	4	Pipe	20	4
Curtain	13	7	Wall	160	4
Bell	18	4	Alarm	16	5
Coffee	78	6	Sugar	34	5
School	492	6	Student	131	7
Parent	15	6	Mother	216	6
Moon	60	4	Star	25	4
Garden	60	6	Painting	59	8
Hat	56	3	Bag	42	3
Farmer	23	6	Wheat	9	5
Nose	60	4	Mouth	103	5
Turkey	9	6	Chicken	37	7
Colour	141	6 (5)	Sound	204	5
House	591	5	Door	312	4
River	165	5	Stream	51	6
Mean	119.47	5.2		94.6	5.2
Range	9–591	3–7		9–312	3–8

Table 16.56. RAVLT.22c; Frequency (Approximate Occurrence per Million) and Length (Number of Letters) of Words, Comparing Rey AVLT Form 1 With Form 4, List B

	Form 1			Form 4	
List B	Frequency	Length	List B	Frequency	Length
Desk	65	4	Bench	35	5
Ranger	2	6	Officer	101	7
Bird	31	4	Cage	9	4
Shoe	14	4	Sock	4	4
Stove	15	5	Fridge°	23	6
Mountain	33	8	Cliff	11	5
Glasses	29	6	Bottle	76	6
Towel	6	5	Soap	22	4
Cloud	28	5	Sky	58	3
Boat	72	4	Ship	83	4
Lamb	7	4	Goat	6	4
Gun	118	3	Bullet	28	6
Pencil	34	6	Paper	157	5
Church	348	6	Chapel	20	6
Fish	35	4	Crab°	2	4
Mean	56.47	4.93		42.33	4.87
Range	2–348	3–8		2–157	3–7

°The actual words were not present in the tables of word frequency.

Table 16.57. RAVLT.22d; Word List for Testing Rey AVLT Recognition (Form 4)[*]

Alarm (A)	Eye (SA)	Soap (B)	Ship (B)	Bottle (B)
Aunt (SA)	Crab (B)	Wall (A)	Car (PA)	Seat (SB)
Bag (A)	Star (A)	Clock (SA)	Mother (A)	Sock (B)
Creek (SA)	Rag (PA)	Sound (A)	Duck (SA)	Tone (SA)
Officer (B)	Bun (PA)	Bench (B)	Wheat (A)	Fridge (B)
Mouth (A)	Cage (B)	Bullet (B)	Floor (SPA)	Rock (SPB)
Arrow (SB)	Cliff (B)	Night (SA)	Sky (B)	Bread (SA)
Student (A)	Sugar (A)	Chapel (B)	Door (A)	Pipe (A)
Hail (PA)	Cream (PA)	Chicken (A)	Bridge (PB)	Ball (PA)
Paper (B)	Stream (A)	Coat (PB)	Painting (A)	Goat (B)

[*]A = words from list A, B = words from list B, P = phonemic associate of words on lists A and B, S = semantic associate of words on lists A and B.

which might cause interference with delayed AVLT testing.

2. The sample had high estimated IQ values, which might limit generalizability of the data.

3. Data were collected in Australia, which may limit its usefulness for clinical interpretive purposes in the United States.

4. Minimal exclusion criteria.

5. Undifferentiated age range.

Other comments

1. The authors concluded that the forms were equivalent. In test–retest conditions, the most reliable were the total number of words learned over the five acquisition trials ($r = 0.77$) and performance on the postinterference trial ($r = 0.70$) (Tables 16.54–16.57).

CONCLUSIONS

A review[*] of the literature on the Rey AVLT suggests high clinical utility of this test due to its sensitivity to disruption in different memory mechanisms reflected in various indices derived from the test performance. Hence the importance of reporting a full range of RAVLT measures in clinical practice and in research,

including delayed recall and recognition (if administered) to assure an optimal use of this test in identifying faulty memory mechanisms. Moreover, thorough description of administration procedure—especially deviations from standard procedure—is of utmost importance for accurate interpretation of test scores.

Due to the considerable effect of age on RAVLT scores, individual sets of data should be referenced to an appropriate age group. Similarly, education, intelligence level, and gender are possible contributing factors in the RAVLT score variance. Therefore, these demographic characteristics should also be of concern for a clinician and investigator alike.

For future research on RAVLT, classification of data into age groups, education/IQ levels, and gender categories would be desirable. Development of new, and validation of existing, alternate forms would aid clinicians and researchers in minimizing carry-over effects in retesting situations. In addition, further studies on different memory mechanisms utilizing concepts adapted from cognitive science would be of great value in understanding underlying cognitive constructs associated with observed RAVLT performance.

[*]Uchiyama et al. reported RAVLT data on a large sample of homosexual/bisexual HIV-seronegative males, originally published in 1995. We did not include this dataset in this book because the authors indicated that a revised dataset is available from them directly. Address further inquiries to Eric Miller, Ph.D.; UCLA/NPI; 760 Westwood Plaza, C8-747; Los Angeles, CA 90024.

VI

MOTOR FUNCTIONS

17

Finger Tapping Test

BRIEF HISTORY OF THE TEST

The Finger Tapping Test (FTT) is one of the original tests introduced by Halstead and is commonly used as a simple measure of motor speed and motor control. Originally, the test was called the Finger Oscillation Test and the number of taps was recorded for the dominant hand only (Russell et al., 1970). Reitan modified the administration of this test to include the performance of both hands. Tapping speed with the dominant hand was one of the 10 measures used in computing the Impairment Index (Halstead, 1947; Reitan, 1955b). In order to take into account impaired performance with the hand contralateral to the brain damage, Rennick modified procedures for computing the Average Impairment Rating to include tapping speed with the most impaired hand, rather than with the dominant hand (Russell et al., 1970).

The interpretation of norms available in the literature is complicated by heterogeneity of the tapping devices and administration techniques. The most frequently used device is a tapping lever mounted with a key-driven counter. The counter rotates when the tapping key is depressed 0.50″. The counter and key are mounted on a board, with the tapping lever located approximately 1.75″ above the surface of the board, and at a 30° angle from the counter. It has been reported that 400 g of pressure is required to depress the lever (Knights and Moule, 1967). This tapper is available from PAR, Inc., and from the Reitan Neuropsychology Laboratory. (See Appendix 1 for ordering information.)

A second finger tapping apparatus, the Digital Tapping Test, is available from Western Psychological Services (WPS, see Appendix 1 for ordering information). This device consists of an electronic self-contained timer with digital readout which automatically begins timing with the first depression of the tapping key and allows for no further recording of taps after exactly 10 seconds have elapsed. This digital finger tapping device requires a static weight of 80 g of pressure to depress the lever and 0.13″ of travel in the key to change the counter. The majority of the studies summarized in this chapter used the standard manual key-driven tapping device that is part of the Halstead-Reitan battery.

The most common administration and scoring technique used in the reviewed studies is based on the instructions for the Halstead-Reitan Battery (Rennick method), in which the Finger Tapping score for each hand is the mean of five consecutive 10-second trials within a range of five taps. A maximum of 10 trials with each hand is allowed, and if the above criterion is not met, the score is the mean of the best five trials (see Lezak, 1995, pp. 680–682; Spreen & Strauss, 1998, for further information). First, all five trials with the preferred hand are completed, which is followed by the nonpreferred hand trials. The majority of authors also refer to the standard description of the procedures specified by Reitan and Wolfson (1985).

It should be noted that some studies used less than five trials per hand, or alternated hands after each trial. There was variability in terms of data recordings as well. Some studies reported performance for the dominant hand only, worse hand only, total for both hands, average of both hands, etc.

The most recent modification of the FTT administration procedure was introduced by Russell and Starkey (1993) as a result of the inclusion of the Finger Tapping Test in their Halstead-Russell Neuropsychological Evaluation System (HRNES). According to their instructions, the subject is to tap, using just the index finger, as fast as possible. Subject is to keep the "heel" of his/her hand on the board and avoid using the whole hand, wrist, or arm. After a brief practice, the subject is instructed to perform six 10-second trials with each hand, in sets of three trials, alternating hands between sets, starting with the dominant hand. A score at least four taps faster or slower than the next highest or lowest score is considered to be an "outlier." This score is eliminated from the calculation of the total score and is replaced with an alternate trial to make a total of six valid trials. This substitution is allowed for two trials only. Fifteen second rest periods are allowed between trials. The total scores represent the average speed for valid trials with each hand and with both hands. The score used in computing an overall index for the entire battery is based on the average performance with the dominant and nondominant hands instead of the worse hand performance used in the earlier versions.

Some studies provide data to allow conversion of raw scores into other units which facilitate comparison between different tests. For example, a normative system for the expanded HRB developed by Heaton et al. (1991) allows conversion of raw scores into scaled score equivalents which can be further converted into T scores, based on the data for a sample of neurologically normal subjects stratified by age, education, and gender.

Golden et al. (1981b) have reported that the Finger Tapping Test is a measure of fine motor control, which is based on motor speed, as well as kinesthetic and visual-motor abilities. It has been suggested that the Finger Tapping Test is one of the most sensitive tests in the Halstead-Reitan Battery for determining brain impairment (Russell et al., 1970). In a factor-analytic study, Lansdell and Donnelly (1977) have reported that tapping performance may be impaired with most, but not necessarily all, types of cerebral damage. Other authors have also noted that brain impairment generally, but not always, results in a compromise in finger tapping speed (Dodrill, 1978a; Haaland et al., 1977; Lezak, 1995).

Golden and his colleagues (Golden, 1978; Golden et al. 1981b) suggested that at the cortical level impaired performance may reflect dysfunction of the premotor and motor strip regions of the frontal lobes or abnormalities of sensory feedback secondary to parietal lobe dysfunction. These authors reported that, in general, the greater the deficit on the finger tapping score, the nearer the lesion is to the area of the precentral gyrus. In addition, they indicated that subcortical disruption of sensory or motor tracts, as well as peripheral damage to the extremities, may result in compromised performance on this measure.

In spite of well-documented sensitivity of the FTT to brain dysfunction, psychometric issues related to the optimal balance of sensitivity and specificity of the test have been widely disputed in the literature. Wheeler and Reitan (1963) have reported 79% hit rates in brain-damaged populations when utilizing a level-of-performance criterion. However, while hit rates across different studies appear to be quite good, the rates of false-positive misclassifications based on the cutoffs proposed by Halstead are unacceptably high (especially for older age groups) (Bornstein, 1986a, 1987b; Heaton et al., 1986; Trahan et al., 1987). In McKeever and Abramson's (1991) study on college students, only 10% and 14% of left-handed vs. right-handed females and 39% and 57% of left-handed vs. right-handed males scored within the nonimpaired range, using original Halstead cutoff criteria. The authors emphasized the need for revising the norms due to the high rate of false-positive "diagnoses," especially for females and left-handers.

In addition to its utility in determining the presence of brain dysfunction, the Finger Tapping Test also provides an index of lateralized dysfunction due to the contralateral effect of cerebral lesions, since independent measures of dominant and nondominant hand performance are customarily obtained.

Bornstein (1986c) has attempted to systematically study the magnitude and variability of these intermanual differences. His results suggest that in a normal sample, for appproximately 30% of the males and 20% of the females, the *nonpreferred hand* was found to be superior to the preferred hand. A study by Trahan et al. (1987) found nonpreferred hand performance to be faster than preferred-hand performance in 14.7% of the subject sample. Similar findings are reported in clinical studies. According to Massman and Doody's (1996) report, 26% of their patients with probable Alzheimer's disease displayed an exaggerated right-hand advantage (associated with higher educational level), whereas 37% demonstrated a reversal of expected asymmetry. The authors emphasized that asymmetry in motor speed correlated significantly with cognitive asymmetries.

In a follow-up on his previous study, Bornstein (1986d) noted that this variability in preferred hand performance frequently results in interpretive difficulties when the commonly used guidline of a 10% preferred-hand superiority is employed. Of note, Fromm-Auch and Yeudall (1983) reported only a 5% difference in favor of preferred hand in males.

Bornstein (1986d) suggests that in the evaluation of lateralized hemisphere lesions, FTT findings have to be supported by nonmotor tasks and by additional instruments measuring motor performance. In this study he evaluated the pattern of motor performance on three motor tests (Finger Tapping Test, Grooved Pegboard Test, and the Hand Dynamometer) which were administered to normal and unilateral brain lesion samples. Interestingly, a large degree of variability was observed across these intermanual measures, whereby "a high percentage (approximately 25 percent) of the normal sample obtained scores more than one standard deviation from the control mean on a single measure" (p. 719). Thus, Bornstein emphasized the importance of consistency in the performance pattern across tasks, rather than use of a "rigid application of 'cookbook' formulas or 'rules of thumb'" (p. 723) in FTT interpretation.

Data on reliability of the FTT vary widely with reliability coefficients ranging from 0.04 to almost perfect values. A majority of the studies, however, report high reliability ratings for different interprobe intervals (Bornstein et al., 1987a; Ruff & Parker, 1993).

RELATIONSHIP BETWEEN FTT PERFORMANCE AND DEMOGRAPHIC FACTORS

Many studies have questioned the feasibility of restricting test interpretation for both males and females to an identical level-of-performance cutoff. Dodrill (1979) has reported considerable sex differences in samples of neurological patients and neurologically intact individuals. Other authors have also reported notable sex differences across demographically diverse samples with males consistently outperforming females by three to five taps (Bornstein, 1985; Echternacht, 1981; Filskov & Catanese, 1986; Fromm-Auch & Yeudall, 1983; Harris et al., 1981; Heaton et al., 1991; Hoffman, 1969; King et al., 1978; McKeever & Abramson, 1991; Morrison et al., 1979; Ruff & Parker, 1993; Trautt et al., 1983).

Empirical investigations also report the effect of other demographic and situational variables on finger tapping speed, such as age (Bornstein, 1986a; Fromm-Auch & Yeudall, 1983; Heaton et al., 1986; Ruff & Parker, 1993; Trahan et al., 1987), education (Bernard, 1989; Bornstein, 1985; Finlayson et al., 1977; Fromm-Auch & Yeudall, 1983; Heaton et al., 1986; Vega & Parsons, 1967), order of test administration (Harris et al., 1981; Neuger et al., 1981), anxiety (King et al., 1978), and personality characteristics (Heaton, 1985).

METHOD FOR EVALUATING THE NORMATIVE REPORTS

Our review of the FTT literature located normative reports and clinical studies reporting control data. In order to adequately evaluate the FTT data, seven key criterion variables were deemed to be critical. The first five relate to *subject* variables, and the remaining two dimensions refer to *procedural* variables.

Subject Variables

Sample Size

Fifty cases have been considered adequate sample size. Although this criterion is somewhat arbitrary, a large number of studies suggest that data based on small sample sizes are highly influenced by individual differences and do not provide a reliable estimate of the population mean.

Sample Composition Description

This criterion addresses adequate information regarding the subject selection criteria, including education or IQ.

Age-Group Intervals

This criterion refers to grouping of the data into limited age intervals.

Reporting of Gender Distribution

Given a reported association between gender and FTT performance, it is preferable that data be stratified by gender.

Description of Hand Preference Assessment

In order to address the issue of lateralization in test performance, assessment procedures for hand preference should be fully described.

Procedural Variables

Description of Administration Procedures

Administration of FTT differs widely among studies. Detailed description of administration procedures allows selection of the most appropriate norms or at least corrections to account for deviation in administration procedure.

Data Reporting

In order to facilitate interpretation of the data, group mean and standard deviation should be presented at minimum.

SUMMARY OF THE STATUS OF THE NORMS

As discussed above, there is a great deal of variability in sample composition, administration, scoring, and interpretation of the FTT. Some of these factors are outlined below.

In addition to normative studies based on "normal" samples, there are a number of clinical comparison studies exploring differences in FTT performance between clinical groups and "normal control" groups (which are sometimes matched on demographic characteristics). Unfortunately, normal control groups are frequently comprised of medical or psychiatric patients. These samples cannot be considered truly "normal" due to possible effects of their illnesses and medication intake on FTT performance. The clinical groups reported in FTT studies represent a wide range of neurological and psychiatric diagnoses (most often brain-injured patients).

The majority of studies present data as the number of taps averaged over five trials for each hand. Some studies, however, present average scores for both hands; total score across both hands; total score across both hands over all trials, cumulatively; raw data converted to *T* scores; or scores for the dominant hand only. Such deviations from the standard method of data reporting are identified in our review of the normative data in the context of each pertinent table. In addition to providing normative data for each hand, several studies report the proportion of subjects falling in the impaired range, or rates of intermanual differences.

Several authors stratify their samples by age, education, and/or gender. Procedures for assessment of handedness are thoroughly described in some studies. Furthermore, some authors divide their samples into groups based on the subjects' handedness pattern.

The majority of investigators recruited mostly young and middle-aged subjects. Only a few studies present data for elderly individuals. Several publications provide test–retest data over varying interprobe intervals. Some studies provide data for left-handed samples. Several studies report data collected abroad including Canada, Australia, Italy, Holland, and Colombia.

Among all the studies available in the literature, we selected for review those investigations based on large, well-defined samples, or studies that offer interesting clinical comparisons or information which is not routinely reported.

Table 17.1 summarizes information provided in the studies described in this chapter.

SUMMARIES OF THE STUDIES

Original Studies

Halstead's (1947) original "control" group included only 28 subjects (eight of whom were females), although 30 sets of scores were presented. Apparently, the reason for this inconsistency was that two subjects took the tests twice (pre- and postlobotomy) and the results of both test administrations were included in the data pool.

Concerning the normative performance of Halstead's control group, Lezak (1995, p. 680) has reported that the mean number of finger taps (per 10-second trial) for these subjects was 50 taps for their right hand and 45 taps for their left. Normative cut scores were obtained by comparing the performance of the control subjects with neurologically impaired individuals. On the basis of this comparison, Halstead (1947) recommended that a cutoff score of 50 (tapping scores of 50 and below are in the brain-damaged range) be utilized as a criterion measure for the dominant hand in differentiating between normal and impaired subjects. The corresponding cutoff for the nondominant hand was set at ≤44.

Methodological concerns are apparent when utilizing these data as a normative reference. For example, the age group interval being assessed was too broad (age range 14–50 years), with an unequal sampling across age ranges. The sample consisted of mostly young people with an average age of 28.3 years. In addition, gender was not adequately represented. Moreover, the sample consisted of inmates and individuals being treated for psychiatric disturbances, thereby confounding normative interpretations. For example, Halstead (1947) noted that "Several gave abnormal scores on the personality tests, thus supporting the psychiatric

diagnoses. Their symptoms at the time of testing ranged from mild to severe headaches; from loss of appetite, easy fatiguability, acute or chronic gastrointestinal disturbance to insomnia and minor disturbances in memory functions" (p. 37).

Reitan (1955b) reported the results of a study designed to assess the validity of Halstead's (1947) Impairment Index. The sample included 50 non-brain-damaged controls (35 males, 15 females) who were matched in pairs with 50 brain-damaged subjects on the basis of race and sex and as closely as possible for chronological age and years of formal education. The mean age of the control subjects was 32.36 (SD = 10.78), and mean education was 11.58 (SD = 2.85). Subjects received neurological examinations before testing and reportedly showed "no signs or symptoms of cerebral damage or dysfunction" (p. 29). The majority of subjects comprising the control group did, however, have various diagnoses such as depression ($N = 17$), paraplegia ($N = 13$), acute anxiety state ($N = 6$), and obsessive-compulsive neurosis ($N = 2$). The author noted that these patients were included to "minimize the possibility that differences in the test results for the brain-damaged and control groups could be attributed to hospitalization, chronic illness, and possible affective disturbances" (p. 29).

Administration procedures followed the Halstead (1947) format. Testing and scoring were completed before the groups were composed or the subjects were matched.

According to the results of this study (for the males only), the mean number of finger taps for the preferred hand was 50.74 (SD = 7.29) for the control group, while for the brain-damaged group it was 45.58 (SD = 7.32). The difference between the means was found to be statistically significant. The data for the nonpreferred hand were not provided. Reitan stated that although further validity studies were needed, the results of this investigation suggested that "the Halstead battery is sufficiently sensitive to the effects of organic brain damage to provide an objective and quantitative basis for detailed study of relationships between brain function and behavior" (p. 35).

These data laid the foundation for extensive research concerning the psychometric proper-

Table 17.1. FT.L; Locator Table for the FT Test.

Study°	Age°°	N	Sample Composition	IQ,°° Education	Country/ Location
FT.1 Fromm-Auch & Yeudall, 1983 page 382	15–17 18–23 24–32 33–40 41–64	111 M 82 F	Normal volunteers	Education 14.8 FSIQ 119.1	Alberta, Canada
FT.2 Bornstein, 1985 page 383	20–39 40–59 60–69	365	178 M 187 F 91.5% R-handed paid volunteers free of neurological or psychiatric illness	Education 12.3 (2.7) Separate data for <HS, ≥HS	Western Canada
FT.3 Villardita et al., 1985 page 383	<25 45–54 55–64 65–74	10 10 10 10	Healthy volunteers	Education 8-13	Catania, Italy
FT.4 Bornstein, 1986a page 383	18–39 40–59 60–69	365	178 M 187 F 91.5% R-handed paid volunteers free of neurological or psychiatric illness	Education 12.3 (2.7) Separate data for <HS, ≥HS	Western Canada
FT.5 Polubinski & Melamed, 1986 page 384	18–24	60 M 60 F	Introductory psychology students. Handedness broken down into firm and mixed groups	College students	Ohio
FT.6 Trahan et al., 1987 page 385	18–32 33–47 48–62 63–91	713	Neurologically intact adults; Sample is stratified by age and gender	—	—
FT.7 Yeudall et al., 1987 page 386	15–20 21–25 26–30 31–40	62 73 48 42	Normal adults; 127 M, 98 F. Sample is strati- fied by age and gender	FSIQ 111.75 109.79 113.95 116.09	Alberta, Canada
FT.8 Bornstein & Suga, 1988 page 387	55–70 62.7 (4.3) 62.3 62.9 63.0	134 46 44 44	49 M, 85 F. Paid volun- teers screened for a history of neurological or psychiatric disorders Divided into three education groups 17 M, 29 F 16 M, 28 F 16 M, 28 F	Education 11.7 (2.9) Ranges: 5–10, 8.5 11–12, 11.7 >12, 15.0	Western Canada
FT.9 Ardila & Rosselli, 1989 page 387	55–60 61–65 66–70 71–75 >75	346	Normal older adults with MMSE scores ≥23	Groups: 0–5 6–12 >12	Bogota, Colombia
FT.10 Heaton et al., 1991 page 387	42.1 (16.8) groups:	486	Volunteers: urban and rural Data collected over 15 years through multi- center collaborative	Education 13.6(3.5) FSIQ 113.8(12.3)	California, Washington, Texas, Oklahoma, *continued*

Table 17.1. (*Continued*)

Study[*]	Age[°°]	N	Sample Composition	IQ,[°°] Education	Country/ Location
	20–34 35–39 40–44 45–49 50–54 55–59 60–64 65–69 70–74 75–80		efforts. Strict exclusion criteria. 65% M Data are presented in *T*-score equivalents for M and F separately in 10 age groupings by six educational groupings	groups: 6–8 9–11 12 13–15 16–17 18+	Wisconsin, Illinois, Michigan, New York, Virginia, Massachusetts, Canada
FT.11 Ruff & Parker, 1993 page 389	16–24 25–39 40–54 55–70	358	Normal volunteers 179 M, 179 F. Data are stratified by gender and age; Separate data presented for L-handers	Education range: 7–22 years	California, Michigan, eastern seaboard
FT.12 Vega & Parsons, 1967 page 390	41.7 (14.8) 40.8 (13.1)	50 50	Brain damaged 44 M, 6 F Control 37 M, 13 F	FSIQ 84.9 (14.8) 99.4 (12.9)	Oklahoma
FT.13 Goldstein & Shelly, 1972 page 391	— 276 156		The study compared brain damaged and non-brain damaged patients who were mostly males. The former sample was further subdivided into right hemisphere, left hemisphere, and diffuse lesion subgroups	—	Topeka, Kansas
FT.14 Goldstein & Braun, 1974 page 391	20–29 30–39 40–49 50–59 60–69 70–79	29 75 47 30 16 12	The sample of neurologically intact Ss was divided into 6 age groups	—	—
FT.15 Finlayson et al., 1977 page 392	All Ss under age 50	51 51	Brain damaged; controls;– healthy Ss, medical & psychiatric patients. All Ss were males	Samples were broken down by education into grade school, HS, university	—
FT.16 Wiens & Matarazzo, 1977 page 393	23.6 24.8	24 24	Normal young men divided into 2 groups	FSIQ 117.5 118.3	Oregon
FT.17 Dodrill, 1978a page 394	27.3 (8.4) 27.3 (9.0)	50 50	The study compares neuropsychological performance of control and epileptic Ss	Education 12.0 12.0	Washington
FT.18 Dodrill, 1978b page 394	Mean age for each group = 41.1	25 25 25 25	Performance was compared for four groups: control R-hemisphere damage L-hemisphere damage Bilateral damage	Mean education for each group = 10.7	Washington

continued

Table 17.1. (*Continued*)

Study°	Age°°	N	Sample Composition	IQ,°° Education	Country/ Location
FT.19 Morrison et al., 1979 page 395	Mode = 19	30 M 30 F	Introductory psychology students	—	Idaho
FT.20 Anthony et al., 1980 page 396	42.7 (15.4) 38.9 (15.8)	150 100	The study compares brain-damaged and normal control Ss	FSIQ 94.8 (16.9) 113.5 (10.8)	Colorado
FT.21 Bak & Greene, 1980 page 396	50-62 67-86	15 15	Healthy active older adults	Education 13.7 (1.91) 14.9 (2.99)	Texas
FT.22 Eckardt & Matarazzo, 1981 page 397	42.2 (10.0) 45.6 (11.1)	91 20	Drug-free alcoholic inpatients were compared to nonalcoholic. All Ss were male V.A. patients. Retest data are provided		California
FT.23 Pirozzolo et al., 1982 page 397	62.7 (8.2)	60 60	The article compares patients w/ Parkinson's disease and matched controls	Education 11.4 (2.8)	—
FT.24 Rounsaville et al., 1982 page 398	27.9 29.2 24.9	72 60 29 59	Opiate addicts Epileptic patients Normal controls Opiate addicts were retested in 6 months	Education 11.5 11.8 11.2	—
FT.25 Yeudall et al., 1982 page 399	14.8 14.5	99 47	Delinquent adolescents Nondelinquent adolescents	FSIQ 95.3 117.1	Alberta, Canada
FT.26 O'Donnell et al., 1983 page 399	20.0 (1.9) 19.2 (2.0) 25.0 (3.5)	30 60 20	The article compares three groups: Normal group Learning disabled Brain damaged patients	FSIQ 117.1 (10.3) 106.4 (9.5) 93.0 (10.5)	—
FT.27 Prigatano et al., 1983 page 400	61.5 (9.9) 59.6 (9.0)	100 25	Hypoxemic patients with COPD. Matched controls	FSIQ 105.3 (12.8) 112.0 (11.0)	Oklahoma City and Winnipeg
FT.28 Heaton et al., 1985 page 400	37.38 (8.28) 32.87 (13.5)	100 100	25 M, 75 F. Multiple sclerosis patients, among them 57 relapsing-remitting course, 43 chronic-progressive form. Mean disease duration = 9.36 years (5.86) 79 M, 21 F. Control Ss with no neurological illness, head trauma or substance abuse	Education 13.71 (2.33) 14.15 (2.84)	Denver
FT.29 Kane et al., 1985 page 401	39.7 (13.5) 38.9 (11.3)	46 44	The study compares brain damaged and control Ss. The latter group consists of medical and non-schizophrenic pyschiatric patients	Education 11.6 (2.0) 12.3 (2.6)	Oklahoma City and Pittsburgh
FT.30 Heaton et al., 1986 page 401	15–81 39.3 (17.5)	207 (UC) 181 (UC	356 M, 197 F. Normal Ss with no history of neurological illness, head trauma, or substance	Education 0–20 13.3 (3.4)	University of Colorado, University of California at *continued*

Table 17.1. (*Continued*)

Study[a]	Age[b]	N	Sample Composition	IQ,[b] Education	Country/ Location
	SD) 165 UW		abuse, 7.2% L-handed		San Diego, University of Wisconsin
FT.31 Alekoumbides et al., 1987 page 402	46.9 (17.2)	123	Mostly inpatients of a large genera hospital without any evidence of brain injury	Mean education 11.4 (3.2)	—
FT.32 Bornstein et al., 1987b page 403	55–70 62.7 (4.3) 60.3 (3.8)	134 94	Control Ss with no history of neurological or psychiatric disease 49 M, 85 F. Patients with neurological confirmation of damage to one or both of the cerebral hemispheres. 47 M, 47 F	Education 11.7 (2.9) 10.6 (4.1)	—
FT.33 Bornstein et al.. 1987a page 403	17-52 32.3 (10.3)	23	9 M, 14 F. Volunteers from a university community. Retest data are provided	VIQ = 105.8 (10.8) PIQ = 105.0 (10.5)	—
FT.34 Russell, 1987 page 404	— 46.19 (12.86)	577 155	Brain damaged patients are compared to controls with negative neurological findings	FSIQ 93.4 111.9	Miami & Cincinnati
FT.35 Thompson et al., 1987 page 405	40.59 (18.27)	426	279 M, 147 F. Normal Ss	Education 13.15 (3.49)	—
FT.36 van den Burg et al., 1987 page 406	37.7 37.4	40 40	MS patients Matched controls	Education according to Dutch educational system 5.0 5.0	Northern Holland
FT.37 Russell & Starkey, 1993 page 406	45.1 (13.0) 46.2 (15.5) 50.5 (14.4) 47.8 (13.8)	176 110 117 319	Data are collected from standardization sample for the HRNES manual. Ss are male VA patients divided into 4 groups: comparison; left-hemisphere damage right-hemisphere damage diffuse brain damage	12.5 (2.8) 11.8 (3.2) 11.8 (3.1) 11.8 (3.3)	Cincinnati & Miami

[a]The study number corresponds to the number provided in the text of the chapter.

[b]Age column and IQ/education column contain information regarding range, and/or mean and standard deviation for the whole sample and/or separate groups, whichever information is provided by the authors.

ties and clinical utility of the FTT. In spite of their historical value, use of these data as normative standard for clinical comparison is not recommended due to the idosyncratic demographic composition of Halstead's and Reitan's samples.

Cutoffs for the FTT based on four performance levels from "Perfectly Normal" to "Severely Impaired" were published by Reitan in the context of his update on the HRB (Reitan, 1985).

The Finger Tapping Test has enjoyed wide popularity among researchers and clinicians. Since its introduction by Halstead and Reitan, over a 100 studies have been published addressing performance on the FTT in normal and clinical samples (usually along with other HRB tests or as part of a battery comprising various neuropsychological tests). The most relevant of those studies are reviewed below.

Normative Studies

[FT.1] Fromm-Auch and Yeudall, 1983

The authors obtained FTT data on 193 Canadian subjects (111 male, 82 female) recruited through posted advertisements and personal contacts. Participants are described as "nonpsychiatric" and "non-neurological". Handedness was determined by the writing hand: 83.4% of the sample were right-handed. Strength of handedness was determined by the Annett Handedness Questionnaire (1970). Means and standard deviations for each hand are reported for the entire sample and for five age groups stratified by age.

Study strengths
  1. Sample composition is well described in terms of IQ, education, gender, geograhpic area, and recruitment procedures.
  2. Some psychiatric and neurological exclusion criteria were used.
  3. The large overall sample size.
  4. Subjects' handedness was established.

  5. Normative data were presented for the entire sample and separately for different age and gender groups.
  6. Means, standard deviations, and ranges are reported.

Considerations regarding use of the study
  1. Sample size for the age group 41–64 is very small, and most cells are well below an N of 50.
  2. The high intellectual and educational level of the sample.
  3. The underrepresentation of older age groups.

Other comments
  1. The article provides a summary of previously published normative data.
  2. Calculation of the educational level included technical or vocational training.
  3. The authors concluded that pronounced effect of gender was seen on all motor tests with females appearing weaker and slower than males. The relationship between age and performance appears to be curvilinear for both genders with the peak of performance in the 33–40-year-old age range.

Table 17.2. FT.1

N	Age	Education	WAIS FSIQ	No. Males	No. Females	Preferred Hand	Nonpreferred Hand
Norms for the Entire Sample							
193	25.4	14.8	119.1	111	82	46.3	43.2
	(8.2)	(3.0)	(8.8)			(6.3)	(5.4)

	Norms for the Sample Stratified by Age and Sex						

		Preferred Hand			Nonpreferred Hand		
Age	N	M	SD	Range	M	SD	Range
Males							
15–17	17	47.6	5.8	38.0–55.6	43.6	4.9	33.4–51.8
18–23	44	49.5	6.9	26.6–64.6	45.4	6.9	26.8–58.6
24–32	31	50.6	6.6	38.2–66.2	46.0	6.1	28.8–55.0
33–40	12	53.4	5.9	39.0–61.0	49.8	4.7	41.0–57.8
41–64	4	44.4	5.8	35.8–48.2	41.4	3.5	36.6–44.4
Age	N	M	SD	Range	M	SD	Range
Females							
15–17	15	42.7	7.9	30.2–54.0	41.1	6.2	31.6–5.10
18–23	30	43.6	7.5	30.6–65.6	41.2	6.5	32.8–61.8
24–32	25	45.2	6.7	31.0–60.0	40.9	5.7	28.6–53.6
33–40	6	45.8	5.5	40.6–55.6	44.3	4.6	40.6–53.2
41–64	6	40.4	4.8	34.2–48.4	38.6	4.8	32.0–46.6

4. The data were collected in Alberta, Canada (Table 17.2).

[FT.2] Bornstein, 1985

The author collected data on 365 Canadian individuals (178 males and 187 females) recruited through posted notices on college campuses and unemployment offices, newspaper ads, and senior citizen groups. Subjects were paid for their participation. Participants ranged in age from 18 to 69 (Mean = 43.3 ± 17.1), and had completed between 5 and 20 years of education (Mean = 12.3 ± 2.7); 91.5% of the sample were right-handed. No other demographic data or exclusion criteria are reported.

Means and standard deviations are reported for each hand. Scores are based on the mean of five trials within five taps of each other to a maximum of 10 trials. When not accomplished, the score is the mean of the best five trials. The sample was stratified by age group (20–39, 40–59, 60–69), level of education (<HS, ≥HS), and gender. Normative data were presented for the preferred and nonpreferred hands for each demographic group separately, as well as for different combinations of demographic strata. Individual group sample sizes ranged form 13 to 86. Hand preference was determined as the hand used for signing the consent form. Subjects were recruited from the general population of a large city in Western Canada.

Study strengths
   1. Very large overall sample size and several individual cells approximate *N*s of 50.
   2. Stratification of the data by age, sex, and educational level.
   3. This dataset is unique in that it reports data for subjects with less than a high school education.
   4. Information on recruitment procedures and geographic area is provided.
   5. Method for determining handedness is specified.
   6. Means and standard deviations are reported.
   7. Test administration procedures are specified.

Considerations regarding use of the study
   1. Individual sample sizes of some cells were

small. It is unclear whether the youngest age included in the study was 18 or 20.
   2. The lack of any reported exclusion criteria (Table 17.3).

[FT.3] Villardita, Cultrera, Cupone and Mejia, 1985

All subjects were healthy volunteers residing in Catania, Italy, with 8 to 13 years of schooling, and scored above 23 on the MMSE. The score is the total number of taps recorded for each hand on two trials. The data are presented in age groupings.

Study strengths
   1. The administration procedure was described.
   2. Means and standard deviations are reported.
   3. Data are presented by age groupings.

Considerations regarding use of the study
   1. Demographic characteristics of the sample such as gender distribution and mean educational level are not presented.
   2. The sample is divided into age groupings. However, the data for 25 to 45 years of age are not presented, and data are not stratified by gender.
   3. Sample sizes are small.
   4. Administration procedures and data reporting deviate from the standard instructions.
   5. Method for determining handedness is not reported.
   6. Exclusion criteria are not adequate (Table 17.4).

[FT.4] Bornstein, 1986a

This paper expands the analysis of the data provided in the Bornstein, (1985), article. The author examined cutoff levels for impairment and the proporion of subjects falling in the impaired range. For the preferred and nonpreferred hands the clinically employed cutoff criteria for males were 50 and 44 taps, respectively. Cutoff criteria used for females were 46 and 40 for each hand, respectively. Performance below these criteria placed subjects into the impaired range. The obtained high proportions of impaired scores are viewed by the authors as suggesting caution in using standard cutoff scores. Base rate issues are discussed from the perspective of the validity of test interpretation.

Table 17.3. FT.2

Data Stratified by Age, Education and Gender for the Whole Sample

Age	Education	No. Males	No. Females	Preferred Hand	Nonpreferred Hand
By Age					
20–39	13.0 (2.3)	107	64	47.2 (6.5)	43.5 (5.4)
40–59	11.9 (2.8)	31	66	40.3 (7.5)	37.8 (5.8)
60–69	11.8 (2.9)	40	57	35.4 (7.7)	33.8 (6.4)
By Education					
48.5 (16.6)	<HS	51	57	39.8 (9.2)	37.6 (7.8)
41.1 (16.8)	≥HS	127	130	43.3 (8.2)	40.3 (7.2)
By Gender					
39.2 (17.2)	12.4 (2.9)	178 Males		46.1 (7.0)	42.6 (6.9)
47.3 (16.1)	12.2 (2.5)	187 Females		38.6 (8.4)	36.5 (6.8)

Data Stratified by Age, Education and Gender for Separate Demographic Groups.

	Males						Females					
	<HS			≥HS			<HS			≥HS		
Age Groups	N	M	SD	N	M	SD	N	M	SD	N	M	SD
Preferred Hand												
20–39	21	49.7	6.0	86	48.5	6.5	13	45.2	6.0	49	44.3	5.8
40–59	13	42.3	5.2	17	43.4	7.9	22	36.3	7.8	43	40.5	7.1
60–69	16	39.1	5.7	23	43.0	4.7	22	29.7	6.2	34	32.2	6.0
Nonpreferred Hand												
20–39		47.0	5.5		44.8	6.4		40.7	5.0		40.6	5.6
40–59		39.8	3.6		39.5	5.8		35.2	5.8		37.8	6.0
60–69		35.2	5.2		39.3	6.2		29.8	5.6		32.0	4.9

The scores are based on the mean of five trials within five taps of each other to a maximum of 10 trials. When not accomplished, the score is the mean of the best five trials.

The sample was stratified by age group (18–39, 40–59, 60–69), level of education (<HS, ≥HS), and gender. A proportion of subjects obtaining scores in the impaired range for each of the above strata was provided for the preferred and nonpreferred hands.

Subjects were recruited from the general population of a large city in western Canada. Those with a history of neurologic or psychiatric illness were excluded from the study.

For the *strengths and considerations on use* of the study see [FT.2] Bornstein, 1985. In addition, in the current study, exclusion criteria and test administration procedures are specified (Tables 17.5 and 17.6).

[FT.5] Polubinski and Melamed, 1986

Subjects were students taking introductory psychology classes. All subjects were right-handed. The Crovitz-Zener test (1962) was used to assess degree of hand dominance based on consistency in hand preference for five unimanual tasks. Subjects with scores of 25 on this test

Table 17.4. FT.3

Age Group	N	Preferred Hand	Nonpreferred Hand
<25	10	93.4[*] (7.9)	90.1 (8.0)
45–54	10	82.8 (11.0)	80.4 (9.2)
55–64	10	70.3 (11.9)	69.5 (9.4)
65–74	10	67.9 (9.9)	69.3 (11.3)

[*]The score is the total number of taps recorded for each hand on two trials.

Table 17.5. FT.4a; Data for the Entire Sample ($N = 365$)

	Mean	Median	Mode	% Classified as Abnormal
Preferred hand (taps)	42.3	43	47	79.9
Nonpreferred hand (taps)	39.5	39.5	39	70.2

formed the firm right-handed groups, while those with scores of ≤24 formed the mixed right-handed groups.

A switch-back design was used, though it remains unclear how many trials were used per each hand. Number of taps in 15-second trials was averaged for each hand.

Study strengths

1. Assessment of handedness was well identified.

2. Information on age, education, handedness, gender, and occupation (college students) is provided.

3. Relatively large sample for restricted age, education, and handedness groups.

4. Means and standard deviations are reported.

Considerations regarding use of the study

1. The study provides data for limited age and education range.

2. No exclusion criteria are reported.

3. High educational level.

4. Nonstandard test administration (e.g., 15

second trials) and exact test procedures are not specified (Table 17.7).

[FT.6] Trahan, Patterson, Quintana and Biron, 1987

Subjects were 713 neurologically intact adults (382 males, 331 females) between the ages of 18 and 91. The score was the mean for three trials for each hand; trials began with the dominant hand and alternated between hands. The authors found no difference between 3-trial and 5-trial scores in a subgroup of 102 adults.

Study strengths

1. The administration procedure is described.

2. The data are are stratified by age and gender.

3. Minimally adequate exclusion criteria.

4. Means and standard deviations are reported.

5. Percentiles and difference scores between hands are reported.

6. Large sample sizes across age groupings.

Table 17.6. FT.4b; The Percent and Proportion of Subjects Obtaining Scores in the Impaired Range for the Stratified Sample

	Preferred Hand			
	Males (<50)°		Females (<46)	
Age	<HS	≥HS	<HS	≥HS
18–39	35 (7/20)	58.6 (51/87)	61.5 (8/13)	50 (23/46)
40–59	100 (13/13)	75 (12/16)	95.5 (21/22)	79.5 (35/44)
60–69	100 (16/16)	91.3 (21/23)	100 (17/22)	100 (33/33)

	Nonpreferred Hand			
	Males (<44)		Females (<40)	
Age	<HS	≥HS	<HS	≥HS
18–39	20 (4/20)	36.8 (32/87)	69.2 (9/13)	43.4 (20/46)
40–59	84.6 (11/13)	81.3 (13/16)	77.3 (17/22)	56.8 (25/44)
60–69	100 (16/16)	73.9 (17/23)	95.4 (21/22)	96.9 (32/33)

°The cutoff criteria for impairment, which differed for males and females, are presented in parentheses.

Table 17.7. FT.5

		N	Age	Education	Right Hand	Left Hand
Men:	Firm	30	19.7	13.3	93.6°	77.6
			(1.4)	(0.7)	(10.1)	(10.0)
	Mixed	30	20.1	13.6	93.5	79.6
			(1.6)	(0.9)	(13.1)	(12.1)
Women:	Firm	38	19.8	13.4	91.1	76.0
			(1.2)	(0.7)	(12.4)	(13.8)
	Mixed	22	19.4	13.3	88.8	74.5
			(0.8)	(0.6)	(9.9)	(11.6)

°Scores are presented for 15-second trials.

Considerations regarding use of the study

1. Sample composition is minimally described.

2. The procedure to determine hand preference was not described.

3. High educational level of the sample.

Other comments

1. The authors concluded that the data revealed significant age-related differences. In addition, males performed faster than females at all age levels.

2. Use of the traditional cutoff suggested by Halstead and Reitan resulted in false-positive rates ranging from 28.0% to 89.5% in the various groups. The percentage of subjects displaying an intermanual difference greater than 10% ranged from 22.9% to 55.2% in the various groups. Reversals (nonpreferred hand faster than preferred hand) were observed in 14.7% of the sample. The data challenge a traditional hypothesis regarding "normal" adult tapping performance (Table 17.8).

[FT.7] Yeudall, Reddon, Gill and Stefanyk, 1987

The authors obtained data on 225 Canadian subjects recruited from posted advertisements in workplaces and personal solicitations. The participants included meat packers, postal workers, transit employees, hospital lab technicians, secretaries, ward aides, student interns, student nurses, and summer students. In addition, high school teachers identified for participation average students in grades 10 through 12. The subjects (127 males and 98 females) did

not report any history of forensic involvement, head injury, neurological insult, prenatal or birth complications, psychiatric problems, or substance abuse. Handedness was determined by the writing hand. Data were gathered by experienced technicians who "motivated the subjects to achieve maximum performance" partially through the promise of detailed explanations of their test performance.

Study strengths

1. Large sample size and individual cells approximate Ns of 50.

2. The data are stratified by age and gender.

3. Data availability for a 15–20-year-old age group.

Table 17.8. FT.6°

Age	N	Preferred Hand	Nonpreferred Hand
18–32			
Males	175	54.58 (5.19)	50.31 (5.38)
Females	221	48.71 (5.52)	44.75 (5.60)
33–47			
Males	145	53.28 (6.29)	48.52 (6.64)
Females	56	49.12 (5.91)	45.07 (5.12)
48–62			
Males	29	52.80 (5.24)	47.98 (5.78)
Females	35	46.84 (6.05)	43.59 (5.92)
63–91			
Males	33	49.23 (8.94)	45.31 (8.43)
Females	19	43.13 (6.69)	41.03 (7.38)

°The score is the mean for three trials for each hand.

4. Adequate medical and psychiatric exclusion criteria.

5. The administration procedure is well described; standard procedure was used.

6. Information regarding handedness, education, IQ, sex, occupation, recruitment procedures, and geographic area is provided.

7. Method for determining handedness was specified.

8. Means and standard deviations are reported.

Considerations regarding use of the study

1. The sample was atypical in terms of its high average intellectual level and high level of education.

Other comments

1. IQ was measured by the WAIS and WAIS-R. WAIS IQ scores were equated to the WAIS-R IQ scores by linear equating.

2. Correlations of the FTT scores with age and education were 0.20 and 0.06 for the preferred hand and 0.22 and 0.08 for the nonpreferred hand. Effect of sex on subjects' performance was also explored. The authors concluded that age effects were not significant for either hand, but there were sex effects for both preferred and nonpreferred hands. Therefore they suggest using the sex norms collapsed across age (Table 17.9).

[FT.8] Bornstein and Suga, 1988

In a more recent publication, the authors reported data on 134 healthy elderly Canadian volunteers, aged 55 to 70, according to three education levels. Nearly two-thirds of the sample were female ($N = 85$). The average age for the sample was 62.7 (± 4.3), and the mean ages of the three educational groups were comparable. Exclusion criteria were history of neurological or psychiatric disease.

Study strengths

1. Large sample size and individual cells approximate Ns of 50.

2. Reporting of data by three educational groups; the study is unique in terms of representation of subjects with less than 12 years of education.

3. Information regarding sex, age, and geographic area is provided.

4. Means and standard deviations are reported.

5. Minimally adequate exclusion criteria.

6. Data are presented in age grouping (i.e., all subjects were 55–70 years old).

Considerations regarding use of the study

1. Procedure for determination of hand preference was not identified.

2. Greater than 12 years of education too large a category.

3. Data collapsed across genders.

Other comments

1. Subjects used in this study represent a subset of subjects used in Bornstein (1985) article (Table 17.10).

[FT.9] Ardila and Rosselli, 1989

The study included 346 normal adults. Subjects had a score of 23 or higher on the MMSE, had no neurological or psychiatric background as determined by a neurological and psychiatric screening, and performed adequately in everyday life activities.

Study strengths

1. The overall sample size is large.

2. The sample was broken down by age and education subgroups.

3. Adequate exclusion criteria.

Considerations regarding use of the study

1. Demographic characteristics are cursorily described.

2. Sample size for each cell is small ($N = 11$ or 12).

3. Standard deviations are not reported.

4. Procedures used to determine hand preference are not described.

5. Data are apparently collapsed across genders.

Other comments

1. The data were collected in Bogota, Colombia (Table 17.11).

[FT.10] Heaton, Grant, and Matthews, 1991

The authors provide normative data from 486 (378 in the base sample and 108 in the validation sample) urban and rural subjects recruited

Table 17.9. FT.7

Data for the Entire Sample (N = 225)

Age Group	N	Age	Education	WAIS-R FSIQ	% Right-Handed	Preferred Hand	Nonpreferred Hand
15–20	62	17.76 (1.96)	12.16 (1.75)	111.75 (10.16)	79.03	46.59 (6.60)	42.51 (5.81)
21–25	73	22.70 (1.40)	14.82 (1.88)	109.79 (9.97)	86.30	47.28 (8.13)	44.38 (7.20)
26–30	48	28.06 (1.52)	15.50 (2.65)	113.95 (10.61)	89.58	50.47 (7.28)	45.64 (6.68)
31–40	42	34.38 (2.46)	16.50 (3.11)	116.09 (9.51)	90.48	50.52 (8.37)	46.54 (6.75)
15–40	225	24.66 (6.16)	14.55 (2.78)	112.25 (10.25)	85.78	48.38 (7.76)	44.54 (6.76)

Data for Females (N = 98)

Age Group	N	Age	Education	WAIS-R FSIQ	% Right-Handed	Preferred Hand	Nonpreferred Hand
15–20	30	17.73 (1.84)	12.10 (1.52)	110.32 (10.64)	73.33	44.77 (7.37)	41.63 (5.69)
21–25	36	22.83 (1.54)	14.53 (1.99)	107.28 (9.14)	83.33	44.36 (7.48)	41.62 (6.82)
26–30	16	28.69 (1.25)	14.94 (2.32)	113.10 (11.37)	93.75	48.14 (6.99)	43.24 (4.44)
31–40	16	33.88 (2.53)	16.19 (2.29)	114.27 (11.32)	87.50	44.35 (5.64)	41.98 (4.65)
15–40	98	24.03 (5.95)	14.12 (2.43)	110.19 (10.46)	82.65	45.10 (7.12)	41.95 (5.76)

Data for Males (N = 127)

Age Group	N	Age	Education	WAIS-R FSIQ	% Right-Handed	Preferred Hand	Nonpreferred Hand
15–20	32	17.78 (2.09)	12.22 (1.96)	113.00 (9.72)	84.38	48.36 (5.31)	43.36 (5.89)
21–25	37	22.57 (1.26)	15.11 (1.74)	112.30 (10.27)	89.19	50.20 (7.78)	47.14 (6.55)
26–30	32	27.75 (1.57)	15.78 (2.79)	114.38 (10.43)	87.50	51.68 (7.24)	46.88 (7.34)
31–40	26	34.69 (2.41)	16.69 (3.55)	117.31 (8.21)	92.31	54.32 (7.52)	49.35 (6.34)
15–40	127	25.15 (6.29)	14.87 (2.99)	113.87 (9.83)	88.19	50.97 (7.26)	46.60 (6.81)

Table 17.10. FT.8

Education	Age	No. Males	No. Females	Preferred Hand	Nonpreferred Hand
5–10	62.3	17	29	34.1 (7.1)	32.8 (5.9)
11–12	62.9	16	28	36.9 (7.9)	35.2 (5.2)
>12	63.0	16	28	37.4 (8.1)	35.4 (7.0)

Table 17.11. FT.9

Age Group/ Schooling	Preferred Hand	Nonpreferred Hand
55–60		
0 to 5	40.9	37.2
6 to 12	44.4	39.2
>12	48.1	46.3
61–65		
0 to 5	39.7	36.2
6 to 12	43.3	39.9
>12	41.7	39.6
66–70		
0 to 5	32.7	31.6
6 to 12	39.8	37.0
>12	40.0	37.5
71–75		
0 to 5	32.4	29.7
6 to 12	36.2	35.2
>12	39.4	36.0
>75		
0 to 5	26.2	26.6
6 to 12	30.0	27.7
>12	33.5	31.3

in several states (California, Washington, Colorado, Texas, Oklahoma, Wisconsin, Illinois, Michigan, New York, Virginia, and Massachusetts) and Canada. Data were collected over a 15-year period through multicenter collaborative efforts.

Sixty-five percent of the sample were males. Mean age for the total sample was 42.06 ± 16.8, and mean educational level was 13.6 ± 3.5. Mean FSIQ, VIQ, and PIQ were 113.8 ± 12.3, 113.9 ± 13.8, and 111.9 ± 11.6, respectively. Exclusion criteria were history of learning disability, neurologic disease, illnesses affecting brain function, significant head trauma, significant psychiatric disturbance (e.g., schizophrenia), and alcohol or other substance abuse.

The FTT was administered according to procedures described by Reitan and Wolfson (1985). Subjects were generally paid for their participation and were judged to have provided their best efforts on the tasks. Average number of taps for five trials per hand were recorded. The normative data, which are not reproduced here, are presented in comprehensive tables in *T*-score equivalents for test scaled scores for males and females separately in 10 age groupings (20–34, 35–39, 40–44, 45–49, 50–54, 55–59, 60–64, 65–69, 70–74, 75–80) by six educational groupings (6–8 years, 9–11 years, 12 years, 13–15 years, 16–17 years, 18+ years).

Study strengths
   1. Large sample size.
   2. Comprehensive exclusion criteria.
   3. Detailed description of the demographic characteristics of the sample in terms of age, education, IQ, geographic area, and gender.
   4. Administration procedures were outlined.
   5. The normative data are presented in comprehensive tables in *T*-score equivalents for males and females separately in 10 age groupings by six educational groupings.

Considerations regarding use of the study
   1. Above average mean intellectual level (which is probably less of an issue given that these are WAIS rather than WAIS-R IQ data).
   2. No information regarding how hand preference was determined.

Other comments
   1. For dominant hand performance, 19% of score variance was accounted for by sex, while 9% was attributable to age and 6% to educational level. A total of 32% of test score variance was accounted for by demographic variables. A similar effect was described for nondominant hand performance, where 20% of score variance was accounted for by sex, while 9% was attributable to age and 6% to educational level. A total of 34% of test score variance was accounted for by demographic variables.

For the sample as a whole, mean number of taps for the dominant hand was 49.9 ± 7.9 and for the nondominant hand was 45.2 ± 7.3.
   2. The interested reader is referred to 1996 critique of Heaton et al. (1991) norms, and Heaton et al.'s 1996 response to this critique.

[FT.11] Ruff and Parker, 1993

The FTT was administered as part of a comprehensive test battery to 358 normal volunteers recruited in California, Michigan, and the eastern seaboard who ranged in age between 16 and 70 years and in education between 7 and 22 years. Subjects were screened for psychiatric hospitalizations, chronic polydrug abuse, or neurological disorders.

The score was the mean number of taps over five 10-second trials with alternating hands starting with the dominant hand. If the criterion was not met, up to two additional trials were given per hand and the highest/lowest scores were eliminated from computation of the mean score.

Study strengths

1. Sample composition was identified in terms of age, education, gender, and geographic area.

2. Assessment of handedness was well described.

3. The test administration procedure was thoroughly described.

4. The data are stratified according to gender and age.

5. Data for a left-hand-dominant sample are reported.

6. The sample sizes for each demographic cell are quite large and approximate Ns of 50.

7. Good exclusion criteria.

8. Means and standard deviations are reported.

Considerations regarding use of the study

1. The data stratified by three educational groups were not presented.

2. High educational level.

Other comments

1. The authors report test–retest reliability for a 6-month interval based on the data for five or more subjects from each of the 12 demographic cells (30% of the sample). The reliability coefficients for women, men and total sample were 0.63, 0.70, 0.70 for the dominant hand, and 0.68, 0.75, 0.76 for the nondominant hand.

2. Effect of age and gender on motor speed was specifically addressed.

3. The authors explored the ratio of dominant/nondominant hand performance rate (Tables 17.12 and 17.13).

Control Groups in Clinical Studies

[FT.12] Vega and Parsons, 1967

The HRB performance for brain-damaged and control groups recruited in Oklahoma was compared. The brain-damaged group included patients with different kinds of CNS dysfunction supported by pathological findings on established diagnostic techniques. This group included 15 patients with right hemisphere damage, 15 with left hemisphere damage, and 20 with diffuse, bilateral, or subcortical damage. The control group included 43 patients hospitalized for causes other than CNS dysfunction and seven nonhospitalized subjects.

Study strengths

1. Group composition was described in terms of age, education, gender, IQ, and geographic area.

2. Sample sizes for each group are sufficient.

3. Means and standard deviations are reported.

Considerations regarding use of the study

1. Data are presented only for the dominant hand.

2. Samples are not separated into age groups.

3. Method for determining hand preference is not identified.

4. The control sample is primarily composed of hospitalized patients.

5. Low educational level.

6. Data are collapsed across genders (Table 17.14).

Table 17.12. FT.11a; Data for the *Left-Hand-Dominant* Sample

	Men (N = 17)		Women (N = 18)	
	M	SD	M	SD
Age	37.9	(18.0)	38.7	(16.1)
Education	13.7	(2.8)	14.1	(2.6)
Dominant hand	53.1	(5.8)	44.7	(4.5)
Nondominant hand	46.7	(13.2)	41.9	(6.2)

Table 17.13. FT.11b; Data for the Whole Sample Stratified by Age and Gender

Gender/Age Group	N	Dominant Hand		Nondominant Hand	
		M	SD	M	SD
Women					
16–24	45	49.5	5.1	45.6	5.1
25–39	45	49.0	4.1	44.6	4.6
40–54	44	47.0	5.6	43.5	5.2
55–70	45	45.7	5.5	40.4	5.2
Total	179	47.8	5.3	43.5	5.4
Men					
16–24	45	52.9	5.1	48.2	4.4
25–39	44	52.7	6.8	48.7	5.7
40–54	45	54.3	5.7	48.9	5.8
55–70	45	53.5	6.4	48.3	5.0
Total	179	53.4	6.0	48.5	5.2
Total/Whole sample	358	50.6	6.3	46.0	5.9

[FT.13] Goldstein and Shelly, 1972

Inpatients at the Topeka Veterans Administration Hospital were used in the study. Subjects came from different services in the hospital and were tested on a referral basis. Most subjects were male adults. Subjects were classified into brain-damaged and non-brain-damaged groups. The former group included patients with cerebral lesion of any etiology, and it was further subdivided into left-hemisphere, right-hemisphere, and diffuse damage subgroups. Subgroups with unilateral lesions included primarily cases of cerebrovascular accidents, head injuries, and neoplasms. Subjects in the control group included general medical and psychiatric patients. Those subjects for who definitive diagnostic differentiation could not be made were dropped.

Study strengths
1. Sample sizes are large.
2. The administration procedure, which con-

forms with the original Halstead instructions, was described.
3. Means and standard deviations are reported.
4. Geographic area is indicated.

Considerations regarding use of the study
1. Demographic characteristics for the samples are not presented such as age, education, gender and IQ.
2. Procedures used to determine hand preference are not described.
3. The control sample consisted of medical and psychiatric inpatients (Table 17.15).

[FT.14] Goldstein and Braun, 1974

The study explores changes in speed of performance on bilateral motor tasks as a function of increased age. Subjects were considered representative of a "normal" population without reported history of neurological difficulties. A sample consisting of 201 men and eight women was divided into six age groups.

Table 17.14. FT.12

	N	Gender	Age	Education	WAIS FSIQ	Dominant Hand
Brain damaged	50	44 M	41.7	10.2	84.9	35.5
		6 F	(14.8)	(3.1)	(14.8)	(11.6)
Control	50	37 M	40.8	11.1	99.4	44.6
		13 F	(13.1)	(3.2)	(12.9)	(9.2)

Table 17.15. FT.13

	N	Dominant Hand	Nondominant Hand
Brain-damaged	276	41.3 (13.4)	37.9 (10.5)
Left	27	31.4 (19.9)	39.3 (7.0)
Right	21	45.5 (11.6)	33.4 (15.2)
Diffuse	228	42.0 (12.1)	38.1 (10.3)
Non-brain-damaged	156	46.8 (10.4)	41.2 (8.8)

Preference of the right hand was endorsed by all but five subjects and was confirmed by a lateral dominance examination. Subjects who indicated mixed dominance were not included.

The procedure generally conforms the original Halstead instructions. It should be noted that the first set of trials established the mean for the preferred hand. Then the procedure was repeated for the nonpreferred hand. Means and standard deviations for each hand, as well as percent reversal, are presented.

Study strengths
1. Overall sample size is quite large, although some individual cell sizes fall below 50.
2. The sample was divided into six age groups.

3. Method for determining handedness was indicated.
4. The test administration procedure was described.
5. Gender of subjects is reported.
6. Minimally adequate exclusion criteria.
7. Means and standard deviations are reported.

Considerations regarding use of the study
1. The sample was comprised primarily of males; male and female data were collapsed.
2. No data on educational level, IQ, or geographic area.

Other comments
1. The authors point to a steady decrease in mean speed for both hands as an expected consequence of the aging process and might be related to diminished function of interhemispheric neural transfer. The number of reversals from the expected difference between two hands became substantial in the group of 70-year-olds (Table 17.16).

[FT.15] Finlayson, Johnson and Reitan, 1977

The data are provided for male brain-damaged and control samples. The control groups included healthy individuals as well as hospitalized medical and psychiatric patients. Brain-damaged groups included patients with neurologically established brain damage. Patients with

Table 17.16. FT.14

Age Group	Mean Age	N	Preferred Hand	Nonpreferred Hand	Percent Reversal°
20–29	24.5	29	54.1 (4.4)	49.0 (4.6)	17
30–39	34.9	75	53.4 (5.4)	47.9 (5.2)	11
40–49	44.7	47	53.3 (4.8)	47.4 (4.5)	9
50–59	53.5	30	50.5 (5.4)	45.2 (4.4)	10
60–69	64.2	16	47.4 (8.6)	43.0 (7.0)	19
70–79	72.2	12	44.5 (7.4)	41.1 (7.5)	25

° Percent reversal indicates percent of subjects who were tapping faster with nonpreferred hand than with preferred hand.

traumatic, neoplastic, and cerebrovascular damage were equally represented in the three brain-damaged groups. Both samples were divided into three groups based on education: University groups included persons with at least 3 years of college; high school groups included those who had completed grade 12 but had not attended college; grade school groups included persons with less than 10 years of education.

Study strengths
1. Sample composition was well described in terms of age, education, gender, and IQ.
2. Data are presented by education groupings (with mean IQs for each education subgrouping reported).

Considerations regarding use of the study
1. It is stated by the authors that the groups did not differ in mean age and subjects were less than 50 years old. However, age ranges were not specified. Data were not separated into age groups.
2. All subjects were males.
3. Raw scores were not reported in the article. The results were converted into *T* scores with a mean of 50 and a SD of 10.
4. Procedures for assessment of hand dominance were not described.
5. The control group included hospitalized medical and psychiatric patients.

6. Small individual cell sizes (Table 17.17).

[FT.16] Wiens and Matarazzo, 1977

The authors collected FTT data on 48 male applicants to a patrolman program in Portland, Oregon, as a part of an investigation of the WAIS and MMPI correlates of the Halstead-Reitan Battery. All subjects passed a medical exam and were judged to be neurologically normal. Subjects were divided into two equal groups which were comparable in age, education and WAIS FSIQ. Group 1 ranged in age from 21 to 27 years and group 2 from 21 to 28 years. Means and standard deviations are provided for each hand.

Study strengths
1. Demographic characteristics of the sample are presented in terms of gender, age, education, IQ, recruitment procedures, and geographic area.
2. Adequate medical exclusion criteria.
3. Means and standard deviations are reported.
4. The data are provided in a restricted age range.

Considerations regarding use of the study
1. Hand preference is not reported.
2. High IQ and educational level.

Table 17.17. FT.15

	N	Age	Education	FSIQ	Dominant Hand (*T* Scores)	Nondominant Hand (*T* Scores)
Brain-Damaged						
Grade school	17	35.53 (8.19)	7.82 (1.63)	87.00 (17.90)	46.35	45.65
High school	17	34.53 (7.07)	12.00 0	92.20 (13.50)	45.41	46.00
University	17	34.76 (9.05)	17.06 (1.78)	103.00 (17.40)	47.00	46.53
Controls						
Grade school	17	34.12 (8.72)	7.94 (1.71)	101.88 (10.23)	51.06	55.77
High school	17	34.37 (7.36)	12.00 0	112.71 (12.21)	54.00	55.81
University	17	35.22 (7.78)	17.35 (1.66)	129.53 (7.58)	55.00	56.10

Table 17.18. FT.16

	N	WAIS FSIQ	Age	Education	Preferred Hand	Nonpreferred Hand
Group 1	24	117.5	23.6	13.7	54.0 (4.6)	48.4 (4.4)
Group 2	24	118.3	24.8	14.0	54.5 (4.0)	50.0 (4.1)

3. Relatively small sample size.
4. All-male sample.

Other comments
1. Correlations for the two groups between WAIS FSIQ and FTT scores were −0.05 and 0.03 for the preferred hand, and −0.11 and −0.44 for the nonpreferred hand. The authors concluded that for the top half of the population in terms of education and IQ, individual differences in scores on the WAIS do not influence performance on the HRB measures (Table 17.18).

[FT.17] Dodrill, 1978a

The study compares epileptic and control groups in the state of Washington. The epileptic sample included subjects with a variety of seizure diagnoses. Mean age of onset of seizure disorder for this group was 12.44 (± 9.69) with mean duration of the disorder of 14.90 years (±9.68). The control group included subjects from the community with no evidence of neurological disorder. Demographic characteristics were comparable for control and epileptic groups. Every control subject was individually matched with an epileptic subject on sex, age (±5 years) and education (±2 years). Of the controls, nine were students, six were housewives, 20 were unemployed, and 15 were employed. Controls were recruited through employment facilities, churches, a community college, a public high school, a volunteer service agency, and a semi-sheltered workshop.

Study strengths
1. Sample composition is well described in terms of age, education, gender, occupation, geographic area, ethnicity, and recruitment procedures.

2. Data are stratified by gender.
3. Means and standard deviations are reported.

Considerations regarding use of the study
1. Procedures used to determine hand preference were not described.
2. Apparently adequate exclusion criteria, although some controls were recruited from sheltered workshops.
3. Undifferentiated age range.
4. Relatively small sample sizes in the gender subgroupings (Table 17.19).

[FT.18] Dodrill, 1978b

Performance on motor tests was compared for four groups: control, right hemisphere damage, left hemisphere damage, and bilateral damage.

All brain-damaged groups included five subjects with intrinsic brain tumors, 11 with a history of head trauma, and nine with cerebrovascular problems.

Control subjects were recruited from community resources in the state of Washington and had no history of injury or disease that involved CNS.

All groups included adults age 15 and over. Across all groups, a subject-by-subject matching procedure was maintained for sex, race (all subjects were Caucasian), age, education, and handedness.

Study strengths
1. Sample composition is well described in terms of age, education, gender, handedness and geographic area.
2. Minimally adequate exclusion criteria for control.
3. Means and standard deviations are reported.

Table 17.19. FT.17

	N	Age	Education	% Male	Race	Preferred Hand	Nonpreferred Hand
Control	50	27.3 (8.4)	12.0 (2.0)	60	98% W		
Males	30					56.0 (5.6)	51.43 (5.7)
Females	20					51.2 (4.0)	48.0 (3.7)
Epileptic	50	27.3 (9.0)	12.0 (1.9)	60	98% W		
Males						46.1 (9.4)	41.7 (8.2)
Females						41.6 (6.4)	36.0 (10.6)

Considerations regarding use of the study

1. Procedures used to determine hand preference were not described.
2. Low educational level.
3. Small sample sizes.
4. Undifferentiated age range.
5. Data are collapsed across genders (Table 17.20).

[FT.19] Morrison, Gregory and Paul, 1979

The study exlored interexaminer reliability for the test–retest conditions of the FTT. Subjects were 60 volunteers from introductory psychology courses with a modal age of 19. All subjects were white and were from rural backgrounds in Idaho; half the sample were male and half were female.

Two conditions were utilized:

1. Subjects were tested by the same examiner twice with one week interval (test–retest condition).

2. Subjects were tested by different examiners twice with 1-week interval (interexaminer condition).

Means and standard deviations for the test–retest and interexaminer conditions are presented.

Study strengths

1. Data are presented for males and females separately.
2. Information on ethnicity, occupation (college students), age, and geographic area is presented.
3. Means and standard deviations are reported.
4. Restricted age grouping.

Considerations regarding use of the study

1. Results are reported only for the dominant hand. Data are averaged over the test and retest conditions.

Table 17.20. FT.18

	N	Age	Education	Gender	% Right Handed	Right Hand	Left Hand
Control	25	41.1	10.7	20 M 5 F	100	53.4 (6.2)	49.6 (5.4)
Right	25	41.1	10.7	20 M 5 F	100	41.8 (9.0)	30.7 (14.3)
Left	25	41.1	10.7	20M 5 F	100	37.0 (17.3)	39.2 (11.5)
Bilateral	25	41.1	10.7	20 M 5 F	100	40.4 (11.2)	34.6 (10.3)

Table 17.21. FT.19; Number of Taps for the Dominant Hand on Test–Retest Trials, Averaged Over Two Probes

	Test–Retest		Interexaminer	
	N	Tapping	N	Tapping
Males	30	51.37	30	54.79
		(4.45)		(3.71)
Females	30	48.52	30	50.37
		(4.97)		(4.63)

2. No exclusion criteria.
3. Relatively small individual cell sizes.
4. Procedures for assessment of hand dominance were not described.

Other comments
1. The authors found significant sex differences with males performing about three taps faster than females (Table 17.21).

[FT.20] Anthony, Heaton and Lehman, 1980

The purpose of the study was to cross-validate two computerized programs designed to determine the presence, location, and process of brain lesions using scores from the Halstead-Reitan Battery and the WAIS. Patients with structural brain lesions and normal controls were compared. The clinical group included subjects with neuroradiologically or neurosurgically confirmed brain damage. The control group consisted of volunteers with no presenting medical or psychiatric problems and with no history of head trauma, brain disease, or substance abuse.

Study strengths
1. Information regarding education, IQ, and age is provided.
2. Sample sizes are large.

3. Adequate exclusion criteria.
4. Means and standard deviations are reported.

Considerations regarding use of the study
1. Procedures used to determine hand preference were not described.
2. Undifferentiated age grouping.
3. The IQ range is high average.
4. No information regarding gender (Table 17.22).

[FT.21] Bak and Greene, 1980

The study investigated the effects of age on different neuropsychological measures in healthy, active older adults in Texas ranging in age between 50 and 86 years. Two age groups were compared: 50–62 and 67–86 years. All subjects were right-handed. Subjects were fluent in English and denied history of CNS disorders, uncorrected sensory deficits or illnesses, or "incapacities" which might affect test results; subjects in poor health were excluded. Four WAIS subtests were administered (Information, Arithmetic, Block Design, Digit Symbol); the mean scores on these measures suggested that IQ levels were within the high average range or higher. Means and standard deviations were reported for each hand.

Study strengths
1. The study provides data on a very elderly age cohort not found in other published normative data.
2. Adequate exclusion criteria.
3. Sample composition is well described in terms of age, gender, education, handedness, and geographic area.
4. Means and standard deviations are reported.

Table 17.22. FT.20

	N	Age	Education	WAIS FSIQ	Dominant Hand	Nondominant Hand
Control	100	38.9	13.3	113.5	52.6	48.2
		(15.8)	(2.6)	(10.8)	(9.1)	(7.6)
Brain damaged	150	42.7	12.5	94.8	43.0	37.4
		(15.4)	(3.1)	(16.9)	(11.6)	(11.6)

Table 17.23. FT.21

Age group	N	Gender	Age	Education	Right Hand	Left Hand
50–62	15	6 M	55.6	13.7	44.53	40.80
		9 F	(4.44)	(1.91)	(6.71)	(4.77)
67–86	15	5 M	74.9	14.9	38.73	36.33
		10 F	(6.04)	(2.99)	(4.13)	(5.93)

Considerations regarding use of the study

1. Procedures for assessment of handedness were not described.

2. Sample sizes are small.

3. The high IQ and educational level.

4. The older age grouping spans nearly two decades and may be too broad for optimal clinical interpretative use.

5. Data are collapsed across sexes (Table 17.23).

[FT.22] Eckardt and Matarazzo, 1981

Performance on neuropsychological tests for drug-free alcoholic inpatients and nonalcoholic medical inpatients was compared. All subjects were male inpatients at V.A. hospitals in California and were between the ages of 21 and 60. No psychoactive medication had been ingested by the patients during the 48 hours prior to the testing.

Alcoholic patients were participants in an inpatient alcoholism treatment program. Mean number of years of abusive drinking was 15.9 (±10.9). Forty-eight percent of subjects had some college education. The alcoholic group was tested within 7 days of their last drink, but only after the subsidence of acute withdrawal. They were retested 12–22 days later.

The nonalcoholic group consisted of medical inpatients from the same hospital who were re-ferred from a variety of services and were neurologically stable during the study. They were assumed to have no recent drinking problem. Sixty percent of this group had some college education. They were also tested twice with the same time elapsing between testings as for the alcoholic group.

Study strengths

1. The sample composition is described in terms of age, geographic area, and gender, with cursory information on education.

2. Test–retest data are available.

3. Means and standard deviations are reported.

Considerations regarding use of the study

1. Procedures used to determine hand preference were not described.

2. Data are provided only for males and only for the dominant hand.

3. Small nonalcoholic medical sample.

4. Controls were medical inpatients.

5. Undifferentiated age range (Table 17.24).

[FT.23] Pirozzolo, Hansch, Mortimer, Webster and Kuskowski, 1982

The study compares performance on neuropsychological measures by Parkinson's disease patients and normal controls.

Patients included in the clinical group had

Table 17.24. FT.22

	N	Age	% Male	Dominant Hand	
				Test	Retest
Alcoholic	91	42.2	100	44.3	48.5
		(10.0)		(8.0)	(7.6)
Nonalcoholic	20	45.6	100	42.1	43.6
		(11.1)		(9.4)	(10.4)

Table 17.25. FT.23

	N	Age	Education	Gender	Right Hand	Left Hand
Parkinson's	60	62.7	11.4	58 M	30.27	30.13
		(8.2)	(2.8)	2 F	(13.76)	(11.64)
Normals	60	—	—	—	50.07	46.73
					(8.75)	(8.43)

the average age of onset of symptoms at age 53.3 years (SD = 11.5) with a mean duration of illness of 9.4 years (SD = 8.1). Patients with a history of CVA, alcoholism, or other neurological disease were excluded from the Parkinson's group. No patients underwent surgical procedures for the relief of symptoms.

Normal volunteers were matched on age, sex, and education to the patient group and satisfactorily completed a brief screening exam by a neurologist.

Study strengths
1. Sample sizes are sufficiently large.
2. Minimally adequate exclusion criteria.
3. Means and standard deviations are reported.

Considerations regarding use of the study
1. No data are reported for mean age, education, or gender distribution for controls, although it is assumed that controls approximate the age, gender, and education of patient data given that controls were matched to patients.
2. Method for determining handedness is not reported.
3. Undifferentiated age range (Table 17.25).

[FT.24] Rounsaville, Jones, Novelly and Kleber, 1982

The study compares FTT performance of two clinical and control groups.

Opiate addicts were evaluated at a drug dependence treatment center 1 to 3 weeks after applying for treatment. This group included subjects who were still using opiates and those recently maintained on methadone or recently detoxified.

The epilepsy group was matched for age, sex, handedness, and education and included individuals meeting the following criteria: (1) a neurological diagnosis of either a partial or partial-complex or absence seizure disorder, with epileptic or epileptiform discharges on a serial EEG examination and without evidence of hysterical components; (2) no evidence of either focal or diffuse abnormalities on computerized axial tomography scan as reported by the neuroradiologist; (3) no history of psychiatric hospitalization or drug or alcohol abuse.

A normal comparison group was chosen to provide demographically matched subjects who were in similar social circumstance to the addicts. A sample of Comprehensive Employment Training Act (CETA) participants was used. Subjects with a history of drug or alcohol abuse or of a neurological disorder were excluded. Urine specimens were taken at the time of testing and screened for alcohol and illicit psychoactive substances.

Study strengths
1. Controls were well described in terms of gender, age, education and percent right-handers.
2. The study provides the data on test–retest over a 6-month period.
3. Adequate exclusion criteria.

Considerations regarding use of the study
1. Standard deviations were not provided.
2. The procedures for assessment of hand dominance were not described.
3. Age ranges were not provided and it is unclear to what extent the sample was homogeneous in terms of age.
4. Sample size for the normal comparison group is small.
5. Low educational level.
6. Data are collapsed across genders.

Table 17.26. FT.24

	N	% Male	Education	% Right-Handed	Age	Dominant Hand	Nondominant Hand
Opiate addicts	72	72	11.5	91	27.9	51.19	46.41
Epileptic	60	67	11.8	87	29.2	47.65	42.58
CETA workers	29	59	11.2	90	24.9	48.48	42.58
Opiate addicts 6-month retest	59	—	—	—	—	50.11	45.51

Other comments

1. Opiate addicts were retested in 6 months. Performance at the retest is presented (Table 17.26).

[FT.25] Yeudall, Fromm-Auch and Davies, 1982

The study compares performance on the HRB for delinquent and nondelinquent adolescents in Canada. The delinquent group included adolescents admitted to the primary residential treatment resource for persistent delinquents with severe behavioral disturbances. The nondelinquent group included adolescents from regular classrooms.

Handedness was measured by Annett Handedness Questionnaire (1970): 88% of the delinquent sample and 83% of the control sample were right-handed.

Study strengths

1. The samples were described in terms of age, gender, IQ, handed, and geographic area.
2. Procedure for assessment of handedness was identified.
3. Means and standard deviations are reported.
4. The control sample is relatively large.
5. Age range was not specified but probably is reasonably restricted.

Considerations regarding use of the study

1. No apparent exclusion criteria.
2. Data are collapsed across genders.
3. High intellectual level of the controls (Table 17.27).

[FT.26] O'Donnell, Kurtz and Ramanaiah, 1983

The study compares neuropsychological test performance of normal, learning disabled, and brain-damaged young adults.

Learning disabled subjects had been initially diagnosed during the primary or secondary grades and continued to exhibit disability through the 12th grade. They had either graduated from high school or were within two semesters of high school graduation.

The brain-damaged group was composed of victims of head trauma. Periods of unconsciousness following their accidents ranged between 2 hours and 210 days, and 89% had been comatose for longer than 1 week. The average length of unconsciousness was 52 days (SD = 53 days). They were tested from 9 to 84 months following their injuries (M = 39.7; SD = 22.1 months), at a time when their medical and neurological conditions had stabilized.

The normal control group consisted mostly of college student volunteers without a history of learning problems, blows to the head, or seizures.

Table 17.27. FT.25

	N	Age	WAIS FSIQ	No. Males	No. Females	Preferred Hand	Nonpreferred Hand
Delinquent	99	14.8	95.3	64	35	40.0 (6.7)	37.0 (5.8)
Nondelinquent	46	14.5	117.1	29	18	42.9 (7.7)	40.2 (6.9)

Study strengths

1. Composition of samples is well described in terms of age (college students), education, gender, handedness, and occupation.

2. Minimally adequate exclusion criteria.

3. Age range is not specified, but appears to be relatively narrow.

4. Means and standard deviations are reported.

Considerations regarding use of the study

1. Data are presented for the dominant hand only.

2. Procedures for assessment of hand dominance were not described.

3. Control sample size is relatively small.

4. Data are collapsed across genders.

5. High IQ and educational level of controls. (Table 17.28)

[FT.27] Prigatano, Parsons, Levin, Wright and Hawryluk, 1983

The study explores neuropsychological functioning in mildly hypoxemic patients with chronic obstructive pulmonary disease (COPD), recruited in Oklahoma and Canada. Patients ranged in age between 30 and 74 years and were not severely hypoxemic based on laboratory reports (mean PaO_2 was 66.3). The controls were matched on age, education, handedness, sex ratio, and social class rating. They were free of physical or emotional illnesses.

Study strengths

1. Samples were described in terms of age, gender, IQ, education, handedness, and geographic area.

2. Minimally adequate exclusion criteria for controls.

3. Means and standard deviations are reported.

Considerations regarding use of the study

1. Procedures for assessment of hand dominance were not described.

2. Small sample size of the control group.

3. Undifferentiated age range.

4. Data are collapsed across genders.

Other comments

1. The authors inferred that mild dysfunction correlated with resting partial pressure of oxygen in chronic obstructive pulmonary disease (COPD) patients (Table 17.29).

[FT.28] Heaton, Nelson, Thompson, Burks and Franklin, 1985

The authors compared performance of multiple sclerosis (MS) patients (with both relapsing-remitting and chronic-progressive course) and controls recruited in Colorado. Patients with relapsing-remitting MS course had been in remission for at least 1 month at the time of testing. Sixty MS patients were on medication at the time of testing. Patients' mean score on Kurtzke's Disability Status Scale (DSS) for measuring neurological disability in MS was 3.10 (± 2.09). A detailed account of neurological and medication status of the patients was given.

Study strengths

1. Control sample size is large.

2. Information on age, education, and geographic area is provided.

3. Means and standard deviations are reported.

Considerations regarding use of the study

1. Data were provided only as total for both hands.

Table 17.28. FT.26

	N	Age	Education	Gender	% Right Handed	WAIS FSIQ	Dominant Hand
Normal controls	30	20.0 (1.9)	13.7 (1.4)	21 M 9 F	90	117.1 (10.3)	51.3 (5.5)
Learning disabled	60	19.2 (2.0)	12.1 (1.1)	52 M 8 F	87	106.4 (9.5)	50.8 (6.3)
Brain damaged	20	25.0 (3.5)	12.7 (1.5)	15 M 5 F	95	93.0 (10.5)	29.7 (16.9)

Table 17.29. FT.27

	N	Age	Education	% Male	% Right Handed	WAIS FSIQ	Dominant Hand	Nondominant Hand
Controls	25	59.6 (9.0)	10.5 (3.3)	84	96	112.0 (11.0)	48.4 (7.7)	42.6 (6.0)
Patients	100	61.5 (7.4)	9.9 (3.1)	85	97	105.3 (12.8)	46.6 (10.0)	41.0 (8.1)

2. No information regarding gender.

3. Undifferentiated age range.

4. No information regarding handedness.

5. No information on exclusion criteria.

6. High educational level of controls (Table 17.30).

[FT.29] Kane, Parsons and Goldstein, 1985

The study compares performance of brain-damaged and control subjects recruited in Oklahoma and Pittsburgh on neuropsychological tests.

The brain-damaged group consisted of subjects with a wide range of brain pathology, which was established by neurological, neuroradiological, neurosurgical examinations or by history. This group included 27 head trauma patients, 12 vascular lesions cases, six dementia cases, and one neoplasm patient ranging from very mildly to severely impaired.

The control group consisted of medical and nonschizophrenic psychiatric patients. Groups were comparable with respect to age and education.

Study strengths

1. Sample composition is described in terms of age, education, and geographic area.

2. Adequate sample size.

3. Means and standard deviations are reported.

Considerations regarding use of the study

1. Procedures used to determine handedness were not described.

2. The data are reported in *T* scores rather than in actual number of taps.

3. The control group consisted of medical and psychiatric patients.

4. No information on gender.

5. Undifferentiated age range (Table 17.31).

[FT.30] Heaton, Grant and Matthews, 1986

The authors obtained data on 356 male and 197 female normal controls in Colorado, California, and Wisconsin as a part of an investigation into the effects of age, education, and sex on Halstead-Reitan Battery performance. Exclusion criteria were history of neurologic illness, significant head trauma, and substance abuse. Subjects ranged in age from 15 to 81, and years of education ranged from 0 to 20 years. The sample was divided into three age categories and three education categories.

Testing was conducted by trained technicians and all participants were judged to have expended their best effort on the task.

Study strengths

1. Large overall sample size and sizes of individual cells.

Table 17.30. FT.28

	N	Age	Education	Total for Both Hands
Normal controls	100	32.7 (13.5)	14.15 (2.84)	104.27 (12.03)
Relapsing-remitting MS	57	—	—	86.71 (13.73)
Chronic-progressive MS	43	—	—	67.12 (18.89)

Table 17.31. FT.29

	N	Age	Education	Dominant Hand	Nondominant Hand
Control	46	38.9	12.3	51.5°	51.5
		(11.3)	(2.6)	(10.1)	(8.5)
Brain damaged	44	39.7	11.6	41.7	44.5
		(13.5)	(2.0)	(10.3)	(9.1)

° The data are reported in T-scores.

2. Sample composition is well described. Information regarding sex, geographic area, age, and education is provided.

3. Generally adequate exclusion criteria.

4. Data are presented in age groupings and education groupings.

Considerations regarding use of the study

1. Standard deviations were not provided, which limits utility of the norms.

2. Procedures for assessment of hand dominance were not described.

3. Results were reported only for males.

4. Age groupings are quite large in terms of age ranges.

Other comments

1. The chapter provides a review of different studies exploring the relationship of neuropsychological test performance with age, education, and sex. The authors concluded that different sets of norms should be used for subjects at different age, educational levels, and gender when determining whether an individual's performance is normal or abnormal (Table 17.32).

[FT.31] Alekoumbides, Charter, Adkins and Seacat, 1987

The authors report data on 123 medical and psychiatric inpatients and outpatients without cerebral lesions or histories of alcoholism or cerebral contusion. The sample included 82 subjects not suffering from psychiatric illness and 32 neurotic and 9 psychotic subjects. In addition to psychiatry services, subjects were also drawn from medicine, neurology, spinal cord injury, and surgery units. Subjects' mean IQ was within the average range; means and

standard deviations for individual age-corrected subtest scores are also reported. This group, characterized as "normal subjects," was recruited from the patient population of a large general hospital and consisted mostly of inpatients. Their ages ranged from 19 to 82 years, and education ranged from 1 to 20 years. Seven percent of all subjects were black and all but one were male. Most subjects were urban residents. The data were collected in Southern California as part of a project on development of standardized scores corrected for age and education for the Halstead-Reitan Battery.

Study strengths

1. Sample composition is well described. Information regarding age, IQ, education, ethnicity, sex, occupational attainment, and geographic area is provided.

2. Sample size is large.

3. Regression equation for computation of age and education-corrected scores is provided.

4. Means and standard deviations are reported.

Table 17.32. FT.30

	N	Dominant Hand	Nondominant Hand
Age Subgroups			
<40	319	53.6	48.8
40–59	134	52.8	47.5
≥60	100	47.9	43.5
Education Subgroups			
<12	132	48.7	44.0
12–15	249	53.3	48.1
≥16	172	53.7	49.0

Table 17.33. FT.31

N	Age	Education	Preferred Hand	Nonpreferred Hand
123	46.9 (17.2)	11.4 (3.2)	43.4 (10.2)	38.5 (9.1)

Considerations regarding use of the study
1. Procedures used to determine hand preference were not described.
2. The sample was heterogeneous in terms of medical diagnoses. Psychiatric patients were included in this sample supposedly representative of "normal" subjects.
3. The wide age range is not partitioned by age groups (Table 17.33).

[FT.32] Bornstein, Paniak and O'Brien, 1987b

The data on a control sample (described in Bornstein, 1985 article) and a brain-damaged sample are reported. The brain-damaged sample is described as "comprised of patients with independent neurodiagnostic confirmation of damage to one or both of the cerebral hemispheres. The principal diagnoses included cerebral atrophy or Alzheimer's disease (24), stroke (21), ruptured aneurism (12), head injury (9), hydrocephalus (6), meningioma (5), glioma (5), multiple sclerosis (3), and a variety of other disorders (9)" (p.316).

Study strengths
1. Sample size is large.
2. Data are provided for males and females separately.
3. Cutoff scores are provided, as well as means and standard deviations.
4. Information on age, gender, and education is provided.

Considerations regarding use of the study
1. Procedures for determination of hand preference were not identified.
2. No exclusion criteria are identified.
3. Undifferentiated age range.

Other comments
1. Classification rates obtained with *conventional* cutoff scores presented in Russell et al. (1970) were examined.
2. The distribution of scores for the two groups was examined to determine the *optimal* cutoff score resulting in the best overall classification rates with the emphasis on accurate classification of normal subjects (Tables 17.34 and 17.35).

[FT.33] Bornstein, Baker, and Douglass, 1987a

The study assessed test–retest reliability of FTT over a period of 3 weeks. Subjects were 14 women and nine men without a positive history of neurological or psychiatric illness. Their age ranged from 17 to 52 (mean = 32.3 ± 10.3),

Table 17.34. FT.32a; Mean Number of Taps for Each Hand

	N	Age	Education	Gender	Preferred Hand	Nonpreferred Hand
Control	134	62.7 (4.3)	11.7 (2.9)	49 M 85 F		
Males					41.9 (5.8)	37.3 (5.4)
Females					33.0 (6.9)	32.7 (5.9)
Brain damaged	94	60.3 (3.8)	10.6 (4.1)	47 M 47 F		
Males					37.7 (11.9)	33.4 (11.0)
Females					30.4 (10.1)	27.7 (8.2)

Table 17.35. FT.32b; Classification Rates Based on Conventional and Optimal Cutoff Scores

		Percent Correctly Classified	
		Control	Brain-Damaged
Cut-off **Conventional**			
Males Preferred	<50	8	95
Males Nonpreferred	<44	10	79
Females Preferred	<46	2	95
Females Nonpreferred	<40	12	93
Optimal			
Males Preferred	≤32	92	29
Males Nonpreferred	≤31	86	45
Females Preferred	≤21	95	26
Females Nonpreferred	≤26	88	48

mean VIQ was 105.8 ± 10.8, and mean PIQ was 105.0 ± 10.5. Subjects were administered the Halstead-Reitan Battery in standard order both on initial testing and again three weeks later.

Study strengths

1. Sample composition was adequately described. Age, VIQ and PIQ, and gender statistics were provided.

2. Information on short-term (3 week) retest data were provided.

3. Minimally adequate exclusion criteria.

4. Means and standard deviations are reported.

Considerations regarding use of the study

1. Sample size is small; only 23 subjects were included.

2. Age range is wide: 17 to 52 years. The effect of age on test–retest change was not explored.

3. Educational levels were not specified.

4. Method of handedness assessment and proportion of right-handers were not identified. It is not clear whether the authors utilized dominant/nondominant comparisons or right/left comparisons.

5. Data are collapsed across genders (Table 17.36).

Means and standard deviations for raw score change over 3 weeks are as follows:

Right hand	−1.1 (± 5.3)
Left hand	0.9 (±2.7)

[FT.34] Russell, 1987

The study compares brain-damaged patients and controls. The brain-damaged sample represents typical neuropsychology patients as seen in V.A. Medical Centers in Miami and Cincinnati with a variety of neurological diagnoses. The control group consists of patients who were suspected of having a neurological condition but who had negative neurological findings. No other exclusion criteria are described.

Tests were administered and scored according to the standard directions given by Russell (1984) with some modification for the FTT test.

Study strengths

1. Information regarding IQ, education, ethnicity, sex, age, and geographic area is provided.

2. Samples are quite large.

3. Means and standard deviations are reported.

Table 17.36. FT.33

N = 23	Dominant	Nondominant
Test 1	44.8 (6.3)	42.5 (6.7)
Test 2 (3 weeks later)	43.5 (7.1)	43.0 (7.1)

4. Test administration procedures are reported.

Considerations regarding use of the study
1. The samples were not separated into age groups.
2. Performance was averaged for two hands.
3. Insufficient exclusion criteria.
4. High mean intellectual level.
5. Method for determining handedness is not reported.
6. Data are mostly collected on males and are collapsed across genders.

Other comments
1. The study explored test parameters for the Rennick Index of the Halstead-Reitan Battery (Table 17.37).

[FT.35] Thompson, Heaton, Matthews and Grant, 1987

The article presents a percentage of 426 normal subjects (279 males and 147 females) scoring in lateralized lesion range using Golden's (1978) guidelines. *Dominant hemisphere dysfunction* was defined as the superiority of nonpreferred hand performance over preferred hand performance. *Nondominant hemisphere dysfunction* was identified when preferred hand performance was at least 20% better than nonpreferred hand performance.

Lateral preference type was assessed based on subjects' performance on the Reitan-Klove Lateral Dominance Exam and the Miles ABC Test of Ocular Dominance (Reitan & Wolfson, 1985). The following groups were identified:

1. *All Right*—subjects who wrote with their right hand and manifested right lateral preference on all hand, eye, and foot measures.
2. *Mixed Right*—subjects who wrote with their right hand but manifested left preference on one or more other hand, eye, or foot measures.
3. *Left*—left-handed subjects.

Intermanual percent difference scores were calculated as preferred hand minus nonpreferred hand divided by preferred hand.

Subjects' mean age was 40.59 years (SD = 18.27) and mean education was 13.15 years (SD = 3.49). They had been screened for history of head trauma, neurological illness, substance abuse, serious psychiatric illness, and peripheral injuries that might affect test performance.

Study strengths
1. A large sample size was used.
2. Lateral preference was thoroughly assessed and three groups were identified.
3. Intermanual differences and a percentage of subjects scoring in the lateralized lesion range were reported.
4. Adequate exclusion criteria.
5. Information on age, education, and gender is reported.

Considerations regarding use of the study
1. Means and SDs for each group were not reported.
2. Data are presented for a wide age range not separated into age groups, which precludes consideration of the effect of age on intermanual differences.

Table 17.37. FT.34

	N	Gender	Age	Education	Race	WAIS FSIQ	Average No. of Taps for Both Hands
Control	155	148 M 7 F	46.19 (12.86)	12.29 (3.00)	147 C° 8 A 0 N	111.9	48.48 (5.70)
Brain-damaged	577	546 M 31 F	—	—	520 C 51 A 6 N	93.4	37.10 (11.64)

°C—Caucasian; A—Afro-American; N—other.

Table 17.38. FT.35°

Groups	N	Dominant Hemisphere Dysfunction	Nondominant Hemisphere Dysfunction	Intermanual Percent Difference Scores
All Right	167	10.18	17.96	10.8 (9.4)
Mixed Right	226	12.05	10.27	8.3 (8.3)
Left	33	18.18	0.00	5.2 (5.9)
Total	426	11.79	12.50	9.0 (8.7)

°The table provides percent of subjects scoring in the lateralized dysfunction range.

Other comments

The authors concluded that age, education, and gender were not significantly related to intermanual difference scores (Table 17.38).

[FT.36] van den Burg, van Zomeren Minderhoud, Prange, and Meijer, 1987

The study compares group of mildly disabled and clinically stable patients with multiple sclerosis and demographically matched controls in northern Holland. Only those MS patients whose DSS scores did not exceed 4, who had no other neurological deficits, and who had no relapse reported in the last 2 months were included in the study (mean DSS score 2.6 ±.9, length of illness 8.7 ±6.2 years). The MS sample consisted of 19 patients with a relapsing-remitting course, 14 patients with a history of bouts with remissions but whose handicap had become gradually progressive, and seven patients with a primary progressive course.

The total number of taps in three 10-second trials for each hand constitutes the total score.

Study strengths

1. Samples were described in terms of gender, age, education, and geographic area.
2. The administration procedure is identified.
3. Means and standard deviations are reported.

4. Sample size approximates .50.

Considerations regarding use of the study

1. Samples are not separated into age intervals. Age ranges are not identified.
2. Subjects' handedness was not determined.
3. Data reporting is not standard: totals for both hands over three trials are reported.
4. Exclusion criteria for controls are not specified.
5. Data are collapsed across genders (Table 17.39).

[FT.37] Russell and Starkey, 1993

This study describes the standardization sample used by the authors in their manual introducing the Halstead Russell Neuropsychological Evaluation System (HRNES) and addressing its psychometric properties. The normative sample consisted of veterans treated at Cincinnati V.A. Hospital between 1968 and 1971 and the Miami V.A. Medical Center between 1971 and 1989. All subjects received neurological examinations. Those subjects who were administered the Halstead tests and the WAIS or WAIS-R were included in the study. Nine percent of the sample were representatives of minority groups.

The total sample was divided into a comparison group and a brain-damaged group. The

Table 17.39. FT.36

	N	Gender	Age	Education	Taps for Both Hands Over 3 Trials
Normal controls	40	16 M	37.4	5.0	339
		24 F	(11.9)	(1.2)	(38)
Multiple Sclerosis	40	14 M	37.7	5.0	295
		26 F	(11.5)	(1.1)	(41)

comparison group included "normal" individuals. No subject in this group had a diagnosis of CNS pathology. Presenting symptoms for the majority of these subjects were neurosis with memory or somatic complaints, or personality disorders with episodes of explosive behavior.

The brain-damaged group was obtained through referrals from the neurology, neurosurgery, and psychiatry departments and from other sections of the hospital. Left-handed patients were not included in this group if they had lateralized lesions. Only those patients whose brain lesion was well corroborated by the follow-up review of the medical records were included in this group.

Patients diagnosed with schizophrenia or severe depression requiring hospitalization, as well as those with evidence of systemic vascular disease, were not included in the sample.

The statistics are reported for four groups of patients: comparison, left-hemisphere damage, right hemisphere damage, and diffuse brain damage.

Study strengths
1. The sample composition is identified in terms of age, education, ethnicity, geographic area, and gender.
2. Sample sizes are large.

3. Means and standard deviations are reported.

Considerations regarding use of the study
1. The data were reported for males only.
2. Procedures used to determine hand preference were not described. Percentage of right-handed subjects in nonlateralized groups was not reported.
3. Classification of subjects in the comparison group as normal is questionable, since they had been suspected of having neurological conditions and were referred for neurological evaluation which yielded negative results.
4. Undifferentiated age range.

Other comments
Test scores can be corrected for age and IQ and converted into scale scores to facilitate comparison with other tests (Table 17.40).

CONCLUSIONS

The large number of studies focusing on the Finger Tapping Test's psychometric properties reflect its wide clinical use. In fact, a recent survey of neuropsychologists identified the Finger Tapping Test as one of the two neuropsychological tests (along with the Category Test) most

Table 17.40. FT.37°

	N	Age	Education	Race°°	Dominant Hand	Nondominant Hand
Comparison	176	45.1 (13.0)	12.5 (2.8)	165 W 11 B 0 N	45.2 (8.9)	39.5 (7.9)
Left hemisphere	110	46.2 (15.5)	11.8 (3.2)	97 W 12 B 1 N	29.4 (22.0)	42.4 (9.7)
Right hemisphere	117	50.5 (14.4)	11.8 (3.1)	112 W 5 B 0 N	44.5 (11.8)	23.8 (19.2)
Diffuse	319	47.8 (13.8)	11.8 (3.3)	283 W 32 B 4 N	41.1 (12.4)	36.4 (10.9)

°The above table provides data for males only; °°W—white; B—black; N—other.

frequently used in the assessment of adults (Sellers & Nadler, 1992).

A review of the FTT research suggests considerable consistency in the data across different studies. A decreasing rate of tapping as a function of advancing age and lower levels of education is well demonstrated. Gender differences, with males outperforming females, are also unequivocal. In addition, the literature review suggests that test performance is highly affected by disruption of sensory or motor tracts and by peripheral damage to the upper extremities. Because finger tapping test performance is affected by many factors, the interpretation of tapping speed as indicative of cortical dysfunction should be made with great caution. Following recommendations by Bornstein (1986b), the accuracy of FTT interpretive conclusions must be confirmed by findings from other motor and nonmotor tasks.

The importance of clinical judgement, rather than "rule of thumb," is especially apparent in view of the controversy surrounding cutoffs for brain impairment. Unacceptably high false-positive rates with the use of the original Halstead cutoffs warrant further research directed at the formulation of revised cutoff scores assuring an optimal balance of sensitivity and specificity, which would differ for various demographic groups. Similarly, an issue of intermanual differences remains highly disputed. A 10% dominant hand superiority criterion is clearly consistent with the *average* performance across the studies presented above. However, a wide range of *individual differences* documented in numerous studies (including high rates of reversal in intermanual defference) suggests that great caution should be taken in the interpretation of dominant–nondominant hand comparisons.

Despite the large body of empirical studies exploring the psychometric properties of the FTT accumulated to date, some aspects of FTT performance are not sufficiently addressed. For example, normative data for older age groups are scarce. Test–retest concordance should be further explored to assess the magnitude of practice effect and to address the issue of test reliability over different interprobe intervals. Similarly, very few studies provide norms for left-handers. Investigation of left-handed groups is a challenging task due to the great variability in cerebral dominance among left-handed individuals, which obscures lateralization assumptions in the interpretation of test results. Since FTT interpretation is based on lateralization assumptions, it is of the utmost importance to report the criteria for assessment of handedness, cutoff scores for subject selection on the basis of their handedness pattern, and the number of left-handed individuals in the sample, if they are included.

18

Grip Strength Test (Hand Dynamometer)

BRIEF HISTORY OF THE TEST

The Smedley Hand Dynamometer or Grip Strength Test is a part of the Lateral Dominance Examination added by Reitan to the Halstead battery. It is a measure of pure motor ability (Russell & Starkey, 1993). According to Spreen and Strauss (1998), this test measures strength or intensity of voluntary grip movements of each hand. The Dynamometer is available from Lafayette Instruments, PAR Inc., and the Reitan Neuropsychological Laboratory (see Appendix 1 for ordering instructions).

There are several variations in administration and scoring of the test that should be taken into consideration when interpreting the norms. The majority of authors refer to the standard description of the procedures specified by Reitan and Wolfson (1985). The most common procedure is as follows: Subjects take the test while standing. After the length of the stirrup is adjusted to the size of the subject's hand, one practice trial is allowed. Subjects grip the dynamometer with the arm fully extended and pointing toward the floor. The score is the average of two consecutive trials within 5 kg for each hand, alternating hands after each trial, starting with the dominant hand. Ten-second rests are allowed between the trials.

Instructions provided by the Lafayette Instrument Company, which manufactures the Dynamometer, allow three trials with each hand, alternating right and left hands with a 10-second rest between trials. Only the highest record for each hand is used in subsequent computations. Additional information on the administration of this test is provided in Lezak (1995, pp. 684–685) and Spreen & Strauss (1998).

The grip strength is most commonly reported in kilograms averaged across all trials for each hand. Some studies, however, provide data allowing conversion of raw scores into other units which facilitate comparison between different tests. For example, a normative system for the expanded HRB developed by Heaton et al. (1991) converts raw scores into scaled score equivalents which can be further converted into T scores adjusted for age, education, and gender.

Performance on the Hand Dynamometer Test reflects the integrity of the motor strip (Swiercinsky, 1978). Sensitivity of this test to brain dysfunction has been demonstrated in many clinical comparison studies (Bornstein, 1986b; Dodrill, 1978b; Strauss & Wada, 1988). The Hand Dynamometer allows comparison of grip strength between both hands and therefore is sensitive to a lateralized lesion in the hemisphere contralateral to the hand demonstrating deviant performance. Generally, the preferred hand is expected to be 10% stronger than the nonpreferred hand (Reitan & Wolfson, 1985), with intermanual differences in excess of 20% being suggestive of brain impairment (Golden, 1978). Use of this criterion in normative studies, however, yielded unacceptably high rates of false positive misclassifications, which is especially true for left-handed individuals (Bornstein, 1986b; Koffler & Zehler, 1985; Thompson et al., 1987). The large number of misclassifications is due to a high rate of variability in intermanual differences reported in the above studies, which obscures interpretative accuracy of the results.

Bornstein (1986b) suggests that in the evaluation of left hemisphere lesions, interpretive consistency of performance on motor tasks has to be supported by nonmotor tasks and by additional instruments measuring motor performance. In this study, he evaluated the pattern of motor performance on three motor tests (Finger Tapping Test, Grooved Pegboard Test, and the Hand Dynamometer) which were administered to normal and unilateral brain lesion samples. Interestingly, a large degree of variability was observed across these intermanual measures, whereby "a high percentage (approximately 25 percent) of the normal sample obtained scores more than one standard deviation from the control mean on a single measure" (p. 719). Thus, the author has emphasized the importance of consistency in performance pattern across tasks, rather than use of a "rigid application of 'cookbook' formulas or 'rules of thumb'" (p. 723) in the test interpretation.

High reliability of the Hand Dynamometer is well documented, with coefficients ranging from .79 to .94 across different studies (see Lezak, 1995, p. 685).

RELATIONSHIP BETWEEN HAND DYNAMOMETER PERFORMANCE AND DEMOGRAPHIC FACTORS

Performance on the Hand Dynamometer varies as a function of several demographic variables; however, it is affected by gender differences more than any other motor test (Heaton et al., 1991). Superiority of males in test performance is documented by Fromm-Auch and Yeudall (1983), Koffler and Zehler (1985), and Yeudall et al. (1987). Dodrill (1979) related gender differences on the tests that have a strong motor component to hand size. Effect of gender on intermanual differences is questionable; Ernst

(1988) reported negative findings, whereas Bornstein (1986c) found gender-related differences in intermanual ratios.

The effect of age on test performance is reported by Bornstein (1986a), Fromm-Auch and Yeudall (1983), Heaton et al. (1996), Koffler and Zehler (1985), and Yeudall et al. (1987), with equivocal findings regarding the timing of the onset of decline in grip strength (after age 40 vs. 60). Effect of education on test performance is questionable: Bornstein (1985) found a considerable effect, whereas Ernst (1988) and Heaton et al. (1991) reported negative findings. Spreen and Strauss (1991) relate Hand Dynamometer performance to subjects' height and weight among other variables. Moffoot et al. (1994) relate grip strength to affective state with lower strength in patients suffering from major depression with melancholia.

METHOD FOR EVALUATING THE NORMATIVE REPORTS

Our review of the Hand Dynamometer literature located six normative reports and 12 clinical studies reporting control data for grip strength. In order to adequately evaluate the Hand Dynamometer data, seven key criterion variables were deemed critical. The first five of these relate to *subject* variables, and the remaining two dimensions refer to *procedural* issues.

Subject Variables

Age Group Intervals

This criterion reflects grouping of the data into limited age intervals.

Gender

Given the strong association between gender and test performance, grip strength data must be stratified by gender.

Sample Size

Fifty cases has been considered adequate sample size. Although this criterion is somewhat arbitrary, a large number of studies suggest that data based on small sample sizes are highly influenced by individual differences and do not provide a reliable estimate of the population mean.

Sample Composition Description

This criterion reflects adequate information regarding subject selection criteria, health status, etc.

Description of Hand Preference Assessment

In order to address the issue of lateralization in test performance, assessment procedures for hand preference should be fully described.

Procedural Variables

Description of Administration Procedures

Administration of the Hand Dynamometer differs among studies. Detailed description of administration procedures allows selection of the most appropriate norms or to make corrections in intepretation of the data to account for deviation in administration procedure.

Data Reporting

In order to facilitate interpretation of the data, group mean and standard deviation should be presented at a minimum.

SUMMARY OF THE STATUS OF THE NORMS

Information presented in the studies reporting data for the Hand Dynamometer differs considerably across studies. Some of these differences will be summarized below.

In addition to normative studies based on "normal" samples, there are a number of clinical comparison studies that explore differences in test performance between clinical groups and "normal control" groups (which are sometimes matched on demographic characteristics). Unfortunately, "normal control" groups are frequently comprised of medical or psychiatric patients. These samples cannot be considered truly "normal" due to possible effects of their illnesses and medication intake on the test performance. The clinical groups reported in these studies represent a wide range of neuro-

logical and psychiatric diagnoses (most often brain-injured patients).

Administration and scoring procedures vary among studies. The majority of the authors report data in kilograms, averaged across all trials for each hand; however, some studies present data in *T* scores or provide scores for the dominant hand only. Such deviations from the standard method of data reporting are identified in our review of the normative data in the context of each pertinent table. In addition to providing normative data for each hand, several studies report the proportion of subjects falling in the impaired range or rates of intermanual differences.

Several authors stratify their samples by age, education, and/or gender. Procedures for assessment of handedness are thoroughly described in some studies. Furthermore, some authors divide their samples into groups based on subjects' handedness pattern.

The majority of studies recruit mostly young and middle-aged subjects. Only a few studies present data for elderly individuals. Several studies provide test–retest data over varying interprobe intervals ranging from 14 weeks to 6 months.

Among all the clinical studies available in the literature, we selected for review those studies based on large, well-defined samples or studies that offer interesting clinical comparisons or some aspects of information which are not routinely reported.

Table 18.1 summarizes information provided in the studies described in this chapter.

SUMMARIES OF THE STUDIES

Normative Studies

[D.1] Fromm-Auch and Yeudall, 1983

The authors obtained data on 193 Canadian subjects (111 male, 82 female) recruited through posted advertisements and personal contacts. Subjects' mean education was 14.8 years and mean FSIQ was 119.1. Participants are described as "nonpsychiatric" and "nonneurological." Handedness was determined by the writing hand: 83.4% of the sample were right-handed. Strength of handedness was de-

Table 18.1. D.L; Locator Table for the Hand Dynamometer

Study[*]	Age[**]	N	Sample Composition	IQ,[**] Education	Country/ Location
D.1 Fromm-Auch & Yeudall, 1983 page 411	15–17 18–23 24–32 33–40 41–64	17 44 31 12 4	Normal volunteers 111 M, 82 F	Education 14.8 WAIS-R FSIQ 119.1	Alberta, Canada
D.2 Bornstein, 1985 page 414	20–39 40–59 60–69	365	178 M, 187 F. 91.5% R-handed paid volunteers free of neurological or psychiatric illness	Education 12.3(2.7) Separate data for <HS, ≥HS	Western Canada
D.3 Koffler & Zehler, 1985 page 415	20–29 30–39 40–49 50–59 60–77	206	Normal sample, 100 M, 106 F, was stratified by age and gender	—	—
D.4 Yeudall et al., 1987 page 416	15–20 21–25 26–30 31–40	62 73 48 42	Normal adults: 127 M, 98 F, sample is stratified by age and gender	FSIQ 111.75 109.79 113.95 116.09	Alberta, Canada
D.5 Ernst, 1988 page 417	65–75	85	Normal elderly: 39 M, 46F	Education 10.4 (3.1)	Queensland, Australia
D.6 Heaton et al., 1991 page 418	42.1 (16.8) groups: 20–34 35–39 40–44 45–49 50–54 55–59 60–64 65–69 70–74 75–80	486	Volunteers: urban and rural. Data collected over 15 years through multi-center collaborative efforts. Strict exclusion criteria. 65% M Data are presented in T-score equivalents for M and F separately in 10 age groupings by 6 educational groupings	Education 13.6 (3.5) FSIQ 113.8(12.3) groups 6–8 9–11 12 13–15 16–17 18+	California, Washington, Texas, Oklahoma, Wisconsin, Illinois, Michigan, New York, Virginia, Massachusetts, Canada
D.7 Matarazzo et al., 1974 page 419	21–28 X = 24	29	Normal young men; Patrolmen applicants	12–16 FSIQ 118	Oregon
D.8 Wiens & Matarazzo, 1977 page 420	23.6 24.8	24 24	Normal young men divided into two groups	FSIQ 117.5 118.3	Oregon
D.9 Dodrill, 1978b page 420	M age for each group = 41.1	 25 25 25 25	Performance was compared for four groups: Control R hemisphere damage L hemisphere damage Bilateral brain damage	M education for each group = 10.7	Washington
D.10 Dodrill, 1979 page 421	 27.51 27.49 24.85 24.89	 47 47 47 47	Non-neurological sample: males females Neurological sample: males females	Education 12.47 12.36 11.74 11.76	Washington

continued

Table 18.1. *(Continued)*

Study[*]	Age[**]	N	Sample Composition	IQ,[**] Education	Country/ Location
D.11 Rounsaville et al., 1982 page 421	27.9	72	Opiate addicts	Education 11.5	—
	29.2	60	Epileptic patients	11.8	
	24.9	29	Normal controls	11.2	
		59	Opiate addicts were retested in 6 months		
D.12 Yeudall et al., 1982 page 422	14.8	99	Delinquent adolescents	FSIQ 95.3	Alberta, Canada
	14.5	46	Nondelinquent adolescents	117.1	
D.13 Prigatano et al., 1983 page 423	61.5 (9.9)	100	Hypoxemic patients with COPD. Matched controls	FSIQ 105.3 (12.8)	Oklahoma City and Winnipeg
	59.6 (9.0)	25		112.0 (11.0)	
D.14 Heaton et al., 1985 page 423	37.38 (8.28)	100	25 M, 75 F; multiple sclerosis patients, among them 57 relapsing-remitting course, 43 chronic-progressive form. Mean disease duration 9.36 years (5.86)	Education 13.71 (2.33)	Denver
	32.67 (13.5)	100	79 M, 21 F Control Ss with no neurological illness, head trauma, or substance abuse	14.15 (2.84)	
D.15 Kane et al., 1985 page 424	39.7 (13.5)	46	The study compares brain damaged and control Ss. The latter group consists of medical and non-schizophrenic psychiatric patients	Education 11.6 (2.0)	Oklahoma City and Pittsburgh
	38.9 (11.3)	43		12.3 (2.6)	
D.16 Heaton et al., 1986 page 424	15–81 39.3 (17.5)	207 (UC) 181 (UCSD) 165 (UW)	356 M, 197 F. Normal Ss with no history of neurological illness, head trauma, or substance abuse, 7.2% L-handed	Education 0–20 13.3 (3.4)	University of Colorado, University of California at San Diego, University of Wisconsin
D.17 Thompson et al., 1987 page 425	40.59 (18.27)	426	279 M, 147 F. Normal Ss	Education 13.15 (3.49)	—
D.18 Russell & Starkey, 1993 page 426			Norms are collected from standardization sample for the HRNES manual. Ss are male VA patients, divided into 4 groups:	Education	Cincinnati and Miami
	45.0 (12.9)	175	comparison	12.5	
	46.4 (15.5)	98	L hemisphere damage	12.0	
	50.5 (14.3)	106	R hemisphere damage	11.9	
	47.6 (13.7)	299	Diffuse brain damage	11.9	

[*]The study number corresponds to the number provided in the text of the chapter.

[*]Age column and IQ/education column contain information regarding range and/or mean and standard deviation for the whole sample and/or separate groups, whichever information is provided by the authors.

termined by the Annett Handedness Question-naire (1970). Means and standard deviations for each hand are reported for the entire sample and for five age groups stratified by age.

Study strengths

1. Sample composition is described in terms of gender, IQ, education, geographic area, and recruitment procedures.

2. Some psychiatric and neurological exclusion criteria were used.

3. The large overall sample size and some individual cells approximate Ns of 50.

4. Subjects' handedness was established.

5. Normative data were presented for the entire sample and separately for different age and gender groups.

6. Means, standard deviations, and ranges are reported.

Considerations regarding use of the study

1. Sample size for the age group 41–64 is very small.

Other comments

1. The article provides a summary of previously published normative data.

2. Calculation of the educational level included technical or vocational training.

3. The authors concluded that pronounced effect of gender was seen on all motor tests with females appearing weaker and slower than males. The relationship between age and performance appears to be curvilinear for both genders with the peak of performance in the 33–40-year-old age range.

4. The data were collected in Alberta, Canada (Table 18.2).

[D.2] Bornstein, 1985

The author collected data on 365 Canadian individuals (178 males and 187 females) recruited through posted notices on college campuses and unemployment offices, newspaper ads, and senior-citizen groups. Subjects were paid for their participation. Participants ranged in age from 18 to 69 (Mean = 43.3 ± 17.1) and had completed between 5 and 20 years of education (Mean = 12.3 ± 2.7); 91.5% of the sample were right-handed. No other demographic data or exclusion criteria are reported.

Means and standard deviations are reported for each hand. The sample was stratified by age group (20–39, 40–59, 60–69), level of education (<HS, ≥HS), and gender. Normative data were presented for the preferred and nonpreferred hands for each demographic group separately, as well as for different combinations of demographic strata. Individual group sample sizes ranged form 13 to 86. Hand preference was determined as the hand used for signing the consent form. Subjects were recruited from

Table 18.2. D.1; Normative Data for the Sample Stratified by Age and Sex

Age	N	Preferred Hand			Nonpreferred Hand		
		M	SD	Range	M	SD	Range
Males							
15–17	17	38.0°	8.4	22.2–51.0	35.8	9.6	21.0–57.5
18–23	43	49.7	9.7	30.0–71.2	46.6	9.9	26.7–73.0
24–32	31	51.8	8.1	37.0–65.5	49.6	7.2	30.5–66.0
33–40	12	52.9	8.3	41.0–67.0	51.2	7.9	36.2–58.7
41–64	4	44.5	10.9	30.5–57.0	47.9	11.9	32.0–58.7
Age	N	M	SD	Range	M	SD	Range
Females							
15–17	15	28.1	5.0	21.0–37.5	26.3	5.2	17.8–33.5
18–23	29	28.8	7.8	8.5–43.8	26.4	6.2	13.5–38.0
24–32	24	34.4	9.2	20.5–64.7	30.2	6.8	20.5–49.5
33–40	6	27.7	3.2	23.0–31.5	28.6	3.1	25.2–33.5
41–64	6	28.0	6.2	18.7–37.5	24.1	6.8	16.7–36.5

°Kilogram average of two trials.

Table 18.3. D.2a; Data for the Whole Sample Stratified by Age, Education, and Gender

Age	Education	No. Males	No. Females	Preferred Hand	Nonpreferred Hand
By Age					
20–39	13.0 (2.3)	107	64	43.1 (12.1)	40.1 (11.4)
40–59	11.9 (2.8)	31	66	34.0 (9.7)	31.5 (10.4)
60–69	11.8 (2.9)	40	57	32.0 (10.0)	29.4 (9.2)
By Education					
48.5 (16.6)	<HS	51	57	35.7 (11.9)	33.7 (11.9)
41.1 (16.8)	≥HS	127	130	38.8 (12.1)	35.8 (11.5)
By Gender					
39.2 (17.2)	12.4 (2.9)	178 Males		47.5 (9.0)	44.3 (8.7)
47.3 (16.1)	12.2 (2.5)	187 Females		28.8 (6.2)	26.5 (6.2)

the general population of a large city in western Canada.

Study strengths

1. Very large overall sample size and several individual cells approximate *N*s of 50.

2. Stratification of the data by age, sex, and educational level.

3. This dataset is unique in that it reports data for subjects with less than a high school education.

4. Information on recruitment procedures and geographic area is provided.

5. Method for determining handedness is specified.

6. Means and standard deviations are reported.

Considerations regarding use of the study

1. Individual sample sizes of some cells were small. It is unclear whether the youngest age included in the study was 18 or 20.

2. The lack of any reported exclusion criteria (Tables 18.3 and 18.4).

[D.3] Koffler and Zehler, 1985

In this study, 206 normal (by self-report) adults, aged 20 to 77, were administered the Hand Dynamometer to obtain normative data. The sample was stratified by age and gender. A Stoelting Dynamometer was used and Reitan's procedure of utilizing the highest reading for each hand was followed. After adjustment for the subjects' hand size, two alternating trials were given, beginning with the dominant hand.

Table 18.4. D.2b; Data for Separate Demographic Groups Stratified by Age, Education and Gender

	Male						Female					
	<HS			≥HS			<HS			≥HS		
Age Group	N	M	SD	N	M	SD	N	M	SD	N	M	SD
Preferred hand												
20–39	21	50.8	11.5	86	49.9	8.4	13	32.7	8.7	50	31.0	5.4
40–59	13	39.8	6.0	17	48.2	7.3	22	27.7	5.9	43	29.8	5.8
60–69	16	38.7	5.9	22	44.5	5.6	22	25.6	5.3	34	25.0	4.9
Nonpreferred hand												
20–39		47.7	11.7		46.4	7.6		31.2	8.0		28.7	5.0
40–59		38.2	6.5		46.4	9.1		24.9	6.7		26.9	5.4
60–69		37.2	5.4		39.3	5.5		24.0	6.0		22.8	4.8

Determination of hand dominance was based on self-report; 87% of subjects were right-handed, 9.7% left-handed, and 3.3% reported mixed dominance.

Study strengths
1. Administration procedure is well described.
2. Data are presented by age and gender.
3. Method for determining handedness is specified.
4. Overall sample size is adequate, though sizes of individual cells are low.
5. Means and standard deviations are reported.

Considerations regarding use of the study
1. Demographic characteristics of the sample are only cursorily described.
2. Medical exclusion criteria are unclear.

Other comments
1. Authors infer that greater strength of grip is demonstrated by males at all ages. Authors caution that use of commonly accepted criteria for detection of lateralized motor dysfunction leads to a large number of false-positive errors (Table 18.5).

[D.4] Yeudall, Reddon, Gill and Stefanyk, 1987

The authors obtained data on 225 Canadian subjects recruited from posted advertisements in workplaces and personal solicitations. The participants included meat packers, postal workers, transit employees, hospital lab technicians, secretaries, ward aides, student interns, student nurses, and summer students. In addition, high school teachers identified for participation average students in grades 10 through 12. The subjects (127 males and 98 females) did not report any history of forensic involvement, head injury, neurological insult, prenatal or birth complications, psychiatric problems, or substance abuse. Handedness was determined by the writing hand. Data were gathered by experienced technicians who "motivated the subjects to achieve maximum performance" partially through the promise of detailed explanations of their test performance. Standard test administration procedures were used.

Table 18.5. D.3

Age/Gender	N	Dominant Hand	Nondominant Hand
20–29			
Men	41	53.8 (7.8)	50.3 (7.4)
Women	39	33.3 (4.7)	30.5 (4.4)
30–39			
Men	23	55.4 (7.1)	53.3 (7.4)
Women	25	33.7 (6.2)	31.1 (5.6)
40–49			
Men	13	50.2 (5.3)	49.2 (7.8)
Women	14	30.7 (5.5)	28.7 (4.3)
50–59			
Men	12	44.3 (5.4)	44.8 (5.8)
Women	13	28.8 (3.6)	25.3 (3.8)
60–77			
Men	11	45.5 (5.4)	41.3 (6.7)
Women	15	28.3 (6.3)	23.5 (5.2)

The results are presented for the whole sample and stratified by age and gender.

Study strengths
1. Large sample size and individual cells approximate Ns of 50.
2. The data are stratified by age and gender.
3. Data availability for a 15-to-20 year-old age group.
4. Adequate medical and psychiatric exclusion criteria.
5. The administration procedure is well described; standard procedure was used.
6. Information regarding education, IQ, sex, occupation, recruitment procedures, and geographic area is provided.
7. Method for determining handedness was specified.
8. Means and standard deviations are reported.

Other comments

1. IQ was measured by the WAIS and WAIS-R. WAIS IQ scores were equated to the WAIS-R IQ scores by linear equating.

2. Correlations of the Dynamometer scores with age and education were 0.25 and 0.16 for the preferred hand and 0.27 and 0.17 for the nonpreferred hand. Effect of sex on subjects' performance was also explored. The authors concluded that age and sex effects were significant for both hands. Therefore they suggest using sex norms stratified by age (Table 18.6).

[D.5] Ernst, 1988

The author collected data on 85 Brisbane (Australian) uncompensated volunteers, aged 65 to 75, recruited from the Queensland State electoral roll. All but one participant were Caucasian

Table 18.6. D.4

Age Group	N	Age	Education	WAIS-R FSIQ	% Right-Handed	Preferred Hand	Nonpreferred Hand
Norms for the Entire Sample (N = 225)							
15–20	62	17.76 (1.96)	12.16 (1.75)	111.75 (10.16)	79.03	37.22 (10.68)	34.57 (10.20)
21–25	73	22.70 (1.40)	14.82 (1.88)	109.79 (9.97)	86.30	40.33 (14.33)	37.74 (13.81)
26–30	48	28.06 (1.52)	15.50 (2.65)	113.95 (10.61)	89.58	45.20 (11.59)	42.19 (11.91)
31–40	42	34.38 (2.46)	16.50 (3.11)	116.09 (9.51)	90.48	45.22 (13.47)	42.82 (12.60)
15–40	225	24.66 (6.16)	14.55 (2.78)	112.25 (10.25)	85.78	41.42 (13.01)	38.76 (12.61)
Age Group	N	Age	Education	WAIS-R FSIQ	% Right-Handed	Preferred Hand	Nonpreferred Hand
Norms for Females (N = 98)							
15–20	30	17.73 (1.84)	12.10 (1.52)	110.32 (10.64)	73.33	30.20 (5.56)	28.07 (4.52)
21–25	36	22.83 (1.54)	14.53 (1.99)	107.28 (9.14)	83.33	29.79 (6.92)	27.22 (6.04)
26–30	16	28.69 (1.25)	14.94 (2.32)	113.10 (11.37)	93.75	33.88 (7.65)	30.25 (6.35)
31–40	16	33.88 (2.53)	16.19 (2.29)	114.27 (11.32)	87.50	32.98 (10.10)	30.10 (6.62)
15–40	98	24.03 (5.95)	14.12 (2.43)	110.19 (10.46)	82.65	31.09 (7.33)	28.43 (5.82)
Age Group	N	Age	Education	WAIS-R FSIQ	% Right-Handed	Preferred Hand	Nonpreferred Hand
Norms for Males (N = 127)							
15–20	32	17.78 (2.09)	12.22 (1.96)	113.00 (9.72)	84.38	43.58 (10.25)	40.46 (10.37)
21–25	37	22.57 (1.26)	15.11 (1.74)	112.30 (10.27)	89.19	51.49 (11.36)	48.56 (10.83)
26–30	32	27.75 (1.57)	15.78 (2.79)	114.38 (10.43)	87.50	51.05 (8.55)	48.35 (9.07)
31–40	26	34.69 (2.41)	16.69 (3.55)	117.31 (8.21)	92.31	52.28 (9.57)	50.15 (8.74)
15–40	127	25.15 (6.29)	14.87 (2.99)	113.87 (9.83)	88.19	49.49 (10.53)	46.75 (10.46)

and all but one was right-handed. Thirty-nine were males and 46 were females. The sample was derived from 518 names randomly selected based on date of birth and residence. These potential subjects were sent information regarding the project and a health questionnaire and asked to participate. Individuals with histories of substance abuse, head trauma, stroke, psychiatric hospitalization, or epilepsy were excluded. A large minority of the subjects (42%) had a history of at least one treated and/or well-controlled chronic illness (10 heart disease, 17 hypertension, five asthma, two emphysema, 10 hypo- or hyperthyroidism, two diabetes). A majority of subjects were currently using prescribed medications (55%) for the above chronic diseases or as a hypertensive preventative. Mean educational level of 10.4 was comparable to the modal educational level for that age range according to the Australian Bureau of Statistics. A wide range of occupations was represented, including unskilled laborers, homemakers, business persons, teachers, etc.

Study strengths

1. Ethnic characteristics, sex, education, handedness, age, recruitment procedures, and geographic area are reported.

2. The authors concluded that significant sex differences were demonstrated for the Dynamometer test for both hands. Therefore, the results are presented separately for males and females.

3. The ratio of dominant/nondominant hands was computed for the entire sample to indicate the strength of lateralization.

4. Relatively large sample size for constricted age range.

5. Good medical and psychiatric exclusion criteria.

6. Means and standard deviations are reported.

Considerations regarding use of the study

1. Procedures used to determine hand preference were not described.

2. Approximately half of the subjects had at least one chronic illness, and over half were taking prescribed medications.

Other comments

1. The authors concluded that, on the average, for their elderly sample, superiority of the preferred hand was approximately 10%. No sex differences were demonstrated on intermanual ratio for grip strength (Table 18.7).

[D.6] Heaton, Grant, and Matthews, 1991

The authors provide data from 486 (378 in the base sample and 108 in the validation sample) urban and rural subjects recruited in several states (California, Washington, Colorado, Texas, Oklahoma, Wisconsin, Illinois, Michigan, New York, Virginia, and Massachusetts) and Canada. Data were collected over a 15-year period through multicenter collaborative efforts.

Sixty-five percent of the sample were males. Mean age for the total sample was 42.06 ± 16.8, and mean educational level was 13.6 ± 3.5. Mean FSIQ, VIQ, and PIQ were 113.8 ± 12.3, 113.9 ± 13.8, and 111.9 ± 11.6, respectively. Exclusion criteria were history of learning disability, neurologic disease, illnesses affecting brain function, significant head trauma, significant psychiatric disturbance (e.g., schizophrenia), and alcohol or other substance abuse.

Table 18.7. D.5

	N	Age	Education	% Right-Handed	Dominant Hand	Nondominant Hand	Dominant/ Nondominant Ratio
Total	85	70.0 (2.6)	10.4 (3.1)	99			1.1 (0.2)
Males	39				41.7 (6.2)	38.5 (5.1)	
Females	46				26.9 (4.0)	23.1 (4.9)	

The Hand Dynamometer Test was administered according to procedures outlined by Reitan and Wolfson (1985). Subjects were generally paid for their participation and were judged to have provided their best efforts on the tasks. Average number of kilograms for two trials for each hand separately was recorded. The normative data, which are not reproduced here, are presented in comprehensive tables in *T*-score equivalents for test scaled scores for males and females separately in 10 age groupings (20–34, 35–39, 40–44, 45–49, 50–54, 55–59, 60–64, 65–69, 70–74, 75–80) by six educational groupings (6–8 years, 9–11 years, 12 years, 13–15 years, 16–17 years, 18+ years).

Study strengths

1. Large sample size.
2. Comprehensive exclusion criteria.
3. Detailed description of the demographic characteristics of the sample.
4. Administration procedures were outlined.
5. The normative data are presented in comprehensive tables in *T*-score equivalents for males and females separately in 10 age groupings by six educational groupings.

Considerations regarding use of the study

1. No information regarding how hand preference was determined.

Other comments

1. For dominant hand performance, 58% of score variance was accounted for by sex, while age and educational level accounted for a negligible amount of unique variance in performance (2% and 1%, respectively). A total of 63% of test score variance was accounted for by demographic variables. For nondominant hand performance, 55% of score variance was accounted for by sex, while age and educational level also accounted for a negligible amount of

unique variance in performance (4% and 1%, respectively). A total of 62% of test score variance was accounted for by demographic variables.

For the sample as a whole, mean score in kilograms for the dominant hand was 43.4 ± 13.1 and for the nondominant hand was 39.7 ± 12.7.

2. The interested reader is referred to 1996 critique of Heaton et al. (1991) norms, and Heaton et al.'s 1996 response to this critique.

Control Groups in Clinical Studies

[D.7] Matarazzo, Wiens, Matarazzo, and Goldstein, 1974

Subjects were 29 normal young men who met strict selection criteria for the Portland Police Department. Subjects ranged in age between 21 and 28 years and their educational level ranged between 12 and 16 years. Subjects participated in initial testing and were retested 14 to 24 weeks later with the median of 20 weeks.

Study strengths

1. Sample composition is described in terms of age, gender, education, IQ, and geographic area.
2. Administration procedure is outlined.
3. Data on test–retest are presented.
4. Adequate exclusion criteria.
5. Means and standard deviations are provided.

Considerations regarding use of the study

1. Procedures for assessment of hand dominance were not described.
2. Sample size is relatively small.
3. Only male subjects were included in the study (Table 18.8).

Table 18.8. D.7

N	Age	Education	WAIS FSIQ	Preferred Hand		Nonpreferred Hand	
				Test	Retest	Test	Retest
29	24	14	118	56.84 (7.66)	55.16 (8.48)	53.59 (6.14)	51.74 (7.20)

[D.8] Wiens and Matarazzo, 1977

The authors collected data on 48 male applicants to a patrolman program in Portland, Oregon, as a part of an investigation of the WAIS and MMPI correlates of the Halstead-Reitan Battery. All subjects passed a medical exam and were judged to be neurologically normal. Subjects were divided into two equal groups which were comparable in age, education, and WAIS FSIQ. Group 1 ranged in age from 21 to 27 years and group 2 from 21 to 28 years. Means and standard deviations are provided for each hand.

Study strengths
1. Demographic characteristics of the sample are presented in terms of gender, age, education, IQ, recruitment procedures, and geographic area.
2. Gender of subjects is reported.
3. Adequate medical exclusion criteria.
4. Means and standard deviations are reported.
5. Relatively large sample size for the restricted age range.

Considerations regarding use of the study
1. The data are provided for a restricted age range.
2. Hand preference is not reported.
3. All-male sample.

Other comments
1. Correlations for the two groups between WAIS FSIQ and Dynamometer scores were −0.38 and 0.03 for the preferred hand and −0.13 and −0.36 for the nonpreferred hand. The authors inferred that for the top half of the population in education and IQ, individual differences in scores on the WAIS do not influence performance on the HRB measures (Table 18.9).

[D.9] Dodrill, 1978b

Performance on motor tests was compared for four groups: control, right hemisphere damage, left hemisphere damage, and bilateral damage.

All brain-damaged groups included five subjects with intrinsic brain tumors, 11 with a history of head trauma, and nine with cerebrovascular problems.

The 25 control subjects were recruited from community resources in Washington and had no history of injury or disease that involved CNS.

All groups included adults age 15 and over. Across all groups, a subject-by-subject matching procedure was maintained for sex, race (all subjects were Caucasian), age, education, and handedness.

The Smedley Hand Dynamometer was used. Two trials were given in alternating fashion for each hand beginning with the right hand. The average of the two trials was used as the final score for each hand.

Study strengths
1. Sample composition was described in terms of age, education, gender, handedness, and geographic area.
2. Administration procedures are well described.
3. Minimally adequate exclusion criteria.
4. Means and standard deviations are reported.

Considerations regarding use of the study
1. Procedures used to determine hand preference were not described.
2. Small sample size.
3. Data are collapsed across genders.
4. Undifferentiated age range.

Table 18.9. D.8

	N	WAIS FSIQ	Age	Education	Preferred Hand	Nonpreferred Hand
Group 1	24	117.5	23.6	13.7	58.1 (7.3)	53.4 (5.5)
Group 2	24	118.3	24.8	14.0	57.5 (6.3)	53.9 (6.2)

Table 18.10. D.9

	N	Age	Education	Gender	% Right-Handed	Right Hand	Left Hand
Control	25	41.1	10.7	20 M 5 F	100	48.1 (13.4)	44.9 (12.2)
Right	25	41.1	10.7	20 M 5 F	100	33.9 (12.1)	21.4 (15.2)
Left	25	41.1	10.7	20 M 5 F	100	31.4 (16.9)	37.2 (12.8)
Bilateral	25	41.1	10.7	20 M 5 F	100	36.2 (9.4)	32.4 (11.8)

Other comments

1. The authors inferred that the Dynamometer correctly identified lateralization of brain lesions in more instances than other motor tests (Table 18.10).

[D.10] Dodrill, 1979

The study explores sex differences on various neuropsychological measures. Subjects included 47 matched pairs of non-neurologic males and females as well as 47 pairs of neurologic patients recruited in Washington. Within each pair, subjects were matched for age (±5 years) and for education (±2 years). All subjects were Caucasian and were older than 16 years of age. In addition, the groups were matched for Hollingshead's two-factor index of social position. Subjects in the neurological group were suffering from various forms of seizure disorders; most exhibited psychomotor seizures in combination with major motor attacks; they were evaluated at a center that specialized in the treatment of seizure disorders. The EEG evaluations revealed abnormal findings in 88 cases.

It is assumed but not stated by the authors that the original Halstead's procedure was followed and the score for the dominant hand was reported.

Study strengths

1. Sample composition is described in terms of age, education, SES, gender, ethnicity, and geographic area.
2. Data are presented for males and females separately.
3. Sample sizes are adequate.

4. Means and standard deviations are reported.

Considerations regarding use of the study

1. The administration procedures are not clearly described.
2. The samples were not divided into age groups. Standard deviations for age and education were not provided.
3. Procedures for assessment of hand dominance were not described.
4. No apparent exclusion criteria.

Other comments

1. The authors reported considerable gender differences on the tests that have very strong motor components, which they related to hand size (Table 18.11).

[D.11] Rounsaville, Jones, Novelly and Kleber, 1982

The study compared performance of two clinical groups and one control group. Opiate addicts were evaluated at a drug dependence treatment center 1 to 3 weeks after applying for treatment. This group included subjects who were still using opiates and those recently maintained on methadone or recently detoxified.

The epilepsy group was matched for age, sex, handedness, and education and included individuals meeting the following criteria: (1) a neurological diagnosis of either a partial or partial-complex or absence seizure disorder, with epileptic or epileptiform discharges on a serial EEG examination and without evidence of hysterical components; (2) no evidence of either focal or diffuse abnormalities on computerized axial tomography scan as reported by the neu-

Table 18.11. D.10

	N	Age	Education	SES	Dynamometer
Non-neurologic					
Males	47	27.51	12.47	49.45	54.13 (9.95)
Females	47	27.49	12.36	47.41	34.00 (5.96)
Neurologic					
Males	47	24.85	11.74	55.30	49.23 (8.86)
Females	47	24.89	11.76	52.78	29.13 (6.14)

roradiologist; (3) no history of psychiatric hospitalization or drug or alcohol abuse.

A normal comparison group of 29 subjects was chosen to provide demographically matched subjects who were in similar social circumstances to the addicts. A sample of Comprehensive Employment Training Act (CETA) participants was used. Subjects with a history of drug or alcohol abuse or of a neurological disorder were excluded. Urine specimens were taken at the time of testing and screened for alcohol and illicit psychoactive substances. The Stoelting Dynamometer was utilized; no other test administration information is provided.

Study strengths
1. Control subjects were described in terms of gender, age, education, and percent right-handed.
2. The study provides the data on test–retest over a 6-month period.
3. Adequate exclusion criteria.

Considerations regarding use of the study
1. Standard deviations were not provided.
2. The testing procedure was scarcely described. The Stoelting Dynamometer was used.
3. The procedures for assessment of hand dominance were not described.

4. Undifferentiated age range.
5. Sample size for the normal comparison group is small.
6. Data were collapsed across genders.

Other comments
1. Opiate addicts were retested in 6 months. Performance at the retest is presented in the table (Table 18.12).

[D.12] Yeudall, Fromm-Auch and Davies, 1982

The study compares performance on the HRB for delinquent and nondelinquent adolescents in Canada. The delinquent group included adolescents admitted to the primary residential treatment resource for persistent delinquents with severe behavioral disturbances. The nondelinquent group included adolescents from regular classrooms.

Handedness was measured by the Annett Handedness Questionnaire (1970): 88% of the delinquent sample and 83% of the control sample were right-handed.

Study strengths
1. The samples were described in terms of age, gender, IQ, handedness, and geographic area.

Table 18.12. D.11

	N	% Male	Education	% Right-Handed	Age	Dominant Hand	Nondominant Hand
Opiate addicts	72	72	11.5	91	27.9	43.31	41.07
Epileptic	60	67	11.8	87	29.2	40.26	37.22
CETA workers	29	59	11.2	90	24.9	41.05	38.18
Opiate addicts 6-month retest	59	—	—	—	—	42.67	40.86

Table 18.13. D.12

	N	Age	WAIS FSIQ	No. Males	No. Females	Preferred Hand	Nonpreferred Hand
Delinquent	99	14.8	95.3	64	35	37.0 (11.0)	35.5 (10.0)
Nondelinquent	46	14.5	117.1	29	18	33.1 (7.8)	30.3 (6.9)

2. The procedure for assessment of handedness was identified.

3. Means and standard deviations are reported.

4. The control sample size is relatively large for a restricted age range.

Considerations regarding use of the study
1. Data were collapsed across genders.
2. No apparent exclusion criteria (Table 18.13).

[D.13] Prigatano, Parsons, Levin, Wright and Hawryluk, 1983

The study, conducted in Oklahoma and Canada, explores neuropsychological functioning in mildly hypoxemic patients with chronic obstructive pulmonary disease (COPD). Patients ranged in age between 30 and 74 years and were not severely hypoxemic based on laboratory reports (mean PaO_2 was 66.3). The controls were matched on age, education, handedness, sex ratio and social class rating. They were free of physical or emotional illnesses.

Study strengths
1. The control sample was described in terms of age, education, gender, IQ, handedness, and geographic area.
2. Minimally adequate exclusion criteria.
3. Means and standard deviations are reported.

Considerations regarding use of the study
1. Procedures for assessment of hand dominance were not described.
2. The data are presented for the dominant hand only.
3. Small sample size.
4. Data were collapsed across genders.
5. Undifferentiated age range.

Other comments
1. The authors inferred that mild grip strength dysfunction correlated with resting partial pressure of oxygen in COPD patients (Table 18.14).

[D.14] Heaton, Nelson, Thompson, Burks and Franklin, 1985

The authors compared performance of multiple sclerosis (MS) patients (with both relapsing-remitting and chronic-progressive course) and controls recruited in Colorado. Patients with relapsing-remitting MS course had been in remission for at least 1 month at the time of testing. Sixty MS patients were on medication at the time of testing. Patients' mean score on Kurtzke's Disability Status Scale (DSS) for measuring neurological disability in MS was 3.10 (±2.09). Detailed account of neurological and medication status of the patients was given.

Table 18.14. D.13

	N	Age	Education	% Male	% Right-Handed	WAIS FSIQ	Dominant Hand
Controls	25	59.6 (9.0)	10.5 (3.3)	84	96	112.0 (11.0)	45.1 (11.4)
Patients	100	61.5 (7.4)	9.9 (3.1)	85	97	105.3 (12.8)	39.7 (10.3)

Table 18.15. D.14

	N	Age	Education	Kilograms for Both Hands
Normal controls	100	32.7 (13.5)	14.15 (2.84)	88.99 (21.42)
Relapsing-remitting MS	57	—	—	59.38 (21.66)
Chronic-progressive MS	43	—	—	54.44 (22.74)

Study strengths

1. Control sample size is large.
2. Information regarding age, education, and geographic area is provided.
3. Means and standard deviations are reported.

Considerations regarding use of the study

1. The data are provided as total for both hands only.
2. No information regarding gender.
3. Undifferentiated age range.
4. No information regarding handedness.
5. No information on exclusion criteria (Table 18.15).

[D.15] Kane, Parsons and Goldstein, 1985

The study compares performance of brain-damaged and control subjects on neuropsychological tests in Oklahoma and Pennsylvania.

The brain-damaged group consisted of subjects with a wide range of brain pathology, which was established by neurological, neuroradiological, or neurosurgical examination or by history. This group included 27 head trauma patients, 12 vascular lesions cases, six dementia cases and one neoplasm patient ranging from very mildly to severely impaired.

The control group consisted of medical and nonschizophrenic psychiatric patients. Groups were comparable with respect to age and education.

Study strengths

1. The sample is described in terms of age, education, and geographic area.
2. Adequate sample size.
3. Means and standard deviations are reported.

Considerations regarding use of the study

1. Procedures used to determine handedness were not described.
2. The data are reported in T scores rather than in kilograms.
3. The control group consisted of medical and psychiatric patients.
4. No information regarding gender.
5. Undifferentiated age range (Table 18.16).

[D.16] Heaton, Grant and Matthews, 1986

The authors obtained data on 356 male and 197 female normal controls in Colorado, California, and Wisconsin as a part of an investigation into the effects of age, education, and sex on Halstead-Reitan Battery performance. Exclusion

Table 18.16. D.15

	N	Age	Education	Dominant Hand	Nondominant Hand
Control	46	38.9 (11.3)	12.3 (2.6)	53.7° (6.5)	55.2 (7.1)
Brain damaged	43	39.7 (13.5)	11.6 (2.0)	49.2 (10.1)	51.3 (8.3)

°The data are reported in T scores.

criteria were history of neurologic illness, significant head trauma, and substance abuse. Subjects ranged in age from 15 to 81, and years of education ranged from 0 to 20 years. The sample was divided into three age categories and three education categories.

Testing was conducted by trained technicians and all participants were judged to have expended their best effort on the task.

Study strengths

1. Large overall sample size and sizes of individual cells.

2. Information regarding sex, geographic area, age, and education is provided.

3. Generally adequate exclusion criteria.

4. Data are grouped by age and education level.

Considerations regarding use of the study

1. Standard deviations were not provided, which limits utility of the norms.

2. Procedures for assessment of hand dominance were not described.

3. Results were reported only for males.

Other comments

1. The chapter provides a review of different studies exploring the relationship of neuropsychological test performance with age, education and sex. The authors concluded that different sets of norms should be used for subjects at different age, educational levels, and gender when determining whether an individual's performance is normal or abnormal (Table 18.17).

Table 18.17. D.16

	N	Dominant Hand	Nondominant Hand
Age Subgroups			
<40	319	51.4	47.8
40–59	134	51.7	46.8
≥60	110	44.3	40.5
Education Subgroups			
<12	132	47.1	43.4
12–15	249	51.1	47.1
≥16	172	51.5	47.1

[D.17] Thompson, Heaton, Matthews and Grant, 1987

The article presents a percentage of 426 normal subjects (279 males and 147 females) scoring in lateralized lesion range using Golden's (1978) guidelines. *Dominant hemisphere dysfunction* was defined as the superiority of nonpreferred hand performance over preferred hand performance. *Nondominant hemisphere dysfunction* was identified when preferred hand performance was at least 20% better than nonpreferred hand performance.

Lateral preference type was assessed based on subjects' performance on the Reitan-Klove Lateral Dominance Exam and the Miles ABC Test of Ocular Dominance (Reitan & Wolfson, 1985). The following groups were identified:

1. *All Right*—subjects who wrote with their right hand and manifested right lateral preference on all hand, eye, and foot measures.

2. *Mixed Right*—subjects who wrote with their right hand but manifested left preference on one or more other hand, eye or foot measures.

3. *Left*—left-handed subjects.

Intermanual percent difference scores were calculated as preferred hand minus nonpreferred hand divided by preferred hand.

Subjects' mean age was 40.59 years (SD = 18.27), and mean education was 13.15 years (SD = 3.49). They had been screened for history of head trauma, neurological illness, substance abuse, serious psychiatric illness, and peripheral injuries that might affect test performance.

Study strengths

1. A large sample size was used.

2. Lateral preference was thoroughly assessed and three groups were identified.

3. Intermanual differences and a percentage of subjects scoring in the lateralized lesion range were reported.

4. Adequate exclusion criteria.

5. Information on age and education is reported.

Table 18.18. D.17; Percent of Subjects Scoring in the Lateralized Dysfunction Range and Intermanual Percent Difference Scores

Groups	N	Dominant Hemisphere Dysfunction	Nondominant Hemisphere Dysfunction	Intermanual Percent Difference Scores
All right	167	19.16	8.98	7.7 (9.8)
Mixed right	226	17.70	19.47	9.1 (12.5)
Left	33	48.48	6.06	−0.2 (12.0)
Total	426	20.66	14.32	7.8 (11.7)

Considerations regarding use of the study

1. Means and SDs for each group were not reported.

2. Data are presented for a wide age range not separated into age groups, which precludes consideration of the effect of age on intermanual differences.

Other comments

The authors concluded that neither age, nor education, nor gender were significantly related to intermanual difference scores (Table 18.18).

[D.18] Russell and Starkey, 1993

This study describes the standardization sample used by the authors in their manual introducing the Halstead Russell Neuropsychological Evaluation System (HRNES) and addressing its psychometric properties. The normative sample consisted of male veterans treated at the Cincinnati V.A. Hospital between 1968 and 1971 and the Miami V.A. Medical Center between 1971 and 1989. All subjects received neurological examinations. Those subjects who were administered the Halstead tests and the WAIS or WAIS-R was included in the study. Nine percent of the sample were representatives of minority groups.

The total sample was divided into a comparison group and a brain-damaged group. The comparison group included "normal" individuals. No subject in this group had a diagnosis of CNS pathology. Presenting symptoms for the majority of these subjects were neurosis with memory or somatic complaints, or personality disorders with episodes of explosive behavior.

The brain-damaged group was obtained through referrals from the neurology, neurosurgery, and psychiatry departments and from other sections of the hospital. Left-handed patients were not included in this group if they had lateralized lesions. Only those patients whose brain lesion was well corroborated by follow-up review of the medical records were included in this group.

Patients diagnosed with schizophrenia or severe depression requiring hospitalization, as well as those with the evidence of systemic vascular disease, were excluded from the sample.

The statistics are reported for four groups of patients: comparison, left hemisphere damage, right hemisphere damage, and diffuse brain damage.

Study strengths

1. The sample composition is described in terms of age, education, ethnicity, geographic area, and gender.

2. Control sample size is large.

3. Means and standard deviations are reported.

Considerations regarding use of the study

1. Procedures used to determine hand preference were not described. Percentage of right-handed subjects in nonlateralized groups was not reported.

2. The data were reported for males only.

3. Classification of subjects in the comparison group as normal is questionable, since they had been suspected of having neurological conditions and were referred for neurological evaluation which yielded negative results.

4. Undifferentiated age range.

Table 18.19. D.18

	N	Age	Education	Race°°	Dominant Hand	Nondominant Hand
Comparison	175	45.0 (12.9)	12.5 (2.8)	164 W 11 B 0 N	45.4 (10.6)	41.9 (10.3)
Left Hemisphere	98	46.4 (15.5)	12.0 (3.0)	86 W 11 B 1 N	25.4 (19.8)	37.5 (10.0)
Right Hemisphere	106	50.5 (14.3)	11.9 (3.0)	102 W 4 B 0 N	36.7 (11.9)	19.2 (18.1)
Diffuse	299	47.6 (13.7)	11.9 (3.2)	263 W 32 B 4 N	37.0 (11.8)	34.3 (12.1)

°Provides data for males only, °°W—white; B—black; N—other.

Other comments

1. Test scores can be corrected for age and IQ and converted into scale scores to facilitate comparison with other tests (Table 18.19).

CONCLUSIONS

A review of the above studies suggests high consistency in the data across different reports. Pronounced gender differences with males outperforming females represent an unequivocal finding. Decline in grip strength associated with advancing age is also frequently reported. Although high sensitivity of this test to brain impairment is well documented, interpretation of test results from the perspective of lateralization of brain damage should be made with caution. A 10% dominant hand superiority criterion is clearly consistent with the average performance across the studies presented above. However, a wide range of *individual differences* documented in numerous studies warrants great caution in interpretation of the dominant/nondominant hand comparisons. In addition to high variability of intermanual differences, peripheral dysfunction might influence test performance (e.g., arthritis, hand or arm orthopedic problems, etc.). Unacceptably high false positive misclassification rates using standard criteria for lateralized impairment warrant further research directed at revision of these criteria.

Some aspects of grip strength variability have not received sufficient attention in the literature. For example, normative data for older age groups are scarce. Test–retest concordance should be further explored to assess the magnitude of any practice effect and to address the issue of test reliability over different interprobe intervals. Since interpretation of the results of this test is based on the assumptions of cerebral lateralization, it is of the utmost importance to report the criteria for assessment of handedness, cutoff scores for subject selection on the basis of their handedness pattern, and number of left-handed individuals in the sample, if they are included.

19

Grooved Pegboard Test

BRIEF HISTORY OF THE TEST

The Grooved Pegboard Test (GPT) acquired its popularity over 30 years ago as part of two neuropsychological batteries. It consists of a metal board with a matrix of slotted holes angled in different directions. The task is to insert 25 metal pegs with ridges along the sides into each hole in sequence. A further description of the test, its applications, and references to the original sources are provided in Lezak (1995, pp. 683–684). Administration and scoring instructions are also provided by Lafayette Instrument Company, which manufactures the pegboard.

Scores represent time in seconds required to complete the matrix with each hand, with higher scores reflecting a lower level of performance. Russell and Starkey (1993) propose a limit of 180 seconds after which the trial is discontinued. According to their modification, the number of pegs not placed within the time limit is prorated into the time score.

Although instructions for the test administration are relatively simple, review of the literature suggests that there is considerable variability in the following aspects of administration and scoring:

1. Administration of practice trials:
   a. The trial starts after instructions are given to the subject; no opportunity for practice is offered.
   b. The subject is allowed to place a certain number of pegs (the number varies for different studies) prior to the actual trial, as practice.

2. Beginning of timing:
   a. An examiner starts timing when he cues the subject to start working on the test.
   b. Timing starts as the subject is dropping the first peg into a slot.

3. Number of trials:
   a. According to the test manual, one trial is administered per hand, starting with the dominant hand.
   b. Two or more trials are administered per hand, alternating dominant and nondominant hands to counteract the practice effect which confounds performance with the nondominant hand; the score is the mean of all trials for each hand.
   c. Two trials are administered per hand in a switch-back design, where the first trial is performed with the dominant hand, the next two trials with the nondominant hand, and the last trial with the dominant hand; the score is the mean of all trials for each hand.

4. Assessment of laterality:
This test is known as a sensitive measure of lateralized brain damage. As such, accurate identification of subjects' handedness is of utmost importance. Unfortunately, the majority of studies do not provide a description of laterality assessment. It is based in most cases on a subjects' self-report of the hand preferred for writing.

Unfortunately, precise test administration procedures are not clearly described by the majority of the authors, which hampers the comparability of the norms generated from different studies.

The GPT measures psychomotor speed, fine motor control, and rapid visual–motor coordination. Motor abilities measured by this test are more complex than those measured by Finger Tapping and Dynamometer. Essentially the GPT is a cognitive–motor task. In contrast, the Finger Tapping and Dynamometer tasks require less task-specific cognitive effort and concentration and can be performed passively. Performance on GPT is also highly dependent on psychomotor speed (Miller et al.; 1990, Lezak, 1995). Axelrod and Milner (1997) found the GPT to be a good predictor of low psychomotor speed in veterans of Operation Desert Storm and Operation Desert Shield who displayed cognitive problems. Harnadek and Rourke (1994) report its sensitivity to nonverbal learning disability. However, most commonly the GPT is used for assessment of lateralized cerebral dysfunction. Use of the original cutoff scores for impairment (Heaton et al., 1986) and intermanual differences in determination of brain dysfunction yields high rates of false-positive misclassifications (Bornstein et al., 1987b). Revised cutoffs were proposed in several studies (Bornstein et al., 1987b; Ryan et al., 1987).

Bornstein (1986b) has evaluated the pattern of motor performance on three motor tests (Finger Tapping Test, Grooved Pegboard Test, and the Hand Dynamometer) which were administered to normal and unilateral brain lesion samples. A large degree of variability was observed across these intermanual measures, whereby "a high percentage (approximately 25 percent) of the normal sample obtained scores more than one standard deviation from the control mean on a single measure" (p. 719). Thus, the author has emphasized the importance of consistency in performance pattern across tasks, rather than use of a "rigid application of 'cookbook' formulas or 'rules of thumb'" (p. 723) in test interpretation.

Reliability of the GPT was addressed in several studies. Ruff and Parker (1993) report reliability coefficients ranging between 0.69 and 0.76 for dominant hand and between 0.68 and 0.78 for the nondominant hand over a 6-month period.

RELATIONSHIP BETWEEN GPT PERFORMANCE AND DEMOGRAPHIC FACTORS

The effect of age on GPT performance was quite pronounced across different studies with slowing associated with advancing age (Bornstein, 1985; Concha et al., 1995; Heaton et al., 1991; Ruff & Parker, 1993; Ryan et al., 1987; Selnes et al., 1991). The effects of education and gender have been reported but are much weaker (Bornstein, 1985; Concha et al., 1995; Heaton et al., 1991; Ryan et al., 1987; Selnes et al., 1991). Polubinski and Melamed (1986) found females to perform faster than males and Thompson et al. (1987) report greater intermanual differences for females compared to males. Ryan and his colleagues (1987) proposed a regression equation to control for the effects of age and education on GPT performance.

METHOD FOR EVALUATING THE NORMATIVE REPORTS

Our review of the grooved pegboard literature located eight normative reports and eight clinical studies reporting control data for the pegboard. In order to adequately evaluate the GPT normative reports, six criterion variables were deemed critical. The first four of these relate to *subjects* variables, and the remaining two dimensions refer to *procedural* issues.

Subject Variables

Age Group Intervals

This criterion reflects the grouping of data into limited age intervals. Age proved to be highly related to performance on this test, which warrants careful attention of investigators to appropriate age grouping of the data.

Sample Size

Fifty cases have been considered adequate sample size. Although this number is somewhat arbitrary, a large number of studies suggest that data based on small sample sizes is highly influenced by individual differences and does not provide a stable estimate of the population mean.

Sample Composition Description

As discussed previously, information regarding medical and psychiatric exclusion criteria is important; it is unclear if gender, educational level, intellectual level, geographic recruitment region, socioeconomic status or occupation, ethnicity, or recruitment procedures are relevant, so until this is determined, it is best that this information be provided.

Description of Hand Preference Assessment

In order to address the issue of lateralization in test performance, assessment procedures for hand preference should be fully described. Without this assessment, assumptions regarding functional lateralization cannot be made.

Procedural Variables

Description of Administration Procedures

As noted above, administration procedures for the GPT differ widely among studies. A detailed description of the administration procedures facilitates selection of the most appropriate norms or allows corrections in interpretation of the data to account for deviations in the administration procedure.

Data Reporting

In order to facilitate interpretation of the data, the group means and the standard deviations should be presented at a minimum.

SUMMARY OF THE STATUS OF THE NORMS

A number of studies have reported normative data for the GPT. Studies vary in subject selection, in description of procedural and subject variables, and in the grouping of obtained data into categories. In addition to normative studies based on "normal" samples, there are a number of clinical comparison studies, exploring differences in GPT performance between clinical groups and "normal control" groups. The clinical groups reported in GPT studies represent a wide range of neurological and psychiatric diagnoses (most often brain-injured patients).

The majority of studies present the data in number of seconds required to complete the matrix with each hand. Several studies report the proportion of subjects falling in the impaired range, or the rates of intermanual differences.

Several authors stratify their samples by age, education, and/or gender. Procedures for the assessment of handedness are described in some studies. Furthermore, some authors divide their samples into groups based on a subject's handedness pattern.

The majority of studies include mostly young and middle-aged subjects. Only a few studies present data for elderly individuals. Several studies provide test–retest data over varying interprobe intervals. Some studies provide data for left-handed samples.

Among all the studies available in the literature, we selected for review those reports based on large, well-defined samples, or studies that offer interesting clinical comparisons or information which is not routinely reported.

Table 19.1 summarizes information provided in the studies described in this chapter.

SUMMARIES OF THE STUDIES

Normative Studies

[GPT.1] Bornstein, 1985

The author collected data on 365 Canadian individuals (178 males and 187 females) recruited through posted notices on college campuses and unemployment offices, newspaper ads, and senior-citizen groups. Subjects were paid for their participation. Participants ranged in age from 18 to 69 (Mean = 43.3 ± 17.1) and had completed between 5 and 20 years of education (Mean = 12.3 ± 2.7); 91.5% of the sample were right-handed. No other demographic data or exclusion criteria are reported.

Means and standard deviations are reported for each hand. The sample was stratified by age

Table 19.1. GPT.L; Locator Table for the GPT

Study[°]	Age[°°]	N	Sample Composition	IQ[°°], Education	Country/ Location
GPT.1 Bornstein, 1985 page 430	20–39 40–59 60–69	385	178 M, 187 F; 91.5% R-handed paid volunteers free of neurological or psychiatric illness	Education 12.3 (2.7) Separate data for <HS, ≥HS	Western Canada
GPT.2 Bornstein, 1986a page 433	18–39 40–59 60–69	365	178 M, 187 F; paid volunteers free of neurological or psychiatric illness; 91.5% R-handed	Education 12.3(2.7) Separate data for <HS, ≥HS	Western Canada
GPT.3 Polubinski & Melamed, 1986 page 434	18–24	60 60	Men Women Students taking introductory psychology class; Handedness broken down into firm and mixed groups	Education College students	Ohio
GPT.4 Ryan et al., 1987 page 434	21–30 31–40 41–50 51–59	55 45 44 38	Blue-collar workers with no history of toxic exposure	Education 12.3(1.4) 11.9(2.2) 11.3(1.8) 11.0(1.8)	Eastern Pennsylvania
GPT.5 Bornstein & Suga, 1988 page 436	55–70 62.7 (4.3) 62.3 62.3 63.0	134	49 M, 85 F. Paid volunteers screened for a history of neurological or psychiatric disorders Divided into 3 education groups 17 M, 29 F 16 M, 28 F 16 M, 28 F	Education 11.7 (2.9) Range 5–10, 8.5 Range 11–12, 11.7 Range >12. 15.0	Western Canada
GPT.6 Heaton et al., 1991 page 436	42.1 (16.8) groups: 20–34 35–39 40–44 45–49 50–54 55–59 60–64 65–69 70–74 75–80	486	Volunteers: urban and rural. Data collected over 15 years through multi-center collaborative efforts. Strict exclusion criteria. 65% M. Data are presented in T score equivalents for M and F separately in 10 age groupings by 6 educational groupings	Education 13.6 (3.5) FSIQ 113.8 (12.3) groups 6–8 9–11 12 13–15 16–17 18+	California, Washington, Texas, Oklahoma, Wisconsin, Illinois, Michigan, New York, Virginia, Massachusetts, Canada
GPT.7 Selnes et al., 1991 page 437	25–34 35–44 45–54	733	Homosexual/bisexual men HIV-1 sero-negative, stratified by age & education	Education <College College >College	MACS centers at Baltimore, Chicago, Los Angeles, & Pittsburgh
GPT.8 Ruff & Parker, 1993 page 438	16-70	360	Normal volunteers, Ss screened for psychiatric hospitalization, chronic poly-drug abuse, or neurological disorders	7-22 yrs.	California, Michigan, Eastern seaboard
GPT.9 Rounsaville et al., 1982 page 439	27.9 29.2 24.9	72 60 29 59	Opiate addicts Epileptic patients Normal controls Opiate addicts were retested in 6 months	Education 11.5 11.8 11.2	

continued

Table 19.1. (*Continued*)

Study[*]	Age[**]	N	Sample Composition	IQ[**], Education	Country/ Location
GPT.10 Heaton et al., 1985 page 441	37.38 (8.28)	100	25 M, 75 F. Multiple sclerosis patients, among them 57 relapsing remitting course, 43 chronic-progressive form. Mean disease duration 9.36 years (5.86)	Education 13.71(2.33)	Denver
	32.87 (13.5)	100	79 M, 21 F. Control Ss with no neurological illness, head trauma or substance abuse	14.15 (2.84)	
GPT.11 Heaton et al., 1986 page 442	15–81 39.3 (17.5)	207 (UC) 181 (UCSD) 165 (UW)	356 M,197 F. Normal Ss with no history of neurological illness, head trauma, or substance abuse, 7.2% left-handed	Education 0–20 13.3 (3.4)	University of Colorado, University of California at San Diego, University of Wisconsin
GPT.12 Bornstein et al., 1987b page 442	55–70 62.7 (4.3)	134	49 M, 85 F. Control Ss, no history of neurological or psychiatric disease	Education 11.7 (2.9)	
	60.3 (3.8)	94	47 M, 47 F. Patients with neuro-diagnostic confirmation of damage to one or both of the cerebral hemispheres	Education 10.6 (4.1)	
GPT.13 Bornstein et al., 1987a page 443	17–52 32.3 (10.3)	23	9 M 14 F. Volunteers from a university community	VIQ = 105.8 (10.8) PIQ = 105.0 (10.5)	
GPT.14 Thompson et al., 1987 page 443	40.59 (18.27)	426	279 M, 147 F. Normal Ss	Education 13.15 (3.49)	
GPT.15 Miller et al., 1990 page 444	Age range 21–72		Homosexual/bisexual men	Education	MACS centers at Baltimore,
	37.20 (7.52)	769	HIV-1 sero-negative	16.36 (2.34)	Chicago, Los Angeles,
	35.66 (6.47)	727	HIV-1 sero-positive asymptomatic	15.70 (2.44)	& Pittsburgh
	36.90 (7.04)	84	HIV-1 sero-positive symptomatic	16.06 (2.50)	
GPT.16 Russell & Starkey, 1993 page 445			Norms are collected from standization sample for the HRNES manual. Ss are VA patients divided	Education	Cincinnati and Miami
	45.5 (14.1)	113	into (1) comparison and (2) brain damaged groups. The latter is	12.8	
	51.5 (15.4)	204	further subdivided based on the lateralization of lesion	12.3	

[*]The study number corresponds to the number provided in the text of the chapter.

[**]Age column and IQ/education column contain information regarding range and/or mean and standard deviation for the whole sample and/or separate groups, whichever information is provided by the authors.

group (20–39, 40–59, 60–69), level of education (<HS, ≥HS), and gender. Normative data were presented for the preferred and nonpreferred hands for each demographic group separately, as well as for different combinations of demographic strata. Individual group sample sizes ranged form 13 to 86. Hand preference was determined as the hand used for signing

the consent form. Subjects were recruited from the general population of a large city in western Canada.

Study strengths

1. Very large overall sample size and several individual cells approximate Ns of 50.

2. Stratification of the data by age, sex, and educational level.

3. This dataset is unique in that it reports data for subjects with less than a high school education.

4. Information on handedness, recruitment procedures, and geographic area is provided.

5. Method for determining handedness is specified.

6. Means and standard deviations are reported.

Considerations regarding use of the study

1. Individual sample sizes of some cells were small. It is unclear whether the youngest age included in the study was 18 or 20.

2. The lack of any reported exclusion criteria.

Other comments

1. It has been established in several studies that performance on GPT varies as a function of age; however, it has only a weak relationship with education and gender. Therefore, norms broken down by age group are most appropriate for use (Tables 19.2 and 19.3).

[GPT.2] Bornstein, 1986a

This paper expands the analysis of the data provided in the Bornstein (1985) article. The author examined cutoff levels for impairment and the proportion of subjects falling in the impaired range. For both preferred and nonpreferred hands the clinically employed cutoff criterion was 66 seconds. Performance time greater than 66 seconds placed subjects into the impaired range. The obtained high proportions of impaired scores are viewed by the authors as suggesting caution in using standard cutoff scores. Base rate issues are discussed from the perspective of the validity of test interpretation.

The administration and scoring were as follows: "The score for the Grooved Pegboard Test was the time required to fill the board according to standard instructions, described in privately published manual developed by Matthews. The preferred hand trial was administered first, and timing of the trial was not interrupted in the event of a dropped peg" (p. 414).

The sample was stratified by age group (18–39, 40–59, 60–69), level of education (<HS, ≥HS), and gender. A proportion of subjects obtaining scores in the impaired range for each of the above strata was provided for the preferred and nonpreferred hands.

Subjects were recruited from the general population of a large city in western Canada. Those with a history of neurologic or psychiatric illness were excluded from the study.

Table 19.2. GPT.1a; Data Stratified by Age, Education, and Gender for the Whole Sample

Age	Education	No. Males	No. Females	Preferred Hand	Nonpreferred Hand
By Age					
20–39	13.0 (2.3)	107	64	60.9 (16.2)	66.2 (17.1)
40–59	11.9 (2.8)	31	66	68.6 (15.0)	74.2 (15.7)
60–69	11.8 (2.9)	40	57	75.5 (14.6)	83.1 (15.5)
By Education					
48.5 (16.6)	<HS	51	57	72.4 (17.7)	78.1 (19.1)
41.1 (16.8)	≥HS	127	130	64.2 (15.5)	70.2 (16.6)
By Gender					
39.2 (17.2)	12.4 (2.9)	178 Males		68.7 (20.8)	74.5 (21.3)
47.3 (16.1)	12.2 (2.5)	187 Females		64.6 (10.8)	70.8 (13.3)

Table 19.3. GPT.1b; Data Stratified by Age, Education, and Gender for Separate Demographic Groups

| | Males | | | | | | Females | | | | | |
| | <HS | | | ≥HS | | | <HS | | | ≥HS | | |
Age Groups	N	M	SD	N	M	SD	N	M	SD	N	M	SD
Preferred Hand												
20–39	21	65.3	8.5	85	62.1	20.8	13	60.4	6.4	49	57.2	9.6
40–59	13	86.8	30.1	17	69.5	11.0	22	66.5	7.0	43	63.9	7.1
60–69	16	84.8	22.3	23	75.7	14.4	22	75.4	12.2	34	70.9	9.2
Nonpreferred Hand												
20–39		71.3	12.2		67.6	20.9		64.1	9.2		62.2	11.8
40–59		91.2	30.0		74.2	12.6		71.1	8.5		70.6	9.5
60–69		93.6	21.7		81.9	13.3		82.0	14.0		79.6	12.6

For the *strengths and considerations on use* of the study see [GPT.1] Bornstein, 1985. In addition, in the current study, exclusion criteria and test administration procedures are specified (Tables 19.4 and 19.5).

[GPT.3] Polubinski and Melamed, 1986

Subjects were students taking introductory psychology classes in Ohio. All subjects were right-handed. The Crovitz-Zener Test (1962) was used to assess degree of hand dominance based on consistency in hand preference for five unimanual tasks. Subjects with score of 25 on this test formed the firm right-handed groups while those with scores of ≤24 formed the mixed right-handed groups.

A switch-back design was used in which the first and the fourth trial were performed with the right hand and the second and the third trials were performed with the left hand.

Study strengths
1. Assessment of handedness was well identified.
2. The test administration procedure was described.
3. Sample composition was described in terms of age, education, handedness, gender, occupation (i.e., students), and geographic area.
4. Relatively large sample for restricted age, education, and handedness groups.
5. Means and standard deviations are reported.

Considerations regarding use of the study
1. No exclusion criteria.

Other comments
1. The authors conclude that women performed faster than men and mixed right-handers performed faster than firm right-handers (Table 19.6).

[GPT.4] Ryan, Morrow, Bromet, and Parkinson, 1987

The paper described the development of the Pittsburgh Occupational Exposures Test Battery (POET). It explored the factor structure of the battery and interrelations among test scores and subjects' age and education.

The article provides the norms for 182 blue-collar workers who do not have a history of exposure to industrial toxins to be used in assessment of the effect of industrial toxins on neuropsychological functioning in clinic.

Table 19.4. GPT.2a; Data for the Entire Sample ($N = 365$)

	Mean	Median	Mode	% Classified as Abnormal
Preferred Hand (seconds)	66.6	65	65	40.8
Nonpreferred Hand (seconds)	72.6	70	75	61.5

Table 19.5. GPT.2b; The Proportions of Subjects Obtaining Scores in the Impaired Range for the Stratified Sample

| | Preferred Hand | | | |
| | Males | | Females | |
Age	<HS	≥HS	<HS	≥HS
18–39	25 (5/20)	19.5(17/87)	23.1 (3/13)	13 (6/46)
40–59	76.9(10/13)	75 (12/16)	55.5(12/22)	27.3(12/44)
60–69	81.2(13/16)	82.6(19/23)	77.3(17/22)	57.6(19/33)

| | Nonpreferred Hand | | | |
| | Males | | Females | |
Age	<HS	≥HS	<HS	≥HS
18–39	60 (12/20)	47.1(41/87)	38.5 (5/13)	26.1(12/46)
40–59	84.6(11/13)	75 (12/16)	59.1(13/22)	65.9(29/44)
60–69	100 (16/16)	87 (20/23)	95.5(21/22)	84.8(28/33)

Subjects were all white, native English-speaking males who had been employed at a heavy industrial plant in Eastern Pennsylvania for at least 1 year. Subjects had no previous exposure to industrial toxins and no history of neurologic or psychiatric disorder or renal or hepatic disease and had restrained from alcohol consumption in the 12 hours prior to testing.

Study strengths

1. Sample composition was described in terms of gender, occupation, education, ethnicity, and geographic area.
2. Sample size was large and most individual cell sizes approach Ns of 50.
3. Testing procedure was well described.

4. Sample was divided into four age groups.
5. Means and standard deviations are reported.
6. Adequate exclusion criteria.

Considerations regarding use of the study

1. Procedures for assessment of hand dominance were not described.

Other comments

1. Since age and education were highly related to the test performance, the authors developed a linear regression procedure that controls for the confounding effect of these variables. The prediction of a test score for each individual is based on the following equations:

Table 19.6. GPT.3

Handedness	N	Age	Education	Right Hand	Left Hand
Men					
Firm	30	19.7	13.3	60.1	67.1
		(1.4)	(0.7)	(7.6)	(9.8)
Mixed	30	20.1	13.6	55.3	60.7
		(1.6)	(0.9)	(5.9)	(5.9)
Women					
Firm	38	19.8	13.4	54.8	60.2
		(1.2)	(0.7)	(6.2)	(6.2)
Mixed	22	19.4	13.3	54.9	60.1
		(0.8)	(0.6)	(6.6)	(7.3)

For the Dominant Hand:

Predicted score = 71.233 + 0.301 (age in years) − 0.904 (years of education)

For the Nondominant Hand:

Predicted Score = 85.929 + 0.151 (age in years) − 1.347 (years of education)

The authors also reported the percent predicted ratio score (ratio of the actual score to the predicted score × 100) that falls at or below the fifth centile for this population. The cutoff values for impairment are as follows: for the dominant hand −130; and for the nondominant hand −128 (Table 19.7).

[GPT.5] Bornstein and Suga, 1988

In a more recent publication, the authors reported data on 134 healthy elderly Canadian volunteers, aged 55 to 70, according to three education levels. Exclusion criteria were history of neurological or psychiatric disorder.

Study strengths
   1. Large sample size and individual cells approximate Ns of 50.
   2. Reporting of data by three educational groups; the study is unique in terms of representation of subjects with less than 12 years of education.
   3. Information regarding sex, age, and geographic area is provided.
   4. Means and standard deviations are reported.
   5. Minimally adequate exclusion criteria.
   6. Reasonably restricted age grouping.

Considerations regarding use of the study
   1. Procedure for determination of hand preference was not identified.
   2. Greater than 12 years education too large a category.

Other comments
   1. Subjects used in this study represent a subset of subjects used in the Bornstein (1985) article (Table 19.8).

[GPT.6] Heaton, Grant, and Matthews, 1991

The authors provide normative data from 486 (378 in the base sample and 108 in the validation sample) urban and rural subjects recruited in several states (California, Washington, Colorado, Texas, Oklahoma, Wisconsin, Illinois, Michigan, New York, Virginia, and Massachusetts) and Canada. Data were collected over a 15-year period through multicenter collaborative efforts.

Sixty-five percent of the sample were males. Mean age for the total sample was 42.06 ± 16.8, and mean educational level was 13.6 ± 3.5. Mean FSIQ, VIQ, and PIQ were 113.8 ± 12.3, 113.9 ± 13.8, and 111.9 ± 11.6, respectively. Exclusion criteria were history of learning disability, neurologic disease, illnesses affecting brain function, significant head trauma, significant psychiatric disturbance (e.g., schizophrenia), and alcohol or other substance abuse.

The GPT was administered according to procedures provided by the test manufacturer. Subjects were generally paid for their participation and were judged to have provided their best efforts on the tasks. Time in seconds to complete the 25-peg placement with each hand separately is reported.

Table 19.7. GPT.4

Age Group	Mean Age	Education	N	Dominant	Nondominant
21–30	26.1 (2.3)	12.3 (1.4)	55	69.7 (11.5)	74.5 (10.9)
31–40	36.8 (2.7)	11.9 (2.2)	45	67.2 (10.2)	72.8 (11.9)
41–50	45.7 (2.9)	11.3 (1.8)	44	76.1 (11.9)	77.1 (9.7)
51–59	54.8 (2.8)	11.0 (1.8)	38	78.7 (13.0)	81.2 (12.9)

Table 19.8. GPT.5

Education	Age	No.		Preferred Hand	Nonpreferred Hand
		Males	Females		
5-10	62.3	17	29	78.5 (19.9)	83.1 (17.2)
11-12	62.9	16	28	74.2 (16.0)	84.2 (20.8)
<12	63.0	16	28	71.9 (14.2)	77.7 (13.7)

The normative data, which are not reproduced here, are presented in comprehensive tables in *T*-score equivalents for test scaled scores for males and females separately in 10 age groupings (20–34, 35–39, 40–44, 45–49, 50–54, 55–59, 60–64, 65–69, 70–74, 75–80) by six educational groupings (6–8 years, 9–11 years, 12 years, 13–15 years, 16–17 years, 18+ years).

Study strengths
1. Large sample size.
2. Comprehensive exclusion criteria.
3. Detailed description of the demographic characteristics of the sample in terms of age, education, IQ, geographic area, and gender.
4. Administration procedures were outlined.
5. The normative data are presented in comprehensive tables in *T*-score equivalents for males and females separately in 10 age groupings by six educational groupings.

Considerations regarding use of the study
1. No information regarding how hand preference was determined.

Other comments
1. For dominant hand performance, 40% of score variance was accounted for by age, while 17% was attributable to educational level; sex accounted for a negligible amount of unique variance in performance (4%). A total of 47% of test score variance was accounted for by demographic variables. For nondominant hand performance, 39% of score variance was accounted for by age, while 13% was attributable to educational level; again sex accounted for a negligible amount of unique variance (3%). A total of 42% of test score variance was accounted for by demographic variables.

For the sample as a whole, mean time in seconds for the dominant hand was 67.3 ± 16.1 and for the nondominant hand was 72.3 ± 17.5.
2. The interested reader is referred to 1996 critique of Heaton et al. (1991) norms, and Heaton et al.'s 1996 response to this critique.

[GPT.7] Selnes, Jacobson, Machado, Becker, Wesch, Miller, Visscher, & McArthur, 1991

The study used subjects from the MACS study. The article presents results of seronegative homosexual and bisexual males for the purpose of establishing normative data for neuropsychological test performance based on a large sample. Handedness was established based on self-report. Standard procedures described by Lafayette Instrument Company were utilized.

The paper reports the percentage of right-handed, ambidextral, and left-handed individuals and race composition (Caucasian, African-American) for age and educational strata.

Study strengths
1. Normative data were stratified by age and education.
2. The demographic composition of the sample is described in terms of gender, sexual orientation, handedness, ethnicity, and geographic area.
3. Means, SDs, as well as scores for percentiles 5 and 10 are presented.
4. Method for detemining handedness is reported.
5. Very large sample size and individual cells exceed *N*s of 50.
6. Administration procedures are specified.

Considerations regarding use of the study
1. No exclusion criteria reported.
2. All male sample.

Table 19.9. GPT.7a

	Handedness			Race (%)	
	R	A	L	Caucasian	African-American
By Age					
25–34	84.8	0.3	14.9	96.4	3.6
35–44	87.2	1.1	11.7	96.6	3.4
45–54	86.6	2.1	11.3	95.9	4.1
By Education					
<College	87.8	0.4	11.8	94.8	5.2
College	85.2	0.0	14.8	96.0	4.0
≥College	85.8	1.3	12.0	96.7	3.3

Other comments

1. The authors point out the significant effect of age on performance on the GPT. Education, however, was not significantly related to performance on this test (Tables 19.9–19.11).

[GPT.8] Ruff and Parker, 1993

The GPT was administered as part of a comprehensive test battery to 360 normal volunteers recruited in California, Michigan, and the eastern seaboard who ranged in age between 16 and 70 years and in education between 7 and 22 years. Subjects were screened for psychiatric hospitalizations, chronic polydrug abuse, or neurological disorders.

Study strengths

1. Sample composition was described in terms of age, gender, education, handedness, and geographic area.

2. Assessment of handedness was well described.

3. The test administration procedure was described.

4. The data are stratified according to gender, education, and age.

5. The data for the left-hand-dominant sample are reported.

6. Means and standard deviations are reported.

7. Adequate exclusion criteria.

Table 19.10. GPT.7b; Data for the Sample Stratified by Age and Education

Age	N	Mean Age	Education	Dominant Hand			Nondominant Hand		
					Percentiles			Percentiles	
				Mean (SD)	5th	10th	Mean (SD)	5th	10th
By Age									
25–34	309	31.0 (2.6)	16.1 (2.2)	62.0 (7.8)	76	72.5	67.0 (9.3)	85	80.5
35–44	290	39.3 (2.9)	16.4 (2.3)	64.4 (8.1)	78	75	69.2 (9.1)	85	82
45–54	97	48.5 (2.6)	16.7 (2.6)	67.9 (9.0)	85	80	73.7 (11.1)	90	86
By Education									
<College	229	36.1 (7.4)	13.7 (1.2)	64.1 (8.5)	77	74	69.6 (10.3)	89	84
College	202	35.6 (7.2)	16.0 (0.0)	64.0 (8.7)	79	75	68.4 (10.3)	87	83
≥College	302	38.4 (7.8)	18.6 (1.3)	63.4 (8.3)	80	75	69.0 (9.1)	85	81

Table 19.11. GPT.7c; Data Broken Down by Age and Education (Personal Communication)

	N	Dominant Hand	Percentile 5%	Percentile 10%	Nondominant Hand	Percentile 5%	Percentile 10%
<Col. 25–34	107	62.4 (7.7)	76	73	69.1 (10.4)	89	83
35–44	93	65.3 (8.4)	78	75	68.5 (8.2)	84	82
45–60	42	65.7 (10.0)	81	77	73.0 (12.2)	93	90
Col. 25–34	104	62.4 (8.4)	76	75	65.6 (8.1)	83	74
35–44	77	65.2 (8.2)	80	77	70.4 (10.5)	92	87
45–60	35	67.1 (10.0)	85	80	73.4 (13.5)	93	86
>Col. 25–34	111	61.1 (7.6)	76	71	66.5 (8.7)	84	80
35–44	150	63.4 (8.4)	78	74	68.8 (9.1)	84	80
45–60	64	66.8 (8.7)	84	79.5	72.3 (8.3)	85	81

8. Large overall sample size although some cells have Ns less than 20.

Other comments

1. The authors report test–retest reliability for a 6-month interval, based on the data for five or more subjects from each of the 12 demographic cells (30% of the sample). The reliability coefficients for women, men, and total sample were 0.76, 0.69, 0.72 for the dominant hand, and 0.78, 0.68, 0.74 for the nondominant hand.

2. Effect of age and gender on motor speed was specifically addressed.

3. The authors explored the ratio of dominant/nondominant hand performance rate (Tables 19.12 and 19.13).

Control Groups in Clinical Studies

[GPT.9] Rounsaville, Jones, Novelly and Kleber, 1982

The study compares GPT performance of two clinical and control groups.

Opiate addicts were evaluated at a drug dependence treatment center 1 to 3 weeks after applying for treatment. This group included subjects who were still using opiates and those recently maintained on methadone or recently detoxified.

The epilepsy group was matched for age, sex, handedness, and education and included individuals meeting the following criteria: (1) a neurological diagnosis of either a partial or partial-complex or absence seizure disorder, with epileptic or epileptiform discharges on a serial EEG examination and without evidence of hysterical components; (2) no evidence of either focal or diffuse abnormalities on computerized axial tomography scan as reported by the neuroradiologist; (3) no history of psychiatric hospitalization or drug or alcohol abuse.

A normal comparison group of 29 subjects was chosen to provide demographically matched subjects who were in similar social circumstance to the addicts. A sample of Comprehensive Employment Training Act (CETA) participants was used. Subjects with a history of drug or alcohol abuse or of a neurological disorder were excluded. Urine specimens were taken at the time of testing and screened for alcohol and illicit psychoactive substances.

Table 19.12. GPT.8a; Data for the *Left-Hand-Dominant* Sample

	Men (N = 17)		Women (N = 18)	
	M	SD	M	SD
Age	37.9	(18.0)	38.7	(16.1)
Education	13.7	(2.8)	14.1	(2.6)
Dominant Hand	70.7	(13.5)	65.6	(11.6)
Nondominant Hand	70.3	(15.7)	73.0	(18.6)

Table 19.13. GPT.8b; Data for the Whole Sample Stratified by Gender, Education, and Age

	Men			Women			Combined Sex		
Age/Education	N	M	SD	N	M	SD	N	M	SD
Dominant Hand									
16–39									
≤12	29	67.8	9.2	30	62.8	8.9	59	65.3	9.3
≥13	60	64.7	10.9	60	57.8	6.2	120	61.2	9.5
All	89	65.7	10.4	90	59.5	7.5	179	62.5	9.6
40–54									
≤12	15	71.9	15.1	14	63.1	4.4	29	67.7	12.0
≥13	30	70.4	10.9	30	63.3	7.4	60	66.8	9.9
All	45	70.9	12.3	44	63.2	6.5	89	67.1	10.6
55–70									
≤12	15	83.7	10.2	15	78.6	11.7	30	81.1	11.1
≥13	30	74.1	13.0	29	75.3	11.3	59	74.7	12.1
All	45	77.3	12.8	44	76.5	11.4	89	76.9	12.1
All Age Levels									
≤12	59	72.9	12.8	59	66.9	11.2	118	69.9	12.3
≥13	120	68.5	12.0	119	63.4	10.7	239	66.0	11.6
All	179	69.9	12.5	178	64.6	10.9	357	67.3	12.0
Nondominant Hand									
16–39									
≤12	29	74.5	10.9	29	66.8	10.7	58	70.7	11.4
≥13	59	67.8	10.8	60	65.2	10.3	119	66.5	10.6
All	88	70.0	11.2	89	65.7	10.4	177	67.9	11.0
40–54									
≤12	15	79.1	14.9	14	69.6	6.5	29	74.5	12.4
≥13	30	73.7	9.9	30	70.8	8.9	60	72.3	9.4
All	45	75.1	11.9	44	70.4	6.5	89	73.0	10.5
55–70									
≤12	15	91.0	12.7	13	84.3	15.3	28	87.9	14.1
≥13	28	83.5	13.4	29	82.0	12.5	59	82.8	12.9
All	43	86.1	13.5	42	82.8	13.3	85	84.5	13.4
All Age Levels									
≤12	59	79.9	14.0	56	71.6	13.1	115	75.8	14.1
≥13	117	73.1	12.9	119	70.7	12.5	238	71.9	12.7
All	176	75.4	13.6	175	71.0	12.7	351	73.2	13.3

Table 19.14. GPT.9

	N	% Male	Education	% Right-Handed	Age	Dominant Hand	Nondominant Hand
Opiate addicts	72	72	11.5	91	27.9	74.51	79.78
Epileptic	60	67	11.8	87	29.2	74.20	81.88
CETA workers	29	59	11.2	90	24.9	70.52	75.59
Opiate addicts 6-month retest	59	—	—	—	—	75.68	81.92

Study strengths

1. Controls were described in terms of gender, age, education, and percent right-handed.
2. The study provides the data on test–retest over a 6-month period.
3. Adequate exclusion criteria.

Considerations regarding use of the study

1. Standard deviations were not provided.
2. The testing procedure was scarcely described.
3. The procedures for assessment of hand dominance were not described.
4. Age ranges were not provided. It is difficult to extrapolate age limits for use of the presented norms.
5. Sample size for the normal comparison group is small.

Other comments

1. Opiate addicts were retested in 6 months. Performance at the retest is presented in the table (Table 19.14).

[GPT.10] Heaton, Nelson, Thompson, Burks and Franklin, 1985

The authors compared performance of multiple sclerosis patients (with both relapsing-remitting and chronic-progressive course) and controls recruited in Colorado. Patients with relapsing-remitting MS course had been in remission for at least 1 month at the time of testing. Sixty MS patients were on medication at the time of testing. Patients' mean score on Kurtzke's Disability Status Scale (DSS) for measuring neurological disability in MS was 3.10 ($\pm$2.09). A detailed account of neurological and medication status of the patients was given.

Study strengths

1. Control sample is large.
2. Information regarding age, education, and geographic area is presented.
3. Means and standard deviations are reported.

Considerations regarding use of the study

1. Data were provided as total for both hands only.
2. No information regarding gender is reported.
3. Undifferentiated age range.
4. No information regarding handedness.
5. No information regarding exclusion criteria.
6. High educational level of controls (Table 19.15).

Table 19.15. GPT.10

	N	Age	Education	Time for Both Hands
Normal controls	100	32.7 (13.5)	14.15 (2.84)	131.40 (18.76)
Relapsing-remitting MS	57	—	—	176.67 (62.41)
Chronic-progressive MS	43	—	—	364.47 (199.64)

[GPT.11] Heaton, Grant and Matthews, 1986

The authors obtained data on 553 normal controls in Colorado, California, and Wisconsin as a part of an investigation into the effects of age, education, and sex on Halstead-Reitan Battery performance. The sample consisted of 356 males and 197 females. Exclusion criteria were history of neurologic illness, significant head trauma, and substance abuse. Subjects ranged in age from 15 to 81 and years of education ranged from 0 to 20 years. The sample was divided into three age categories and three education categories.

Testing was conducted by trained technicians and all participants were judged to have expended their best effort on the task.

Study strengths
1. Large overall sample size and sizes of individual cells.
2. Information regarding sex, geographic area, age, and education is provided.
2. Generally adequate exclusion criteria.

Considerations regarding use of the study
1. Standard deviations were not provided, which limits utility of the norms.
2. Procedures for assessment of hand dominance were not described.

Other comments
1. The chapter provides a review of different studies exploring the relationship of neuropsychological test performance with age, education, and sex. The authors concluded that different sets of norms should be used for subjects at different age, educational levels, and gender when determining whether an individual's performance is normal or abnormal (Table 19.16).

[GPT.12] Bornstein, Paniak and O'Brien, 1987b

Data for a control sample recruited in Canada (described in Bornstein, 1985, article) and a brain-damaged sample are reported. The brain-damaged sample is described as "comprised of patients with independent neurodiagnostic confirmation of damage to one or both of the cerebral hemispheres. The principal diagnoses included: cerebral atrophy or Alzheimer's disease (24), stroke (21), ruptured aneurysm (12), head injury (9), hydrocephalus (6), meningioma (5), glioma (5), multiple sclerosis (3), and a variety of other disorders (9)" (p. 316).

Table 19.16. GPT.11

	N	Dominant Hand	Nondominant Hand
Age Subgroups			
<40	319	61.1	65.7
40–59	134	68.1	74.7
≥60	100	85.1	90.0
Education Subgroups			
<12	132	74.6	79.3
12–15	249	66.0	71.3
16+	172	62.3	67.6

Study strengths
1. Sample size is large.
2. Data are provided for males and females separately.
3. Cutoff criteria are provided, as well as means and standard deviations.
4. Information on age, gender, education, and geographic area is reported.

Considerations regarding use of the study
1. Procedures for determination of hand preference were not identified.
2. No exclusion criteria.
3. Undifferentiated age range.

Other comments
1. Classification rates obtained with *conventional* cutoff scores were examined: The cutoff for the preferred hand was based on Rennick unpublished data and for the nonpreferred hand on Heaton et al. (1986) data, suggesting expected 5-second difference between preferred and nonpreferred hands.
2. The distribution of scores for the two groups was examined to determine the *optimal* cutoff score resulting in the best overall classification rates with the emphasis on accurate classification of normal subjects (Tables 19.17 and 19.18).

Table 19.17. GPT.12a; Time for Each Hand

	N	Age	Education	Gender	Preferred	Nonpreferred
Control	134	62.7	11.7	49 M	74.8	81.6
		(4.3)	(2.9)	85 F	(16.6)	(17.1)
Brain Damaged	94	60.3	10.6	47 M	139.2	143.6
		(3.8)	(4.1)	47 F	(81.2)	(84.5)

[GPT.13] Bornstein, Baker and Douglass, 1987a

The study assessed test–retest reliability of GPT over a period of 3 weeks. Subjects were 14 women and nine men in Canada without a positive history of neurological or psychiatric illness. Their age ranged from 17 to 52 (Mean = 32.3 ± 10.3), mean VIQ was 105.8 ± 10.8, and mean PIQ was 105.0 ± 10.5. Subjects were administered the Halstead-Reitan Battery in standard order both on initial testing and again 3 weeks later.

Study strengths
1. Sample composition was adequately described. Age, VIQ, PIQ, gender statistics, and geographic area were provided.
2. Information on short-term (3 week) retest data were provided.
3. Minimally adequate exclusion criteria.
4. Means and standard deviations are reported.

Considerations regarding use of the study
1. Sample size is small; only 23 subjects were included.
2. Age range is wide: 17 to 52 years. The effect of age on test–retest change was not explored.

3. Method of handedness assessment and proportion of right-handers were not identified. It is not clear whether the authors utilized dominant/nondominant comparisons or right/left comparisons.
4. Information on educational level is not reported.

Other comments
Test–retest reliability of GPT over a period of 3 weeks was assessed (Table 19.19).
Means and standard deviations for raw score change over 3 weeks are as follows:

Right hand	−2.8 ± 6.1
Left hand	0.3 ± 6.4

[GPT.14] Thompson, Heaton, Matthews and Grant, 1987

The article presents a percentage of 426 normal subjects (279 males and 147 females) scoring in lateralized lesion range using Golden's (1978) guidelines. *Dominant hemisphere dysfunction* was defined as the superiority of nonpreferred hand performance over preferred hand performance. *Nondominant hemisphere dysfunction* was identified when preferred hand perfor-

Table 19.18. GPT.12b; Classification Rates Based on Conventional and Optimal Cutoff Scores

		Percent Correctly Classified	
		Control	Brain-Damaged
Cutoff Conventional			
Preferred	≥67	34	100
Nonpreferred	≥72	28	97
Cutoff Optimal			
Preferred	≥92	89	73
Nonpreferred	≥99	91	60

Table 19.19. GPT.13

N = 23	Dominant	Nondominant
Test 1	56.6 (5.9)	59.3 (6.6)
Test 2 (3 weeks later)	58.8 (8.9)	58.8 (6.6)

mance was at least 20% better than nonpreferred hand performance.

Lateral preference type was assessed based on subjects' performance on the Reitan-Klove Lateral Dominance Exam and the Miles ABC Test of Ocular Dominance (Reitan & Wolfson, 1985). The following groups were identified:

1. *All Right*—subjects who wrote with their right hand and manifested right lateral preference on all hand, eye, and foot measures.
2. *Mixed Right*—subjects who wrote with their right hand but manifested left preference on one or more other hand, eye, or foot measures.
3. *Left*—left-handed subjects.

Intermanual percent difference scores were calculated as preferred hand minus nonpreferred hand divided by preferred hand.

Subjects' mean age was 40.59 years (SD = 18.27) and mean education was 13.15 years (SD = 3.49). They had been screened for history of head trauma, neurological illness, substance abuse, serious psychiatric illness, and peripheral injuries that might affect test performance.

Study strengths
1. A large sample size was used.
2. Lateral preference was thoroughly assessed and three groups were identified.

3. Intermanual differences and a percentage of subjects scoring in the lateralized lesion range were reported.
4. Adequate exclusion criteria.
5. Information on age and education is reported.

Considerations regarding use of the study
1. Means and SDs for each group were not reported.
2. Data are presented for a wide age range not separated into age groups, which precludes consideration of the effect of age on intermanual differences.

Other comments
1. Authors concluded that females tend to show greater disparity between preferred and nonpreferred hand performance (M = 9.8%, SD = 11.8) than males (M = 6.7%, SD = 12.1). Age and education were not significantly related to intermanual difference scores (Table 19.20).

[GPT.15] Miller, Selnes, McArthur, Satz, Becker, Cohen, Sheridan, Machado, Van Gorp and Visscher, 1990

The article describes the results obtained for homosexual/bisexual males recruited in the MACS study, an epidemiologic project designed to assess the natural history of HIV-1 infection. The study uses large sample sizes to explore the effect of HIV serostatus and symptom status on cognitive and motor functioning. Handedness was established based on self-report. Test administration procedure followed that outlined by Lezak (1983).

The paper reports the percentage of right-handed, ambidextral and left-handed individu-

Table 19.20. GPT.14; The Table Provides Percent of Subjects Scoring in the Lateralized Dysfunction Range

Groups	N	Dominant Hemisphere Dysfunction	Nondominant Hemisphere Dysfunction	Intermanual Percent Difference Scores
All right	167	20.96	14.97	−8.2 (11.3)
Mixed right	226	25.89	18.75	−7.9 (12.8)
Left	33	36.36	6.06	−4.4 (10.8)
Total	426	24.76	16.27	−7.8 (12.1)

Table 19.21. GPT.15a; Demographic Characteristics of the Sample

| | %Handedness | | | Race | | | | CES Depression | |
	R	A	L	W	B	H	O	Scale	CD4
Seronegative	87	0	13	92	2	4	2	9.08 (9.03)	970.42 (332.46)
Asymptomatic Seropositive	86	0	14	91	2	6	2	9.44 (9.27)	561.90 (277.98)
Symptomatic Seropositive	90	1	8	90	2	5	3	15.21 (11.19)	277.22 (269.45)

als, race composition (white, black, Hispanic, other), CES Depression Scale scores (with SDs), and CD4 cells/mm^3 count (with SDs).

Study strengths
1. Sample sizes are large.
2. The demographic characteristics of each sample are meticulously described in terms of gender, sexual orientation, handedness, ethnicity, age, education, and geographic area.
3. Method for determining handedness was described.
4. Means and standard deviations are reported.
5. Test administration procedures are reported.

Considerations regarding use of the study
1. The study recruited subjects ranging in age from 21 to 72. Data are presented for all ages combined.
2. No exclusion criteria reported.
3. All-male sample.
4. High educational level (Tables 19.21 and 19.22).

[GPT.16] Russell and Starkey, 1993

This study describes the standardization sample used by the authors in their manual introducing the Halstead Russell Neuropsychological Evaluation System (HRNES) and addressing its psychometric properties. The normative sample consisted of veterans treated at the Cincinnati V.A. Hospital between 1968 and 1971, and the Miami V.A. Medical Center between 1971 and 1989. All subjects received neurological examination. Those subjects who were administered the Halstead tests and the WAIS or WAIS-R were included in the study. Nine percent of the sample were representatives of minority groups.

The total sample was divided into a comparison group and a brain-damaged group. The comparison group included "normal" individuals. No subject in this group had a diagnosis of CNS pathology. Presenting symptoms for the majority of these subjects were neurosis with memory or somatic complaints, or personality disorders with episodes of explosive behavior.

The brain-damaged group was obtained through referrals from the neurology, neurosurgery, and psychiatry departments and from

Table 19.22. GPT.15b; Data for Each Hand

	N	Age	Education	Dominant Hand	Nondominant Hand
Seronegative	769	37.20 (7.52)	16.36 (2.34)	64.28 (9.10)	69.28 (9.91)
Asymptomatic Seropositive	727	35.66 (6.47)	15.70 (2.44)	63.39 (9.17)	68.90 (12.52)
Symptomatic Seropositive	84	36.90 (7.04)	16.06 (2.50)	66.57 (11.42)	73.27 (16.39)

other sections of the hospital. Left-handed patients were not included in this group if they had lateralized lesions. Only those patients whose brain lesion was well corroborated by the follow-up review of the medical records were included in this group.

Patients diagnosed with schizophrenia or severe depression requiring hospitalization as well as those with the evidence of systemic vascular disease were not included in the sample.

The statistics are reported for four groups of patients: comparison, left hemisphere damage, right hemisphere damage, and diffuse brain damage.

Study strengths

1. The sample composition is described in terms of age, education, ethnicity, and geographic area.
2. Control sample size is large.
3. Means and standard deviations are reported.

Considerations regarding use of the study

1. Procedures used to determine hand preference were not described. Percentage of right-handed subjects in nonlateralized groups was not reported.
2. The classification of these subjects as normal is questionable, since they had been suspected of having neurological conditions and

were referred for neurological evaluation which yielded negative results.

3. Undifferentiated age range.

Other comments

Test scores can be corrected for age and IQ and converted into scale scores to facilitate comparison with other tests (Table 19.23).

CONCLUSIONS

Despite the wide variability in administration procedures for the GPT, there is high consistency in the data across different studies. Decline in performance is clearly associated with advancing age. The effects of education and, specifically, gender, are more equivocal. Peripheral (orthopedic and muscular) problems impacting performance on the test must also be considered. Because GPT performance is affected by several factors, its interpretation as an indicator of cortical dysfunction should be made with great caution. Following recommendations by Bornstein (1986b), the diagnostic accuracy rests on the consistency of findings across different tasks and different functional domains.

Given the unacceptably high false positive rates with the use of original cutoffs for impairment, further research should be directed at

Table 19.23. GPT.16

	N	Age	Education	Race	Gender	Dominant Hand	Nondominant Hand
Comparison	113	45.5 (14.1)	12.8 (2.9)	106 W° 7 B 0 N	95 M 18 F	74.4 (24.4)	78.4 (25.9)
Brain damaged	204	51.5 (15.4)	12.3 (3.0)	169 W 31 B 4 N	194 M 10 F		
Left hemisphere	38					119.9 (42.3)	107.0 (37.9)
Right hemisphere	36					116.1 (40.9)	144.2 (39.8)
Diffuse	130					124.5 (39.2)	127.7 (37.8)

°W—white; B—black; N—other.

the formulation of revised cutoff scores to improve this test's specificity.

Despite the large body of empirical studies exploring the psychometric properties of the GPT accumulated to date, some aspects of performance are not sufficiently addressed. For example, normative data for older age groups are scarce. Since interpretation of the results is based on assumptions of cerebral lateralization, it is of utmost importance to report the criteria for the assessment of handedness, cutoff scores for subject selection on the basis of their handedness pattern, and the number of left-handed individuals in the sample (if they are included).

VII

CONCEPT FORMATION
AND REASONING

20

Category Test

BRIEF HISTORY OF THE TEST

The Category Test was developed by Halstead (1947) to assess the ability to "abstract" categorization parameters such as size, shape, number, position, brightness, and color. The original test apparatus consisted of a boxed screen placed in front of the subject on which were presented visual stimuli in groups of four; the task was to identify which of the four stimuli differed from the other designs by pressing one of four corresponding keys located on a pad below the screen. Feedback was provided in the form of a "chime" for correct responses and a "raspberry buzzer" for incorrect answers. Halstead's (1947) original test included 336 items organized into nine subtests, while the version employed by Reitan (Reitan & Wolfson, 1985) was reduced to 208 stimuli in seven subgroups. The Halstead version is no longer in use and the data presented in this chapter refer to the Reitan edition of the Category Test. A recent survey of neuropsychologists identified the Category Test as one of the two neuropsychological tests (along with the Finger Oscillation Test) most frequently used in the assessment of adults (Sellers & Nadler, 1992).

The Category Test involves several different abilities, including attention and concentration, learning and memory, and visuospatial skills, as well as concept formation, abstraction of similarities and differences among stimuli, and modification of problem-solving hypotheses in responses to feedback. The majority of the re-cent studies on the construct validity of the Category Test describe it as a measure of different aspects of reasoning (Johnstone et al., 1997; Kelly et al., 1992; Perrine, 1993; Shute & Huertas, 1990). However, Leonberger et al. (1991) emphasize visual concentration and visual memory as important determinants of the Category Test performance, while Boyle (1988) views this test as a measure of intelligence.

Golden and colleagues (1981a) suggest that the Category test is sensitive to a prefrontal lobe disturbance as well as diffuse dysfunction. Adams and colleagues (1993, 1995) explored the association between Category Test performance and frontal tissue glucose metabolism rates. The authors attribute Category Test's sensitivity to reasoning, concept formation, and abstraction to involvement of three frontal subdivisions in information processing: cingulate gyrus and the dorsolateral and orbitomedial aspects of frontal lobes (Adams et al., 1993; Adams et al., 1995). Other authors, however, do not relate Category Test performance to any localized brain area (Bornstein, 1986b; Choca et al., 1997).

Specific test administration instructions are provided in Reitan's (1979) *Manual for Administration of Neuropsychological Test Batteries for Adults and Children* and in Reitan and Wolfson's (1985) *The Halstead-Reitan Neuropsychological Test Battery*. Snow (1987) cites concerns regarding lack of standardization of test administration. He points out that the test manual dictates that the examiner assist the subject, but the nature and extent of the help to be offered is not specified. He quotes the following passage from the manual: "it may become necessary to urge [the patient] to study the pictures carefully, to ask for . . . description . . . , to urge them to try to notice and remember how the pictures change . . . , and to try to think of the possible reason when a correct answer occurs" (pp. 26–27).

Halstead (1947) comments that although several methods of scoring Category Test performances were considered, he settled on a single score: total number of errors. He recommended a cutoff of greater than 80 errors as the criterion score in computing his impairment index, while Reitan (Reitan & Wolfson, 1985) uses a criterion score of 50 for his shortened test. Given the significant association between Category Test scores and demographic factors and IQ, a single cutoff would not appear to be appropriate, particularly in older subjects. For example, Ernst (1987) documented in his sample of 65–75-year-olds a misclassification rate of 84% on a booklet version of the Category Test. Dodrill (1987) documented a 22.5% misclassification rate in a young control sample. Logue and Allen (1971) recommend that "ultimate interpretation of the significance of critical data on the Category test rests often not only on the standard cutoff of 50 but also on a subjective evaluation by the psychologist as to whether the score is to be reasonably expected by a normal subject of this general level of intelligence" (p. 1095). Similarly, Bornstein and colleagues (1987a) emphasize that cutoff scores may be useful but only if considered in the context of other neuropsychological information obtained in a test battery, and if age, education, and other appropriate adjustments are made.

Charter (1994) examined frequency of random responding on the Category Test using the formula approximating binomial distribution for a large sample, based on observed score and a probability of guessing. Frequencies of random responses for the 90%, 95%, and 99% confidence intervals presented in this article are summarized in Table 20.1.

Charter's review of different studies reported in the literature suggested that no normative subjects' scores fall in the random range.

Of some concern, a low relationship between Category Test scores and activities of daily living (as measured by the Scale of Competence in Independent Living Skills; SCILS) in a sample of geriatric patients was reported by Searight et al. (1989). The authors report correlation coefficients between Category Test scores and measures of 16 activities of daily living ranging between -0.03 and 0.37. Correlation between the Category Test score and the total SCILS score was relatively low (0.30).

The item analysis reported by Laatsch and Choca (1991) revealed an uneven progression of the item difficulty in successive subtests. In addition, all items on subtests I and II were found to be too easy to yield useful information (see Choca et al., 1997).

Alternate Formats

Several authors have observed that a major negative aspect of the Category Test for clinical use is the extensive amount of time which may be required for test administration (Golden et al., 1981a). Some patients may complete the task in 2 hours or more, and the associated fatigue may result in random responding. Rest periods alleviate fatigue, but these breaks may compromise performance on subtest 7 because it involves recall of earlier strategies.

To address the problem of lengthy administration, at least eight shortened versions of the Category Test have been developed. Some formats have involved administration of three or

Table 20.1. CT.Charter

	90%		95%		99%	
	Low	High	Low	High	Low	High
Full test	146	167	145	169	141	173
Subtests II, VII	13	19	12	19	12	21
Subtests III–VI	26	35	26	36	24	38

four of the seven subtests (Calsyn et al., 1980; Moehle et al., 1988), while other formats have used selected items from five or six subtests (Boyle, 1975, 1986; Gregory et al., 1979; Russell & Levy, 1987) or have split the test in half using even vs. odd items (Kilpatrick, 1970). Kilpatrick documented high correlations between number of errors on odd items, even items, and all items ($r = 0.90$ to 0.99). Calsyn et al. (1980; cf. Dunn, 1985; Golden et al., 1981; Taylor et al., 1984) found that scores based on administration of the first four subtests of the Category Test had high correlations with the total score ($r = 0.83$ to 0.89) and accounted for 77% to 79% of total score variance. They suggest that full test scores can be approximated by multiplying the shortened version score by 1.4 and adding 14. Inclusion of information regarding age, education, and gender have not increased the predictive accuracy of this short form (Pierce et al., 1990). Taylor and colleagues (Taylor et al., 1984) were able to corroborate a high correlation between the Calsyn short version and complete test format ($r - 0.91$) but note that use of the short form resulted in a substantially higher misclassification of normals as brain damaged, and subjects with right-sided focal lesions tended to be misidentified as normal. Dunn et al. (1985) suggest that the following equation may lead to more accurate estimates of full Category Test scores in a geriatric population: (short form score $\times 1.6$) + 22.

Moehle and colleagues (1988), using multiple regression analyses, reported that a short form composed of subtests 4, 6, and 3 accounted for the highest percentage of long-form score variance (77%) and is the "psychometrically soundest short form." Their analyses indicated that the Calsyn short form accounted for only 62% of full-form score variance. Moehle et al. (1988) recommend a cutoff of 26 (which represents the score 1 standard deviation below the mean for their brain-damaged sample) for use with their short form. They suggest some caution in the use of their version because all their subjects on whom the analyses were based were administered the entire Category Test. The authors question whether there are unknown order effects or if some subtests (i.e., I and II) have an influence on subsequent subtest performance.

Other investigators have opted to retain at least five or six of the seven subtests from the Reitan version of the Category Test but to shorten some of the subtests (Boyle, 1975, 1986; Gregory et al. 1979; Russell & Levy, 1987). Taylor et al. (1990) argue that "because the Category Test is designed to be a test of abstract reasoning and requires the subject to make conceptual shifts among several principles, the same number of principles and the same number of conceptual shifts should be required on a shortened version of the Category Test" (p. 486).

Boyle (1975, 1986) created two parallel 84-item forms of the Category Test involving half the items from subtests 1–4 and 7, and 20 items from subtests 5 and 6. The 84-item version discriminated between a normal and neurologic population, and using cutoffs of 38 and 39 errors, only 6% to 13% of the brain-damaged subjects were misclassified, while 20%–22% of the non-brain-damaged subjects were misidentified.

Gregory et al. (1979) developed a 120-item test version employing all subtest 1 items, the first 16 items from subtest 2, and the first 32 items from subtests 3 through 6. While Gregory and colleagues suggest that a cutoff score of 35 best corresponded to the full test cutoff of 51 in their brain-damaged subjects vs. college students, Sherrill (1985) found that a cutoff of 29 was a better predictor of the long-form cutoff in his heterogeneous, neuropsychiatric population.

Russell and Levy (1987) developed a 95-item Category Test format which was composed of five items from subtest 1, 10 items from subtest 2, and 20 items from subtests 3–6. Items from subtests 5 and 6 were reorganized so that subtest 5 included only pure quantitative items and subtest 6 consisted of complex counting items. A full Category Test score was calculated by multiplying the short-version score by 2.2. A correlation of 0.97 was obtained between the abbreviated and full test scores in a neurologic population.

Sherrill (1985) found that the Gregory et al. (1979) 120-item version and the Calsyn et al. (1980) 108-item version were highly correlated with each other (0.968) and that while both were highly correlated with the standard format

(0.943–0.981), the 120-item version had the highest correlation with the full test and the smallest standard error of estimate (+7.5), suggesting that it was the overall best predictor of the full test score. Sherrill (1985) suggests that the 120-item version is probably the most attractive short-form alternative to the 208-item test, particularly for high-functioning subjects, since it includes subtest 5; a wide variation in scores occurs on this subtest in this population.

Taylor et al. (1990) compared the Gregory et al. (1979), Calsyn et al. (1980), and Russell and Levy (1987) short forms and reported that the Russell and Levy version and the Gregory version were better predictors of total test scores than the Calsyn version and that while the Russell version had only 95 items, it performed comparably to the 120-item Gregory format. Taylor and colleagues (1990) recommend the following equation for the Russell format in calculating the predicted total Category Test score: (No. short-form errors × 2.73) − 4.49. These authors suggest that the Russell and Levy (1987) formula of short-form errors × 2.2 tends to overestimate total test errors.

While efforts to shorten the Category Test are commendable, a major concern involves the fact that all of the shortened versions have been based on analyses derived from administration of the entire Category Test. To our knowledge, no published reports have actually administered a shortened version, and it is unknown if some subtests (i.e., I and II) have an influence on subsequent subtest performance, or if unique order effects emerge if subtests are given out of order (Moehle et al., 1988). Moehle and colleagues (1988) rightly express caution in the use of their shortened version for these reasons. Snow (1987) reminds that any shortening of a test necessitates compilation of new normative data; "for example, the process of shortening the Category Test may make it less fatiguing, and hence less demanding. Short forms may therefore be less able to discriminate patients with subtle brain dysfunction. Further, when short forms are developed, it is often the case that little work is done in validating the findings obtained with the newer versions of the test. Instead, the old cutting scores continued to be used, with short-form scores merely being prorated to their equivalent lengthier versions. Clearly, when a test is shortened, new norms will be required" (p. 258).

In addition to the length of time required for administration, the lack of portability and cumbersome nature of the Category Test apparatus have been a drawback (Slay, 1984; Wood & Strider, 1980). Slay (1984) provides instructions for constructing a portable Category test for the clinician "with a modicum of workshop skills." Several investigators have developed paper and pen, card, or booklet forms of the Category Test (Adams & Trenton, 1981; DeFilippis et al., 1979; Kimura, 1981; Wood & Strider, 1980). The DeFilippis (DeFillippis et al., 1979) version in particular appears to be in much wider usage than the original slide-projector format.

Adams and Trenton (1981) devised a laminated booklet test form which provides visual feedback as to the correctness of a response, although the practicality of this method is somewhat in doubt; "the answer sheet was treated by touching each correct answer with a swab containing dimenthylglyoxine. The subject was given a felt tip pen that was treated chemically with nickel chloride in aqueous ammonia. If the subject responded to an item correctly, the circle on the answer sheet would immediately turn red. An incorrect response resulted in a green circle" (p. 299). The high modified split-half Spearman-Brown coefficient documented between the slide format Category Test and the paper and pen version did not significantly differ from the coefficient obtained for the slide version, and the two test forms were judged to be equivalent.

Wood and Strider (1980) report a similar shortened version of the Category Test using a latent image transfer sheet. When a developer pen is applied to the correct rectangle on the answer sheet, the rectangle darkens, providing feedback as to the correctness of the response. No significant difference in performance across psychiatric groups was found between this version and the original Reitan format.

Kimura (1981) also developed a card version of the Category Test in which the patient provides verbal responses to which the examiner responds "Right" or "Wrong". No significant differences in test performance were noted between groups of neurologic patients.

Finally, DeFilippis et al. (1979) created a

booklet form in which the Category Test slides were reproduced onto 8.5″ × 11″ sheets which were then placed into notebooks. A piece of cardboard with the numbers 1 through 4 was placed below the notebook and subjects were instructed to point to the appropriate number for each sheet. The examiner provided feedback as to the correctness of a response by saying "Correct" or "Incorrect." The booklet format was highly correlated with the original slide version, and no effect of test version was documented in patients and normals administered both formats. MacInnes et al. (1983) report data validating the use of the Calsyn et al. (1980) short form in conjunction with the DeFilippis booklet format.

A comprehensive summary of the history and current perspectives on the Category Test is offered by Choca et al. (1997).

RELATIONSHIP BETWEEN CATEGORY TEST PERFORMANCE AND DEMOGRAPHIC FACTORS

Corrigan et al. (1987) summarize much of the available literature on the relationship of IQ, education, and age to Category Test scores, and the interested reader is referred to this publication.

A highly consistent relationship has been documented between age and Category Test scores in both normal and patient (brain damaged, psychiatric, medical) samples (Alekoumbides et al., 1987; Anthony et al., 1980; Bigler et al., 1981a; Boyle, 1986; Choca et al., 1997; Corrigan et al., 1987; Ernst et al., 1987; Fitzhugh et al., 1964; Heaton et al., 1986, 1991; Mack & Carlson, 1978; Prigatano & Parsons, 1976; Reed & Reitan, 1963b; Seidenberg et al., 1984; Vega & Parsons, 1967). However, Willis et al. (1988) did not find relationship between age and performance on the orignal version of the Category Test in a sample of 154 healthy elderly individuals. It should noted that the age range of their subjects was quite narrow: 65 to 79 years old.

A negative correlation frequently has been noted between education and Category Test scores, particularly in normal as compared to patient groups. Several investigators have reported associations between education and Cat-

egory Test performance in normal individuals (Anthony et al., 1980; Boyle, 1986; Choca et al., 1997; Ernst, 1987; Finlayson et al., 1977; Heaton et al., 1986, 1991; Prigatano & Parsons, 1976; Vega & Parsons, 1967; Warner et al., 1987; Yeudall et al., 1987). However, the relationship between education and Category Test performance has been equivocal in patient groups, with some authors documenting a significant correlation (Alekoumbides et al., 1987; Boyle, 1986; Lin & Rennick, 1974; Seidenberg et al., 1984), and other failing to detect an association (Corrigan et al., 1987; Finlayson et al., 1977; Prigatano & Parsons, 1976; Vega & Parsons, 1967). Seidenberg et al. (1984), using a multivariate approach, reported that education was a more influential variable in Category Test performance than age, however, the age range of their subjects was very attenuated (range = 15 to 52).

A consistent negative relationship has been observed between Category Test scores and IQ in both normal and patient groups, although reports have differed as to whether VIQ or PIQ is more tied to the Category Test performance. For example, several studies have indicated that Category Test scores are more associated with PIQ (Corrigan et al., 1987; Cullum et al., 1984; Goldstein & Shelly, 1972; Lansdell and Donnelly, 1977), while other publications have documented a stronger association between VIQ or WAIS verbal factor scores and Category Test performance (Shore et al., 1971; Yeudall et al., 1987). Corrigan et al. (1987) point out that the correlations with PIQ have been relatively consistent across studies, suggesting the presence of a reliable relationship; however, the correlation with VIQ has varied widely, and inexplicably, across studies.

In general, no significant sex differences have been noted in Category Test performance (Dodrill, 1979; Fromm-Auch & Yeudall, 1983; Heaton et al., 1986, 1991; Kupke, 1983; Pauker, 1980; Seidenberg et al., 1984; Yeudall et al., 1987), although Ernst (1987) reported that in his elderly sample men performed slightly better than women on the booklet version of the test.

Handedness (Gregory & Paul, 1980; Seidenberg et al., 1984) and socioeconomic status (Seidenberg et al., 1984) do not appear to be related to Category Test scores. However, health status is moderately related to Category Test performance as reported by Willis et al. (1988).

A recent article by Arnold et al. (1994) documents a significant effect of acculturation on the original version of the Category Test performance for a sample of Mexican-American subjects, with more acculturated individuals demonstrating higher performance.

METHOD FOR EVALUATING THE NORMATIVE REPORTS

Our review of the literature located seven Category Test normative reports for adults published since 1965 (Dodrill, 1987; Ernst, 1987; Fromm-Auch & Yeudall, 1983; Harley et al., 1980; Heaton et al., 1991; Pauker, 1980; Yeudall et al., 1987), as well as the original Halstead (1947) and Reitan (1955b, 1959) normative data and three interpretive guides (Logue & Allen, 1971; Reitan & Wolfson, 1985; Russel et al., 1970). Hundreds of other studies have also reported control subject data, and we have included discussion of nine of those investigations which involved some unique feature, such as large sample size (>100), retest data, elderly population, or non-English-speaking sample (Alekoumbides et al., 1987; Anthony et al., 1980; Bornstein et al., 1987a; El-Sheikh et al., 1987; Heaton et al., 1986; Klove & Lochen, in Klove, 1974; Mack & Carlson 1978; Russell, 1987; Wiens & Matarazzo, 1977).

Russell and Starkey (1993) developed the Halstead-Russell Neuropsychological Evaluation System (HRNES), which includes the Category Test among 22 tests. In the context of this system, individual performance is compared to that of 576 brain-damaged subjects and 200 subjects who were initially suspected of having brain damage but had negative neurological findings. Data were partitioned into seven age groups and three educational/IQ levels. This study will not be reviewed in this chapter because the "normal" group consisted of the V.A. patients who presented with symptomatology requiring neuropsychological evaluation. For further discussion of the HRNES system see Lezak (1995, pp. 714–715).

Of note, few relevant manuscripts have emerged since the 1980s, perhaps due either to the publication of Heaton et al.'s (1991) comprehensive normative tables, or to the escalating use in research and clinical practice of flexible neuropsychological test protocols which include newer tasks rather than traditional fixed neuropsychological batteries.

In order to adequately evaluate the Category Test normative reports, six key criterion variables were deemed critical. The first five of these relate to *subject* variables, and the one remaining dimension refers to *procedural* issues.

Minimal requirements for meeting criterion variables were as follows:

Subject Variables

Sample Size

As discussed in previous chapters, a minimum of at least 50 subjects per grouping interval is optimal.

Sample Composition Description

As discussed previously, information regarding medical and psychiatric exclusion criteria is important; it is unclear if geographic recruitment region, sex, socioeconomic status or occupation, ethnicity, handedness, and recruitment procedures are relevant, so until this is determined, it is best that this information be provided.

Age-Group Intervals

Given the association between age and Category Test performance, information regarding age of the normative sample is critical and normative data should be presented by age intervals.

Reporting of IQ Levels

Given the relationships between Category Test performance and IQ, data should be presented by IQ intervals or at least information regarding intellectual level should be provided. In addition, given some evidence that PIQ may be more related to Category Test performance than is VIQ, information on PIQ and VIQ separate from FSIQ is desirable.

Reporting of Education Levels

Given a possible, although minor, association between education level and Category Test scores, it is preferable that information regarding highest educational level completed be reported.

Procedural Variables

Data Reporting

Means and standard deviations, and preferably ranges, for total Category Test errors are required.

SUMMARY OF THE STATUS OF THE NORMS

All but eight datasets had total sample sizes larger than 100 (Bornstein et al., 1987a; El-Sheikh et al., 1987; Halstead, 1947; Klove & Lochen, in Klove, 1974; Mack & Carlson, 1978; Reitan, 1955b, 1959; Wiens & Matarazzo, 1977). Only two publications consistently had at least 50 subjects in individual subject groupings (Ernst, 1987; Heaton et al., 1986), although some reports had some subgroups which met this criterion (Fromm-Auch & Yeudall, 1983; Harley et al., 1980; Pauker, 1980; Yeudall et al., 1987).

Nine of the studies summarized in this chapter present Category Test data according to circumscribed age ranges (Ernst, 1987; Fromm-Auch & Yeudall, 1983; Harley et al., 1980; Heaton et al., 1986, 1991; Mack & Carlson, 1978; Pauker, 1980; Wiens & Matarazzo, 1977; Yeudall et al., 1987). Information on IQ levels is reported in all but five studies (El-Sheikh et al., 1987; Ernst, 1987; Heaton et al., 1986; Klove & Lochen, in Klove, 1974; Russell, 1985), and one report presented Category Test data in age-by-IQ groupings (Pauker, 1980). Similarly, educational level was also indicated in all but two studies (Bornstein et al., 1987a; Pauker, 1980), and Heaton et al. (1986, 1991) organized data by educational levels. Information on gender composition of the samples was available in all but three reports (Anthony et al., 1980; Harley et al., 1980; Klove & Lochen, in Klove, 1974); three datasets included only male (Wiens & Matarazzo, 1977) or nearly all male (Alekoumbides et al., 1987; Russell, 1987) populations, and one dataset was composed primarily of females (Mack & Carlson, 1978).

Ernst (1987) and Heaton et al. (1991) presented data separately for males and females.

Information on other subject variables was provided less frequently; data on handedness were indicated in three studies (Dodrill, 1987; Fromm-Auch & Yeudall, 1983; Yeudall et al., 1987); occupation or socioeconomic status was described in five reports (Alekoumbides et al., 1987; Dodrill, 1987; Halstead, 1947; Wienes & Matarazzo, 1977; Yeudall et al., 1987); and information regarding ethnicity was presented in three datasets (Alekoumbides et al., 1987; Dodrill, 1987; Russell, 1987). Exclusion criteria were judged to be adequate in only eight publications (Anthony et al., 1980; Bornstein et al., 1987a; Dodrill, 1987; Fromm-Auch & Yeudall, 1983; Heaton et al., 1991; Pauker, 1980; Wiens & Matarazzo, 1977; Yeudall et al., 1987). Geographic recruitment areas were specified in all but three publications (Bornstein et al., 1987a; Dodrill, 1987; Mack & Carlson, 1978). Eleven datasets were obtained in the United States (Alekoumbides et al., 1987; Anthony et al., 1980; Halstead, 1947; Harley et al., 1980; Heaton et al., 1986, 1991; Klove & Lochen, in Klove, 1974; Reitan, 1955b, 1959; Russell, 1987; Wiens & Matarazzo, 1977), three in Canada (Fromm-Auch & Yeudall, 1983; Pauker, 1980; Yeudall et al., 1987), one in Norway (Klove & Lochen, in Klove, 1974), one in Egypt (El-Sheikh et al., 1987), and one in Australia (Ernst, 1987).

Total mean number of errors was reported in all datasets, and standard deviations were indicated in all but three studies (Halstead, 1947; Heaton et al., 1986; Klove & Lochen, in Klove, 1974). Ranges for number errors were presented in four publications (Bornstein et al., 1987a; Fromm-Auch & Yeudall, 1983; Halstead, 1947; Harley et al., 1980), and means and standard deviations for individual subtest scores are provided in two publications (Ernst, 1987; Mack & Carlson, 1978). Some studies reported supplementary Category Test scores such as IQ-equivalent scores (Dodrill, 1987), test–retest data (Bornstein et al., 1987; El-Sheikh et al., 1987), T-score equivalents for raw scores (Harley et al., 1980), and T-score equivalents corrected for age, education, and sex (Heaton et al., 1991).

Table 20.2 summarizes information provided in the studies described in this chapter.

Table 20.2. CT.L; Locator Table for the CT

Study°	Age°°	N	Sample Composition	IQ,°° Education	Country/ Location
CT.1 Halstead, 1947 page 460	15–50	28	14 Ss without psychiatric diagnosis, no history of brain injury. 14 Ss with psychiatric diagnosis	Education 7–18 IQ 70–140	Chicago
CT.2 Reitan, 1955b; 1959 page 460	32.36 (10.78)	50	35 M, 15 F, volunteers. Ss hospitalized with paraplegia and neurosis were included	Education 11.58 (2.85) FSIQ 112.6 (14.3)	Indiana
CT.3 Reitan & Wolfson, 1985 page 461			No information is provided regarding the normmative sample. Cutoffs for "severity ranges" (perfectly normal, normal, mildly normal, impaired and seriously impaired) are presented		
CT.4 Harley, et al., 1980 page 461	55–79 55–59 60–64 65–69 70–74 75–79	193 56 45 35 37 20	V.A. hospitalized patients. T score equivalents are reported	Education 8.8	Wisconsin
CT.5 Pauker, 1980 page 462	19–71 19–34 35–52 53–71	363	Volunteers fluent in English. 152 M, 211 F. Ss had no physical disability, sensory deficit, current medical illness, brain disorder, or alcoholism. Data are presented in age × IQ cells	WAIS IQ 89–102 103–112 113–122 123–143	Toronto
CT.6 Fromm-Auch & Yeudall, 1983 page 464	15–64 25.4 (8.2) 15–17 18–23 24–32 33–40 41–64	193 32 75 57 18 10	111 M, 82 F. Participants described as non-psychiatric and non-neurological. 83% are R-handed. Ss classified in 5 age groupings	Education 8–26 years 14.8 (3.0) FSIQ 119.1 (8.8)	Canada
CT.7 Dodrill, 1987 page 465	27.73 (11.04)	120	60 M, 60 F volunteers. Data for various intelligence levels are presented	Education 12.28 (2.18) FSIQ 100 (14.35)	Washington
CT.8 Ernst, 1987 page 465	65–75 69.6 (2.7)	110	51 M, 59 F volunteers	Education 10.3	Brisbane, Australia
CT.9 Yeudall et al., 1987 page 466	15–40 15–20 21–25 26–30 31–40	225 62 73 48 42	Volunteers, 127 M, 98 F classified in 4 age groupings; 88% were R-handed	Education 14.55 (2.78) FSIQ 112.25 (10.25)	Canada
CT.10 Heaton et al., 1991 page 467	42.1 (16.8) Groups: 20–34 35–39 40–44 45–49 50–54 55–59 60–64 65–69	486	Volunteers: urban and rural. Data collected over 15 years through multi-center collaborative efforts. Strict exclusion criteria. 65% M. Data are presented in T score equivalents for M and F separately in 10 age groups by 6 educational groups	Education 13.6 (3.5) Groups: 6–8 9–11 12 13–15 16–17 ≥18 FSIQ 113.8 (12.3)	California, Washington, Texas, Oklahoma, Wisconsin, Illinois, Michigan, New York, Virginia Massachusetts, Canada

continued

Table 20.2. (*Continued*)

Study[a]	Age[b]	N	Sample Composition	IQ,[b] Education	Country/Location
	70–74 75–80				
CT.11 Klove & Lochen (in Klove, 1974) page 468	31.6 32.1	22 22	American and Norwegian controls	Education 11.1 12.2 FSIQ 109.3 111.9	Wisconsin, Norway
CT.12 Wien & Matarazzo, 1977 page 469	23.6 24.8	48	All male, neurologically normal. Divided into two groups. Random sample of 29 were retested 14 to 24 weeks later	Education 13.7 14.0 FSIQ 117.5 118.3	Portland, Oregon
CT.13 Mack & Carlson, 1978 page 469	60–80 69.76 (4.87) 20–37 25.03 (3.70)	41 40	Older Ss: 3 M, 38 F no history of neurological impairment. Younger Ss: 9 M, 31 F; no screening for neurological impairment was conducted. Computerized administration was used	Older Ss Education 14.05 (3.39) FSIQ 119.90 (15.14) Younger Ss Education 15.43 (2.65) FSIQ 113.76 (4.89)	
CT.14 Anthony et al., 1980 page 470	38.88 (15.80)	100	Normal volunteers, no history of medical or psychiatric problems, head injury, brain disease, or substance abuse	Education 13.33 (2.56) FSIQ 113.5 (10.8)	Colorado
CT.15 Heaton, et al., 1986 page 471	15–81 39.3 (17.5) <40 40–59 ≥60	553 319 134 100	356 M,197 F. Exclusion criteria included history of neurologic illness, significant head trauma, and substance abuse. Sample was divided into 3 age groups and 3 education groups. % classification as normal is provided	Education 0–20 13.3 (3.4) <12 (132) 12–15 (249) ≥16(172)	Colorado, California, Wisconsin
CT.16 Alekoumbides et al., 1987a page 471	19–82 46.85 (17.17)	112	Ss were medical and psychiatric V.A. patients without cerebral lesions or histories of alcoholism or cerebral contusions. All Ss except for one were male	Education 1–20 11.43(3.20) FSIQ 105.9 (13.5)	S. California
CT.17 Bornstein et al., 1987a page 472	17–52 32.3 (10.3)	23	Volunteers: 9 M, 14 F. No history of neurological or psychiatric illness. Test–retest data are provided	VIQ 88–128 105.8 (10.8) PIQ 85–121 105.0(10.5)	
CT.18 El-Sheikh et al., 1987 page 473	17–24 20.6	32	Ss were undergrads and graduate students; 54 M, 58 F with no history of brain damage. Test–retest data are provided		Cairo, Egypt
CT.19 Russell, 1987 page 473	46.19 (12.86)	155	Patients in V.A. hospitals. 148 M, 7 F; Ss were suspected of having neuro- logical disorders, but had negative findings	Education 12.29(3.00) FSIQ 111.9	Cincinnati & Miami

[a]The study number corresponds to the number provided in the text of the chapter.

[b]Age column and IQ/education column contain information regarding range and/or mean and standard deviation for the whole sample and/or separate groups, whichever information is provided by the authors.

SUMMARIES OF THE STUDIES

Given that the use of the Category Test has typically been within the context of the Halstead-Reitan Battery, the Halstead (1947) and Reitan (1955b, 1959; Reitan & Wolfson, 1985) data and interpretation recommendations will be reported first, followed by a summary of the other interpretation formats, and then the normative publications will be presented in ascending chronological order. The chapter will conclude with a review of Category Test control data reported in various clinical studies.

Original Studies

[CT.1] Halstead, 1947

The author obtained Category Test data on 28 control subjects in Chicago, more than half of whom had psychiatric diagnoses. The 14 subjects without psychiatric diagnoses were nine male and five female civilians ranging in age from 15 to 50 (Mean = 25.9), without history of brain injury. The eight subjects who carry diagnoses of mild psychoneurosis were male soldiers ranging in age from 22 to 38 (Mean = 29.6); some had had combat experience but none had a history of head injury. The last six subjects ranged in age from 27 to 39 and included a depressed military prisoner facing execution, a severely depressed female with suicidal and homicidal impulses tested prior to lobotomy, and a suicidal/homicidal female and a suicidal male tested pre- and *post*lobotomy. Educational level ranged from 7 to 18 years, and the following occupations were represented: artist, entertainer, farmer, housewife, semiskilled and unskilled laborers, professional, secretary, teacher, technician, trade, and student. Ethnic background included American, Balkan, English, French, German, Irish, Polish, Scandinavian, and Scotish. IQ levels ranges from 70 to 140.

Mean errors are reported for the total group and each control "subgroup," as well as individual scores for each subject. The Category Test criterion score used in calculating the Impairment Index was greater than 80 errors.

Study strengths
1. Information provided regarding IQ, education, occupation, ethnicity, geographic recruitment area, age, and gender.

Considerations regarding use of the study
1. Small sample size including use of two subjects twice.
2. Inclusion of subjects with psychiatric diagnoses and postlobotomy.
3. No reporting of standard deviations.
4. Undifferentiated age range (Table 20.3).

[CT.2] Reitan, 1955b (see also Reitan, 1959)

The author obtained Category Test scores on 50 subjects in Indiana who had apparently been referred for neuropsychological testing and "who had received neurological examinations before testing and showed no signs or symptoms of cerebral damage or dysfunction. . . . None . . . had positive anamnestic findings" (p. 29), but some were hospitalized with paraplegia or neurosis. The sample included 35 men and 15 women, mean age was 32.36 ± 10.78, and mean educational level was 11.58 ± 2.85. Mean WAIS VIQ, PIQ, and FSIQ were 110.82 ± 14.46, 112.18 ± 14.23, and 112.64 ± 14.28, respectively.

Study strengths
1. Information regarding IQ, educational level, sex, age, and geographic recruitment area.
2. Adequate sample size.
3. Means and standard deviations are reported.

Considerations regarding use of the study
1. Undifferentiated age range.
2. Insufficient medical and psychiatric exclusion criteria; the sample included subjects hospitalized with spinal cord injuries and psychiatric disorders.
3. High average IQ (Table 20.4).

Table 20.3. CT.1; Mean Number of Errors for the Total Group and for Three "Subgroups"

	N	No. of Errors
Total	28	36.72
Civilian	14	26.8 (10–46)
Military	8	50.8 (29–75)
Miscellaneous	6	34.8 (16–93)

Table 20.4. CT.2

N	Age	Education	VIQ	PIQ	FSIQ	No. of Errors
50	32.36 (10.78)	11.58 (2.85)	110.82 (14.46)	112.18 (14.23)	112.64 (14.28)	32.38 (12.62)

Interpretive Guides

In constructing their neuropsychological key approach, *Russell, Neuringer, and Goldstein, 1970,* devised six rating equivalents of Category Test raw error scores based primarily on "rules of thumb" recommended by P. M. Rennick. Russell (1984) subsequently modified the ratings as reflected in Table 20.5.

Logue and Allen (1971) published a predictor table plotting the expected number of Category Test errors for nine WAIS FSIQ values based on Reitan's 1959 Wechsler-Bellevue and Category Test scores on control subjects. "Use of the table . . . allows a direct comparison of scores actually obtained from a given client on the WAIS and on the Category Test. Where the relationship is not at the predicted level, the examiner can have more confidence that the obtained category score is not an artifact of limited or superior intelligence " (p. 1096). The authors caution that the expected Category Test scores at the highest IQ values are probably unrealistically low (Table 20.6).

[CT.3] Reitan and Wolfson, 1985

The authors provide general guidelines for Category Test score interpretation in the form of "severity ranges": "perfectly normal (or better than average)," "normal," "mildly impaired," and "seriously impaired." They list the number of errors which correspond to each severity range. No other information is provided such as score means or standard deviations, or any data regarding the normative sample on which these guidelines were developed.

Considerations regarding use of the study

The authors argued that these norms were meant as "general guidelines" and that "exact percentile ranks corresponding with each possible score are hardly necessary because the other methods of inference are used to supplement normative data in clinical interpretation of results of individual subjects" (p. 977). However, we maintain that more precise scores as well as separate normative data for different age, IQ, and educational levels are necessary to avoid false positive errors in diagnosis.

It is not clear how the cutoffs depicted below were developed; they do not match the cutoffs cited by Halstead (1947). The authors report that a cutoff of 50 was recommended by Halstead in computing the Impairment Index, but examination of Halstead's (1947) manuscript revealed that his cutoff was greater than 80, not greater than 50. It appears that Reitan derived his cutoff by computing the ratio of errors to total items for the Halstead administration and applied the same ratio to his 208-item version (e.g., $80/336 = 50/208$) (Table 20.7).

Normative Studies

[CT.4] Harley, Leuthold, Matthews, and Bergs, 1980

The authors collected Category Test data on 193 V.A.-hospitalized patients in Wisconsin ranging in age from 55 to 79. Exclusion criteria included FSIQ less than 80, active psychosis, unequivocal neurological disease or brain damage, and serious visual or auditory acuity prob-

Table 20.5. CT.Russell°

	Rating equivalent of raw scores						
	0	1	2	3	4	5	6
Errors	0–25	26–52	53–78	79–104	105–130	131–156	>5 Er-col II

°A score of 156 is considered a random score.

Table 20.6. CT.L&A

WAIS FSIQ	Predicted Category Test Score
140	10
130	15
120	21
110	26
100	32
90	37
80	43
70	48
60	54

lems. Patients with diagnosis of chronic brain syndrome *were* included. Patient diagnoses were as follows: chronic brain syndrome unrelated to alcoholism, psychosis, alcoholic, neurotic, and personality disorder. Mean educational level was 8.8 years. The sample was divided into five age groupings: 55–59 (*n* = 56), 60–64 (*n* = 45), 65–69 (*n* = 35), 70–74 (*n* = 37), and 75–79 (*n* = 20). Mean educational level and percent of sample included in each of the diagnostic classifications are reported for each of the diagnostic classifications and for each age grouping. The authors also provide test data on a subgroup of 160 subjects equated for percent diagnosed with alcoholism across the five age groupings. The "alcohol-equated sample" was developed "to minimize the influence that cognitive or motor/sensory differences uniquely attributable to alcohol abuse might have upon group test performance levels" (p. 2). This subsample remained heterogeneous regarding representation of the other diagnostic categories.

Mean errors and standard deviations are provided by age groupings for the total and alcohol-equated samples. In addition, *T*-score equivalents for raw scores are reported as well as "percentage of best raw score," which indicated where a raw score falls within the range of raw scores for that age grouping. We repro-

Table 20.7. CT.3; Severity Ranges (Based on the Number of Errors)

Normal	Perfectly Normal	0–25	Impaired	Mildly	46–65
	Normal	26–45		Seriously	≥66

duce only the mean, standard deviation, and range for total errors due to space considerations.

Study strengths
1. Large sample size and many individual cells approximate *N*s of 50.
2. Reporting of data on IQ, educational level, and geographic recruitment area.
3. Data presented in age groupings.
4. Means and standard deviations are reported.

Considerations regarding use of the study
1. The presence of substantial neurologic (chronic brain syndrome), substance abuse, and major psychiatric disorders in the sample.
2. Low educational level, although IQ levels are average.
3. No information regarding sex, although given that data were obtained in a V.A. setting, the sample is likely all or nearly all male.
4. The presence of odd variability across scores, with the 75–79-year-olds outperforming the younger age groups, and the 60–64-year-olds outperforming the 55–59-year-olds.

Other comments
The scores for the two oldest age groups are identical in the whole sample and alcohol-equated group because these two groups did not have overrepresentation of alcoholics, so they did not need to be adjusted (Table 20.8).

[CT.5] Pauker, 1980
The author obtained Category Test scores on 363 Toronto citizens fluent in English recruited through announcements and notices. Subjects ranged in age from 19 to 71 and included 152 men and 211 women. Exclusion criteria consisted of significant physical disability, sensory deficit, current medical illness, using of medication that might affect test performance, history of actual or suspected brain disorder, and alcoholism. The MMPI profiles "could not suggest severe disturbance" or include more than three clinical scales with *T* scores greater than or equal to 70 or an F scale score greater than 80.

The Category Test was administered accord-

Table 20.8. CT.4; Means, Standard Deviations, and Ranges for the Number of Errors per Five Age Intervals for the Whole Sample and for the Alcohol-Equated Sample

N	Age	WAIS			Education	Errors
		FSIQ	VIQ	PIQ		
Total Sample						
56	55–59	98.57	99.39	97.00	10.1	64.13
		(11.43)	(12.92)	(10.65)		(28.47)
		80–129	77–131	72–129		19–115
45	60–64	98.58	101.27	95.00	9.8	59.78
		(9.93)	(11.42)	(9.82)		(19.68)
		80–121	78–123	78–116		30–110
35	65–69	97.51	100.37	93.66	8.7	72.65
		(11.18)	(12.51)	(10.20)		(28.96)
		80–130	80–135	68–120		22–141
37	70–74	100.41	102.95	97.24	8.8	85.60
		(9.92)	(11.81)	(10.08)		(36.27)
		82–125	80–133	75–114		21–162
20	75–79	101.75	101.40	102.15	6.5	69.60
		(10.18)	(11.40)	(9.95)		(26.89)
		81–119	77–117	83–119		19–110
Alcohol-Equated Sample						
47	55–59	99.00	100.00	98.00	10.1	65.43
		(11.73)	(13.02)	(11.13)		(28.51)
		80–129	77–131	72–129		20–115
33	60–64	96.00	99.00	93.00	9.3	63.42
		(9.43)	(11.33)	(9.30)		(19.24)
		80–117	78–123	78–112		34–110
23	65–69	99.00	102.00	95.00	8.8	71.68
		(12.06)	(13.06)	(11.52)		(31.14)
		80–130	80–135	68–120		22–141
37	70–74	100.00	103.00	97.00	8.8	85.60
		(9.92)	(11.81)	(10.08)		(36.27)
		82–125	80–133	75–114		21–162
20	75–79	102.00	101.00	102.00	6.5	69.60
		(10.18)	(11.40)	(9.95)		(26.89)
		81–119	77–117	83–119		19–110

ing to Reitan's guidelines. Means and standard deviations for total errors are reported for the sample as a whole and for three age groupings (19–34, 35–52, 53–71) by four WAIS IQ levels (89–102, 103–112, 113–122, 123–143). Individual cell sample sizes ranged from four to 60. Age-by-IQ categories were determined "in a compromise between what would be desirable and what the obtained sample characteristics and size dictated" (p. 1). No differences in Cat-

egory Test performance between men and women were documented.

Study strengths
1. Large sample size, although individual cell sizes are substantially less than 50.
2. Presentation of the data in age-by-IQ groupings.
3. Adequate medical and psychiatric exclusion criteria.

4. Information regarding sex, recruitment procedures, and geographic recruitment area.

5. Means and standard deviations are reported.

Considerations regarding use of the study

1. No information regarding education.

2. Subjects were recruited in Canada, raising questions regarding usefulness for clinical interpretive purposes in the United States.

3. The age-by-IQ cell representing subjects aged 53 to 71 with IQs of 89 to 102 contained only four subjects; Pauker comments that this category "should not be considered to be of any more than interest value" (p. 2).

4. IQ levels below the average range not represented (Table 20.9).

[CT.6] Fromm-Auch and Yeudall, 1983

The authors obtained Category Test data on 193 Canadian subjects (111 male, 82 female) recruited through posted advertisements and personal contacts. Participants are described as "nonpsychiatric" and "non-neurological." Eighty-three percent of the sample were right-handed and mean age was 25.4 ± 8.2 (range = 15 to 64). Mean years of education were 14.8 ± 3.0 (range = 8–26) and included technical and university training. Mean WAIS FSIQ, VIQ, and PIQ were 119.1 ± 8.8 (range = 98 to 142), 119.8 ± 9.9 (range = 95 to 143), and 115.6 ± 9.8 (range = 89 to 146), respectively. Of note, no subjects obtained a FSIQ which was lower

than the average range. Subjects were classified into five age groupings: 15–17 ($n = 32$), 18–23 ($n = 75$), 24–32 ($n = 57$), 33–40 ($n = 18$), and 41–64 ($n = 10$).

Mean errors, standard deviations, and ranges are reported for each age grouping. No sex differences were documented and male and female data were collapsed. The authors suggest that a cutoff of 50 errors is only appropriate for the subjects less than 40 years of age.

Study strengths

1. Large overall sample size and some individual cells approximate Ns of 50.

2. Presentation of the data by age groupings.

3. Information regarding mean IQ, educational levels, handedness, sex, recruitment procedures, and geographical recruitment area.

4. Some psychiatric and neurological exclusion criteria.

5. Means and standard deviations are reported.

Considerations regarding use of the study

1. The high intellectual and educational level of the sample.

2. An age grouping of 41 to 64 with 10 subjects would not appear to be particularly useful.

3. Subjects were recruited in Canada, raising questions regarding usefulness for clinical interpretive purposes in the United States.

4. At least one subject in the 18–23-year-old group scored particularly poorly, causing the

Table 20.9. CT.5; Means and Standard Deviations for Total Errors for the Whole Sample and for Three Age Groups by Four WAIS IQ Levels

Age	WAIS IQ				
	89–102	103–112	113–122	123–143	89–143
19–34	$n = 21$	$n = 53$	$n = 60$	$n = 28$	$n = 162$
	61.67	40.08	29.82	23.64	36.24
	(18.95)	(17.47)	(14.26)	(11.93)	(19.33)
35–52	$n = 20$	$n = 34$	$n = 56$	$n = 25$	$n = 135$
	75.80	59.06	42.77	37.52	50.79
	(24.12)	(17.03)	(15.25)	(18.79)	(21.98
53–71	$n = 4$	$n = 15$	$n = 27$	$n = 20$	$n = 66$
	90.00	63.80	58.85	47.60	58.45
	(15.25)	(14.99)	(18.17)	(20.96)	(20.59)
19–71	$n = 45$	$n = 102$	$n = 143$	$n = 73$	$n = 363$
	70.47	49.89	40.37	34.96	45.69
	(22.69)	(19.76)	(18.69)	(19.58)	(22.37)

Table 20.10. CT.6; Mean Number of Errors, Standard Deviations, and Ranges for Each Age Grouping

N	Age	Category Errors
32	15–17	35.8 (16.2) 16–68
74	18–23	35.9 (21.2) 9–106
56	24–32	30.5 (13.6) 10–68
18	33–40	36.3 (14.3) 11–67
10	41–64	53.0 (21.0) 29–96

mean to be artificially low and the standard deviation to be excessively large for this age grouping (Table 20.10).

[CT.7] Dodrill, 1987

The author collected Category Test data on 120 subjects in Washington during the years 1975–1976 ($n = 81$) and 1986–1987 ($n = 39$). Half of the sample was female and 10% were minorities (six African-American, three native American, two Asian-American, one unknown). Eighteen were left-handed and occupational status included 45 students, 37 employed, 26 unemployed, 11 homemakers, and one retiree. Subjects were recruited from various sources including schools, churches, employment agencies, and community service agencies, and they either were paid for their participation or offered an interpretation of their abilities. Exclusion criteria included history of "neurologically relevant disease (such as meningitis or encephalitis)," alcoholism, birth complications "of likely neurological significance," oxygen deprivation, peripheral nervous system injury, psychotic or psychotic-like disorders, or head injury associated with unconsciousness, skull fracture, persisting neurological signs, or diagnosis of concussion or contusion. Of note, one-third of potential participants failed to meet the

above medical and psychiatric criteria, resulting in a final sample of 120. Mean age was $27.73 + 11.04$ and mean years of education was $12.28 + 2.18$. The subjects tested in the 1970s were administered the WAIS and the subjects assessed in the 1980s were administered the WAIS-R; WAIS scores were converted to WAIS-R equivalents by subtracting seven points from the VIQ, PIQ, and FSIQ. Mean FSIQ, VIQ, and PIQ scores were 100.00 ± 14.35, 100.92 ± 14.73 and 98.25 ± 13.39, respectively. IQ scores ranged from 60 to 138 and reflected a normal distribution.

Mean errors and standard deviation are reported as well as IQ-equivalent scores for various levels of intelligence. Using Reitan's cutoff of 50/51 errors, 22.5% of a subgroup of the sample were misclassified as brain damaged.

Study strengths
1. Large sample size.
2. Comprehensive exclusion criteria (although the appropriateness of including individuals with WAIS-R scores falling in the mentally deficient range could be questioned).
3. Information regarding age, education, IQ, occupation, sex ratio, handedness, ethnicity, recruitment procedures, and geographic area.
4. IQ equivalent scores provided.
5. Data for different IQ levels provided.
6. Means and standard deviations are reported.

Considerations regarding use of the study
1. Undifferentiated age range.
2. On the IQ-equivalent scores, the two highest IQ groups have poorer scores than the 115–120 IQ groups (Table 20.11).

[CT.8] Ernst, 1987

The author obtained Category Test data on 110 primarily Caucasian (99%) residents of Brisbane, Australia, aged 65 to 75. Fifty-nine were female and 51 were male, and mean educational level was 10.3 years; men and women did not differ in years of education. Subjects were recruited primarily through random selection from the Queensland State electoral roll ($n = 97$), with the remainder ($n = 13$) solicited through senior-citizen centers. Exclusion crite-

Table 20.11. CT.7; The Table Provides Mean Number of Errors and Standard Deviations for the Whole Sample and for Various Levels of Intelligence

N	Age	Education	FSIQ	VIQ	PIQ	Category Errors
120	27.73	12.28	100.00	100.92	98.25	35.74
	(11.04)	(2.18)	(14.35)	(14.73)	(13.39)	(22.76)

N	FSIQ	Category Errors	N	FSIQ	Category Errors
7	130	29	60	95	36
18	125	23	48	90	41
34	120	21	33	85	47
64	115	22	19	80	54
93	110	26	10	75	70
101	105	30		70	77
75	100	33			

ria included history of significant head trauma or neurologic disease. Nearly one-half of the sample were diagnosed with at least one chronic disease (hypertension = 33, heart disease = 9, thyroid dysfunction = 7, asthma = 5, emphysema = 2, diabetes = 1) for which they were receiving treatment and which was described as well controlled. Sixty-six of the subjects were receiving medications, primarily for the diseases listed above.

All subjects were administered the Trailmaking Test first, and half of the subjects were also administered the TPT prior to the Booklet Category Test. Mean errors and standard deviations for each of the seven subtests as well as total errors are reported. Using a cutoff of 51 errors, 84% of the sample were classified as impaired. Men obtained fewer errors than women on subtests 3 and 4 and on total errors. No differences in Category Test scores emerged between subjects with and without chronic disease. Educational level appeared to be related to scores on subtests 4, 5, and 7 and total errors. No differences in test performance were documented between those subjects who were or were not administered the TPT prior to the Category Test.

Study strengths
1. Large sample size in a restricted age range.
2. Presentation of the data by sex.
3. Information regarding education, geographic recruitment area, recruitment procedures, and ethnicity.

4. Information regarding test administration order effects.
5. Means and standard deviations are reported.

Considerations regarding use of the study
1. Approximately half of the subjects had at least one chronic illness, and over half were taking prescribed medications.
2. No information regarding IQ.
3. Low mean educational level.
4. Data were collected in Australia and may be unsuitable for clinical use in the United States (Table 20.12).

[CT.9] Yeudall, Reddon, Gill, and Stefanyk, 1987

The authors obtained Category Test data on 225 Canadian subjects recruited from posted advertisements in workplaces and personal solicitations. The participants included meat packers, postal workers, transit employees, hospital lab technicians, secretaries, ward aides, student interns, student nurses, and summer students. In addition, high school teachers identified for participation average students in grades 10 through 12. Exclusion criteria included evidence of "forensic involvement," head injury, neurological insult, prenatal or birth complications, psychiatric problems, or substance abuse. Subjects were classified into four age groupings: 15–20, 21–25, 26–30, and 31–40. Information regarding percent right-handers, mean years of education, and mean WAIS/WAIS-R FSIQ, VIQ, and PIQ are re-

Table 20.12. CT.8; Mean Number of Errors and Standard Deviations for Each of the Seven Subtests as Well as Total Errors for Each Gender Separately

| N | Sex | Category Test | | | | | | | |
		I	II	III	IV	V	VI	VII	Total
51	Male	0.1	0.5	19.9	13.7	16.5	10.6	5.8	66.7
		(0.6)	(0.7)	(10.0)	(11.1)	(7.5)	(7.1)	(2.6)	(27.3)
59	Female	0.2	0.5	25.4	20.5	17.8	12.4	6.7	83.3
		(0.6)	(0.8)	(7.3)	(10.6)	(6.5)	(5.7)	(2.3)	(21.6

ported for each age grouping for males and females separately and combined. For the sample as a whole, 88% were right-handed and had completed an average of 14.87 ± 2.99 years of schooling. The mean FSIQ, VIQ, and PIQ were 113.98 ± 9.83, 114.77 ± 10.34, and 108.50 ± 10.34, respectively.

Category Test data were gathered by experienced testing technicians who "motivated the subjects to achieve maximum performance" partially through the promise of detailed explanations of their test performance.

Means and standard deviations for total errors are presented for each age grouping and each age-by-sex grouping.

No significant relationships were found between Category Test scores and sex. Age effects were also not significant, although the authors note that variance effects with age were significant, and they recommend use of age norms. A significant negative association was found between Category Test scores and education, particularly in males, but education accounted for less than 10% of test score variance. Significant negative correlations were documented between test scores and VIQ and PIQ, again particularly in males, but only VIQ accounted for more than 10% of score variance. Because no significant differences were found between men and women, only the combined sample data are reproduced below.

Study strengths
1. Large sample size and individual cells approximate Ns of 50.
2. Grouping data by age.
3. Data availability for a 15–20-year-old age group.
4. Adequate medical and psychiatric exclusion criteria.

5. Information regarding handedness, education, IQ, sex, occupation, and geographic recruitment area, and recruitment procedures.
6. Means and standard deviations are reported.

Considerations regarding use of the study
1. The sample was atypical in terms of its high average intellectual level and high level of education.
2. The data were obtained on Canadian subjects, which may limit their usefulness for clinical interpretation in the United States due to possible subtle cultural differences.
3. Examination of the data reveals odd, unpredicted variability, with the 21–25-year-olds performing more poorly than the 26–30-year-olds (Table 20.13).

[CT.10] Heaton, Grant, and Matthews, 1991

The authors provide normative data on the Category Test from 486 urban and rural subjects recruited in several states (California, Washington, Colorado, Texas, Oklahoma, Wisconsin, Illinois, Michigan, New York, Virginia, and Massachusetts) and Canada. Data were collected over a 15-year period through multicenter collaborative efforts; the authors trained the test administrators and supervised data collection. Exclusion criteria included history of learning disability, neurologic disease, illness affecting brain function, significant head trauma, significant psychiatric disturbances (e.g., schizophrenia), and alcohol or other substance abuse. Mean age for the total sample was 42.0 ± 16.8, and mean educational level was 13.6 ± 3.5. Sixty-five percent of the sample were males. Mean WAIS FSIQ, VIQ, and PIQ were 113.8 ± 12.3, 113.9 ± 13.8, and 111.9 ± 11.6, respectively.

Subjects were generally paid for their partic-

Table 20.13. CT.9; The Table Provides Mean Number of Errors for the Whole Sample and for Each Age Group

N	Age	Education	% Right-Handed	FSIQ	VIQ	PIQ	Category Errors
62	15–20	12.16 (1.75)	79.09	111.75 (10.16)	111.18 (10.92)	108.30 (10.47)	33.88 (18.25)
73	21–25	14.82 (1.88)	86.03	109.79 (9.97)	110.48 (10.43)	105.88 (11.20)	35.10 (19.82)
48	26–30	15.50 (2.65)	89.58	113.95 (10.61)	114.40 (11.45)	110.28 (8.72)	30.52 (14.00)
42	31–40	16.50 (3.11)	90.48	116.09 (9.51)	117.76 (9.32)	109.72 (11.45)	36.28 (13.66)
225	15–40	14.55 (2.78)	85.78	112.25 (10.25)	112.60 (10.86)	108.13 (10.63)	33.97 (17.20)

ipation, and were judged to have provided their best efforts on the tasks. The Category Test was administered according to Reitan and Wolfson's (1985) instructions. A *T*-score system with demographic correction was developed on 378 subjects and cross-validated on 108 subjects. Total number of errors was the performance parameter employed. Age accounted for 38% of the variance in test scores, and education was associated with 20% of score variance: Sex did not account for any score variance. These demographic variables in combination were associated with 43% of score variance. Extensive *T*-score tables corrected for age, education, and sex are provided, and the interested reader is referred directly to the handbook for these data. The comprehensive tables present *T*-score equivalents for test scaled scores for males and females separately in 10 age groupings (20–34, 35–39, 40–44, 45–49, 50–54, 55–59, 60–64, 65–69, 70–74, 75–80) by six educational groupings (6–8 years, 9–11 years, 12 years, 13–15 years, 16–17 years, 18+ years). For the sample as a whole, mean errors was 39.6 ± 25.6.

Study strengths
1. Large sample size.
2. *T* scores corrected for age, education, and sex.
3. Adequate exclusion criteria.
4. Information regarding IQ and geographic recruitment area.

Considerations regarding use of the study
1. Above average mean intellectual level (which is probably less of an issue given that this is WAIS rather than WAIS-R IQ data).

Other comments
1. The interested reader is referred to 1996 critique of Heaton et al. (1991) norms, and Heaton et al.'s 1996 response to this critique.

Control Groups in Clinical Studies

[CT.11] Klove and Lochen (in Klove, 1974)

The authors obtained Category Test data on 22 American controls from Wisconsin and 22 Norwegian controls as a part of a validation study on the ability of the Halstead-Reitan Battery to detect brain damage. The mean age, educational level, and IQ for the American subjects were 31.6, 11.1, and 109.3, respectively, and the mean age, educational level, and IQ for the Norwegian subjects were 32.1, 12.2, 111.9, respectively. Category Test scores are presented in terms of mean errors for each group.

Study strengths
1. This publication is unique in providing Category Test data on a Norwegian population.
2. Information regarding educational level, IQ, age, and geographic recruitment area reported.

Table 20.14. CT.11

	N	Age	Education	IQ	Category Errors
Americans	22	31.6	11.1	109.3	34.6
Norwegians	22	32.1	12.2	111.9	45.5

Considerations regarding use of the study

1. The small sample size.
2. Undifferentiated age ranges.
3. No standard deviations reported.
4. No exclusion criteria specified and no information regarding gender distribution of the sample is provided (Table 20.14).

[CT.12] Wiens and Matarazzo, 1977

The authors collected Category Test data on 48 male applicants to a patrolman program in Portland, Oregon, as part of an investigation of the WAIS and MMPI correlates of the Halstead-Reitan Battery. All subjects passed a medical exam and were judged to be neurologically normal. Subjects were divided into two equal groups which were comparable in age (23.6 vs. 24.8), education (13.7 vs. 14.0), and WAIS FSIQ (117.5 vs. 118.3). A random subsample of 29 of the applicants was readministered the Category Test 14 to 24 weeks following the original administration. Means and standard deviations for Category Test total errors are reported for both the original testing and retest. One of the 29 subjects obtained a score higher than Reitan's suggested cutoff of 50/51 errors. No significant correlations were observed between Category Test scores and FSIQ, VIQ, or PIQ in either control group (Wiens & Matarazzo, 1977).

Study strengths

1. Information on test/retest performance.
2. Relatively large sample size for the small age range.
3. Adequate medical exclusion criteria.
4. Information provided regarding educational level, IQ, sex, and geographic recruitment area.
5. Means and standard deviations are reported.

Considerations regarding use of the study

1. High IQ level.
2. High educational level.
3. The standard deviations differ markedly between the two control groups, suggesting either unusual variability in scores for the first group or unusual lack of variability in the second group, or an error in reporting the data.
4. All-male sample (Table 20.15).

[CT.13] Mack and Carlson, 1978

The authors obtained Category Test data on 41 older (range 60–80) and 40 young (range 20–37) subjects as a part of an investigation into the neuropsychological effects of aging. Older subjects with histories of neurological impairment or "signs or symptoms of diseases with neurological significance (or which predispose subjects to possible neurological disorder)" were excluded. No screening for neurological

Table 20.15. CT.12; Mean Number of Errors and Standard Deviations for Two Equal Subject Groups[°]

			WAIS			Category Errors	
N	Age	Education	FSIQ	VIQ	PIQ	Test	Retest
24	23.6 (21–27)	13.7 (12–16)	117.5 (8.3)	117.4 (8.4)	115.4 (10.5)	23.5 (21.3)	
24	24.8 (21–28)	14.0 (12–16)	118.3 (6.8)	116.4 (6.9)	118.2 (8.6)	22.8 (11.8)	
29	24 (21–28)	14 (12–16)	118	116	118	22.83 (19.15)	11.21 (9.32)

[°]Test–retest data are also provided for 29 subjects who were assessed twice.

impairment was conducted in the younger sample, which was drawn from a university student body and hospital staff. The older sample included three men and 38 women; mean educational level was 14.05 ± 3.39 years and mean WAIS FSIQ was 119.90 ± 15.14. The young sample consisted of 31 female and nine male subjects, and mean years of education and mean IQ (based on Shipley scores in 17 subjects) were 15.43 ± 2.65 and 113.76 ± 4.89, respectively.

The Category Test was computer administered according to standard instructions with the exception that after subjects made a response by pressing a button, they could change their response. Once they were satisfied with a response they pushed an "0" key which was followed by feedback on the correctness of the response and the slide projector advanced to the next trial. The authors concluded that this modification had little effect given that few subjects corrected an initial choice.

Total mean errors and standard deviations are provided as well as mean errors and standard deviations for subtests III, IV, V, VI, and VII. The elderly subjects performed significantly more poorly than young controls and comparable to a middle-aged brain damaged sample. The elderly sample showed particular difficulty on subtests II and IV relative to the younger sample.

Study strengths
1. Data are presented in the age groupings.
2. Adequate exclusion criteria in the older subjects.
3. Information regarding education, IQ, sex, and (in the younger subjects) occupation.
4. Data for several individual subtests as well as total errors.

5. Means and standard deviations are reported.

Considerations regarding use of the study
1. No exclusion criteria for the younger subjects.
2. IQ data not available for all subjects and two IQ measures used.
3. Minor alterations in test administration format (computer-assisted).
4. Relatively small sample size and relatively large age range within each age grouping.
5. High educational and intellectual levels.
6. Samples are primarily female (Table 20.16).

[CT.14] Anthony, Heaton, and Lehman, 1980

The authors amassed Category Test data on 100 normal volunteers from Colorado as a part of a cross-validation of two objective, computerized interpretative programs for the Halstead-Reitan Battery. Subjects had no history of medical or psychiatric problems, head trauma, brain disease, or substance abuse. In addition, for 85% of the controls, normal EEGs and neurological exams were obtained; in the remaining 15% of the subjects it appeared that this information was not available. Mean age was 38.88 ± 15.80 and mean years of education were 13.33 ± 2.56. Mean WAIS FSIQ, VIQ, and PIQ were 113.54 ± 10.83, 113.24 ± 11.59, and 112.26 ± 10.88, respectively. Category Test data are presented in terms of mean number of errors and standard deviation. Subjects incorrectly identified as brain damaged (according to the Russell et al., 1970, system) were older, less educated, and less intelligent than subjects correctly classified as non–brain damaged.

Table 20.16. CT.13; Mean Number of Errors and Standard Deviations for the Whole Test and for The Subtests III–VII for Two Age Groups

						Subtest			
N	Age	Education	IQ	III	IV	V	VI	VII	Total
40	25.03	15.43	113.76	14.95	10.00	12.55	7.00	3.72	48.82
	(3.70)	(2.65)	(14.89)	(11.93)	(9.54)	(6.55)	(5.39)	(2.92)	(27.93)
41	69.76	14.05	119.90	25.07	23.46	19.22	15.32	7.93	91.73
	(4.87)	(3.39)	(15.14)	(10.74)	(8.57)	(6.34)	(7.51)	(2.62)	(26.26)

Table 20.17. CT.14

N	Age	Education	WAIS			Category Errors
			FSIQ	VIQ	PIQ	
100	38.88	13.33	113.54	113.24	112.26	32.59
	(15.80)	(2.56)	(10.83)	(11.59)	(10.88)	(21.80)

Study strengths
1. Large sample size.
2. Adequate exclusion criteria.
3. Information regarding education, IQ, age, and geographic recruitment area.
4. Means and standard deviations are reported.

Considerations regarding use of the study
1. The large undifferentiated age grouping.
2. The IQ range is high average.
3. No information regarding sex (Table 20.17).

[CT.15] Heaton, Grant, and Matthews, 1986

The authors obtained Category Test data on 553 normal controls in Colorado, California, and Wisconsin as a part of an investigation into the effects of age, education, and sex on Halstead-Reitan Battery performance. Nearly two-thirds of the sample were male (males = 356, females = 197). Exclusion criteria included history of neurological illness, significant head trauma, and substance abuse. Subjects ranged in age from 15 to 81 years (Mean = 39.3 ± 17.5), and mean years of education was 13.3 ± 3.4 with a range of 0 to 20 years. The sample was divided into three age categories (<40, 40–59, and ≥0) with sizes of 319, 134, and 100, respectively, and classified into three education categories (<12 years, 12 to 15 years, ≥6 years) with sizes of 132, 249, and 172, respectively.

Testing was conducted by trained technicians and all participants were judged to have expended their best effort on the task. Mean errors are reported for the six subgroups, as well as percent classified as normal using Russell et al.'s (1970) criteria. Approximately 30% of the test score variance was accounted for by educational level. Significant group differences were found across the three age groups and the three educational levels, and a significant age-by-

education interaction was documented. No significant differences in performance were found between males and females.

Study strengths
1. Large size of overall sample and individual cells.
2. Information regarding education, sex, age, and geographic recruitment area.
3. Data are grouped by age as well as education level.

Considerations regarding use of the study
1. No reporting of standard deviations.
2. Means for individual WAIS subtest scaled scores reported but not overall IQ scores (Table 20.18).

[CT.16] Alekoumbides, Charter, Adkins, and Seacat, 1987

The authors report Category Test data on 112 medical and psychiatric inpatients and outpatients without cerebral lesions or histories of alcoholism or cerebral contusion, from V.A. hospitals in Southern California, as a part of their development of standardized scores corrected for age and education for the Halstead-Reitan Battery. Among the 41 psychiatric patients, nine were diagnosed as psychotic and 32 were neurotic. In addition to Psychiatry Services, patients were also drawn from medicine (n = 57), neurology (n = 22), spinal cord injury (n = 9), and surgery (n = 6) units. Mean age was 46.85 ± 7.17 (ranging from 19 to 82), and mean years of education were 11.43 ± 3.20 (ranging from 1 to 20). Frequency distributions for age and years of education are provided. Mean WAIS FSIQ, VIQ, and PIQ were within the average range (105.89 ± 13.47, 107.03 ± 14.38, and 103.31 ± 13.02, respectively). Means and standard deviations for individual age-corrected subtest scores are also reported. All subjects ex-

Table 20.18. CT.15°

N	Age	Education	WAIS Mean SS	Category Errors	% Classified Normal
319	<40		11.9	29.3	89.0
134	40–59		11.2	42.6	70.2
100	≥60		9.7	66.4	31.0
132		<12	9.5	53.8	49.2
249		12–15	11.2	38.6	76.7
172		≥16	12.9	28.9	89.0

°Mean number of errors for the six subgroups as well as percent of subjects classified as normal using Russell et al.'s (1970) criteria. Mean scaled scores for the WAIS subtests are also reported.

cept one were male; the majority were Caucasian (93%), with 7% African-American. The mean score on a measure of occupational attainment was 11.29.

No differences were found in test performances between the two psychiatric groups and the nonpsychiatric group and the data were collapsed. Mean errors and standard deviation are presented. Both age and educational level had significant associations with Category Test scores in the expected direction, and regression equation information to allow correction of raw scores for age and education is included.

Study strengths
1. Large sample size.
2. Information regarding age, IQ, education, ethnicity, sex, occupational attainment, and geographic recruitment area.
3. Regression equation data for computation of age- and-education-corrected scores.
4. Means and standard deviations are reported.

Considerations regarding use of the study
1. Data were collected on medical and psychiatric patients.
2. Undifferentiated age range (mitigated by the regression equation information).
3. Nearly all male sample (Table 20.19).

[CT.17] Bornstein, Baker, and Douglass, 1987a

The authors collected Category test–retest data on 23 volunteers (14 women, nine men) who ranged in age from 17 to 52 (Mean = 32.3 ± 10.3), as part of an examination of the short-term retest reliability of the Halstead-Reitan Battery. Exclusion criteria consisted of a positive history of neurological or psychiatric illness. Mean verbal IQ was 105.8 ± 10.8 (range = 88 to 128) and mean performance IQ was 105.0 ± 10.5 (range 85 to 121).

Subjects were administered the Halstead-Reitan Battery in standard order both on initial testing and again 3 weeks later. Mean, standard deviation, and range for total errors for both testing sessions are provided, as well as raw score change and standard deviation, median raw score change, and mean percent of change. Significant improvement in performance over the 3-week period was documented. Correlations of such demographic variables as age and education with mean percent of change and mean change were small, with education accounting for up to 7% of variance and age accounting for up to 4% of variance.

Study strengths
1. Information on short-term (3-week) retest data.

Table 20.19. CT.16

N	Age	Education	WAIS			Category Errors
			FSIQ	VIQ	PIQ	
112	46.85	11.43	105.89	107.03	103.31	62.04
	(17.17)	(3.20)	(13.47)	(14.38)	(13.02)	(28.16)

Table 20.20. CT.17; Means, Standard Deviations, and Ranges for Total Number of Errors for Both Testing Sessions°

N	Age	VIQ	PIQ	Test	Retest
23	32.3	105.8	105.0	46.7	23.8
	(10.3)	(10.8)	(10.5)	(25.3)	(19.0)
				16–112	4–56

Raw Score Change	Median Raw Score Change	Mean % of Change
23.5	22	46

°Raw score change, median raw score change, and mean percent of change from the test to the retest are also reported.

2. Information on IQ level, sex, and age.
3. Minimally adequate exclusion criteria.
4. Means and standard deviations are reported.

Considerations regarding use of the study
1. Undifferentiated age range.
2. Relatively small sample size.
3. No information regarding education (Table 20.20).

[CT.18] El-Sheikh, El-Nagdy, Townes, and Kennedy, 1987

The authors report Category Test data on 32 undergraduate and graduate Egyptians at the American University in Cairo as a part of their cross-cultural investigation of the Luria-Nebraska and Halstead-Reitan Battery. No subject had a history of known brain damage. Participants were described as "Arabic and English-speaking." Category Test instructions were translated in Egyptian colloquial Arabic by the first author and checked by two independent judges fluent in both Arabic and English. In the case of disagreement between these two judges, a third judge was consulted.

The Category Test was administered in English to 23 subjects and in Arabic to nine subjects and readministered 2 weeks later. Mean errors and standard deviation are reported. No differences in performance were found between subjects administered the test in English or Arabic. A significant practice effect was documented over the 2-week interval.

Study strengths
1. Data obtained on an Arabic sample.
2. Information on test–retest scores.

3. Information regarding educational level, age, and geographic recruitment area.
4. Means and standard deviations are reported.

Considerations regarding use of the study
1. Small sample size.
2. Minimal exclusion criteria.
3. No information regarding intellectual level.
4. Undifferentiated age range, although it can be assumed it is fairly restricted (Table 20.21).

[CT.19] Russell, 1987

The author obtained Category Test data on 155 controls during the years 1968 to 1982 in V.A. hospitals in Cincinnati and Miami for his development of a reference scale method for neuropsychological test batteries. The 148 male and seven female subjects were suspected of having neurological disorders but had "negative neurological findings." No other exclusion criteria were described. Mean age was 46.19 ± 12.86 and the mean years of education were 12.29 ± 3.00. All but eight of the participants were Caucasian; the remainder were African-American. Mean WAIS FSIQ, VIQ, and PIQ were 111.9, 112.3, and 109.90, respectively.

Table 20.21. CT.18; The Table Provides Mean Number of Errors and Standard Deviations for the Total Sample for the Two Testing Probes

N	Age	Test	Retest
32	20.6	29.5	9.84
		(18.78)	(6.37)

Table 20.22. CT.19

N	Age	Education	WAIS			Category Errors
			FSIQ	VIQ	PIQ	
155	46.19	12.29	111.9	112.3	109.9	52.11
	(12.86)	(3.00)				(26.31)

Mean errors and standard deviations are provided.

Study strengths

1. Large sample size.
2. Information regarding IQ, education, ethnicity, sex, age, and geographic recruitment area.
3. Means and standard deviations are reported.

Considerations regarding use of the study

1. Undifferentiated age range.
2. Insufficient exclusion criteria; all subjects were suspected of having neurological disorders.
3. High mean intellectual level.
4. Mostly male sample (Table 20.22).

CONCLUSIONS

A large number of studies document the popularity of the Category Test in clinical assessment. The major drawbacks of the original version of the test are its length and a lack of portability. In order to overcome these problems, more recent modifications focus on development of short forms and creation of the booklet formats of the test. Despite the greater convenience offered by these modified versions, their psychometric properties are not yet sufficiently assessed. The studies address reliability and validity of the short forms based on the analyses of extrapolated items from the full version of the test, rather than on the data for the actual short version of the test. This suggests caution in using these data in diagnostic decision-making and prompts further investigations of the psychometric properties of this test. Correspondence between the original version and the booklet version of the test also deserves more attention. Further research also needs to focus on standardization of instructions for the test.

The clinical utility of the Category Test would also be improved by adjusting cutoff criteria relative to subjects' age, education, and intelligence level. Consideration of demographic factors in assigning subjects into impaired vs. nonimpaired groups would improve specificity of the Category Test. This would reduce excessively high rates of misclassification of "normal" subjects in the impaired range reported in the literature.

REFERENCES*

Abikoff, H., Alvir, J., Hong, G., Sukoff, R., Orazio, J., Solomon, S., & Saravay, S. (1987). Logical Memory Subtest of the Wechsler Memory Scale: Age and education norms and alternate-form reliability of two scoring systems. *Journal of Clinical and Experimental Neuropsychology, 9*(4), 435–448.

Abraham, E., Axelrod, B.N., & Ricker, J.H. (1996). Application of the oral Trail Making Test to a mixed clinical sample. *Archives of Clinical Neuropsychology, 11*(8), 697–701.

Adams, R.L., & Trenton, S.L. (1981). Development of a paper-and-pen form of the Halstead Category Test. *Journal of Consulting and Clinical Psychology, 49*(2), 298–299.

Adams, R.L., Boake, C., & Crain, C. (1982). Bias in a neuropsychological test classification related to education, age, and ethnicity. *Journal of Consulting and Clinical Psychology, 50*(1), 143–145.

Akshoomoff, N.A., & Stiles, J. (1995a). Developmental trends in visuospatial analysis and planning: I. Copying a complex figure. *Neuropsychology, 9*(3), 364–377.

Akshoomoff, N.A., & Stiles, J. (1995b). Developmental trends in visuospatial analysis and planning: II. Memory for a complex figure. *Neuropsychology, 9*(3), 378–389.

Albert, M.S., Heller, H.S., & Milberg, W. (1988). Changes in naming ability with age. *Psychology and Aging, 3*(2), 173–178.

Alekoumbides, A., Charter, R.A., Adkins, T.G., & Seacat, F. (1987). The diagnosis of brain damage by the WAIS, WMS, and Reitan battery utilizing standardized scores corrected for age and education. *The International Journal of Clinical Neuropsychology, 9*(1), 11–28.

American Psychological Association (1992). Ethical principles of psychologists and code of conduct. *American Psychologist, 47,* 1597–1611.

Anastasi, A. (1988). Norms and the interpretations of test scores. In A. Anastasi (Ed.), *Psychological Testing* (6th ed.). New York: MacMillan, (pp. 71– 108).

Andrew, J.M. (1977). Delinquents and the Tapping Test. *Journal of Clinical Psychology, 33*(3), 786–790.

Annett, M. (1970). A classification of hand preference by association analysis. *British Journal of Psychology, 61,* 303–321.

Anschutz, L., Camp, C.J., Markley, R.P., & Kramer, J.J. (1985). Maintenance and generalization of mnemonics for grocery shopping by older adults. *Experimental Aging Research, 11*(3–4), 157–160.

Anthony, W.Z., Heaton, R.K., & Lehman, R.A.W. (1980). An attempt to cross-validate two actuarial systems for neuropsychological test interpretation. *Journal of Consulting and Clinical Psychology, 48*(3), 317–326.

Ardila, A., & Rosselli, M. (1989). Neuropsychological characteristics of normal aging. *Developmental Neuropsychology, 5*(4), 307–320.

Ardila, A., Rosselli, M., & Rosas, P. (1989). Neuropsychological assessment in illiterates: Visuospatial and memory abilities. *Brain and Cognition, 11*(2), 147–166.

Arima, J.K. (1965). Performance of normal males on the Halstead Tactual Performance Test under severe environmental stress. *Perceptual and Motor Skills, 21,* 83–90.

Armstrong, C., Onishi, K., Robinson, K., D'Esposito, M., Thompson, H., Rostami, A., & Grossman, M. (1996). Serial position and temporal cue effects in multiple sclerosis: Two subtypes of defective memory mechanisms. *Neuropsychologia, 34*(9), 853–862.

*Unpublished manuscripts and personal communications (as indicated in the text) are not included in the list of references.

Arnett, J.A., & Labovitz, S.S. (1995). Effect of physical layout in performance of the Trail Making Test. *Psychological Assessment, 7*(2), 220–221.

Arnold, B.R., Montgomery, G.T., Castaneda, I., & Longoria, R. (1994). Acculturation and performance of Hispanics on selected Halstead-Reitan neuropsychological tests. *Assessment, 1*(3), 239–248.

Axelrod, B.N., & Henry, R.R. (1992). Age-related performance on the Wisconsin Card Sorting, Similarities, and Controlled Oral Word Association Tests. *The Clinical Neuropsychologist, 6*(1), 16–26.

Axelrod, B.N., & Milner, I.B. (1997). Neuropsychological findings in a sample of Operation Desert Storm veterans. *Journal of Neuropsychiatry and Clinical Neurosciences, 9*(1), 23–38.

Bak, J.S., & Greene, R.L. (1980). Changes in neuropsychological functioning in an aging population. *Journal of Consulting and Clinical Psychology, 48*(3), 395–399.

Barr, A., & Brandt, J. (1996). Word-list generation deficits in dementia. *Journal of Clinical and Experimental Neuropsychology, 18*(6), 810–822.

Bayles, K.A., & Tomoeda, C.K. (1983). Confrontation naming impairment in dementia. *Brain and Language, 19,* 98–112.

Bayles, K.A., Salmon, D.P., Tomoeda, C.K., Jacobs, D., Caffrey, J.T., Kaszniak, A.W., & Tröster, A.I. (1989). Semantic and letter category naming in Alzheimer's patients: A predictable difference. *Developmental Neuropsychology, 5*(4), 335–347.

Bechtoldt, H.P., Benton, A.L., & Fogel, M.L. (1962). An application of factor analysis in neuropsychology. *Psychological Record, 12,* 147–156.

Becker, J.T. (1988). Working memory and secondary memory deficits in Alzheimer's Disease. *Journal of Clinical and Experimental Neuropsychology, 10*(6), 739–753.

Becker, J.T., Huff, F.J., Nebes, R.D., Holland, A., & Boller, F.H. (1988). Neuropsychological function in Alzheimer's disease: Patterns of impairment and rate of progression. *Archives of Neurology, 45,* 263–268.

Bench, C.J., Frith, C.D., Grasby, P.M., Friston, K.J., Paulseu, E., Frackowiak, R.S.J., & Dolan, R.J. (1993). Investigations of the functional anatomy of attention using the Stroop test. *Neuropsychologia, 31,* 907–922.

Bennett-Levy, J. (1984). Determinants of performance on the Rey-Osterrieth Complex Figure test: An analysis, and a new technique for single-case assessment. *British Journal of Clinical Psychology, 23,* 109–119.

Benton, A.L. (1967). Problems of test construction in the field of aphasia. *Cortex, 3,* 32–58.

Benton, A.L. (1968). Differential behavioral effects in frontal lobe disease. *Neuropsychologia, 6,* 53–60.

Benton, A.L., & Hamsher, K. (1978). *Multilingual Aphasia Examination Manual.* Iowa City: University of Iowa.

Benton, A.L., Hamsher, K., & de S. Sivan, A.B. (1994). *Multilingual Aphasia Examination.* Iowa City: AJA Associates.

Bernard, L.C. (1989). Halstead-Reitan Neuropsychological Test performance of black, Hispanic, and white young adult males from poor academic backgrounds. *Archives of Clinical Neuropsychology, 4,* 267–274.

Bernard, L.C. (1990). Prospects for faking believable memory deficits on neuropsychological tests and the use of incentives in simulation research. *Journal of Clinical and Experimental Neuropsychology, 12,* 715–728.

Bernard, L.C. (1991). The detection of faked deficits on the Rey Auditory Verbal Learning Test: The effect of serial position. *Archives of Clinical Neuropsychology, 6,* 81–88.

Bernard, L.C., Houston, W., & Natoli, L. (1993). Malingering on neuropsychological memory tests: Potential objective indicators. *Journal of Clinical Psychology, 49,* 45–53.

Berry, D.T.R., & Carpenter, G.C. (1992). Effect of four different delay periods on recall of the Rey-Osterrieth Complex Figure by older persons. *The Clinical Neuropsychologist, 6*(1), 80–84.

Berry, D.T.R., Allen, R.S., & Schmitt, F.A. (1991). Rey-Osterrieth Complex Figure: Psychometric characteristics in a geriatric sample. *The Clinical Neuropsychologist, 5*(2), 143–153.

Bigler, E., Steinman, D., & Newton, J. (1981a). Clinical assessment of cognitive deficit in neurologic disorder. I: Effects of age and degenerative disease. *Clinical Neuropsychology, 3*(3), 5–13.

Bigler, E.D., Steinman, D.R., & Newton, J.S. (1981b). Clinical assessment of cognitive deficit in neurologic disorder. II: Cerebral trauma. *Clinical Neuropsychology, 3*(3), 13–18.

Bigler, E., Rosa, L., Schultz, F., Hall, S., & Harris, J. (1989). Rey-Auditory Verbal Learning and Rey-Osterrieth Complex Figure Design performance in Alzheimer's Disease and closed head injury. *Journal of Clinical Psychology, 45*(2), 277–280.

Binder, L.M. (1982). Constructional strategies on complex figure drawings after unilateral brain damage. *Journal of Clinical Neuropsychology, 4*(1), 51–58.

Binder, L.M., Villanueva, M.R., Howieson, D., & Moore, R.T. (1993). The Rey AVLT recognition memory task measures motivational impairment after mild head trauma. *Archives of Clinical Neuropsychology, 8,* 137–147.

Binetti, G., Magni, E., Padovani, A., Cappa, S.F., Bianchetti, A., & Trabucchi, M. (1996). Executive dysfunction in early Alzheimer's disease. *Journal of Neurology, Neurosurgery and Psychiatry, 60,* 91–93.

Blachstein, H., Vakil, E., & Hoffien, D. (1993). Impaired learning in parients with closed-head injuries: An analysis of components of the acquisition process. *Neuropsychology, 7*(4), 530–535.

Bleecker, M.L., Bolla-Wilson, K., Agnew, J., & Meyers, D.A. (1988). Age-related sex differences in verbal memory. *Journal of Clinical Psychology, 44*(3), 403–411.

Boll, T.J., & Reitan, R.M. (1973). Effect of age on performance on the Trail Making Test. *Perceptual and Motor Skills, 36,* 691–694.

Bolla, K.I., Lindgren, K.N., Bonaccorsy, C., & Bleecker, M.L. (1990). Predictors of verbal fluency (FAS) in the healthy elderly. *Journal of Clinical Psychology, 46*(5), 623–628.

Bolla-Wilson, K., & Bleecker, M.L. (1986). Influence of verbal intelligence, sex, age, and education on the Rey Auditory Verbal Learning Test. *Developmental Neuropsychology, 2*(3), 203–211.

Bolter, J.F., Hutcherson, W.L., & Long, C.J. (1984). Speech Sounds Perception Test: A rational response strategy can invalidate the test results. *Journal of Consulting and Clinical Psychology, 52*(1), 132–133.

Boone, K.B. (in press). Clinical neuropsychological assessment of executive functions: Impact of age, education, gender, intellectual level, and vascular status on executive test scores. In B.L. Miller, & J. Cummings (Eds.), *The Frontal Lobes.* Guilford Press.

Boone, K.B., & Rausch, R. (1989). Seashore Rhythm Test performance in patients with unilateral temporal lobe damage. *Journal of Clinical Psychology, 45*(4), 614–618.

Boone, K.B., Miller, B.L., Rosenberg, L., Durazo, A., McIntyre, H., & Weil, M. (1988). Neuropsychological and behavioral abnormalities in an adolescent with frontal lobe seizures. *Neurology, 38,* 583–586.

Boone, K.B., Miller, B.L., Lesser, I.M., Hill, E., & D'Elia, L. (1990). Performance on frontal lobe tests in healthy, older individuals. *Developmental Neuropsychology, 6*(3), 215–223.

Boone, K.B., Ananth, J., Philpott, L., Kaur, A., & Djenderedjian, A. (1991). Neuropsychological characteristics of nondepressed adults with obsessive-compulsive disorder. *Neuropsychiatry, Neuropsychology, and Behavioral Neurology, 4,* 96–109.

Boone, K.B., Miller, B.L., Lesser, I.M., Mehringer, C.M., Hill-Gutierrez, E., Goldberg, M.A., & Berman, N.G. (1992). Neuropsychological correlates of white-matter lesions in healthy elderly subjects: A threshold effect. *Archives of Neurology, 49,* 549–554.

Boone, K.B., Lesser, I.M., Hill-Gutierrez, E.H., Berman, N.G., & D'Elia, L.F. (1993a). Rey-Osterrieth complex figure performance in healthy, older adults: Relationship to age, education, sex and IQ. *The Clinical Neuropsychologist, 7*(1), 22–28.

Boone, K.B., Miller, B.L., & Lesser, I.M. (1993b). Frontal lobe cognitive functions in aging: Methodologic considerations. *Dementia, 4,* 232–236.

Boone, K.B., Lesser, I.M., Miller, B.L., Wohl, M., Berman, N., Lee, A., Palmer, B., & Back, C. (1995). Cognitive functioning in older depressed outpatients: Relationship of presence and severity of depression to neuropsychological test scores. *Neuropsychology, 9*(3), 390–398.

Boone, K.B., Ponton, M.O., Gorsuch, R.L., Gonzales, J.J., & Miller, B.L. (in press). Factor analysis of four measures of prefrontal lobe functioning. *Archives of Clinical Neuropsychology.*

Borkowski, J., Benton, A., & Spreen, O. (1967). Word fluency and brain damage. *Neuropsychologia, 5,* 135–140.

Bornstein, R.A. (1982a). Reliability of the Speech Sounds Perception Test. *Perceptual and Motor Skills, 55,* 203–210.

Bornstein, R.A. (1983a). Construct validity of the Knox Cube Test as a neuropsychological measure. *Journal of Clinical Neuropsychology, 5*(2), 105–114.

Bornstein, R.A. (1983b). Reliability and item analysis of the Seashore Rhythm Test. *Perceptual and Motor Skills, 57,* 571–574.

Bornstein, R.A. (1985). Normative data on selected neuropsychological measures from a nonclinical sample. *Journal of Clinical Psychology, 41*(5), 651–658.

Bornstein, R.A. (1986a). Classification rates obtained with "standard" cut-off scores on selected neuropsychological measures. *Journal of Clinical and Experimental Neuropsychology, 8*(4), 413–420.

Bornstein, R.A. (1986b). Contribution of various neuropsychological measures to detection of frontal lobe impairment. *International Journal of Clinical Neuropsychology, 8*(1), 18–22.

Bornstein, R.A. (1986c). Normative data on intermanual differences on three tests of motor performance. *Journal of Clinical and Experimental Neuropsychology, 8*(1), 12–20.

Bornstein, R.A. (1986d). Consistency of intermanual discrepancies in normal and unilateral brain lesion patients. *Journal of Consulting and Clinical Psychology, 54*(5), 719–723.

Bornstein, R.A. (1990). Neuropsychological test batteries in neuropsychological assessment. In

A.A. Boulton, G.B. Baker, & M. Hiscock (Eds.), *Neuromethods-17; Neuropsychology.* Clifton, NJ: Humana Press.

Bornstein, R.A., & Leason, M. (1984). Item analysis of Halstead's Speech-Sounds Perception Test: Quantitative and qualitative analysis of errors. *Journal of Clinical Neuropsychology, 6*(2), 205–214.

Bornstein, R.A., & Suga, L.J. (1988). Educational level and neuropsychological performance in healthy elderly subjects. *Developmental Neuropsychology, 4*(1), 17–22.

Bornstein, R.A., Weizel, M., & Grant, C.D. (1984). Error pattern and item order on Halstead's Speech Sounds Perception Test. *Journal of Clinical Psychology, 40*(1), 266–270.

Bornstein, R.A., Baker, G.B., & Douglass, A.B. (1987a). Short-term retest reliability of the Halstead-Reitan Battery in a normal sample. *Journal of Nervous and Mental Disease, 175*(4), 229–232.

Bornstein, R.A., Paniak, C., & O'Brien, W. (1987b). Preliminary data on classification of normal and brain-damaged elderly subjects. *The Clinical Neuropsychologist, 1*(4), 315–323.

Borod, J.C., Goodglass, H., & Kaplan, E. (1980). Normative data on the Boston Diagnostic Aphasia Examination, Parietal Lobe Battery, and the Boston Naming Test. *Journal of Clinical Neuropsychology, 2*(3), 209–215.

Botwinick, J. (1981). Neuropsychology of aging. In S. Filskov, & T. Boll (Eds.), *Handbook of Clinical Neuropsychology.* New York: Wiley.

Bowden, S., & Bell, R. (1992). Relative usefulness of the WMS and WMS-R: A comment on D'Elia et al. (1989). *Journal of Clinical and Experimental Neuropsychology, 14*(2), 340–346.

Bowles, N.L., & Poon, L.W. (1985). Aging and retrieval of words in semantic memory. *Journal of Gerontology, 40*(1), 71–77.

Boyd, J.L. (1981). A validity study of the Hooper Visual Organization Test. *Journal of Consulting and Clinical Psychology, 49,* 15–19.

Boyd, J.L. (1982a). Reply to Rathbun and Smith: Who made the Hooper blooper? *Journal of Consulting and Clinical Psychology, 50,* 284–285.

Boyd, J.L. (1982b). Reply to Woodward. *Journal of Consulting and Clinical Psychology, 50*(2), 289–290.

Boyle, G.J. (1975). Shortened Halstead Category Test. *Australian Psychologist, 10*(1), 81–84.

Boyle, G.J. (1986). Clinical neuropsychological assessment: Abbreviating the Halstead Category Test of brain dysfunction. *Journal of Clinical Psychology, 42*(4), 615–625.

Boyle, G.J. (1988). What does the neuropsychological category test measure? *Archives of Clinical Neuropsychology, 3,* 69–76.

Bradford, D.T. (1992). *Interpretive Reasoning and the Halstead-Reitan Tests.* Brandon, VT: Clinical Psychology.

Brebion, G., Smith, M.J., Gorman, J.M., & Amador, X. (1996). Reality monitoring failure in schizophrenia: The role of selective attention. *Schizophrenia Research, 22,* 173–180.

Breteler, M.M., van Amerongen, N.M., van Swieten, J.C., Claus, J.J., Grobbee, D.E., van Gijn, J., Hofman, A., & van Harskamp, F. (1994). Cognitive correlates of ventricular enlargement and cerebral white matter lesions on magnetic resonance imaging. The Rotterdam Study. *Stroke, 25,* 1109–1115.

Brooks, D.N. (1972). Memory and head injury. *The Journal of Nervous and Mental Disease, 155*(5), 350–355.

Brouwers, P., Cox, C., Martin, A., Chase, T., & Fedio, P. (1984). Differential perceptual-spatial impairment in Huntington's and Alzheimer's dementias. *Archives of Neurology, 41,* 1073–1076.

Brown, J. (1958). Some tests of the decay theory of immediate memory. *Quarterly Journal of Experimental Psychology, 10,* 12–21.

Buchanan, R.W., Strauss, M.E., Kirkpatrick, B., Holstein, C., Breier, A., & Carpenter, W.T. (1994). Neuropsychological impairments in deficit vs. nondeficit forms of schizophrenia. *Archives of General Psychiatry, 51,* 804–811.

Butters, N., Granholm, E., Salmon, D.P., & Grant, I. (1987). Episodic and semantic memory: A comparison of amnesic and demented patients. *Journal of Clinical and Experimental Neuropsychology, 9,* 479–497.

Cahn, D.A., Salmon, D.P., & Butters, N. (1995). Detection of dementia of the Alzheimer's Type in a population-based sample: Neuropsychological test performance. *Journal of International Neuropsychological Society, 1*(3), 252–260.

Cahn, D.A., Marcotte, A.C., Stern, R.A., Arruda, J.E., Akshoomoff, N.A., & Leshko, I.C. (1996). The Boston Qualitative Scoring System for the Rey-Osterrieth Complex Figure: A study of children with Attention Deficit Hyperactivity Disorder. *The Clinical Neuropsychologist, 10*(4), 397–406.

Caine, E.D. (1986). The neuropsychology of depression: The pseudodementia syndrome. In I. Grant & K.M. Adams, eds., *Neuropsychological Assessment of Neuropsychiatric Disorders.* New York: Oxford University Press, pp. 221–243.

Calsyn, D.A., O'Leary, M.R., & Chaney, E.F. (1980). Shortening the Category test. *Journal of Consulting and Clinical Psychology, 48*(6), 788–789.

Canadian Study of Health and Aging Working Group (1994). The Canadian Study of Health and Aging:

Study methods and prevalence of dementia. *Canadian Medical Association Journal, 150,* 899–913.

Caplan, B., & Shechter, J. (1995). The role of nonstandard neuropsychological assessment in rehabilitation: History, rationale, and examples. In L.A. Cushman, & M.J. Scherer (Eds.), *Psychological Assessment in Medical Rehabilitation.* APA, Washington DC.

Carr, E.K., & Lincoln, N.B. (1988). Inter-rater reliability of the Rey figure copying test. *British Journal of Clinical Psychology, 27,* 267–268.

Casey, M.B., Winner, E., Hurwitz, I., & DaSilva, D. (1991). Does processing style affect recall of the Rey-Osterrieth or Taylor Complex Figures? *Journal of Clinical and Experimental Neuropsychology, 13,* 600–606.

Cattell, J. (1886). The time it takes to see and name objects. *Mind, 11,* 63–65.

Cauthen, N. (1977). Extension of the Wechsler Memory Scale norms to the older age groups. *Journal of Clinical Psychology, 33,* 208–212.

Cauthen, N. (1978a). Normative data for the Tactual Performance Test. *Journal of Clinical Psychology, 34*(2), 456–460.

Cauthen, N. (1978b). Verbal fluency: Normative data. *Journal of Clinical Psychology, 32*(1), 126–129.

Cavalli, M., De Renzi, E., Faglioni, P., & Vitale, A. (1981). Impairment of right brain-damaged patients on a linguistic cognitive task. *Cortex, 17,* 546–556.

Cermak, L.S., & Butters, N. (1972). The role of interference and encoding in the short-term memory deficits of Korsakoff patients. *Neuropsychologia, 10,* 89–95.

Charter, R.A. (1994). Determining random responding for the Category, Speech-Sounds Perception, and Seashore Rhythm Tests. *Journal of Clinical and Experimental Neuropsychology, 16*(5), 744–748.

Charter, R.A., & Webster, J.S. (1997). Psychometric structure of the Seashore Rhythm Test. *The Clinical Neuropsychologist, 11*(2), 167–173.

Charter, R.A., Adkins, T.G., Alekoumbides, A., & Seacat, G.F. (1987). Reliability of the WAIS, WMS, and Reitan Batteries: Raw scores and standardized scores corrected for age and education. *International Journal of Clinical Neuropsychology, 9*(1), 28–32.

Chavez, E.L., Schwartz, M.M., & Brandon, A. (1982). Effects of sex of subjects and method of block presentation on the Tactual Performance Test. *Journal of Consulting and Clinical Psychology, 50*(4), 600–601.

Chelune, G., Bornstein, R.., & Prifitera, A. (1989). The Wechsler Memory Scale-Revised: Current status and applications. In J. Rosen, P. McReynolds,

& G. Chelune (Eds.), *Advances in psychological assessment.* New York: Plenum Press.

Chen, H., & Ho, C. (1986). Developmental study of the reversed Stroop effect in Chinese-English bilinguals. *Journal of General Psychology, 113,* 121–125.

Chervinsky, A.B., Mitrushina, M., & Satz, P. (1992). Comparison of four methods of scoring the Rey-Osterrieth Complex Figure Drawing Test on four age groups of normal elderly. *Brain Dysfunction, 5,* 267–287.

Chiulli, S., Yeo, R., Haaland, K., & Garry, P. (1989). Complex figure copy and recall in the elderly. *Journal of Clinical and Experimental Neuropsychology, 11,* 95.

Chiulli, S.J., Haaland, K.Y., Ellis, H.C., & Rhodes, J.M. (1985, February). *Recall and recognition memory with a variant of the Rey Auditory Verbal Learning Test in a clinically depressed population.* Paper presented at the 13th Annual Convention of the International Neuropsychology Society, San Diego, CA.

Chiulli, S.J., Haaland, K.Y., LaRue, A., & Garry, P.J. (1995). Impact of age on drawing the Rey-Osterrieth Figure. *The Clinical Neuropsychologist, 9*(3), 219–224.

Choca, J.P., Laatsch, L., Wetzel, L., & Agresti, A. (1997). The Halstead Category Test: A fifty year perspective. *Neuropsychology Review, 7*(2), 61–75.

Clark, C., & Klonoff, H. (1988). Reliability and construct validity of the six-block Tactual Performance Test in an adult sample. *Journal of Clinical and Experimental Neuropsychology, 10*(2), 175–184.

Cohn, N.B., Dustman, R.E., & Bradford, D.C. (1984). Age-related decrements in Stroop Color Test performance. *Journal of Clinical Psychology, 40,* 1244–1250.

Colombo, F., & Assal, G. (1992). Adaptation francaise du test de denomination de Boston. Versions abregees. *European Review of Applied Psychology, 42*(1), 67–73.

Comalli, P.E., Wapner, S., & Werner, H. (1962). Interference effects of Stroop Color-Word Test in childhood, adulthood, and aging. *Journal of Genetic Psychology, 100,* 47–53.

Concha, M., Selnes, O.A., McArthur, J.C., & Nance-Sproson, T. (1995). Normative data for a brief neuropsychological test battery in a cohort of injecting drug users. *International Journal of the Addictions, 30*(7), 823–841.

Connor, A., Franzen, M., & Sharp, B. (1988). Effects of practice and differential instructions on Stroop Performance. *The International Journal of Clinical Neuropsychology, 10,* 1–4.

Corrigan, J.D., Agresti, A.A., & Hinkeldey, N.S. (1987a). Psychometric characteristics of the Category Test: Replication and extension. *Journal of Clinical Psychology, 43*(3), 368–376.

Corrigan, J.D., & Hinkeldey, N.S. (1987b). Relationships between parts A and B of the Trail Making Test. *Journal of Clinical Psychology, 43*(4), 402–409.

Corrigan, J.D., Agresti, A.A., & Hinkeldey, N.S. (1987). Psychometric characteristics of the Category Test: Replication and extension. *Journal of Clinical Psychology, 43*(3), 368–376.

Corwin, J., & Bylsma, F.W. (1993). Psychological examination of traumatic encephalopathy. The Complex Figure Copy Test. *The Clinical Neuropsychologist, 7*, 4–21.

Craik, F.I., Byrd, M., & Swanson, J.M. (1987). Patterns of memory loss in three eldery samples. *Psychology and Aging, 2*, 79–86.

Crawford, J.R., Stewart, L.E., & Moore, J.W. (1989). Demonstration of savings on the AVLT and development of a parallel form. *Journal of Clinical and Experimental Neuropsychology, 11*(6), 975–981.

Crockett, D.J., Hadjistavropoulos, T., & Hurwitz, T. (1992). Primacy and recency effects in the assessment of memory using the Rey Auditory Verbal Learning Test. *Archives of Clinical Neuropsychology, 7*, 97–107.

Crossen, J.R., & Wiens, A.N. (1994). "Comparison of Auditory-Verbal Learning Test (AVLT) and California Verbal Learning Test (CVLT) in a sample of normal subjects". *Journal of Clinical and Experimental Neuropsychology, 16*(2), 190–194.

Crossley, M., D'Arcy, C., & Rawson, N.S.B. (1997). Letter and category fluency in community-dwelling Canadian seniors: A comparison of normal participants to those with dementia of the Alzheimer or vascular type. *Journal of Clinical and Experimental Neuropsychology, 19*(1), 52–62.

Crosson, B., Hughes, C., Roth, D., & Monkowski, P. (1984a). Review of Russell's (1975) Norms for the Logical Memory and Visual Reproduction subtests of the Wechsler Memory Scale. *Journal of Consulting and Clinical Psychology, 52*(4), 635–641.

Crosson, B., Hughes, C., Roth, D., & Monkowski, P. (1984b). *Use of errors and correct ideas in scoring Wechsler Memory Scale stories.* Paper presented at the meeting of the International Neuropsychological Society, Houston, TX.

Crovitz, H.F., & Zener, K. (1962). A group-test for assessing hand-and-eye dominance. *American Journal of Psychology, 75*, 271–276.

Cullum, C.M., Steinman, D.R., & Bigler, E.D. (1984). Relationship between fluid and crystallized cognitive functions using Category Test and WAIS scores. *The International Journal of Clinical Neuropsychology, 6*(3), 172–174.

Cullum, C., Butters, N., Tröster, A., & Salmon, D. (1990). Normal aging and forgetting rates on the Wechsler Memory Scale–Revised. *Archives of Clinical Neuropsychology, 5*, 23–30.

Cullum, C.M., Filley, C.M., & Kozora, E. (1995). Episodic memory function in advanced aging and early Alzheimer's Disease. *Journal of International Neuropsychological Society, 1*(1), 100–103.

Daigneault, S., Braun, C.M.J., & Whitaker, H.A. (1992). Early effects of normal aging on perseverative and non-perseverative prefrontal measures. *Developmental Neuropsychology, 8*, 99–114.

Davies, A.D. (1968). The influence of age on Trail Making Test performance. *Journal of Clinical Psychology, 24*, 96–98.

Davis, R.D., Adams, R.E., Gates, D.O., & Cheramie, G.M. (1989). Screening for learning disabilities: A neuropsychological approach. *Journal of Clinical Psychology, 45*(3), 423–429.

D'Elia, L.F., Satz, P., & Schretlen, D. (1989). Wechsler Memory Scale: A critical appraisal of the normative studies. *Journal of Clinical and Experimental Neuropsychology, 11*(4), 551–568.

D'Elia, L., Satz, P., Uchiyama, C., & White, T. (1994). *Color Trails Test, Professional Manual.* Odessa, FL: PAR.

DeFilippis, N.A., McCampbell, E., & Rogers, P. (1979). Development of a booklet form of the Category Test: Normative and validity data. *Journal of Clinical Neuropsychology, 1*(4), 339–342.

Delaney, R.C., Prevey, M.L., Cramer, J., & Mattson, R.H. (1992). Test-retest comparability and control subject data for the Rey-Auditory Verbal Learning Test and Rey-Osterrieth/Taylor Complex Figures. *Archives of Clinical Neuropsychology, 7*(6), 523–528.

Delis, D.C., Kramer, J.H., Kaplan, E., & Ober, B.A. (1987). *California Verbal Learning Test Manual.* San Antonio: Harcourt Brace Jovanovich.

Demick, J., & Harkins, D. (1997). *Role of cognitive style in the driving skills of young, middle-aged, and older adults.* American Association of Retired Persons (AARP) Andrus Foundation Final Grant Report, Washington, DC.

Demick, J., & Wapner, S. (1985, August). *Age differences in processes underlying sequential activity (Stroop color-word test).* Eastern Psychological Association annual meeting, Los Angeles, CA.

Demick, J., Salas-Passeri, J., & Wapner, S. (1986, August). *Age differences among preschoolers in processes underlying sequential activity,* Eastern Psychological Association annual meeting, New York, N.Y.

Denman, S. (1984). *Denman Neuropsychology Memory Scale.* Charleston, SC: Privately published.

desRosiers, G., & Ivison, D. (1986). Paired associate learning: Normative data for differences between high and low associate word pairs. *Journal of Clinical and Experimental Neuropsychology, 8*(6), 637–642.

Dodrill, C.B. (1978a). A neuropsychological battery for epilepsy. *Epilepsia, 19,* 611–623.

Dodrill, C.B. (1978b). The Hand Dynamometer as a neuropsychological measure. *Journal of Consulting and Clinical Psychology, 46*(6), 1432–1435.

Dodrill, C.B. (1979). Sex differences on the Halstead-Reitan Neuropsychological Battery and on other neuropsychological measures. *Journal of Clinical Psychology, 35*(2), 236–241.

Dodrill, C.B. (1987). *What's normal: Presidential address.* Paper presented at the first annual meeting of the Pacific NW Neurological Association, Seattle, WA.

Dujovne, B.E., & Levi, B.I. (1971). The psychometric structure of the Wechsler Memory Scale. *Journal of Clinical Psychology, 27,* 351–354.

Duley, J.F., Wilkins, J.W., Hamby, S.L., Hopkins, D.G., Burwell, R.D., & Barry, N.S. (1993). Explicit scoring criteria for the Rey-Osterrieth and Taylor Complex Figures. *The Clinical Neuropsychologist, 7*(1), 29–38.

Dunn, E.J., Margolis, R.B., & Taylor, J.M. (1985). Short forms of the Category Test: Applications for geriatric patients. *International Journal of Clinical Neuropsychology, 7*(1), 29–31.

Dyer, F.N. (1973). The Stroop phenomenon and its use in the study of perceptual, cognitive, and response processes. *Memory and Cognition, 1,* 106–120.

Echternacht, R. (1981). Neuropsychological assessment of motor functioning: The Finger Tapping Test: Data on an adult female inpatient psychiatric population. *Clinical Neuropsychology, 3*(2), 8–9.

Eckardt, M.J., & Matarazzo, J.D. (1981). Test-retest reliability of the Halstead impairment index in hospitalized alcoholic and nonalcoholic males with mild to moderate neuropsychological impairment. *Journal of Clinical Neuropsychology, 3*(3), 257–269.

Elfgren, C.I., Ryding, E., & Passant, U. (1996). Performance on neuropsychological tests related to single photon emission computerised tomography findings in frontotemporal dementia. *British Journal of Psychiatry, 169,* 416–422.

El-Sheikh, M., El-Nagdy, S., Townes, B.D., & Kennedy, M.C. (1987). The Luria-Nebraska and Halstead-Reitan neuropsychological test batteries: A cross-cultural study in English and Arabic. *International Journal of Neuroscience, 32,* 757–764.

Elwood, R.W. (1991). Factor structure of the Wechsler Memory Scale-Revised (WMS-R) in a clinical sample: A methodological reappraisal. *The Clinical Neuropsychologist, 5,* 329–337.

Elwood, R.W. (1995). The California Verbal Learning Test: Psychometric characteristics and clinical application. *Neuropsychology Review, 5*(3), 173–201.

Ernst, J. (1987). Neuropsychological problem-solving skills in the elderly. *Psychology and Aging, 2*(4), 363–365.

Ernst, J. (1988). Language, grip strength, sensory-perceptual, and receptive skills in a normal elderly sample. *The Clinical Neuropsychologist, 2*(1), 30–40.

Ernst, J., Warner, M.H., Townes, B.D., Peel, J.H., & Preston, M. (1987). Age group differences on neuropsychological battery performance in a neuropsychiatric population: An international descriptive study with replications. *Archives of Clinical Neuropsychology, 2,* 1–12.

Eson, M.E., Yen, J.K., & Bourke, R.S. (1978). Assessment of recovery from serious head injury. *Journal of Neurology, Neurosurgery, and Psychiatry, 41,* 1036–1042.

Estes, W.K. (1974). Learning theory and intelligence. *American Psychologist, 29,* 740–749.

Fabian, M.S., & Parsons, O.A. (1983). Differential improvement of cognitive functions in recovering alcoholic women. *Journal of Abnormal Psychology, 92*(1), 87–95.

Fabian, M.S., Jenkins, R.L., & Parsons, O.A. (1981). Gender, alcoholism and neuropsychological functioning. *Journal of Consulting and Clinical Psychology, 49*(1), 138–140.

Fabry, J. (Pers. Comm.). *A Primer of the Rey Auditory Verbal Learning Test.* White Bear Press: Omaha, NE.

Farmer, A. (1990). Performance of normal males on the Boston Naming Test and The Word Test. *Aphasiology, 4*(3), 293–296.

Farver, P.F., & Farver, T.B. (1982). Performance of normal older adults on tests designed to measure parietal lobe functions. *The American Journal of Occupational Therapy, 36*(7), 444–449.

Fastenau, P. (1996). An elaborated administration of the Wechsler Memory Scale-Revised. *The Clinical Neuropsychologist, 10*(4), 425–434.

Fastenau, S. & Adams, K.M. (1996). Book review: Heaton, Grant and Matthews' comprehensive norms: An overzealous attempt. *Journal of Clinical and Experimental Neuropsychology, 18*(3), 444–448.

Faust, D., Ziskin, J., & Hiers, J. (1991). *Brain Damage Claims: Coping with neuropsychological evidence.* Volumes 1&2. LA: Law and Psychology Press.

Feinstein, A., Brown, R., & Ron, M. (1994). Effects of practice of serial tests of attention in healthy subjects. *Journal of Clinical and Experimental Neuropsychology, 16,* 436–447.

Ferraro, F.R. & Bercier, B. (1996). Boston Naming Test performance in a sample of Native American elderly adults. *Clinical Gerontologist, 17*(1), 58–60.

Fillenbaum, G.G., Huber, M., & Taussig, I.M. (1997). Performance of elderly white and African American community residents on the abbreviated CERAD Boston Naming Test. *Journal of Clinical and Experimental Neuropsychology, 19*(2), 204–210.

Filskov, S.B., & Catanese, R.A. (1986). Effects of sex and handedness on neuropsychological testing. In S.B. Filskov, & T.J. Boll (Eds.), *Handbook of Clinical Neuropsychology* (Vol. 2). New York: John Wiley.

Finlayson, M.A.J., Johnson, K.A., & Reitan, R.M. (1977). Relationship of level of education to neuropsychological measures in brain-damaged and non-brain-damaged adults. *Journal of Consulting and Clinical Psychology, 45*(4), 536–542.

Fisher, L.M., Freed, D.M., & Corkin, S. (1990). Stroop Color-Word Test Performance in patients with Alzheimer's disease. *Journal of Clinical and Experimental Neuropsychology, 12,* 745–758.

Fitz, A.G., Conrad, P.M., Hom, D.L., Sarff, P., & Majovski, L.V. (1992). Hooper Visual Organization Test performance in lateralized brain injury. *Archives of Clinical Neuropsychology, 7,* 243–250.

Fitzhugh, K.B., Fitzhugh, L.C., & Reitan, R.M. (1964). Influence of age upon measures of problem solving and experimental background in subjects with longstanding cerebral dysfunction. *Journal of Gerontology, 19,* 132–134.

Flanagan, J.L., & Jackson, S.T. (1997). Test-retest reliability of three aphasia tests: Performance of non-brain damaged older adults. *Journal of Communication Disorders, 30,* 33–43.

Fleming, K., Goldberg, T.E., Gold, J.M., & Weinberger, D.R. (1995). Verbal working memory dysfunction in schizophrenia: Use of a Brown-Peterson paradigm. *Psychiatry Research, 56,* 155–161.

Flicker, C., Ferris, S., Crook, T., & Bartus, R. (1987). Implications of memory and language dysfunction in the naming deficit of senile dementia. *Brain and Language, 31,* 187–200.

Folstein, M., Folstein, S., & McHugh, P. (1975). Mini-Mental State: A practical method for grading the cognitive state of patients for the clinician. *Journal of Psychiatric Research, 12,* 189–198.

Fox, D.D. (1994). Normative problems for the Wechsler memory scale-revised logical memory test when used in litigation. *Archives of Clinical Neuropyschology, 9*(3), 211–214.

Frank, E.M., McDade, H.L., & Scott, W.K. (1996). Naming in dementia secondary to Parkinson's, Huntington's, and Alzheimer's diseases. *Journal of Communication Disorders, 29,* 183–197.

Franzen, M.D., Robbins, D.E., & Sawicki, R.F. (1989). *Reliability and Validity in Neuropsychological Assessment.* New York: Plenum Press.

Franzen, M.D., Haut, M.W., Rankin, E., & Keefover, R. (1995). Empirical Comparison of alternate forms of the Boston Naming Test. *The Clinical Neuropsychologist, 9*(3), 225–229.

Frith, C.D., Friston, K.J., Herold, S., Silbersweig, D., Fletcher, P., Cahill, C., Dolan, R.J., Frackowiak, R.S.J., & Liddle, P.F. (1995). Regional brain activity in chronic schizophrenic patients during the performance of a verbal fluency task. *British Journal of Psychiatry, 167,* 343–349.

Fromm-Auch, D., & Yeudall, L.T. (1983). Normative data for the Halstead-Reitan neuropsychological tests. *Journal of Clinical Neuropsychology, 5*(3), 221–238.

Fukui, T., Sugita, K., Sato, Y., Takeuchi, T., & Tsukagoshi, H. (1994). Cognitive functions in subjects with incidental cerebral hyperintensities. *European Neurology, 34,* 272–276.

Fuld, P.A. (1981). *The Fuld Object Memory Test.* Chicago, IL: The Stoelting Instrument.

Fuller, K.H., Gouvier, W.D., & Savage, R.M. (1997). Comparison of list B and list C of the Rey Auditory Verbal Learning Test. *The Clinical Neuropsychologist, 11*(2), 201–204.

Furry, C.A., & Baltes, P.B. (1973). The effect of age differences in ability-extraneous performance variables on the assessment of intelligence in children, adults, and the elderly. *Journal of Gerontology, 28,* 73–80.

Gaddes, W.H., & Crockett, D.J. (1975). Spreen-Benton aphasia tests: Normative data as a measure of normal language development. *Brain and Language, 2*(3), 257–280.

Ganguli, M., Seaberg, E., Belle, S., Fischer, L., & Kuller, L.H. (1993). Cognitive impairment and the use of health services in an elderly rural population: The MoVIES Project. *Journal of the American Geriatrics Society, 41,* 1065–1070.

Geffen, G., Moar, K.J., O'Hanlon, A.P., Clark, C.R., & Geffen, L.B. (1990). Performance measures of 16- to 86-Year-old males and females on the Auditory Verbal Learning Test. *The Clinical Neuropsychologist, 4*(1), 45–63.

Geffen, G.M., Butterworth, P., & Geffen, L.B. (1994). Test-retest reliability of a new form of the Auditory Verbal Learning Test (AVLT). *Archives of Clinical Neuropsychology, 9*(4), 303–316.

Gerson, A. (1974). Validity and reliability of the

Hooper Visual Organization Test. *Perceptual and Motor Skills, 39,* 95–100.

Gilandas, A.J., Touyz, S., Beumont, P.J.V., & Greenberg, H.P. (1984). *Handbook of Neuropsychological Assessment.* Sydney, Australia: Grune and Stratton.

Gilleard, E., & Gilleard, C. (1989). A comparison of Turkish and Anglo-American normative data on the Wechsler Memory Scale. *Journal of Clinical Psychology, 45*(1), 114–117.

Giovagnoli, A.R., & Avanzini, G. (1996). Forgetting rate and interference effects on a verbal memory distractor task in patients with temporal lobe epilepsy. *Journal of Clinical and Experimental Neuropsychology, 18,* 259–264.

Glennerster, A., Palace, J., Warburton, D., & Oxbury, S. (1996). Memory in myasthenia gravis: Neuropsychological tests of central cholinergic function before and after effective immunologic treatment. *Neurology, 46*(4), 1138–1142.

Golden, C. (1978). *Stroop Color and Word Test: Manual for Clinical and Experimental Uses.* Chicago, IL: Stoelting.

Golden, C.J., Kuperman, S.K., MacInnes, W.D., & Moses, J.A. (1981). Cross-validation of an abbreviated form of the Halstead Category test. *Journal of Consulting and Clinical Psychology, 49,* 606–607.

Golden, C.J., MacInnes, W.D., Kuperman, S.K., & Moses, J.A. (1981a). Cross-validation of an abbreviated form of the Halstead Category test. *Journal of Consulting and Clinical Psychology, 49*(4), 606–607.

Golden, C.J., Hammeke, T.A., & Purisch, A.D. (1978). Diagnostic validity of a standardized neuropsychological battery derived from Luria's neuropsychological tests. *Journal of Consulting and Clinical Psychology, 46*(6), 1258–1265.

Golden, C.J., Osmon, D.C., Moses, J.A., Jr., & Berg, R.A. (1981b). *Interpretation of the Halstead-Reitan Neuropsychological Test Battery: A Casebook Approach.* New York: Grune & Stratton.

Goldstein, S.G., & Braun, L.S. (1974). Reversal of expected transfer as a function of increased age. *Perceptual and Motor Skills, 38,* 1139–1145.

Goldstein, G., & Shelly, C.H. (1972). Statistical and normative studies of the Halstead neuropsychological test battery relevant to a neuropsychiatric hospital setting. *Perceptual and Motor Skills, 34,* 603–620.

Gordon, N.G. (1972). The Trail Making Test in neuropsychological diagnosis. *Journal of Clinical Psychology, 28,* 167–169.

Gordon, N.G., & O'Dell, J.W. (1983). Sex differences in neuropsychological performance. *Perceptual and Motor Skills, 56,* 126.

Goul, W.R., & Brown, M. (1970). Effects of age and intelligence on Trail Making Test performance and validity. *Perceptual and Motor Skills, 30,* 319–326.

Graf, P., & Uttl, B. (1995). Component processes of memory: Changes across the adult lifespan. *Swiss Journal of Psychology, 54*(2), 113–130.

Graf, P., Uttl, B., & Tuokko, H. (1995). Color- and Picture-Word Stroop Tests: Performance changes in old age. *Journal of Clinical and Experimental Neuropsychology, 17,* 390–415.

Greene, R.L., & Farr, S.P. (1985, August). *Multiple regression of moderator variables on Trail Making Test performance.* Paper presented at the Annual meeting of the American Psychological Association, Los Angeles, CA.

Gregory, R., & Paul, J. (1980). The effects of handedness and writing posture on neuropsychological test results. *Neuropsychologia, 18,* 231–235.

Gregory, R.J., Paul, J.J., & Morrison, M.W. (1979). A short form of the Category Test for adults. *Journal of Clinical Psychology, 35*(4), 795–798.

Greiffenstein, M.F., Baker, W.J., & Gola, T. (1994). Validation of malingered amnesia measures with a large clinical sample. *Psychological Assessment, 6*(3), 218–224.

Guilford, J.P. (1965). *Fundamental Statistics in Psychology and Education,* New York: McGraw-Hill.

Guilmette, T.J., & Rasile, D. (1995). Sensitivity, specificity, and diagnostic accuracy of three verbal memory measures in the assessment of mild brain injury. *Neuropsychology, 9*(3), 338–344.

Haaland, K.Y., Cleeland, C.S., & Carr, D. (1977). Motor performance after unilateral hemisphere damage in patients with tumor. *Archives of Neurology, 34,* 556–559.

Haaland, K., Linn, R., Hunt, W., & Goodwin, J. (1983). A normative study of Russel's variant of the Wechsler Memory Scale in a healthy elderly population. *Journal of Consulting and Clinical Psychology, 51*(6), 878–881.

Halstead, W.C. (1947). *Brain and Intelligence.* Chicago, IL: University of Chicago Press.

Hamby, S.L., Wilkins, J.W., & Barry, N.S. (1993). Organizational quality on the Rey-Osterrieth and Taylor Complex Figure tests: A new scoring system. *Psychological Assessment, 5*(1), 27–33.

Harley, J.P., Leuthold, C.A., Matthews, C.G., & Bergs, L.E. (1980). *T-score norms: Wisconsin Neuropsychological Test Battery.* Unpublished manuscript.

Harnadek, M.C.S., & Rourke, B.P. (1994). Principal identifying features of the syndrome of nonverbal learning disabilities in children. *Journal of Learning Disabilities, 27*(3), 144–154.

Harris, M., Cross, H., & VanNieuwkerk, R. (1981). The effects of state depression, induced depression and sex on the Finger Tapping and Tactual Performance Tests. *Clinical Neuropsychology,* 3(4), 28–34.

Hawkins, K.A., Sledge, W.H., Orleans, J.F., Quinlan, D.M., Rakfeldt, J., & Hoffman, R.E. (1993). Normative implications of the relationship between reading vocabulary and Boston Naming Test performance. *Archives of Clinical Neuropsychology,* 8, 525–537.

Hayes, W.L. (1963). *Statistics.* New York: Rinehart & Winston.

Hays, J.R. (1995). Trail Making Test norms for psychiatric patients. *Perceptual and Motor Skills,* 80(1), 187–194.

Heaton, R.K. (1985). *Importance of demographic variables in interpreting scores on the Halstead-Reitan battery.* Paper presented at the 13th Annual Meeting of the International Neuropsychological Society, San Diego, CA.

Heaton, R.K., Vogt, A.T., Hoehn, M.M., Lewis, J.A., Crowley, T.J., & Stallings, M.A. (1979). Neuropsychological impairment with schizophrenia vs. acute and chronic cerebral lesions. *Journal of Clinical Psychology,* 35(1), 46–53.

Heaton, R.K., Nelson, L.M., Thompson, D.S., Burks, J.S., & Franklin, G.M. (1985). Neuropsychological findings in relapsing-remitting and chronic-progressive multiple sclerosis. *Journal of Consulting and Clinical Psychology,* 53(8), 103–110.

Heaton, R.K., Grant, I., & Matthews, C.G. (1986). Differences in neuropsychological test performance associated with age, education, and sex. In I. Grant, & K. Adams (Eds.), *Neuropsychological Assessment of Neuropsychiatric Disorders.* New York: Oxford University Press.

Heaton, R., Grant, I., & Matthews, C. (1991). *Comprehensive Norms for an Expanded Halstead-Reitan Neuropsychological Battery: Demographic Corrections, Research Findings, and Clinical Applications.* Odessa, FL: Psychological Assessment Resources.

Heaton, R.K., Ryan, L., Grant, I., & Matthews, C.G. (1996). Demographic influences on neuropsychological test performance. In I. Grant, & K.M. Adams (Eds.), *Neuropsychological Assessment of Neuropsychiatric Disorders* (2nd ed.). New York: Oxford University Press.

Heaton, R., Matthews, C., Grant, I., & Avitable, N. (1996). Demographic corrections with comprehensive norms: an overzealous attempt or a good start? *Journal of Clinical and Experimental Neuropsychology,* 18(3), 449–458.

Heilbronner, R.L., Henry, G.K., Buck, P., Adams, R.L., & Fogle, T. (1991). Lateralized brain damage and performance on Trail Making A and B, Digit Span forward and backward, and TPT memory and location. *Archives of Clinical Neuropsychology,* 6, 251–258.

Hemsley, D. (1974). Relationship between two tests of visual retention. *Perceptual and Motor Skills,* 39, 1132–1134.

Henderson, V.W., Mack, W., Freed, D.M., Kempler, D., & Andersen, E.S. (1990). Naming consistency in Alzheimer's disease. *Brain and Language,* 39, 530–538.

Heubrock, D. (1995). Error analysis in neuropsychological assessment of verbal memory and learning. *European Journal of Psychological Assessment,* 11(1), 21–28.

Hilgert, L.D., & Treloar, J.H. (1985). The relationship of Hooper Visual Organization Test to sex, age and intelligence of elementary school children. *Measurement and Evaluation in Counseling and Development,* 17(4), 203–206.

Hodges, J.R., Salmon, D.P., & Butters, N. (1991). The nature of the naming deficit in Alzheimer's and Huntington's Disease. *Brain,* 114, 1547–1558.

Hoffman, D.T. (1969). Sex differences in preferred finger tapping rates. *Perceptual and Motor Skills,* 29, 676.

Hom, J., & Reitan, R.M. (1990). Generalized cognitive function after stroke. *Journal of Clinical and Experimental Neuropsychology,* 12, 644–654.

Hooper, H.E. (1958, 1983). *Hooper Visual Organization Test (VOT).* Los Angeles, CA: Western Psychological Services.

Houx, P., Jolles, J., & Vreeling, F. (1993). Stroop interference: Aging effects assessed with the Stroop Color-Word test. *Experimental Aging Research,* 19, 209–224.

Hsieh, S., & Riley, N. (1997, November). *Neuropsychological performance in the People's Republic of China: Age and educational norms for four attention tasks.* Presented at the National Academy of Neuropsychology, Las Vegas, NV.

Huff, F.J., Collins, C., Corkin, S., & Rosen, T.J. (1986a). Equivalent forms of the Boston Naming Test. *Journal of Clinical and Experimental Neuropsychology,* 8(5), 556–562.

Huff, F.J., Corkin, S., & Growdon, J.H. (1986b). Semantic impairment and anomia in Alzheimer's disease. *Brain and Language,* 28, 235–249.

Hugdahl, K., & Franzon, M. (1985). Visual half-field presentations of incongruent color-words reveal mirror-reversal of language lateralization in dextral and sinistral subjects. *Cortex,* 21, 359–374.

Huhtaniemi, P., Haier, R.J., Fedio, P., & Buchsbaum, M.S. (1983). Neuropsychological characteristic of college males who show attention dysfunction. *Perceptual and Motor Skills, 57*, 399–406.

Hulicka, I.M. (1966). Age differences in Wechsler Memory Scale scores. *Journal of Genetic Psychology, 190*, 135–145.

Ingraham, L., Chard, F., Wood, M., & Mirsky, A. (1988). An Hebrew language version of the Stroop test. *Perceptual and Motor Skills, 67*, 187–192.

Inman, V.W., & Parkinson, S.R. (1983). Differences in Brown-Peterson recall as a function of age and retention interval. *Journal of Gerontology, 38*, 58–64.

Isaacs, B., & Kennie, A.T. (1973). The Set Test as an aid to the detection of dementia in old people. *British Journal of Psychiatry, 123*, 467–470.

Ivinskis, A., Allen, S., & Shaw, E. (1971). An extension of Wechsler Memory Scale norms to lower age groups. *Journal of Clinical Psychology, 27*, 354–357.

Ivison, D. (1977). The Wechsler Memory Scale: Preliminary findings toward an Australian standardization. *Australian Psychologist, 12*, 303–312.

Ivison, D. (1986). Anna Thompson and the American Liner New York: Some normative data. *Journal of Clinical and Experimental Neuropsychology, 8*(3), 317–320.

Ivnik, R.J., Sharbrough, F.W., & Laws, E.R. (1987). Effects of anterior temporal lobectomy on cognitive function. *Journal of Clinical Psychology, 43*, 128–137.

Ivnik, R.J., Malec, J.F., Tangalos, E.G., Petersen, R.C., Kokmen, E., & Kurland, L.T. (1990). The Auditory-Verbal Learning Test (AVLT): Norms for ages 55 and older. *Psychological Assessment: A Journal of Consulting and Clinical Psychology, 2*, 304–312.

Ivnik, R., Smith, G., Tangalos, E., Petersen, R., Kokmen, E., & Kurland, L. (1991). Wechsler Memory Scale: IQ-dependent norms for persons ages 65 to 97 years. *Psychological Assessment, 3*(2), 156–161.

Ivnik, R.J., Malec, J.F., Smith, G.E., Tangalos, E.G., Petersen, R.C., Kokmen, E., & Kurland, L.T. (1992a). Mayo's older Americans normative studies: WAIS-R norms for ages 56 to 97. *The Clinical Neuropsychologist, 6* (Supplement), 1–30.

Ivnik, R., Malec, J., Smith, G., Tangalos, E., Petersen, R., Kokman, E., & Kurland, L. (1992b). Mayo's older Americans normative studies: WMS-R norms for ages 56 to 94. *The Clinical Neuropsychologist, 6* (Supplement), 49–82.

Ivnik, R.J., Malec, J.F., Smith, G.E., Tangalos, E.G., Petersen, R.C., Kokmen, E., & Kurland, L.T. (1992c). Mayo's older Americans normative studies: Updated AVLT norms for ages 56 to 97. *The Clinical Neuropsychologist, 6*, 83–104.

Ivnik, R., Smith, G., Malec, J., Tangalos, E., & Parisi, J. (1993). Comparison of Wechsler vs. Mayo summary scores in a clinical sample. *Journal of Clinical Psychology, 49*(4), 534–542.

Ivnik, R.J., Malec, J.F., Smith, G.E., Tangalos, E.G., & Petersen, R.C. (1996). Neuropsychological tests' norms above age 55: COWAT, BNT, MAE Token, WRAT-R Reading, AMNART, STROOP, TMT, and JLO. *The Clinical Neuropsychologist, 10*(3), 262–278.

Jackson, S.T., & Tompkins, C.A. (1991). Supplemental aphasia tests: Frequency of use and psychometric properties. *Clinical Aphasiology, 20*, 91–99.

Jacobs, D.M., Sano, M., Dooneief, G., Marder, K., Bell, K., & Stern, Y. (1995). Neuropsychological detection and characterization of preclinical Alzheimer's disease. *Neurology, 45*, 957–962.

Janowsky, J.S., & Thomas-Thrapp, L.J. (1993). Complex figure recall in the elderly: A deficit in memory or constructional strategy? *Journal of Clinical and Experimental Neuropsychology, 15*(2), 159–169.

Janowsky, J.S., Shimamura, A.P., Kritchevsky, M., & Squire, L.R. (1989). Cognitive impairment following frontal lobe damage and its relevance to human amnesia. *Behavioral Neuroscience, 103*, 548–560.

Jarvis, P.E., & Barth, J.T. (1984). Halstead-Reitan Test Battery: An interpretive Guide. PAR: Odessa, FL.

Jensen, A. (1965). Scoring the Stroop Test. *Acta Psychologica, 24*, 398–408.

Jensen, A., & Rohwer, W. (1966). The Stroop Color-Word Test: A review. *Acta Psychologica, 25*, 36–93.

Johnstone, B., & Wilhelm, K.L. (1997). The constract validity of the Hooper Visual Organization Test. *Assessment, 4*(3), 243–248.

Johnstone, B., Holland, D., & Hewett, J.E. (1997). The construct validity of the Category Test: Is it a measure of reasoning or intelligence? *Psychological Assessment, 9*(1), 28–33.

Kane, R.L., Parsons, O.A., & Goldstein, G. (1985). Statistical relationships and discriminative accuracy of the Halstead-Reitan, Luria-Nebraska, and Wechsler IQ scores in the identification of brain damage. *Journal of Clinical and Experimental Neuropsychology, 7*(3), 211–223.

Kaplan, E. (1988). A process approach to neuropsychological assessment. In T. Boll, & B.K. Bryant (Eds.) *Clinical Neuropsychology and Brain Function: Research, Measurement and Practice* (Vol. 7). Washington, DC: APA.

Kaplan, E., Goodglass, H., & Weintraub, S. (1978). *The Boston Naming Test, Experimental Edition.* Boston: Kaplan and Goodglass.

Kaplan, E., Goodglass, H., & Weintraub, S. (1983). *The Boston Naming Test*. Philadelphia: Lea and Febiger.

Kaplan, E., Fein, D., Morris, R., & Delis, D.C. (1991). *WAIS-R as a neuropsychological instrument: WAIS-R-NI Manual*. New York: The Psychological Corporation.

Karzmark, P., Heaton, R.K., Grant, I., & Matthews, C.G. (1984). Use of demographic variables to predict overall level of performance on the Halstead-Reitan battery. *Journal of Consulting and Clinical Psychology, 52*(4), 663–665.

Karzmark, P., Heaton, R.K., Lehman, R.A.W., & Crouch, J. (1985). Utility of the Seashore Tonal Memory Test in neuropsychological assessment. *Journal of Clinical and Experimental Neuropsychology, 7*(4), 367–374.

Kear-Colwell, J.J., & Heller, M. (1978). A normative study of the Wechsler Memory Scale. *Journal of Clinical Psychology, 34*(2), 437–442.

Keenan, P.A., Ricker, J.H., Lindamer, L.A., Jiron, C.C., & Jacobson, M.W. (1996). Relationship between WAIS-R Vocabulary and Performance on the California Verbal Learning Test. *The Cliinical Neuropsychologist, 10*(4), 455–458.

Kelly, M.D., Kundert, D.K., & Dean, R.S. (1992). Factor analysis and matrix invariance of the HRNB-C Category Test. *Archives of Clinical Neuropsychology, 7*, 415–418.

Kennedy, K.J. (1981). Age effects on Trail Making Test performance. *Perceptual and Motor Skills, 52*, 671–675.

Kilpatrick, D.G. (1970). The Halstead Category test of brain dysfunction: Feasibility of a short form. *Perceptual and Motor Skills, 30*, 577–578.

Kimura, S.D. (1981). A card form of the Reitan-modified Halstead Category test. *Journal of Consulting and Clinical Psychology, 49*(1), 145–146.

King, G.D., Hannay, H.J., Masek, B.J., & Burns, J.W. (1978). Effects of anxiety and sex on neuropsychological tests. *Journal of Consulting and Clinical Psychology, 46*(2), 375–376.

King, M.C. (1981). Effects of non-focal brain dysfunction on visual memory. *Journal of Clinical Psychology, 37*(3), 638–643.

Kirk, U. (1992). Evidence for early acquisition of visual organization ability: A developmental study. *The Clinical Neuropsychologist, 6*(2), 171–177.

Kirk, U., & Kelly, M.S. (1986). *Scoring scale for the Rey-Osterrieth Complex Figure*. Paper presented at the meeting of the International Neuropsychological Society, Denver.

Kirshner, H.S., Webb, W.G., & Kelly, M.P. (1984). The naming disorder of dementia. *Neuropsychologia, 22*, 23–30.

Klein, M., Ponds, R.W.H.M., Houx, P.J., & Jolles, J. (1997). Effect of test duration on age-related differences in Stroop interference. *Journal of Clinical and Experimental Neuropsychology, 19*, 77–82.

Klicpera, C. (1983). Poor planning as a characteristic of problem-solving behavior in dyslexic children: A study with the Rey-Osterrieth Complex Figure Test. *Acta Paedopsychiatrica, 49*, 73–82.

Klonoff, H., & Kennedy, M. (1965). Memory and perceptual functioning in octogenarians and nonagenarians in the community. *Journal of Gerontology, 20*, 328–333.

Klonoff, H., & Kennedy, M. (1966). A comparative study of cognitive functioning in old age. *Journal of Gerontology, 21*, 239–243.

Klove, H. (1974). Validation studies in adult clinical neuropsychology. In R.M. Reitan, & L.A. Davison (Eds.), *Clinical Neuropsychology: Current Status and Applications*. Washington, DC: Winston (pp. 211–236).

Knesevich, J.W., LaBarge, E., & Edwards, D. (1986). Predictive value of the Boston Naming Test in mild senile dementia of the Alzheimer type. *Psychiatry Research, 19*, 155–161.

Knights, R.M., & Moule, A.D. (1967). Normative and reliability data on finger and foot tapping in children. *Perceptual and Motor Skills, 25*, 717–720.

Koffler, S.P., & Zehler, D. (1985). Normative data for the hand dynamometer. *Perceptual and Motor Skills, 61*, 589–590.

Kohn, S.E., & Goodglass, H. (1985). Picture-naming in aphasia. *Brain and Language, 24*, 266–283.

Koss, E., Ober, B.A., Delis, D.C., & Friedland, R.P. (1984). The Stroop Color-Word Test: Indicator of dementia severity. *International Journal of Neuroscience, 24*, 53–61.

Kozora, E., & Cullum, C.M. (1995). Generative naming in normal aging: Total output and qualitative changes using phonemic and semantic constraints. *The Clinical Neuropsychologist, 9*(4), 313–320.

Kramer, J.H., Delis, D.C., & Daniel, M. (1988). Sex differences in verbal learning. *Journal of Clinical Psychology, 44*(6), 907–915.

Kuehn, S.M., & Snow, W.G. (1992). Are the Rey and Taylor figures equivalent? *Archives of Clinical Neuropsychology, 7*, 445–448.

Kupke, T. (1983). Effect of subject sex, examiner sex, and test apparatus on Halstead Category and Tactual Performance Tests. *Journal of Consulting and Clinical Psychology, 51*(4), 624–626.

Laatsch, L., & Choca, J. (1991). Understanding the Halstead Category Test by using item analysis. *Psychological Assessment: A Journal of Consulting and Clinical Psychology, 3*, 701–704.

LaBarge, E., Edwards, D., & Knesevich, J.W. (1986). Performance of normal elderly on the Boston Naming Test. *Brain and Language, 27*, 380–384.

LaBarge, E., Balota, D.A., Storanalt, M., & Smith, D.S. (1992). An analysis of confrontation naming errors in senile dementia of the Alzheimer type. *Neuropsychology, 6*(1), 77–95.

Lacy, M.A., Gore, Jr., P.A., Pliskin, N.H., Henry, G.K., Heilbronner, R.L., & Hamer, D.P. (1996). Verbal fluency task equivalence. *The Clinical Neuropsychologist, 10*(3), 305–308.

Lafleche, G., & Albert, M.S. (1995). Executive function deficits in mild Alzheimer's disease. *Neuropsychology, 9*(3), 313–320.

Lansdell, H., & Donnelly, E.F. (1977). Factor analysis of the Wechsler Adult Intelligence Scale subtests and the Halstead-Reitan Category and Tapping Tests. *Journal of Consulting and Clinical Psychology, 45*, 412–416.

Leckliter, I.N., & Matarazzo, J.D. (1989). The influence of age, education, IQ, gender, and alcohol abuse on Halstead-Reitan Neuropsychological Test Battery performance. *Journal of Clinical Psychology, 45*(4), 485–512.

Leng, N.R.C., & Parkin, A.J. (1989). Aetiological variation in the amnesic syndrome: comparisons using the Brown-Peterson task. *Cortex, 25*, 251–259.

Leonberger, F.T., Nicks, S.D., Goldfader, P.R., & Munz, D.C. (1991). Factor analysis of the Wechsler Memory Scale-Revised and the Halstead-Reitan Neuropsychological Battery. *The Clinical Neuropsychologist, 5*, 83–88.

Lewis, S., Campbell, A., Takushi-Chinen, R., Brown, A., Dennis, G., Wood, D., Weir, R. (1997). Visual Organization Test performance in an African American population with acute unilateral cerebral lesions. *International Journal of Neuroscience, 91*(3–4), 295–302.

Lezak, M.D. (1982). *The test-retest stability and reliability of some tests commonly used in neuropsychological assessment.* Paper presented at the meeting of the International Neuropsychological Society, Deauville, France.

Lezak, M.D. (1987). Norms for growing older. *Developmental Neuropsychology, 3*, 1–12.

Lezak, M.D. (1995). *Neuropsychological Assessment.* New York: Oxford University Press.

Lezak, M.D. (1976). *Neuropsychological assessment.* New York: Oxford University Press.

Lezak, M.D. (1983). Neuropsychological Assessment. New York: Oxford University Press.

Liberman, J.N., Stewart, W., Selnes, O., & Gordon, B. (1994). Rater agreement for the Rey Osterrieth Complex Figure test. *Journal of Clinical Psychology, 50*(4), 615–624.

Libon, D.J., Glosser, G., Malamut, B.L., Kaplan, E., Goldberg, E., Swenson, R., & Sands, L.P. (1994). Age, executive functions, and visuospatial functioning in healthy older adults. *Neuropsychology, 8*, 38–43.

Lichtenberg, P., & Christensen, B. (1992). Extended normative data for the Logical Memory subtest of the Wechsler Memory Scale—Revised: responses from a sample of cognitively intact elderly medical patients. *Psychological Reports, 71*, 745–746.

Lichtenberg, P.A., Ross, T., & Christensen, B. (1994). Preliminary normative data on the Boston Naming Test for an older urban population. *The Clinical Neuropsychologist, 8*(1), 109–111.

Liddle, P.F., Friston, K.J., Frith, C.D., & Frackowiak, R.S.J. (1992). Cerebral blood flow and mental processes in schizophrenia. *Journal of the Royal Society of Medicine, 85*, 224–227.

Lin, Y.G., & Rennick, P.M. (1974). Correlations between performance on the Category Test and the Wechsler Adult Intelligence Scale in an epileptic sample. *Journal of Clinical Psychology, 31*(1), 62–65.

Locascio, J.L., Growdon, J.H., & Corkin, S. (1995). Cognitive test performance in detecting, staging, and tracking Alzheimer's disease. *Archives of Neurology, 52*, 1087–1099.

Logue, P.E., & Allen, K. (1971). WAIS-predicted Category Test scores with the Halstead Neuropsychological Battery. *Perceptual and Motor Skills, 33*, 1095–1096.

Loring, D.W., Lee, G.P., & Meador, K.J. (1988). Revising the Rey-Osterrieth: Rating right hemisphere recall. *Archives of Clinical Neuropsychology, 3*, 239–247.

Loring, D.W., Martin, R.L., Meador, K.J., & Lee, G.P. (1990). Psychometric construction of the Rey-Osterrieth Complex Figure: Methodological considerations and interrater reliability. *Archives of Clinical Neuropsychology, 5*, 1–14.

Lucas, M.D., & Sonnenberg, B.R. (1996). Neuropsychological trends in the Parkinsonism-Plus Syndrome: A pilot study. *Journal of Clinical and Experimental Neuropsychology, 18*(1), 88–97.

Luria, A.R. (1980). *Higher Cortical Functions in Man.* New York: Basic Books.

Lyness, S.A., Eaton, E.M., & Schneider, L.S. (1994). Cognitive performance in older and middle-aged depressed outpatients and controls. *Journal of Gerontology: Psychological Sciences, 49*, P129–P136.

MacInnes, W.D., McFadden, J.M., & Golden, C.J. (1983). A short-portable version of the Category Test. *International Journal of Neuroscience, 18*, 41–44.

Mack, J.L., & Carlson, N.J. (1978). Conceptual deficits and aging: The Category Test. *Perceptual and Motor Skills, 46,* 123–128.

Mack, W.J., Freed, D.M., Williams, B.W., & Henderson, V.W. (1992). Boston Naming Test: Shortened versions for use in Alzheimer's disease. *Journal of Gerontology, 47,* P154–P158.

MacLeod, C. (1991). Half century of research on the Stroop effect: An integrative review. *Psychological Bulletin, 109,* 163–203.

Madison, L.S., George, C., & Moeschler, J.B. (1986). Cognitive functioning in the fragile-X syndrome: A study of intellectual, memory and communication skills. *Journal of Mental Deficiency Research, 30,* 129–148.

Maj, M., Janssen, R., Satz, P., Zaudig, M., Starace, F., Boor, D., Sughondhabirom, B., Bing, E., Luabeya, M., Ndetei, D., Reidel, R., Schulte, G., & Sartorius, N. (1991). The World Health Organization's cross-cultural study on neuropsychiatric aspects of infection with the human immunodeficiency virus (HIV-1): Preparation and pilot phase. *British Journal of Psychiatry, 159,* 351–356.

Maj, M., D'Elia, L., Satz, P., Jansses, R., Zaudig, M., Uchiyama, C., Starace, F., Galderisi, S., & Chervinsky, A. (1993). Evaluation of two new neuropsychological tests designed to minimize cultural bias in the assessment of HIV-1 seropositive persons: A WHO study. *Archives of Clinical Neuropsychology, 8,* 123–135.

Majdan, A., Sziklas, V., & Jones-Gotman, M. (1996). Performance of healthy subjects and patients with resection from the anterior temporal lobe on matched tests of verbal and visuoperceptual learning. *Journal of Clinical and Experimental Neuropsychology, 18*(3), 416–430.

Malec, J., Ivnik, R., Smith, G., Tangalos, E., Petersen, R., Kokmen, E., & Kurland, L. (1992). Mayo's older americans normative studies: Utility of corrections for age and education for the WAIS-R. *The Clinical Neuropsychologist, 6* (Suppl), 31–47.

Marcopulos, B.A., McLain, C.A., & Giuliano, A.J. (1997). Cognitive impairment or inadequate norms? A study of healthy, rural, older adults with limited education. *The Clinical Neuropsychologist, 11*(2), 111–131.

Margolin, D., Pate, D.S., Friedrich, F.J., & Elia, E. (1990). Dysnomia in dementia and in stroke patients: Different underlying cognitive deficits. *Journal of Clinical and Experimental Neuropsychology, 12*(4), 597–612.

Margolis, R.B., & Scialfa, C.T. (1984). Age differences in Wechsler Memory Scale performance. *Journal of Clinical Psychology, 40*(6), 1442–1449.

Marie, R.M., Rioux, P., Eustache, F., Travere, J.M., et al. (1995). Clues and functional neuroanatomy of verbal working memory: A study about the resting brain glucose metabolism in Parkinson's disease. *European Journal of Neurology, 2,* 83–94.

Martin, A., & Fedio, P. (1983). Word production and comprehension in Alzheimer's Disease: The breakdown of semantic knowledge. *Brain and Language, 19,* 124–141.

Martin, N.J., & Franzen, M.D. (1989). The effect of anxiety on neuropsychological function. *International Journal of Neuropsychology, 11,* 1–8.

Mason, C.F., & Ganzler, H. (1964). Adult norms for the Shipley Institute of Living Scale and Hooper Visual Organization Test based on age and education. *Journal of Gerontology, 19,* 419–424.

Massman, P.J., & Doody, R.S. (1996). Hemispheric asymmetry in Alzheimer's Disease is apparent in motor functioning. *Journal of Clinical and Experimental Neuropsychology, 18*(1), 110–121.

Matarazzo, J.D. (1990). Psychological assessment versus psychological testing. *American Psychologist, 45*(9), 999–1017.

Matarazzo, J.D., Wiens, A.N., Matarazzo, R.G., & Goldstein, S.G. (1974). Psychometric and clinical test-retest reliability of the Halstead impairment index in a sample of healthy, young, normal men. *The Journal of Nervous and Mental Disease, 158*(1), 37–49.

Matthews, C.G. (1974). Application of neuropsychological test methods in mentally retarded subjects. In R.M. Reitan & L.A. Davison (Eds.), *Clinical neuropsychology: Current status and applications.* Washington: Hemisphere Publishing.

Mattis, S. (1976). Mental status examination for organic mental syndrome in the elderly patient. In L. Bellak & T. Karasu (Eds.), *Geriatric psychiatry.* New York: Grune and Stratton.

Mattis, S. (1988). *Dementia Rating Scale.* Odessa, FL: Psychological Assessment Resources.

McCarthy, D. (1972). *Manual for the McCarthy Scales for Children's Abilities.* New York: The Psychological Corporation.

McIntosh, D.E., Dunham, M.D., Dean, R.S., & Kundert, D.K. (1995). Neuropsychological characteristics of learning disabled/gifted children. *International Journal of Neuroscience, 83*(1-2), 123–130.

McKay, S.E., Golden, C.J., & Wolf, B.A. (1983). Effects of age and education on the Luria-Nebraska neuropsychological battery performance of selected populations. *International Journal of Neuroscience, 21,* 25–38.

McKeever, W.F., & Abramson, M. (1991). Halstead and Halstead-Reitan norms for Finger Tapping Test are severely biased against females and left-handers. *Journal of Clinical and Experimental Neuropsychology, 13*(1), 91.

McKinzey, R.K., Curley, J.F., & Fish, J.M. (1985). False negatives, Canter's background interference procedure, the Trail Making Test, and epileptics. *Journal of Clinical Psychology, 41*, 812–820.

Meyers, J.E., & Lange, D. (1994). Recognition subtest for the Complex Figure. *The Clinical Neuropsychologist, 8*(2), 153–166.

Meyers, J.E., & Meyers, K.R. (1992). *A training manual for the clinical scoring of the Rey-Osterrieth Complex Figure and the recognition subtest.* Published by John E. Meyers, Marian Health Center, Department of Psychology, Sioux City, Iowa.

Meyers, J.E., & Meyers, K.R. (1995). Rey Complex Figure Test under four different administration procedures. *The Clinical Neuropsychologist, 9*(1), 63–67.

Miceli, G., Caltagirone, C., Gainotti, G., Masullo, C., & Siweri, M.C. (1981). Neuropsychological correlates of localized cerebral lesions in nonaphasic braindamaged patients. *Journal of Clinical Neuropsychology, 3*, 53–63.

Mickanin, J., Grossman, M., Onishi, K., Auriacombe, S., & Clark, C. (1994). Verbal and nonverbal fluency in patients with probable Alzheimer's disease. *Neuropsychology, 8*, 385–394.

Miller, E. (1984). Verbal fluency as a function of a measure of verbal intelligence and in relation to different types of cerebral pathology. *British Journal of Clinical Psychology, 23*, 53–57.

Miller, E. (1985). Possible frontal impairments: A test using a measure of verbal fluency. *British Journal of Clinical Psychology, 24*, 211–212.

Miller, E.N., Selnes, O.A., McArthur, J.C., Satz, P., Becker, J.T., Cohen, B.A., Sheridan, K., Machado, A.M., VanGorp, W.G., & Visscher, B. (1990). Neuropsychological performance in HIV-1-infected homosexual men: The Multicenter AIDS Cohort Study (MACS). *Neurology, 40*(2), 197–204.

Miller, B.L., Lesser, I.M., Boone, K.B., Hill, E., Mehringer, C.M., & Wong, K. (1991). Brain lesions and cognitive function in late-life psychosis. *British Journal of Psychiatry, 158*, 76–82.

Milner, B. (1962). Laterality effects in audition. In V.B. Mountcastle (Ed.), *Interhemispheric relations and cerebral dominance.* Baltimore: Johns Hopkins University Press.

Milner, B. (1964). Some effects of frontal lobectomy in man. In J.M. Warren, & K.A. Akert (Eds.), *The Frontal Granular Cortex and Behavior.* New York: McGraw-Hill, (pp. 331–334).

Milner, B. (1970). Memory and the medial temporal regions of the brain. In K.H. Pribram, & D.E.

Broadbent (Eds.), *Biology of Memory.* New York: Academic Press (pp. 29–50).

Milner, B. (1971). Disorders of learning and memory after temporal lobe lesions in man. *Clinical Neurosurgery, 19*, 421–446.

Milner, B. (1975). Psychological aspects of focal epilepsy and its neurosurgical management. *Advances in Neurology, 8*, 299–321.

Mitrushina, M., & Satz, P. (1991a). Effect of repeated administration of a neuropsychological battery in the elderly. *Journal of Clinical Psychology, 47*(6), 790–801.

Mitrushina, M., & Satz, P. (1991b). Changes in cognitive functioning associated with normal aging. *Archives of Clinical Neuropsychology, 6*, 49–60.

Mitrushina, M., & Satz, P. (1995). Repeated testing of normal elderly with the Boston naming test. *Aging: Clinical & Experimental Research, 7*, 123–127.

Mitrushina, M., Satz, P., & Van Gorp, W. (1989). Some putative cognitive precursors in subjects hypothesized to be at-risk for dementia. *Archives of Clinical Neuropsychology, 4*, 323–333.

Mitrushina, M., Satz, P., & Chervinsky, A.B. (1990). Efficiency of recall on the Rey-Osterrieth Complex Figure in normal aging. *Brain Dysfunction, 3*, 148–150.

Mitrushina, M., Satz, P., Chervinsky, A., & D'Elia, L. (1991). Performance of four age groups of normal elderly on the Rey Auditory-Verbal Learning Test. *Journal of Clinical Psychology, 47*(3), 351–357.

Mitrushina, M., D'Elia, L., Satz, P., Uchiyama, C., Mathews, A., & Harker, J. (1993). A comparison of selective attention deficits in normal elderly and AIDS patients. *Developmental Brain Dysfunction, 6*, 324–328.

Mitrushina, M., Drebing, C., Uchiyama, C., Satz, P., Van Gorp, W., & Chervinsky, A. (1994). The pattern of deficit in different memory components in normal aging and dementia of Alzheimer's type. *Journal of Clinical Psychology, 50*(4), 591–596.

Mitrushina, M., Fogel, T., D'Elia, L., Uchiyama, C., & Satz, P. (1995a). Performance on motor tasks as an indication of increased behavioral asymmetry with advancing age. *Neuropsychologia, 33*(3), 359–364.

Mitrushina, M., Uchiyama, C., & Satz, P. (1995b). Heterogeneity of cognitive profiles in normal aging: Implications for early manifestations of Alzheimer's Disease. *Journal of Clinical and Experimental Neuropsychology, 17*(3), 374–382.

Mittenberg, W., Seidenberg, M., O'Leary, D.S., & DiGiulio, D.V. (1989). Changes in cerebral functioning associated with normal aging. *Journal of Clinical and Experimental Neuropsychology, 11*, 918–932.

Mittenberg, W., Burton, D., Darrow, E., & Thompson, G. (1992). Normative data for the WMS-R: 25 to 34 year olds. *Psychological Assessment, 4*(3), 363–368.

Moehle, K.A., Fitzhugh-Bell, K.B., Engleman, E., & Hennon, D. (1988). Statistical and diagnostic adequacy of a short form of the Halstead Category Test. *International Journal of Neuroscience, 42,* 107–112.

Moffoot, A.P.R., O'Carroll, R.E., Bennie, J., Carroll, S., Dick, H., Ebmeier, K.P., & Goodwin, G.M. (1994). Diurnal variation of mood and neuropsychological function in major depression with melancholia. *Journal of Affective Disorders, 32,* 257–269.

Monsch, A.U., Bondi, M.W., & Butters, N. (1994). A comparison of category and letter fluency in Alzheimer's disease. *Neuropsychology, 8,* 25–30.

Moore, J.L., & Hannay, H.J. (1981). Verbal-performance IQ-discrepancy and Rhythm Test performance. *Perceptual and Motor Skills, 52,* 819–826.

Moore, J.L., & Hannay, H.J. (1982). Verbal-performance IQ discrepancy and perception of rhythm and timbre. *Neuropsychologia, 20*(6), 661–668.

Morris, J.C., Heyman, A., Mohs, R.C., Hughes, S.P., van Belle, G., Fullenbaum, G., Mellits, E.D., Clark, C., & the CERAD investigators, (1989). The Consortium to Establish a Registry for Alzheimer's Disease (CERAD). Part 1. Clinical and neuropsychological assessment of Alzheimer's disease. *Neurology, 39,* 1159–1165.

Morrison, M.W., Gregory, R.J., & Paul, J.J. (1979). Reliability on the Finger Tapping Test and a note on sex differences. *Perceptual and Motor Skills, 48,* 139–142.

Moses, J.A. (1985). Internal consistency of standard and short forms of three itemized Halstead-Reitan Neuropsychological Battery tests. *International Journal of Clinical Neuropsychology, 7*(3), 164–166.

Mungas, D. (1983). Differential clinical sensitivity of specific parameters of the Rey Auditory-Verbal Learning Test. *Journal of Consulting and Clinical Psychology, 51*(6), 848–855.

Murphy, K.R., & Davidshofer, C.O. (1991). *Psychological Testing: Principles and Applications* (2nd ed.). Englewood Cliffs, New Jersey: Prentice Hall.

Mutchnick, M.G., Ross, L.K., & Long, C.J. (1991). Decision strategies for cerebral dysfunction: IV. Determination of cerebral dysfunction. *Archives of Clinical Neuropsychology, 6*(4), 259–270.

Nabors, N.A., Vangel, S.J., Lichtenberg, P.A., & Walsh, P. (1997). Normative and clinical utility of the Hooper Visual Organization Test with geriatric medical inpatients. *Journal of Clinical Gerontology, 3*(3), 191–198.

Nadler, J.D., Grace, J., White, D.A., Butters, M.A., & Malloy, P.F. (1996). Laterality differences in quantitative and qualitative Hooper performance. *Archives of Clinical Neuropsychology, 11*(3), 223–229.

Nebes, R.D. (1989). Semantic memory in Alzheimer's disease. *Psychological Bulletin, 106,* 377–394.

Nebes, R.D., & Brady, C.B. (1990). Preserved organization of semantic attributes in Alzheimer's Disease. *Psychology and Aging, 5,* 574–579.

Nebes, R.D., Martin, D.C., & Horn, L.C. (1984). Sparing of semantic memory in Alzheimer's Disease. *Journal of Abnormal Psychology, 93,* 321–330.

Nehemkis, A.M., & Lewinsohn, P.M. (1972). Effects of left and right cerebral lesions on the naming process. *Perceptual and Motor Skills, 35,* 787–798.

Neils, J., Baris, J.M., Carter, C., Dell'aira, A.L., Nordloh, S.J., Weiler, E., & Weisiger, B. (1995). Effects of age, education, and living environment on Boston Naming Test performance. *Journal of Speech and Hearing Research, 38,* 1143–1149.

Neils, J., Brennan, M.M., Cole, M., Boller, F., & Gerdeman, B. (1988). The use of phonemic cueing with Alzheimer's Disease patients. *Neuropsychologia, 26,* 351–354.

Nelson, H.E. (1982). *National Adult Reading Test (NART) Test Manual.* Berkshire: NFER-Nelson.

Neuger, G.J., O'Leary, D.S., Berent, S., Fishburne, F.J., Giordani, B., Boll, T.J., & Barth, J.T. (1981). Order effects on the Halstead-Reitan Neuropsychological Test Battery and allied procedures. *Journal of Consulting and Clinical Psychology, 49,* 722–730.

Newcombe, F. (1969). *Missile Wounds of the Brain.* London: Oxford University Press.

Nicholas, L.E., Brookshire, R.H., MacLennan, D.L., Schumacher, J.G., & Porrazzo, S.A. (1989). Revised administration and scoring procedures for the Boston Naming Test and norms for non-brain-damaged adults. *Aphasia, 5*(6), 569–580.

Nicholas, M., Obler, L., Albert, M., & Goodglass, H. (1985). Lexical retrieval in healthy aging. *Cortex, 21,* 595–606.

Nicholas, M., Obler, L., Au, R., & Albert, M.L. (1996). On the nature of naming errors in aging and dementia: A study of semantic relatedness. *Brain and Language, 54,* 184–195.

Nielsen, H., Knudsen, L., & Daugbjerg, O. (1989). Normative data for eight neuropsychological tests based on a Danish sample. *Scandinavian Journal of Psychology, 30,* 37–45.

Norris, M.P., Blankenship-Reuter, L., Snow-Turek, A.L., & Finch, J. (1995). Influence of depression on verbal fluency performance. *Aging and Cognition, 2*(3), 206–215.

Ober, B.A., Dronkers, N.F., Koss, E., Delis, D.C., & Friedland, R.P. (1986). Retrieval from semantic memory in Alzheimer-type dementia. *Journal of Clinical and Experimental Neuropsychology, 8,* 75–92.

O'Donnell, P.O., Kurtz, J., & Ramanaiah, N.V. (1983). Neuropsychological test findings for normal, learning-disabled and brain-damaged young adults. *Journal of Consulting and Clinical Psychology, 51*(5), 726–729.

Osterrieth, P.A. (1944). Le test de copie d'une figure complexe. *Archives de Psychologie, 30,* 206–356.

Osterrieth, P.A. (1993). The complex figure copy test. *The Clinical Neuropsychologist, 7*(1), 3–21.

Ostrosky-Solis, F., Canseco, E., Quintanar, L., Navarro, E., & Meneses, S. (1985). Sociocultural effects in neuropsychological assessment. *International Journal of Neuroscience, 27,* 53–66.

Otto, M.W., Bruder, G.E., Fava, M., Delis, D.C., Quitkin, F.M., & Rosenbaum, J.F. (1994). Norms for depressed patients for California Verbal Learning Test: Associations with depression severity and self-report of cognitive difficulties. *Archives of Clinical Neuropsychology, 9,* 81–88.

Pachana, N.A., Boone, K.B., Miller, B.L., Cummings, J.L., & Berman, N. (1996). Comparison of neuropsychological functioning in Alzheimer's disease and frontotemporal dementia. *Journal of the International Neuropsychological Society, 2,* 505–510.

Paivio, A., Yuille, J.C., & Madigan, S.A. (1968). Concreteness, imagery, and meaningfulness values for 925 nouns. *Journal of Experimental Psychology (Monograph Supplement), 76,* 1–25.

Panek, P.E., Rush, M.C., & Slade, A.L. (1984). Locus of the age-Stroop interference relationship. *The Journal of Genetic Psychology, 145*(2), 209–216.

Paolo, A.M., Cluff, B.R., & Ryan, J.J. (1996). Influence of perceptual organization and naming abilities on the Hooper Visual Organization Test. *Neuropsychiatry, Neuropsychology, and Behavioral Neurology, 9*(4), 254–257.

Pardo, J.V., Pardo, P.J., Janer, K.W., & Raichle, M.E. (1990). The anterior cingulate cortex mediates processing selection in the Stroop attentional conflict paradigm. *Proceedings of the National Academy of Science, 87,* 256–259.

Parkin, A.J., & Lawrence, A. (1994). A dissociation in the relation between memory tasks and frontal lobe tests in the normal elderly. *Neuropsychologia, 32,* 1523–1532.

Parkin, A.J., & Walter, B.M. (1991). Aging, short-term memory and frontal dysfunction. *Psychobiology, 19,* 175–179.

Parkinson, S.R., Inman, V.W., & Dannenbaum, S.E. (1985). Adult age differences in short-term forgetting. *Acta Psychologica, 60,* 83–101.

Parks, R.W., Loewenstein, D.A., Dodrill, K.L., Barker, W.W., Yoshii, F., Chang, J.Y., Emran, A., Apicella, A., Sheramata, W.A., & Duara, R. (1988). Cerebral metabolic effects of a Verbal Fluency Test: A PET scan study. *Journal of Clinical and Experimental Neuropsychology, 10,* 565–575.

Parks, R.W., Levine, D.S., Long, D.L., Crockett, D.J., Dalton, I.E., Weingartner, H., Fedio, P., Coburn, K.L., Siler, G., Matthews, J.R., & Becker, R.E. (1992). Parallel distributed processing and neuropsychology: A neural network model of Wisconsin Card Sorting and Verbal Fluency. *Neuropsychology Review, 3*(2), 213–233.

Parsons, O.A., Maslow, H.I., Morris, F., & Denny, J.P. (1964). Trail Making Test performance in relation to certain experimenter, test and subject variables. *Perceptual and Motor Skills, 19,* 199–206.

Pauker, J.D. (1980). *Norms for the Halstead-Reitan Neuropsychological Test Battery based on a nonclinical adult sample.* Address presented at the meeting of the Canadian Psychological Association, Calgary, Alberta, Canada.

Peaker, A., & Stewart, L.E. (1989). Rey's Auditory Verbal Learning Test—a review. In J.R. Crawford, & D.M. Parker (Eds.), *Developments in Clinical and Experimental Neuropsychology.* New York: Plenum Press.

Peirson, A.R., & Jansen, P. (1997). Comparability of the Rey-Osterrieth and Taylor forms of the Complex Figure Test. *The Clinical Neuropsychologist, 11*(3), 244–248.

Pendleton, M.G., Heaton, R.K., Lehman, R.A.W., & Hulihan, D. (1982). Diagnostic utility of the Thurstone Word Fluency Test in neuropsychological evaluations. *Journal of Clinical Neuropsychology, 4,* 307–317.

Perlmuter, L.C., Tun, P., Sizer, N., McGlinchey, R.E., & Nathan, E.M. (1987). Age and diabetes related changes in verbal fluency. *Experimental Aging Research, 13,* 9–14.

Perret, E. (1974). The left frontal lobe of man and the suppression of habitual responses in verbal categorical behaviour. *Neuropsychologia, 12,* 323–330.

Perrine, K. (1993). Differential aspects of conceptual processing in the Category Test and Wisconsin Card Sorting Test. *Journal of Clinical and Experimental Neuropsychology, 15,* 461–473.

Peterson, L.R., & Peterson, M.J. (1959). Short-term

retention of individual verbal items. *Journal of Experimental Psychology, 58,* 193–198.

Pierce, T.W., Elias, M.F., Keohane, P.J., Podraza, A.M., Robbins, M.A., & Schultz, N.R. (1990). Validity of a short form of the Category Test in relation to age, education and gender. *Experimental Aging Research, 15*(3), 137–141.

Piersma, H.L. (1986). Wechsler Memory Scale performance in geropsychiatric patients. *Journal of Clinical Psychology, 42*(2), 323–327.

Pirozzolo, F.J., Hansch, E.C., Mortimer, J.A., Webster, D.D., & Kuskowski, M.A. (1982). Dementia in Parkinson disease: A neuropsychological analysis. *Brain and Cognition, 1,* 71–83.

Polubinski, J.P., & Melamed, L.E. (1986). Examination of the sex difference on a Symbol Digit Substitution Test. *Perceptual and Motor Skills, 62,* 975–982.

Ponton, M.O., Satz, P., Herrera, L., Ortiz, F., Urrutia, C.P., Young, R., D'Elia, L.F., Furst, C.J., & Namerow, N. (1996). Normative data stratified by age and education for the Neuropsychological Screening Battery for Hispanics (NeSBHIS): Initial report. *Journal of International Neuropsychological Society, 2*(2), 96–104.

Portin, R., Saarijarvi, S., Joukamaa, M., & Salokangas, R.K.R. (1995). Education, gender and cognitive performance in a 62-year-old normal population: results from the Turva Project. *Psychological Medicine, 25,* 1295–1298.

Powell, G.E. (1979). The relationship between intelligence and verbal and spatial memory. *Journal of Clinical Psychology, 35*(2), 335–340.

Power, D.G., Logue, P.E., McCarty, S.M., Rosenstiel, A.K., & Ziezat, H.A. (1979). Inter-rater reliability of the Russell revision of the Wechsler Memory Scale: An attempt to clarify some ambiguities in scoring. *Journal of Clinical Neuropsychology, 1,* 343–345.

Price, L.J., Fein, G., & Feinberg, I. (1980). *Neuropsychological Assessment of Cognitive Function in the Elderly.* In L.W. Poon (ed.), Aging in the 1980's. Washington, DC: American Psychological Association Press.

Prigatano, G.P. (1978). Wechsler Memory Scale: A selective review of the literature. *Journal of Clinical Psychology, 34,* 816–832.

Prigatano, G.P., & Parsons, O.A. (1976). Relationship of age and education to Halstead test performance in different patient populations. *Journal of Consulting and Clinical Psychology, 44*(4), 527–533.

Prigatano, G.P., Parsons, O.A., Levin, D.C., Wright, E., & Hawryluk, G. (1983). Neuropsychological test performance in mildly hypoxemic patients with chronic obstructive pulmonary disease. *Journal of Consulting and Clinical Psychology, 51*(1), 108–116.

Puckett, J.M., & Lawson, W.M. (1989). Absence of adult age differences in forgetting in Brown-Peterson task. *Acta Psychologica, 72,* 159–175.

Pujol, J., Vendrell, P., Dues, J., Kulisevsky, J., Marti-Valalta, J.L., Garcia, C., Junque, C., & Capdevila, A. (1996). Frontal lobe activation during word generation studied by functional MRI. *Acta Neurologica Scandinavica, 93,* 403–410.

Query, W.T., & Berger, R.A. (1980). AVLT memory scores as a function of age among general medical, neurologic and alcoholic patients. *Journal of Clinical Psychology, 36*(4), 1009–1012.

Query, W.T., & Megran, J. (1983). Age-related norms for AVLT in a male patient population. *Journal of Clinical Psychology, 39*(1), 136–138.

Query, W.T., & Megran, J. (1984). Influence of depression and alcoholism on learning, recall and recognition. *Journal of Clinical Psychology, 40*(4), 1097–1100.

Randolph, C., Braun, A.R., Goldberg, T.E., & Chase, T.N. (1993). Semantic fluency in Alzheimer's, Parkinson's and Huntington's Disease: Dissociation of storage and retrieval failures. *Neuropsychology, 7,* 82–88.

Rapport, L.J., Dutra, R.L., Webster, J.S., Charter, R., & Morrill, B. (1995). Hemispatial deficits on the Rey-Osterrieth Complex Figure drawing. *The Clinical Neuropsychologist, 9*(2), 169–179.

Rapport, L.J., Charter, R.A., Dutra, R.L., Farchione, T.J., & Kingsley, J.J. (1997). Psychometric properties of the Rey-Osterrieth Complex Figure: Lezak-Osterrieth versus Denman scoring systems. *The Clinical Neuropsychologist, 11*(1), 46–53.

Rathbun, J., & Smith, A. (1982). Comment on the validity of Boyd's validation study of the Hooper Visual Organization Test. *Journal of Consulting and Clinical Psychology, 50,* 281–283.

Reader, M.J., Harris, E.L., Schuerholz, L.J., & Denckla, M.B. (1994). Attention Deficit Hyperactivity Disorder and executive dysfunction. *Developmental Neuropsychology, 10*(4), 493–512.

Reddon, J.R., Schopflocher, D., Gill, D.M., & Stefanyk, W.O. (1989). Speech Sounds Perception Test: Nonrandom response locations form a logical fallacy in structure. *Perceptual and Motor Skills, 69,* 235–240.

Reed, H.B.C., & Reitan, R.M. (1962). The significance of age in the performance of a complex psychomotor task by brain-damaged and non-brain-damaged subjects. *Journal of Gerontology, 17,* 193–196.

Reed, H.B.C., & Reitan, R.M. (1963a). A comparison of the effects of the normal aging process with the effects of organic brain damage on adaptive abilities. *Journal of Gerontology, 18,* 177–179.

Reed, B.C., & Reitan, R.M. (1963b). Changes in psychological test performance associated with the normal aging process. *Journal of Gerontology, 18,* 271–274.

Regard, M., & Landis, T. (1994). The "smiley": A graphical expression of mood in right anterior cerebral lesions. *Neuropsychiatry, Neuropsychology, and Behavioral Neurology, 7*(4), 303–307.

Reitan, R.M. (1955a). Certain differential effects of left and right cerebral lesions in human adults. *The Journal of Comparative and Physiological Psychology, 48,* 474–477.

Reitan, R.M. (1955b). Investigation of the validity of Halstead's measures of biological intelligence. *Archives of Neurology and Psychiatry, 73,* 28–35.

Reitan, R.M. (1955c). The relation of the Trail Making Test to organic brain damage. *Journal of Consulting Psychology, 19*(5), 393–394.

Reitan, R.M. (1955d). The distribution according to age of a psychologic measure dependent upon organic brain functions. *Journal of Gerontology, 10,* 338–340.

Reitan, R.M. (1958). Validity of the Trail Making Test as an indicator of organic brain damage. *Perceptual and Motor Skills, 8,* 271–276.

Reitan, R.M. (1959). The comparative effects of brain damage on the Halstead impairment index and the Wechsler-Bellevue scale. *Journal of Clinical Psychology, 15,* 281–285.

Reitan, R.M. (1964). Psychological deficits resulting from cerebral lesions in man. In J.M. Warren & K.A. Akert (Eds.), *The frontal granular cortex and behavior.* New York: McGraw-Hill.

Reitan, R.M. (1979). *Manual for Administration of Neuropsychological Test Batteries for Adults and Children.* Tucson, AZ: Neuropsychology Laboratory.

Reitan, R.M. (1985). *The Halstead-Reitan Neuropsychological Test Battery.* Tucson, AZ: Neuropsychology Press.

Reitan, R.M., & Wolfson, D. (1985). *The Halstead-Reitan Neuropsychological Test Battery. Theory and Clinical Interpretation.* Tucson, AZ: Neuropsychology Press.

Reitan, R.M., & Wolfson, D. (1989). The Seashore Rhythm Test and brain functions. *The Clinical Neuropsychologist, 3*(1), 70–78.

Reitan, R.M., & Wolfson, D. (1993). *The Halstead-Reitan Neuropsychological Test Battery: Theory and Clinical Interpretation* (2nd ed). Tucson, AZ: Neuropsychology Press.

Reitan, R.M., & Wolfson, D. (1995). Influence of age and education on neuropsychological test results. *The Clinical Neuropsychologist, 9*(2), 151–158.

Rey, A. (1941). L'examen psychologique dans les cas d'encephalopathie traumatique. *Archives de Psychologie, 28,* 286–340.

Rey, A. (1964). *L'examen clinique en psychologie.* Paris: Presses Universitaires de France.

Rey, G.J., & Benton, A.L. (1991). *Examen de Afasia Multilingue.* Iowa City: AJA.

Rey, A., & Osterrieth, P.A. (1993). Translations of excerpts from Andre Rey's Psychological examination of traumatic encephalopathy and P.A. Osterrieth's The Complex Figure Copy Test. *The Clinical Neuropsychologist, 7*(1), 4–21.

Richardson, E.D., & Marottoli, R.A. (1996). Education-specific normative data on common neuropsychological indices for individuals older than 75 Years. *The Clinical Neuropsychologist, 10*(4), 375–381.

Ricker, J.H., & Axelrod, B.N. (1995). Hooper Visual Organization Test: Effects of object naming ability. *The Clinical Neuropsychologist, 9*(1), 57–62.

Ripich, D.N., Petrill, S.A., Whitehouse, P.J., & Ziol, E.W. (1995). Gender differences in language of AD patients: A longitudinal study. *Neurology, 45,* 299–302.

Rosen, W.G. (1980). Verbal fluency in aging and dementia. *Journal of Clinical Neuropsychology, 2*(2), 135–146.

Rosenberg, S., Ryan, J.J., & Prifitera, A. (1984). Rey Auditory-Verbal Learning Test performance of patients with and without memory impairment. *Journal of Clinical Psychology, 40*(3), 785–787.

Ross, T.P., Lichtenberg, P.A., & Christensen, B.K. (1995). Normative data on the Boston naming test for elderly adults in a demographically diverse medical sample. *The Clinical Neuropsychologist, 9*(4), 321–325.

Rosselli, M., & Ardila, A. (1991). Effects of age, education, and gender on the Rey-Osterrieth Complex Figure. *The Clinical Neuropsychologist, 5,* 370–376.

Rosser, A., & Hodges, J.R. (1994). Initial letter and semantic category fluency in Alzheimer's Disease, Huntington's Disease, and Progressive Supranuclear Palsy. *Journal of Neurology, Neurosurgery, and Psychiatry, 57*(11), 1389–1394.

Roth, E., Davidoff, G., Thomas, P., Doljanac, R., Dijkers, M., Berent S., Morris, J., & Yarkony, G. (1989). A controlled study of neuropsychological deficits in acute spinal cord injury patients. *Paraplegia, 27*(6), 480–489.

Rounsaville, B.J., Jones, C., Novelly, R.A., & Kleber, H. (1982). Neuropsychological functioning in opiate addicts. *The Journal of Nervous and Mental Disease, 170*(4), 209–216.

Ruff, R.M., & Parker, S.B. (1993). Gender- and age-specific changes in motor speed and eye-hand coordination in adults: Normative values for the Finger Tapping and Grooved Pegboard Tests. *Perceptual and Motor Skills, 76,* 1219–1230.

Ruff, R.M., Light, R.H., Parker, S.B., & Levin, H.S. (1996). Benton Controlled Oral Word Association Test: Reliability and updated norms. *Archives of Clinical Neuropsychology, 11*(4), 329–338.

Russell, E.W. (1974). The effect of acute lateralized brain damage on Halstead's biological intelligence factors. *The Journal of Clinical Psychology, 90,* 101–107.

Russell, E.W. (1975). A multiple scoring method for the assessment of complex memory functions. *Journal of Consulting and Clinical Psychology, 43,* 800–809.

Russell, E.W. (1984). Theory and development of pattern analysis methods related to the Halstead-Reitan Battery. In P.E. Logue & J.M. Schear (Eds.), *Clinical neuropsychology, a multidisciplinary approach* (pp. 50–98). Springfield, IL: Charles C. Thomas.

Russell, E.W. (1985). Comparison of the TPT 10 and 6 hole form board. *Journal of Clinical Psychology, 41*(1), 68–81.

Russell, E.W. (1987). A reference scale method for constructing neuropsychological test batteries. *Journal of Clinical and Experimental Neuropsychology, 9*(4), 376–392.

Russell, E.W., & Levy, M. (1987). Revision of the Halstead Category Test. *Journal of Consulting and Clinical Psychology, 55*(6), 898–901.

Russell, E., & Starkey, R. (1993). *Halstead-Russell Neuropsychological Evaluation System (HRNES).* Los Angeles, CA: Western Psychological Services.

Russell, E.W., Neuringer, C., & Goldstein, G. (1970). *Assessment of Brain Damage: A Neuropsychological Key Approach.* New York: Wiley.

Ryan, J.J., & Geisser, M.E. (1986). Validity and diagnostic accuracy of an alternate form of the Rey Auditory Verbal Learning Test. *Archives of Clinical Neuropsychology, 1,* 209–217.

Ryan, J.J., Larsen, J., & Prifitera, A. (1982). Short form of the Speech Sounds Perception Test: Further considerations. *Clinical Neuropsychology, 4*(3), 97–98.

Ryan, J.J., Morris, J., Yaffa, S., & Peterson, L. (1981). Test-retest reliability of the Wechsler Memory Scale, Form I. *Journal of Clinical Psychology, 37*(4), 847–848.

Ryan, J.J., Rosenberg, S.J., & Mittenberg, W. (1984). Factor analysis of the Rey Auditory-Verbal Learn-

ing Test. *the International Journal of Clinical Neuropsychology, 6*(4), 239–241.

Ryan, J.J., Geisser, M.E., Randall, D.M., & George-miller, R.J. (1986). Alternate form reliability and equivalency of the Rey Auditory Verbal Learning Test. *Journal of Clinical and Experimental Neuropsychology, 8*(5), 611–616.

Ryan, C.M., Morrow, L.A., Bromet, E.J., & Parkinson, D.K. (1987). Assessment of neuropsychological dysfunction in the workplace: Normative data from the Pittsburgh Occupational Exposures Test Battery. *Journal of Clinical and Experimental Neuropsychology, 9*(6), 665–679.

Ryan, J.J., Paolo, A.M., & Brungardt, T.M. (1990). Standardization of the Wechsler Adult Intelligence Scale–Revised for persons 75 years and older. *Psychological Assessment, 2,* 404–411.

Ryan, J.J., Paolo, A.M., & Skrade, M. (1992). Rey Auditory Verbal Learning Test performance of a federal corrections sample with acquired immunodeficiency syndrome. *International Journal of Neuroscience, 64,* 177–181.

Sacks, T.L., Clark, C.R., Pols, R.G., & Geffen, L.B. (1991). Comparability and stability of performance of six alternate forms of the Dodrill-Stroop Color-Word Test. *The Clinical Neuropsychologist, 5,* 220–225.

Salthouse, T.A., & Fristoe, N. (1995). A process analysis of adult age effects on a computer-administered Trail Making Test. *Neuropsychology, 9,* 518–528.

Salthouse, T.A., Fristoe, N., & Rhee, S.H. (1996). How localized are age-related effects on neuropsychological measures? *Neuropsychology, 10*(2), 272–285.

Samuels, I., Butters, N., & Fedio, P. (1972). Short term memory disorders following temporal lobe removals in humans. *Cortex, 8,* 283–298.

Satz, P. (1988). Neuropsychological testimony: Some emerging concerns. *The Clinical Neuropsychologist, 2,* 89–100.

Satz, P. (1993). Brain reserve capacity on symptom onset after brain injury: A formulation and review of evidence for threshold theory. *Neuropsychology, 7,* 273–295.

Satz, P., & Mogel, S. (1962). An abbreviation of the WAIS for clinical use. *Journal of Clinical Psychology, 18,* 77–79.

Savage, R.M., & Gouvier, W.D. (1992). Rey Auditory-Verbal Learning Test: The effects of age and gender, and norms for delayed recall and story recognition trials. *Archives of Clinical Neuropsychology, 7,* 407–414.

Schaie, K.W. (1983). The Seattle longitudinal study: A 21-year exploration of psychometric intelligence in adulthood. In K.W. Schaie (Ed.), *Longitudinal Studies of Adult Psychological Development.* New York: The Guilford Press (pp. 64–135).

Schaie, K.W., & Strother, C.R. (1968a). Cognitive and personality variables in college graduates of advanced age. In G.A. Talland (Ed.), *Human Aging and Behavior.* New York: Academic Press.

Schaie, K.W., & Strother, C.R. (1968b). A cross-sectional study of age changes in cognitive behavior. *Psychological Bulletin, 70,* 671–680.

Schaie, K.W., & Parham, I.A. (1977). Cohort-sequential analyses of adult intellectual development. *Developmental Psychology, 13*(6), 649–653.

Schear, J. M. (1984). Neuropsychological assessment of the elderly in clinical practice. In P. E. Logue, & J. M. Schear (Eds.), *Clinical Neuropcychology: A multidisciplinary approach.* Springfield, IL: Charles C. Thomas.

Schear, J.M. (1986). Utility of half-credit scoring of Russell's revision of the Wechsler Memory Scale. *Journal of Clinical Psychology, 42*(5), 783–787.

Schear, J.M., Skenes, L.L., & Larson, V.D. (1988). Effect of simulated hearing loss on speech sounds perception. *Journal of Clinical and Experimental Neuropsychology, 10*(5), 597–602.

Schonfield, A.D., Davidson, H., & Jones, H. (1983). An example of age-associated interference in memorizing. *Journal of Gerontology, 38,* 204–210.

Schreiber, D.J., Goldman, H., Kleinman, K.M., Goldfader, P.R., & Snow, M.Y. (1976). The relationship between independent neuropsychological and neurological detection and localization of cerebral impairment. *The Journal of Nervous and Mental Disease, 162*(5), 360–365.

Schreiber, H., Rothmeier, J., Becker, W., Jurgens, R., Born, J., Stolz-Born, G., Westphal, K.P., & Kornhuber, H.H. (1995). Comparative assessment of saccadic eye movements, psychomotor and cognitive performance in schizophrenics, their first-degree relatives and control subjects. *Acta Psychiatrica Scandinavica, 91,* 195–201.

Schwartz, M.S., & Ivnik, R.J. (1980, September). *Wechsler Memory Scale I: Toward a more objective and systematic scoring system for the Logical Memory and Visual Reproduction subtests.* Paper presented at the meeting of the Americal Psychological Association, Montreal, Canada.

Searight, H.R., Dunn, E.J., Grisso, T., Margolis, R.B., & Gibbons, J.L. (1989). The relation of the Halstead-Reitan Neuropsychological Battery to ratings of everyday functioning in a geriatric sample. *Neuropsychology, 3,* 135–145.

Seashore, C.E., Lewis, D., & Saetveit, J.G. (1960). *Seashore Measures of Musical Talents.* New York: The Psychological Corporation.

Seidel, W.T. (1994). Applicability of the Hooper Visual Organization Test to pediatric population: Preliminary findings. *The Clinical Neuropsychologist, 8,* 59–68.

Seidenberg, M., Gamache, M.P., Smith, M., Sackellares, J.C., Beck, N.C., Giordani, B., Berent, S., & Boll, T. (1984). Subject variables and performance on the Halstead Neuropsychological Test Battery: A multivariate analysis. *Journal of Consulting and Clinical Psychology, 52*(4), 658–662.

Seidman, L.J., Benedict, K.B., Biederman, J., Bernstein, J.H. et al. (1995). Performance of children with ADHD on the Rey-Osterrieth Complex Figure: A pilot neuropsychological study. *Journal of Child Psychology and Psychiatry and Allied Disciplines, 36*(8), 1459–1473.

Seidman, L.J., Biederman, J., Faraone, S.V., & Weber, W. (1997). Toward defining a neuropsychology of Attention Deficit-Hyperactivity Disorder: Performance of children and adolescents from a large clinically referred sample. *Journal of Consulting and Clinical Psychology, 65*(1), 150–160.

Sellers, A.H., & Nadler, J.D. (1992). A survey of current neuropsychological assessment procedures used for different age groups. *Psychotherapy in Private Practice, 11*(3), 47–57.

Selnes, O.A., Jacobson, L., Machado, A.M., Becker, J.T., Wesch, J., Miller, E.N., Visscher, B., & McArthur, J.C. (1991). Normative data for a brief neuropsychological screening battery. *Perceptual and Motor Skills, 73,* 539–550.

Shapiro, D.M., & Harrison, D.W. (1990). Alternate forms of the AVLT: A procedure and test of form equivalency. *Archives of Clinical Neuropsychology, 5,* 405–410.

Sherer, M., Parsons, O.A., Nixon, S.J., & Adams, R.L. (1991). Clinical validity of the Speech-Sounds Perception Test and the Seashore Rhythm Test. *Journal of Clinical and Experimental Neuropsychology, 13*(5), 741–751.

Sherrill, R.E. (1985). Comparison of three short forms of the Category Test. *Journal of Clinical and Experimental Neuropsychology, 7*(3), 231–238.

Shimamura, A.P., Salmon, D.P., Squire, L.R., & Butters, N. (1987). Memory dysfunction and word priming in dementia and amnesia. *Behavioral Neuroscience, 101,* 347–351.

Shore, C., Shore, H., & Pihl, R.O. (1971). Correlations between performance on the category test and the Wechsler Adult Intelligence Scale. *Perceptual and Motor Skills, 32,* 70.

Shorr, J., Delis, D., & Massman, P. (1992). Memory for the Rey-Osterrieth Figure: Perceptual clustering, encoding, and storage. *Neuropsychology, 6,* 43–50.

Shum, D., Murray, R., & Eadie, K. (1997). Effect of speed of presentation on administration of the Logical Memory subtest of the Wechsler Memory Scale-Revised. *The Clinical Neuropsychologist, 11*(2), 188–191.

Shure, G.H., & Halstead, W.C. (1958). Cerebral localization of intellectual processes. *Psychological Monographs: General and Applied, 72*(12), 1–40.

Shute, G.E., & Huertas, V. (1990). Developmental variability in frontal lobe function. *Developmental Neuropsychology, 6*(1), 1–11.

Shuttleworth, E.C., & Huber, S.J. (1988). The naming disorder of dementia of Alzheimer type. *Brain and Language, 34*, 222–234.

Skelton-Robinson, M., & Jones, S. (1984). Nominal dysphasia and the severity of senile dementia. *British Journal of Psychiatry, 145*, 168–171.

Slay, D.K. (1984). A portable Halstead-Reitan category test. *Journal of Clinical Psychology, 40*(4), 1023–1027.

Smith, G.E., Ivnik, R.J., Malec, J.F., Petersen, R.C., Kokmen, E., Tangalos, E.G., & Kurland, L.T. (1992). Mayo's older Americans normative studies (MOANS): Factor structure of a core battery. *Psychological Assessment, 4*(3), 382–390.

Smith, S., Murdoch, B., & Chenery, H. (1989). Semantic abilities in dementia of the Alzheimer's type. *Brain and Language, 36*, 314–324.

Snodgrass, J.G. (1984). Concepts and their surface representations. *Journal of Verbal Learning and Verbal Behavior, 23*, 3–22.

Snodgrass, J.G., & Vanderwart, M. (1980). A standardized set of 260 pictures: Norms for name agreement, image agreement, familiarity and visual complexity. *Journal of Experimental Psychology: Human Learning and Memory, 6*, 174–215.

Snow, W.G. (1987). Standardization of test administration and scoring criteria: Some shortcomings of current practice with the Halstead-Reitan Test Battery. *The Clinical Neuropsychologist, 1*(3), 250–262.

Snyder, K.A., & Harrison, D.W. (1997). The Affective Auditory Verbal Learning Test. *Archives of Clinical Neuropsychology, 12*(5), 477–482.

Snyder, K.A., Harrison, D.W., & Shenal, B.V. (1998). The Affective Auditory Verbal Learning Test: Peripheral arousal correlates. *Archives of Clinical Neuropsychology, 13*(3), 251–258.

Sovcikova, E., & Bronis, M. (1985). Evaluation of mental workload by Stroop Colour-Word Test. *Studia Psychologica, 27*, 245–248.

Spreen, O., & Benton, A.L. (1969). *Neurosensory Center Comprehensive Examination for Aphasia: Manual of directions.* Victoria, BC: Neuropsychology Laboratory, University of Victoria.

Spreen, O., & Strauss, E. (1991). *A Compendium of Neuropsychological Tests.* New York: Oxford University Press.

Spreen, O., & Strauss, E. (1998). *A Compendium of Neuropsychological Tests.* New York: Oxford University Press.

Squire, L.R., & Shimamura, A.P. (1986). Characterizing amnesic patients for neurobehavioral study. *Behavioral Neuroscience, 100*, 866–877.

Stallings, G., Boake, C., & Sherer, M. (1995). Comparison of the California Verbal Learning Test and the Rey Auditory Verbal Learning Test in head-injured patients. *Journal of Clinical and Experimental Neuropsychology, 17*(5), 706–712.

Stanton, B.A., Jenkins, C.D., Savageau, J.A., & Zyzanski, S.J. (1984). Age and educational differences on the Trail Making Test and Wechsler Memory Scales. *Perceptual and Motor Skills, 58*, 311–318.

Steinmeyer, C.H. (1986). A meta-analysis of Halstead-Reitan test performances of non-brain damaged subjects. *Archives of Clinical Neuropsychology, 1*, 301–307.

Stern, Y., Andrews, H., Pittman, J., Sano, M., Tatemichi, T., Lantigua, R., & Mayeux, R. (1992). Diagnosis of dementia in a heterogeneous population. *Archives of Neurology, 49*, 453–460.

Stern, R., Singer, E., Duke, L., Singer, N., Morey, C.E., & Daughtrey, E.W. (1994). The Boston Qualitative Scoring System for the Rey-Osterrieth Complex Figure: Description and interrater reliability. *The Clinical Neuropsychologist, 8*, 309–322.

Storandt, M., & Hill, R.D. (1989). Very mild senile dementia of the Alzheimer type: II. Psychometric test performance. *Archives of Neurology, 46*, 383–386.

Strauss, E., & Spreen, O. (1990). A comparison of the Rey and Taylor figures. *Archives of Clinical Neuropsychology, 5*, 417–420.

Strauss, E., & Wada, J. (1988). Hand preference and proficiency and cerebral speech dominance determined by the carotid amytal test. *Journal of Clinical and Experimental Neuropsychology, 10*, 169–174.

Strickland, T., D'Elia, L., James, R., & Stein, R. (1997). Stroop Color-Word performance of African Americans. *The Clinical Neuropsychologist, 11*, 87–90.

Stroop, J. (1935). Studies of interference in serial verbal reactions. *Journal of Experimental Psychology, 18*, 643–662.

Stuss, D.T., Ely, P., Hugenholtz, H., Richard, M.T., LaRochelle, S., Poirier, C.A., & Bell, I. (1985). Subtle neuropsychological deficits in patients with good recovery after closed head injury. *Neurosurgery, 17*(1), 41–47.

Stuss, D.T., Stethem, L.L., & Poirier, C.A. (1987).

Comparison of three tests of attention and rapid information processing across six age groups. *The Clinical Neuropsychologist, 1,* 139–152.

Stuss, D.T., Stethem, L.L., & Pelchat, G. (1988). Three tests of attention and rapid information processing: An extension. *The Clinical Neuropsychologist, 2,* 246–250.

Stuss, D.T., Kaplan, E.F., Benson, D.F., Weir, W.S., Chiulli, S., & Sarazin, F.F. (1982). Evidence for the involvement of orbitofrontal cortex in memory functions: An interference effect. *Journal of Comparative and Physiological Psychology, 96,* 913–925.

Swerdlow, N.R., Filion, D., Geyer, M.A., & Braff, D.L. (1995). "Normal" personality correlates of sensorimotor, cognitive, and visuospatial gating. *Biological Psychiatry, 37,* 286–299.

Swiercinsky, D.P. (1978). *Manual for the Adult Neuropsychological Evaluation.* Springfield, IL: Charles C. Thomas.

Tamkin, A.S., & Hyer, L.A. (1984). Testing for cognitive dysfunction in the aging psychiatric patient. *Military Medicine, 149*(7), 397–399.

Tamkin, A.S., & Jacobsen, R. (1984). Age-related norms for the Hooper Visual Organization Test. *Journal of Clinical Psychology, 40*(6), 1459–1463.

Taylor, D.J., Hunt, C., & Glaser, B. (1990). A cross-validation of the revised Category Test. *Psychological Assessment: A Journal of Consulting and Clinical Psychology, 2*(4), 486–488.

Taylor, E.M. (1959). *Psychological Appraisal of Children With Cerebral Defects.* Cambridge, MA: Harvard University Press.

Taylor, J.M., Goldman, H., Leavitt, J., & Kleinman, K.N. (1984). Limitations of the brief form of the Halstead Category Test. *Journal of Clinical Neuropsychology, 6*(3), 341–344.

Taylor, H.C., & Russell, J.T. (1939). The relationship of validity coefficients to the practical effectiveness of tests in selection: Discussion and tables. *Journal of Applied Psychology, 23,* 565–578.

Taylor, L.B. (1969). Localization of cerebral lesions by psychological testing. *Clinical Neurosurgery, 16,* 269–287.

Taylor, L.B. (1979). Psychological assessment of neurosurgical patients. *Functional Neurosurgery,* 165–180.

Thompson, L.L., & Heaton, R.K. (1989). Comparison of different versions of the Boston Naming Test. *The Clinical Neuropsychologist, 3*(2), 184–192.

Thompson, L.L., & Heaton, R.K. (1991). Pattern of performance on the Tactual Performance Test. *The Clinical Neuropsychologist, 5*(4), 322–328.

Thompson, L.L., & Parsons, O.A. (1985). Contribution of the TPT to adult neuropsychological assessment: A review. *Journal of Clinical and Experimental Neuropsychology, 7*(4), 430–444.

Thompson, L.L., Heaton, K.R., Matthews, C.G., & Grant, I. (1987). Comparison of preferred and nonpreferred hand performance on four neuropsychological motor tasks. *The Clinical Neuropsychologist, 1*(4), 324–334.

Thorndike, E.L., & Lorge, I. (1944). *The Teacher's Word Book of 30,000 words.* New York: Teacher's College, Columbia University.

Thurstone, L. (1944). *A Factorial Study of Perception.* Chicago, IL: University of Chicago Press.

Thurstone, L.L., & Thurstone, T.G. (1962). Primary mental abilities (Rev.) Chicago: Science Research Associates.

Tierney, M.C., Nores, A., Snow, W.G., Fisher, R.H., Zorzitto, M.L., & Reid, D.W. (1994). Use of the Rey Auditory Verbal Learning Test in differentiating normal aging from Alzheimer's and Parkinson's dementia. *Psychological Assessment, 6,* 129–134.

Toglia, M.P., & Battig, W.F. (1978). *Handbook of Word Norms.* Hillsdale, NJ: Lawrence Erlbaum.

Tombaugh, T.N., & Hubley, A.M. (1991). Four studies comparing the Rey-Osterrieth and Taylor complex figures. *Journal of Clinical and Experimental Neuropsychology, 13,* 587–599.

Tombaugh, T.N., & Hubley, A.M. (1997). The 60-item Boston Naming Test: Norms for cognitively intact adults aged 25 to 88 years. *Journal of Clinical and Experimental Neuropsychology, 19*(6), 922–932.

Tombaugh, T.N., Hubley, A.M., Faulkner, P., & Schmidt, J.P. (1990). *The Rey-Osterrieth and Taylor complex figures: comparative studies, modified figures and normative data for the Taylor figure.* Paper presented at the 18th Annual Meeting of the International Neuropsychology Society, Orlando, FL.

Tombaugh, T.N., Faulkner, P., & Hubley, A.M. (1992a). Effects of age on the Rey-Osterrieth and Taylor complex figures: Test-retest data using an intentional learning paradigm. *Journal of Clinical and Experimental Neuropsychology, 14,* 647–661.

Tombaugh, T.N., Schmidt, J.P., & Faulkner, P. (1992b). A new procedure for administering the Taylor Complex Figure: Normative data over a 60-year age span. *The Clinical Neuropsychologist, 6*(1), 63–79.

Tomer, R., & Levin, B.E. (1993). Differential effects of aging on two verbal fluency tasks. *Perceptual and Motor Skills, 76,* 465–466.

Toshima, T., Toma, C., Demic, J., & Wapner, S. (1992). Age and cross-cultural differences in processes underlying sequential cognitive activity. In

B. Wilpert, H. Motoaki, & J. Misumi (Eds.), *General psychology and environmental psychology: Proceedings of the 22nd International Congress of Applied Psychology* (p. 189). Hillsdale, N.J.: Lawrence Erlbaum Associates.

Toshima, T., Demick, J., Miyatani, M., Ishii, S., & Wapner, S. (1996). Cross-cultural differences in processes underlying sequential cognitive activity. *Japanese Psychological Research, 38*(2), 90–96.

Trahan, D.E., Patterson, J., Quintana, J., & Biron, R. (1987). *The Finger Tapping Test: A reexamination of traditional hypotheses regarding normal adult performance.* Paper presented to the 15th Annual Meeting of the International Neuropsychological Society, Washington, DC.

Trahan, D., Quintana, J., Willingham, A., & Goethe, K. (1988). The Visual Reproduction subtest: Standardization and clinical validation of a delayed recall procedure. *Neuropsychology, 2*(1), 29–39.

Trautt, G.M., Chavez, E.L., Brandon, A.D., & Steyaert, J. (1983). Effects of test anxiety and sex of subject on neuropsychological test performance: Finger Tapping, Trail Making, Digit Span, and Digit Symbol Tests. *Perceptual and Motor Skills, 56,* 923–929.

Trenerry, M., Crosson, B., DeBoe, J., & Leber, W. (1989). *Stroop Neuropsychological Screening Test, Manual.* Odessa, FL: Psychological Assessment Resources (PAR).

Trichard, C., Martinot, J.L., Alagille, M., Masure, M.C., Hardy, P., Ginestet, D., & Feline, A. (1995). Time course of prefrontal lobe dysfunction in severely depressed inpatients: A longitudinal neuropsychological study. *Psychological Medicine, 25,* 79–85.

Tuokko, H., & Woodward, T.S. (1996). Development and validation of a demographic correction system for neuropsychological measures used in the Canadian Study of Health and Aging. *Journal of Clinical and Experimental Neuropsychology, 18*(4), 479–616.

Tupler, L.A., Welsh, K.A., Asare-Aboagye, Y., & Dawson, D.V. (1995). Reliability of the Rey-Osterrieth Complex Figure in use with memory-impaired patients. *Journal of Clinical and Experimental Neuropsychology, 17,*(4), 566–579.

Uzzell, B.P., & Oler, J. (1986). Chronic low-level mercury exposure and neuropsychological functioning. *Journal of Clinical and Experimental Neuropsychology, 8*(5), 581–593.

Vakil, E., & Blachstein, H. (1993). Rey Auditory-Verbal Learning Test: Structure analysis. *Journal of Clinical Psychology, 49,* 883–890.

Vakil, E., & Blachstein, H. (1994). A supplementary measure in the Rey AVLT for assessing incidental learning of temporal order. *Journal of Clinical Psychology, 50*(2), 240–245.

Vakil, E., & Blachstein, H. (1997). Rey AVLT: Developmental norms for adults and the sensitivity of different memory measures to age. *The Clinical Neuropsychologist, 11*(4), 356–369.

Van den Burg, W., van Zomeren, A.H., Minderhoud, J.M. et al., (1987). Cognitive impairment in patients with multiple sclerosis and mild physical disability. *Archives of Neurology, 44,* 494–501.

Vanderploeg, R.D., Schinka, J.A., & Retzlaff, P. (1994). Relationships between measures of auditory verbal learning and executive functioning. *Journal of Clinical and Experimental Neuropsychology, 16*(2), 243–250.

Van Gorp, W.G., Satz, P., Kiersch, M.E., & Henry, R. (1986). Normative data on the Boston naming test for a group of normal older adults. *Journal of Clinical and Experimental Neuropsychology, 8*(6), 702–705.

Van Gorp, W.G., Satz, P., Miller, E., & Visscher, E. (1989). Neuropsychological performance in HIV-1 immunocompromised patients: A preliminary report. *Journal of Clinical and Experimental Neuropsychology, 11*(5), 763–773.

Van Gorp, W.G., Satz, P., & Mitrushina, M. (1990). Neuropsychological processes associated with normal aging. *Developmental Neuropsychology, 6*(4), 279–290.

Vega, A., & Parsons, O.A. (1967). Cross-validation of the Halstead-Reitan Tests for brain damage. *Journal of Consulting Psychology, 31,* 619–625.

Verma, S.K., Pershad, D., & Khanna, R. (1993). Hooper's Visual Organization Test: Item analysis on Indian subjects. *Indian Journal of Clinical Psychology, 20*(1), 5–10.

Veroff, A.E. (1980). The neuropsychology of aging: Qualitative analysis of visual reproductions. *Psychological Research, 41,* 259–268.

Villardita, C., Cultrera, S., Cupone, V., & Mejia, R. (1985). Neuropsychological test performances and normal aging. International Workshop: Psychiatry in aging and dementia. *Archives of Gerontology and Geriatrics, 4*(4), 311–319.

Visser, R.S.H. (1973). *Manual of the Complex Figure Test (CFT).* Amsterdam, Netherlands: Swets & Zeitlinger B.V.

Waber, D.P., & Holmes, J.M. (1985). Assessing children's copy productions of the Rey-Osterrieth Complex Figure. *Journal of Clinical and Experimental Neuropsychology, 7*(3), 264–280.

Waber, D.P., & Holmes, J.M. (1986). Assessing children's memory productions of the Rey-Osterrieth Complex Figure. *Journal of Clinical and Experimental Neuropsychology, 8,* 563–580.

Waber, D., Bernstein, J., & Merola, J. (1989). Remembering the Rey-Osterrieth Complex Figure: A dual-code, cognitive neuropsychological model. *Developmental Neuropsychology, 5,* 1–15.

Waber, D.P., Isquith, P.K., Kahn, C.M., & Romero, I. (1994). Metacognitive factors in the visuospatial skills of long-term survivors of acute lymphoblastic leukemia: An experimental approach to the Rey-Osterrieth Complex Figure Test. *Developmental Neuropsychology, 10*(4), 349–367.

Wallace, J.L. (1984). Wechsler Memory Scale. *The International Journal of Clinical Neuropsychology, 6*(3), 216–226.

Wang, P.J. (1977). Visual organization ability in brain damaged adults. *Perceptual and Motor Skills, 45,* 723–728.

Warner, M.H., Ernst, J., Townes, B.D., Peel, J.H., & Preston, M. (1987). Relationships between IQ and neuropsychological measures in neuropsychiatric populations: Within-laboratory and cross-cultural replications using WAIS and WAIS-R. *Journal of Clinical and Experimental Neuropsychology, 9*(5), 545–562.

Warrington, E. (1984). *Recognition Memory Test—Faces.* Windsor, England: NFER-Nelson.

Wechsler, D. (1945). A standardized Memory Scale for clinical use. *Journal of Psychology, 19,* 87–95.

Wechsler, D. (1987). *Wechsler Memory Scale—Revised.* San Antonio, TX: The Psychological Corporation. Harcourt Brace Jovanovich.

Wechsler, D. (1997). *WMS-III. Administration and Scoring Manual.* San Antonio: The Psychological Corporation. Harcourt Brace Jovanovich.

Wechsler, D., & Stone, C. (1945). *Wechsler Memory Scale Manual.* San Antonio, TX: The Psychological Corporation.

Weingartner, H., Burns, S., Diebel, R., & LeWitt, P.A. (1984). Cognitive impairments in Parkinson's disease: Distinguishing between effort-demanding and automatic cognitive processes. *Psychiatry Research, 11,* 223–235.

Weinstein, C., Kaplan, E., Casey, M., & Hurwitz, I. (1990). Delineation of female performance on the Rey-Osterrieth Complex Figure. *Neuropsychology, 4,* 117–127.

Welch, L.W., Doineau, D., Johnson, S., & King, D. (1996). Educational and gender normative data for the Boston Naming Test in a group of older adults. *Brain and Language, 53,* 260–266.

Wentworth-Rohr, I., Mackintosh, R.M., & Fialkoff, B.S. (1974). The relationship of Hooper VOT score to sex, education, intelligence and age. *Journal of Clinical Psychology, 30*(1), 73–75.

Wetzel, L., & Murphy, G.S. (1991). Validity of the use of a discontinue rule and evaluation of discriminability of the Hooper visual organization test. *Neuropsychology, 5*(2), 119–122.

Wheeler, L., & Reitan, R.M. (1963). Discriminant functions applied to the problem of predicting cerebral damage from behavioral tests: a cross-validation study. *Perceptual and Motor Skills, 16,* 681–701.

Whelihan, W.M., & Lesher, E.L. (1985). Neuropsychological changes in frontal functions with aging. *Developmental Neuropsychology, 1,* 371–380.

White, A.J. (1984). Cognitive impairment of acute mountain sickness and acetazolamide. *Aviation, Space and Environmental Medicine, 55,* 589–603.

Wiens, A.M., & Matarazzo, J.D. (1977). WAIS and MMPI correlates of the Halstead-Reitan Neuropsychology Battery in normal male subjects. *The Journal of Nervous and Mental Disease, 164*(2), 112–121.

Wiens, A.N., McMinn, M.R., & Crossen, J.R. (1988). Rey Auditory-Verbal Learning Test: Development of norms for healthy young adults. *The Clinical Neuropsychologist, 2*(1), 67–87.

Wiens, A.N., Tindall, A.G., & Crossen, J.R. (1994). California Verbal Learning Test: A normative data study. *The Clinical Neuropsychologist, 8*(1), 75–90.

Williams, B.W., Mack, W., & Henderson, V.W. (1989). Boston Naming Test in Alzheimer's Disease. *Neuropsychologia, 27*(8), 1073–1079.

Williams, J., Rickert, V., Hogan, J., Zolten, A., Satz, P., D'Elia, L., Asarnow, R., Zaucha, K., & Light, R. (1995). Children's color trails. *Archives of Clinical Neuropsychology, 10*(3), 211–223.

Willis, L., Yeo, R., Thomas, P., & Garry, P.G. (1988). Differential declines in cognitive function with aging: The possible role of health status. *Developmental Neuropsychology, 4*(1), 23–28.

Wood, F.B., Ebert, V., & Kinsbourne, M. (1982). The episodic-semantic memory distinction in memory and amnesia: Clinical and experimental observations. In L. Cermak (Ed.), *Memory and Amnesia.* Hillsdale, N.J.: Lawrence Erlbaum.

Wood, W.D., & Strider, M.A. (1980). Comparison of two methods of administering the Halstead Category Test. *Journal of Clinical Psychology, 36*(2), 476–479.

Woodward, A.C. (1982). The Hooper Visual Organization Test: A case against its use in neuropsychological assessment. *Journal of Consulting and Clinical Psychology, 50*(2), 286–288.

Worrall, L.E., Yiu, E.M-L., Hickson, L.M.H., & Barnett, H.M. (1995). Normative data for the Boston naming test for Australian elderly. *Aphasiology, 9*(6), 541–551.

Yamazaki, A. (1985). Interference in the Stroop color-naming task. *Japanese Journal of Psychology, 56,* 185–191.

Yesavage, J.A., Brink, T.L., Rose, T.L., Lum, O., Huang, V., Adey, M., & Leiter, V.O. (1983). Development and validity of a Geriatric Depression Scale: A preliminary report. *Journal of Psychiatric Research, 17,* 37–49.

Yeudall, L.T., Fromm-Auch, D., & Davies, P. (1982). Neuropsychological impairment of persistent delinquency. *Journal of Nervous and Mental Disease, 170*(5), 257–265.

Yeudall, L.T., Reddon, J.R., Gill, D.M., & Stefanyk, W.O. (1987). Normative data for the Halstead-Reitan Neuropsychological Tests stratified by age and sex. *Journal of Clinical Psychology, 43*(3), 346–367.

Yeudall, L. T., Fromm, D., Reddon, J. R., & Stefanyk, W. O. (1986). Normative data stratified by age and sex for 12 neuropsychological tests. *Journal of Clinical Psychology, 43,*(3) 918–946.

Ylikoski, R., Ylikoski, A., Erkinjuntti, T., Sulkava, R., Raininko, R., & Tilvis, R. (1993). White matter changes in healthy elderly persons correlate with attention and speed of mental processing. *Archives of Neurology, 50,* 818–824.

Young, K.L., & Delay, E.R. (1993). Seashore Rhythm Test: Comparison of signal detection theory and standard scoring procedures. *Archives of Clinical Neuropsychology, 8,* 111–121.

Appendix 1: Where to buy the tests

Several of the tests mentioned in this book are available from more than one distributor. An asterisk placed before the name of the test indicates that the company listed at left is also the primary publisher of the test.

TEST PUBLISHER/DISTRIBUTOR	TEST NAME
Allpoints Publications 1137 Second Street, #109 Santa Monica, CA 90403-5000 1-310-399-8999 [FAX orders only]	°Color Trails (Children's version) °Stroop (Comalli /Kaplan versions in Spanish) °WHO-UCLA Test Battery
Boston Neuropsychological Foundation P.O. Box 476 Lexington, MA 02173 1-781-862-1207 [Phone orders] 1-781-861-6230 [FAX orders]	°Stroop (Comalli /Kaplan versions in English)
Lafayette Instrument 3700 Sagamore Parkway North P.O. Box 5729 Lafayette, IN 47903 1-800-428-7545 [Phone orders] 1-317-423-4111 [FAX orders]	°Lafayette Hand Dynamometer °Grooved Pegboard Test
Psychological Assessment Resources PAR P.O. Box 998 Odessa, FL 33556 1-800-331-TEST [Phone orders] 1-800-383-6595 [24-hours order line] 1-800-727-9329 [FAX orders]	°Color Trails Test (Adult versions) Grooved Pegboard Test Finger Tapping Test Lafayette Hand Dynamometer Boston Naming Test—Revised °Rey Complex Figure & Recognition °Intermediate Booklet Category Test °Portable Tactual Performance Test °Stroop Test (Trenerry et al.) Stroop Color & Word Test (Golden)

TEST PUBLISHER/DISTRIBUTOR	**TEST NAME**
The Psychological Corporation 555 Academic Court San Antonio, TX 78204-2498 1-800-211-8378 [Phone orders] 1-800-232-1223 [FAX orders]	Boston Naming Test—Revised Rey Complex Figure & Recognition °Wechsler Memory Scale—Revised °Wechsler Memory Scale—III
Reitan Neuropsychology Laboratory 2920 4th Street Tuscon, AZ 85775-1336 1-520-882-2022 [Phone orders] 1-520-884-0040 [FAX orders]	°Category Test °Finger Tapping Test °Tactual Performance Test °Rhythm Test (Seashore) °Speech-Sounds Perception Test Trail Making Test (1945 version) Hand Dynamometer
Riverside Publishing 425 Spring Lake Drive Itasca, IL 60143 1-800-323-9540 [Phone orders] 1-630-467-7192 [FAX orders]	Boston Naming Test—Revised Stroop Color & Word Test (Golden) Lafayette Hand Dynamometer Grooved Pegboard Test
Western Psychological Services 12031 Wilshire Blvd. Los Angeles, CA 90025-1251 1-800-648-8857 [Phone orders] 1-310-478-7838 [FAX orders]	°Short Category Test, Booklet Format Stroop Color & Word Test (Golden) °Hooper Visual Organization Test Rey Auditory Verbal Learning Test

Appendix 2a: Subject Instructions for ACT According to Boone et al. (1990), Boone (1998)

The examiner instructs the patient: "I'm going to say three letters and I want you to say them back to me. Ready? QLX . . ."

Administer first five trials. Write down patient's responses in the response column. In the next column, indicate the number of correct responses (i.e., 0, 1, 2, or 3). If more than one or two errors are present, the test should be discontinued. If they cannot repeat the letters reliably, this would point to a linguistic or hearing problem, in which case frontal lobe functioning cannot be assessed with this test.

"Now I'm going to say three letters, and then I'm going to say a number. After I say the number, I want you to count backwards outloud by threes from the number. For example, if the number was 100, you would say, '100, 97, 94', etc. After a few seconds of counting I will stop you and I will want you to tell me the letters. In other words, you have to do two things at once—hold the letters in mind while you are counting backwards by threes. It is a difficult task and it is normal to make mistakes. Let's try one, XCP 194 . . . starting counting".

The numbers in the "delay" column indicate for how many seconds the person should count backwards by threes. Begin timing when the patient actually says a number outloud. You may allow the patient to attempt to consolidate the information for approximately 1–2 seconds prior to their actual commencement of counting; do not allow more time than this.

A perseveration is scored if the person says a letter that is *incorrect* and one which was said in the trial directly preceding the current one; a total of 57 perseverations are possible. A sequence error occurs when the patient says the letters out of sequence; a total of 20 sequence errors are possible.

Appendix 2b: Auditory Consonant Trigrams (Boone et al., 1990; Boone, 1998)

Stimulus	Starting Number	Delay (Seconds)	Responses	# Correct	Perseveration	Sequence
QLX	—	0				
SZB	—	0				
HJT	—	0				
GPW	—	0				
DLH	—	0				
XCP	194	18				
NDJ	75	9				
FXB	28	3				
JCN	180	9				
BGQ	167	18				
KMC	20	3				
RXT	188	18				
KFN	82	9				
MBW	47	3				
TDH	141	9				
LRP	51	3				
ZWS	117	18				
PHQ	89	9				
XGD	158	18				
CZQ	91	3				

Number Correct:

0″ Delay	_____	/15
3″ Delay	_____	/15
9″ Delay	_____	/15
18″ Delay	_____	/15
TOTAL	_____	/60

Appendix 2c: Subject Instructions for ACT According to Stuss et al. (1987, 1988)

The examiner starts by saying: "I am going to say three letters and when I am through, I am going to knock like this. When I do I want you to say the letters back to me." The examiner says letters outloud at the rate of 1 per second and records the patient's answers.

After the five trials with "0" delay, the examiner continues the test. "This time, I am going to say three letters followed immediately by a number. As soon as you get the number, I want you to start counting backward outloud until I knock as before." (Examiner demonstrates by knocking on the desk). "When I knock, I want you to recall the three letters. Do you have any questions?"

If the instructions are clearly understood, the examiner starts with the delayed trials. If not understood, repeat with examples. For this part of the test there are three delayed recall conditions, which are "3," "9," and "18" randomly alternating. All trials are presented independently of the patient's performance.

The examiner says the letters and the numbers and immediately starts the stopwatch until the corresponding delay recall period elapses. He then knocks on the desk and records the letters reported by the patient.

SUPPLEMENTARY INSTRUCTIONS

On this test, it is important to maintain interference conditions. The examiner must make sure that the patient is counting during the delayed period. Some patients tend to repeat the letters after the examiner instead of starting counting immediately. In this instance, the patient should be told not to repeat the letters, but to start counting as soon as he hears the number. The examiner may have to encourage him to count outloud by counting with him at the beginning, or if the patient hesitates.

Some patients have great difficulty counting by threes backwards. In such cases, the patient is asked to count backward by ones instead. However, this procedure is nonstandard and should be noted.

On this test, only one presentation for each trial is allowed.

SCORING

For each trial, the letters given by the patient are recorded verbatim (i.e., in the order reported by the patient) in the first column of the score sheet. The number of correct letters identified is noted in the second column. The number of correct letters for each delayed condition over 15 is registered at the bottom of the score sheet. The summation of these subscores constitutes the total score of the test over 60.

Appendix 2d: Auditory Consonant Trigrams (Stuss et al., 1987, 1988)

Stimulus	Starting Number	Delay (Seconds)	Responses	Number Correct	Correct Sequence	Correct Position	Perseveration Number	Occurred
QLX	—	0					B (4)	
SZB	—	0					C (4)	
HJT	—	0					D (4)	
GPW	—	0					F (2)	
DLH	—	0					G (3)	
XCP	194	18					H (4)	
NDJ	75	9					J (3)	
FXB	128	36					K (2)	
JCN	180	9					L (3)	
BGQ	167	18					M (2)	
KMC	120	36					N (3)	
RXT	188	18					P (4)	
KFN	82	9					Q (4)	
MBW	147	36					R (2)	
TDH	141	9					S (2)	
LRP	151	36					T (3)	
ZWS	117	18					W (3)	
PHQ	89	9					X (5)	
XGD	158	18					Z (3)	
CZQ	191	36						

	1st Two	Last Two
Number Correct		
0″ Delay ____		
9″ Delay ____	____	____
18″ Delay ____	____	____
36″ Delay ____	____	____
TOTAL ____	____	____

TOTAL CORR. SEQ.: ——
TOTAL CORR. POS.: ——
PERSEV. SINGLE: ——
PERSEV. DOUBLE: ——
PERSEV. TRIPLE ——

Appendix 3: WHO-UCLA Auditory Verbal Learning Test: Instructions and Test Forms

GENERAL INSTRUCTIONS FOR EXAMINERS

Instructions to Subjects: The instructions to subjects are printed on the test form. Be sure to indicate before Trial II that the subject should try to remember as many words as he can, *". . .including the words you remembered on the first trial."* After the last trial (Trial V), you should remember to tell the subject that *"I want you to try to remember as many of those words as possible because I'm going to ask you about them again a little later."* These instructions are printed on the test form for "Recall Following Interference."

Instructions to Examiners: Use a clipboard to hold the test forms out of the subject's view. Read the words at the rate of approximately 1 word per second. On the last word, drop the pitch of your voice to indicate that you are finished. If necessary, prompt the subject to begin recall. In general, you should not look at the subject while reading the list or while recording his responses since this kind of eye contact makes many people nervous.

Code all responses by placing a check mark in the relevant box. Place additional check marks when items are repeated. If the subject gives a word that is not on the list, record the intrusion in the spaces provided below the 15-item list. At the end of each trial write down the total numbers of correct responses, repetitions, and intrusions.

If the subject makes an intrusion, wait until he indicates that he is finished, then prompt the subject by saying, *"You said ____, ____ was not on the list."*

If the subject makes an intrusion that may reflect poor hearing on the part of the subject, or poor pronunciation on the part of the examiner (such as saying "Pie" instead of "Eye"), count the item as correct the first time, and correct the subject by saying, *"You said Pie, the correct word is Eye."* If the subject continues to produce the same intrusion on subsequent trials, correct the subject in the same manner, but score the response as an intrusion. Make allowances for translation and pronunciation difficulties on the part of nonnative speakers of the language being used for test administration.

If a subject asks if a particular response is correct, answer him truthfully. If a subject asks if he has already said a particular word, again, answer truthfully, but count the word as a repetition if he has already said it once. In general, feel free to answer any of the subject's questions about the task, including the number of trials, and the number of words on the list.

If the subject is not producing at least 10 responses by the third trial, encourage the subject to try a little longer.

ACQUISITION TRIALS

Trial I: *"The next task may seem a bit difficult in the beginning, but usually it gets easier as we* go along. I am going to read for you a long list of words. Once I'm done, I'd like to see how many of the words you can recall. You can repeat the words in any order that you prefer; you don't have to use the same order that I use. Then, I am going to read the same list for you a few more times, to see how many of the words you can eventually learn. Ready?"

Trial II: "That was a good beginning. Now I'm going to read the same list again, and again I would like to see how many of the words you can recall, including the words you remembered on the first trial. Again, listen very carefully. Ready?"

Trials III–V: "Very good. I'm going to read the list again. Again, listen carefully and try to remember as many words as you can. Ready?"

	Trial I	Trial II	Trial III	Trial IV	Trial 5	
Arm						Arm
Cat						Cat
Axe						Axe
Bed						Bed
Plane						Plane
Ear						Ear
Dog						Dog
Hammer						Hammer
Chair						Chair
Car						Car
Eye						Eye
Horse						Horse
Knife						Knife
Clock						Clock
Bike						Bike

Correct: ———— ———— ———— ———— ————
Repeats: ———— ———— ———— ———— ————
Instructions: ———— ———— ———— ———— ————

INTERFERENCE LIST, RECALL FOLLOWING INTERFERENCE

Instructions for Trial VI: After Trial V of the primary word list, say "Very good. I want you to try to remember as many of those words as possible because I'm going to ask you about them again a little later." Then say, "Now I am going to read for you a different list of words. Once again, when I'm done, I'd like to see how many of the words you can recall. Ready?" Read the interference list (boot, monkey, etc.), and record responses under Trial VI. Unlike earlier trials, you should not correct any intrusions that the subject makes.

Instructions for Trial VII: After the subject has recalled as much as possible from the inter-ference list, say, *"Now I'd like to see how many words you can recall from the first list—the one we went through five times. Tell me as many words as you can remember from the first list."* Record responses under Trial VII.

	Trial VI
Boot	
Monkey	
Bowl	
Cow	
Finger	
Dress	
Spider	
Cup	
Bee	
Foot	
Hat	
Butterfly	
Kettle	
Mouse	
Hand	

	Trial VII
Arm	
Cat	
Axe	
Bed	
Plane	
Ear	
Dog	
Hammer	
Chair	
Car	
Eye	
Horse	
Knife	
Clock	
Bike	

Correct: _____   _____

Repeats: _____   _____

Intrusions: _____   _____

30-MINUTE DELAYED RECALL AND RECOGNITION

Instructions for Trial VIII: Without reading the list again, say: *"Remember the long list of words I read to you five times? I'd like you now to tell me as many of the words from that list as you can remember."* Do not correct the subject if he/she makes any intrusions.

Instructions for Trial IX: Immediately following the delayed recall say, *"Next I would like to see how many of the words you can recognize. Say Yes if you hear a word you think was part of the original list we went through five times. If you think that the word is not from that* list, *say No. Make sure you only say Yes to those words you are sure you remember as being a part of that list we went through five times."* Read the words in order from left to right. Circle the word if the subject says 'Yes.' If the subject hesitates and fails to answer within a few seconds, say *"If you are not sure, just make your best guess."* Words from the original list are capitalized.

Scoring: 'Correct Recognitions' is the total number of circled words that are capitalized. 'False Identifications' is the total number of circled words that are *not* capitalized.

	Trial VIII
Arm	
Cat	
Axe	
Bed	
Plane	
Ear	
Dog	
Hammer	
Chair	
Car	
Eye	
Horse	
Knife	
Clock	
Bike	

Trial IX—Oral Recognition		
mirror	HORSE	truck
HAMMER	leg	EYE
KNIFE	DOG	fish
candle	table	EAR
motorcycle	CAT	BIKE
AXE	lips	snake
CLOCK	tree	stool
CHAIR	ARM	bus
PLANE	nose	BED
turtle	sun	CAR

Correct Recognitions: _____

False Identifications: _____

Correct   _____

Repeats: _____

Copyright Acknowledgments

chological measures. *Journal of Clinical and Experimental Neuropsychology, 8*(4), 413–420.

Tables 4.6, 12.5, 13.6, 14.8, 17.2 , 18.2, 20.10 reprinted from:
Fromm-Auch & Yeudall (1983). Normative data for the Halstead-Reitan neuropsychological tests. *Journal of Clinical Neuropsychology, 5*(3), 221–238.

Tables 16.16–16.19 reprinted from:
Geffen, Moar, O'Hanlon, Clark, & Geffen (1990). Performance measures of 16- to 86-year old males and females on the Auditory Verbal Learning Test. *The Clinical Neuropsychologist, 4*(1), 45–63.

Tables 4.18, 4.19, 6.5, 6.6, 8.12, 8.13, 9.14, 9.15 reprinted from:
Ivnik, Malec, Smith, Tangalos, & Petersen, (1996). Neuropsychological tests' norms above age 55: COWAT, BNT, MAE Token, WRAT-R Reading, AMNART, Stroop, TMT, and JLO. *The Clinical Neuropsychologist, 10*(3), 262–278.

Tables 15.36–15.39 reprinted from:
Marcopulos, McLain, & Giuliano (1997). Cognitive impairment or inadequate norms? A study of healthy, rural, older adults with limited education. *The Clinical Neuropsychologist, 11*(2), 111–131.

Tables 4.20, 4.21, 11.2, 11.3, 15.35 reprinted from:
Richardson & Marottoli (1996). Education-specific normative data on common neuropsychological indicies for individuals older that 75 years. *The Clinical Neuropsychologist, 10*(4), 375–381.

Tables 4.14, 7.4, 7.5 reprinted from:
Stuss, Stethem, & Pelchat (1988). Three tests of attention and rapid information processing: An extension. *The Clinical Neuropsychologist, 2,* 246–250.

Tables 8.18, 8.19 reprinted from:
Tombaugh & Hubley (1997). The 60-item Boston Naming Test: Norms for cognitively intact adults aged 25 to 88 years. *Journal of Clinical and Experimental Neuropsychology, 19*(6), 922–932.

Tables 16.9–16.11 reprinted from:
Wiens, McMinn, & Crossen (1988). Rey Auditory-Verbal Learning Test: Developmental norms for healthy young adults. *The Clinical Neuropsychologist, 2*(1), 67–87.

Reprinted with permission from **American Psychological Association:**

Tables 16.20–16.26 reprinted from:
Ivnik, R.J., Malec, J.F., Tangalos, E.G., Petersen, R.C., Kokmen, E., & Kurland, L.T. (1990). The Auditory-Verbal Learning Test (AVLT): Norms for ages 55 and older. *Psychological Assessment, 2,* 304–312.

Tables 15.26, 15.27 reprinted from:
Ivnik, R.J., Smith, G., Tangalos, E.G., Petersen, R.C., Kokmen, E., & Kurland, L.T. (1991). Wechsler Memory Scale: IQ-dependent norms for persons aged 65 to 97 years. *Psychological Assessment, 3*(2), 156–161.

Table 8.2 reprinted from:
LaBarge, E., Balota, D., Storandt, M., & Smith, D. (1992). An analysis of confrontation naming errors in senile dementia of the Alzheimer type. *Neuropsychology, 6*(1), 77–95.

Reprinted with permission from **Mayo Foundation:**

Tables 16.39–16.50 reprinted from:
Ivnik, R.J., Malec, J.F., Smith, G.E., Tangalos, E.G., Petersen, R.C., Kokmen, E., & Kurland, L.T. (1990). Mayo's older Americans normative studies: Updated AVLT norms for ages 56–97. *The Clinical Neuropsychologist, 6* (Supplement), 83–104.

Name Index

Subject Index